Essentials of OCT in Ocular Disease

Amar Agarwal, MS, FRCS, FRCOphth
Professor and Head
Dr. Agarwal's Group of Eye Hospitals and Eye Research Centre
Chennai, Tamil Nadu
India

Dhivya Ashok Kumar, MD, FICO
Consultant Ophthalmologist and Head of R & D
Dr. Agarwal's Group of Eye Hospitals and Eye Research Centre
Chennai, Tamil Nadu
India

Thieme
New York • Stuttgart • Delhi • Rio de Janeiro

Thieme Medical Publishers, Inc.
333 Seventh Avenue
New York, New York 10001

Executive Editor: William Lamsback
Managing Editor: Elizabeth Palumbo
Director, Editorial Services: Mary Jo Casey
Editorial Assistant: Mohammad Ibrar
International Production Director: Andreas Schabert
Vice President, Editorial and E-Product Development: Vera Spillner
International Marketing Director: Fiona Henderson
International Sales Director: Louisa Turrell
Director of Sales, North America: Mike Roseman
Senior Vice President and Chief Operating Officer: Sarah Vanderbilt
President: Brian D. Scanlan

Library of Congress Cataloging-in-Publication Data

Essentials of OCT in ocular disease / [edited by] Amar Agarwal, Dhivya Ashok Kumar.
p. ; cm.
Includes bibliographical references and index.
ISBN 978-1-62623-098-9 (hardcover) – ISBN 978-1-62623-099-6 (electronic)
I. Agarwal, Amar, editor. II. Kumar, Dhivya Ashok, editor.
[DNLM: 1. Eye Diseases–diagnosis. 2. Eye Diseases–surgery.
3. Tomography, Optical Coherence–methods. WW 141]
RE46
617.7–dc23

2014032079

Thieme Publishers New York
333 Seventh Avenue, New York, NY 10001 USA
+1 800 782 3488, customerservice@thieme.com

Thieme Publishers Stuttgart
Rüdigerstrasse 14, 70469 Stuttgart, Germany
+49 [0]711 8931 421, customerservice@thieme.de

Thieme Publishers Delhi
A-12, Second Floor, Sector-2, Noida-201301
Uttar Pradesh, India
+91 120 45 566 00, customerservice@thieme.in

Thieme Publishers Rio de Janeiro, Thieme Publicações Ltda.
Edifício Rodolpho de Paoli, 25º andar
Av. Nilo Peçanha, 50 - Sala 2508,
Rio de Janeiro 20020-906 Brasil
+55 21 3172-2297 / +55 21 3172-1896

Cover design: Thieme Publishing Group
Typesetting by DiTech Process Solutions

Printed in India by Replika Press Pvt. Ltd. 5 4 3 2 1

ISBN 978-1-62623-098-9

Also available as an e-book:
eISBN 978-1-62623-099-6

Important note: Medicine is an ever-changing science undergoing continual development. Research and clinical experience are continually expanding our knowledge, in particular our knowledge of proper treatment and drug therapy. Insofar as this book mentions any dosage or application, readers may rest assured that the authors, editors, and publishers have made every effort to ensure that such references are in accordance with **the state of knowledge at the time of production of the book.**

Nevertheless, this does not involve, imply, or express any guarantee or responsibility on the part of the publishers in respect to any dosage instructions and forms of applications stated in the book. **Every user is requested to examine carefully** the manufacturers' leaflets accompanying each drug and to check, if necessary in consultation with a physician or specialist, whether the dosage schedules mentioned therein or the contraindications stated by the manufacturers differ from the statements made in the present book. Such examination is particularly important with drugs that are either rarely used or have been newly released on the market. Every dosage schedule or every form of application used is entirely at the user's own risk and responsibility. The authors and publishers request every user to report to the publishers any discrepancies or inaccuracies noticed. If errors in this work are found after publication, errata will be posted at www.thieme.com on the product description page.

Some of the product names, patents, and registered designs referred to in this book are in fact registered trademarks or proprietary names even though specific reference to this fact is not always made in the text. Therefore, the appearance of a name without designation as proprietary is not to be construed as a representation by the publisher that it is in the public domain.

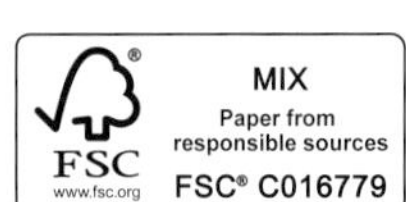

This book is dedicated to
Thomas Oetting

Contents

Foreword ix

Preface x

Acknowledgments xi

About the Editors xii

Contributors xiv

Video Contents xviii

Part 1. Basics

1 **History, Principles, and Instrumentation of Optical Coherence Tomography** 2
Dhivya Ashok Kumar and Amar Agarwal

2 **Time-Domain and Fourier-Domain Optical Coherence Tomography** 9
Dhivya Ashok Kumar and Amar Agarwal

3 **Ultrahigh-Resolution Optical Coherence Tomography for Imaging of Ocular Surface Tumors** 16
Juan C. Murillo, Anat Galor, and Carol L. Karp

4 **Phase-Variance Optical Coherence Tomography** 25
Scott M. McClintic, Dae Yu Kim, Jeff Fingler, Susan Garcia, Robert J. Zawadzki, Lawrence S. Morse, Susanna S. Park, Scott E. Fraser, John S. Werner, Jason P. Ruggiero, and Daniel M. Schwartz

5 **Swept-Source Optical Coherence Tomography** 32
Cong Ye and Vishal Jhanji

Part 2. Anterior-Segment Optical Coherence Tomography

6 **Visante Anterior-Segment Optical Coherence Tomography in the Evaluation of Patients for Refractive Surgery** 38
Amin Ashrafzadeh and Roger F. Steinert

7 **Anterior-Segment Exploration with Optical Coherence Tomography** 53
Georges Baikoff

8 **Corneal Inflammation and Optical Coherence Tomography** 63
Dhivya Ashok Kumar and Amar Agarwal

9 **Optical Coherence Tomography in Corneal Ectasia** 68
Otman Sandali, Vincent Borderie, and Laurent Laroche

10 **Spectral-Domain Anterior-Segment Optical Coherence Tomography in Refractive Surgery** 74
Karolinne Maia Rocha and Ronald R. Krueger

11 **Descemet Membrane Detachment: Classification and Management** 82
Soosan Jacob and Amar Agarwal

12 **Optical Coherence Therapy in Endothelial Keratoplasty** 89
Yuri McKee, Evan D. Schoenberg, and Francis Price, Jr.

13 **Spectral-Domain Optical Coherence Tomography Evaluation of Pre-Descemet Endothelial Keratoplasty Graft** 100
Ashvin Agarwal, Dhivya Ashok Kumar, and Amar Agarwal

Part 3. Cataract Surgery

14 **Optical Coherence Tomography Analysis in Cataract Surgery** 108
Richard Packard

15 **Optical Coherence Tomography Analysis of Wound Architecture in Sub-1-mm Cataract Surgery (700-µm Cataract Surgery)** 115
Dhivya Ashok Kumar and Amar Agarwal

16 **Intraocular Lens Tilt** 119
Kaladevi Satish, Dhivya Ashok Kumar, and Amar Agarwal

17 **Glued Intraocular Lens Position: An Optical Coherence Tomography Assessment** 124
Athiya Agarwal, Dhivya Ashok Kumar, and Amar Agarwal

18 **Use of Optical Coherence Tomography in Femtosecond Laser Lens and Cornea Surgery** . 130
Jason Philip Brinton and George O. Waring IV

Part 4. Optical Coherence Tomography in Retinal Diseases

19 **Optical Coherence Tomography Diagnosis of Retinal Diseases** 144
Mandeep Lamba, Soosan Jacob, and Amar Agarwal

20 **Vitreomacular Traction and Optical Coherence Tomography Classification** 154
Mehreen Adhi and Jay S. Duker

21 **Optical Coherence Tomography Diagnosis of Macular Pathologies** 161
J. Fernando Arevalo, Andres F. Lasave, and Fernando A. Arevalo

22 **Optical Coherence Tomography and Anti-Vascular Endothelial Growth Factor Therapy** 182
Mariana R. Thorell and Philip J. Rosenfeld

Part 5. Miscellaneous

23 **Optical Coherence Tomography for Imaging Anterior-Chamber Inflammatory Reaction in Uveitis** 194
Dhivya Ashok Kumar and Amar Agarwal

24 **Optical Coherence Tomography for Imaging the Subtenon Space, Sclera, and Choroid** 199
Soundari Sivagnanam, Dhivya Ashok Kumar, Amar Agarwal, and Rekha S. Bainchincholemath

25 **Optical Coherence Tomography and Glaucoma** 208
Jullia Ann Rosdahl and Sanjay Asrani

26 **Optical Coherence Tomography in Intraocular Tumors** 215
Santosh G. Honavar, Tika Siburt, and Carol L. Shields

27 **Optical Coherence Tomography–Assisted Anterior-Segment Surgery** 231
Gabor B. Scharioth

28 **Optical Coherence Tomography in Neurophthalmology** 234
Dhivya Ashok Kumar and Amar Agarwal

Index 239

Foreword

It is my distinct honor and privilege to write the foreword for this new textbook, *Essentials of OCT in Ocular Disease*. As in his other very practical and comprehensive textbooks, Dr. Agarwal has assembled an outstanding group of contributors who are all experts in this field. Their approach and experience in using this technology to improve the quality of care for patients are uniquely presented in each chapter and will provide an outstanding resource for all clinicians.

Dr. Agarwal is not only a prolific writer and contributor to our profession, but also an extremely astute and skilled anterior segment clinician and surgeon. After my personal visit to his hospital in Chennai, India, I was impressed with his clinical acumen and innovative spirit in approaching anterior-segment diseases of the eye. His understanding of ocular disease and thoughtful approach to patients with complex ophthalmic medical and surgical problems are reflected in this textbook.

I congratulate Dr. Agarwal and his colleagues for bringing us another comprehensive and beautifully written and illustrated textbook on an integral part of ophthalmic clinical care. I highly recommend it as a definitive resource for learning both the basics and the subtleties of this important technology.

Richard L. Abbott, MD
Thomas W. Boyden Endowed Chair
Health Sciences Clinical Professor of Ophthalmology
Department of Ophthalmology
University of California San Francisco
and
Research Associate
Francis I. Proctor Foundation
San Francisco, California

Preface

As well stated by one of our yesteryear leaders, "Live as if you were to die tomorrow, learn as if you were to live forever," learning is a continuous process. We all know that the more we read, the more we come to recognize that we know less. Books have always been a strong and standard medium in promoting and transferring information in every field, even in this Internet era. This book on ocular optical coherence tomography (OCT) is one such effort in providing for widespread acquaintance and understanding of OCT in ophthalmology. The main objective of the book is to provide postgraduates, general ophthalmologists, and ophthalmology specialists with an understanding of OCT's usefulness so that they can apply this imaging modality to various clinical scenarios in patient treatment. The book contains chapters by distinguished experts from their specific fields. High-resolution images with corresponding video illustrations will surely emit interest among the readers. This book comprises chapters on recent innovative applications of OCT, such as femtosecond-assisted cataract surgery with OCT, anterior-chamber inflammation, intraocular lens position, glued intraocular lens, pre-Descemet endothelial keratoplasty, and choroid evaluation. This text covers almost all fields in ophthalmology, from the anterior to the posterior segment of the eye. We are convinced this book will be an awakener in ocular imaging using OCT.

Acknowledgments

Nothing in this world moves without Him, and so also this book was only written by Him.

About the Editors

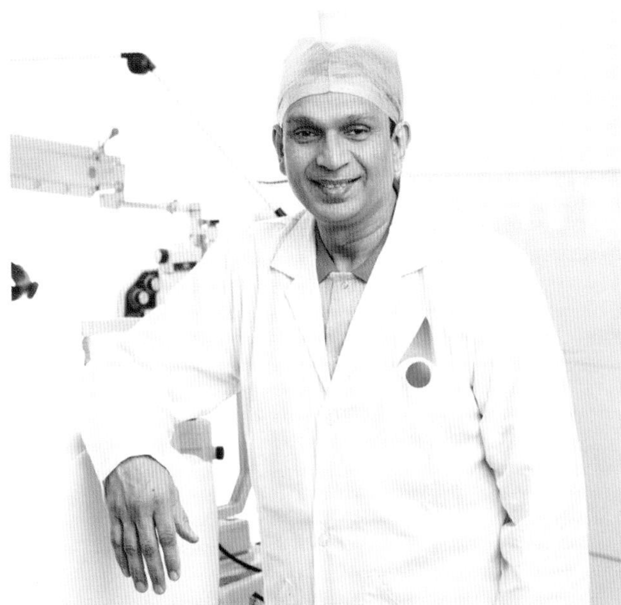

Professor Amar Agarwal, MS, FRCS, FRCOphth
Chairman and Managing Director
Dr. Agarwal's Group of Eye Hospitals and Eye Research Centre
Chennai, Tamil Nadu
India

Past President, International Society of Refractive Surgery (ISRS)

Secretary General, Indian Intraocular Implant and Refractive Society (IIRSI)

Professor Amar Agarwal is the pioneer of phakonit (phako with a needle incision) technology. This technique became popularized as bimanual phaco, microincision cataract surgery, or microphaco. He was the first to remove cataracts through a 0.7-mm tip using a technique called microphakonit and initiated no-anesthesia cataract surgery and sleeveless phacotip-assisted levitation, previously known as FAVIT ("fallen vitreous"), a new technique to remove dropped nuclei. A sleeveless extrusion cannula to lift dropped intraoperative lens (IOL) was also started in Dr. Agarwal's Group of Eye Hospitals. The air pump, which was a simple idea of using an aquarium fish pump to increase the fluid into the eye in bimanual phaco and coaxial phaco, has helped prevent surge and has been the basis for various techniques of forced infusion for small-incision cataract surgery. Dr. Agarwal also discovered a new refractive error called aberropia. He was the first to do a combined surgery of microphakonit (700-µm cataract surgery) using a 25-gauge vitrectomy in the same patient, thus using the smallest possible incisions for cataracts and vitrectomy. He was the first surgeon to implant a new mirror telescopic IOL (LMI) for patients suffering from age-related macular degeneration, as well as the first in the world to implant a glued IOL, in which a posterior-chamber IOL is fixed in an eye using fibrin glue, without any capsules. He modified the Malyugin ring for small pupil cataract surgery as the Agarwal modification of the Malyugin ring for miotic pupil cataract surgeries with posterior capsular defects. Dr. Agarwal's Eye Hospital was the first to do anterior-segment transplantation in a 4-month-old child with anterior staphyloma. He also developed the technique of IOL scaffold, in which a three-piece IOL is injected into an eye between the iris and the nucleus to prevent the nucleus from falling down in posterior capsular ruptures. He combined glued IOL and IOL scaffold in cases of posterior chamber rupture where there is no iris or capsular support and termed the technique glued IOL scaffold. The first performance of glued endocapsular ring in cases of subluxated cataract was at Dr. Agarwal's Eye Hospital.

Pre-Descemet endothelial keratoplasty, or PDEK, was started by Prof. Agarwal. In this procedure, the Pre-Descemet layer and the Descemet membrane with endothelium are transplanted en bloc in patients with diseased endothelium. Dr. Agarwal's Eye Hospital also was first to perform CACXL, or contact lens–assisted collagen cross-linking, a new technique for cross-linking thin corneas, and worked on E-DMEK, in which an endoilluminator is used to assist in DMEK surgeries. He was first to combine PDEK and glued IOL in the same patient.

Professor Agarwal has received many awards for his work in ophthalmology, the most significant being the Casebeer Award (International Society of Refractive Surgery), the Barraquer Award (Keratomileusis Study Group), and the Kelman Award (Hellenic Society). He has performed more than 150 live surgeries at various conferences. His videos have won many awards at the film festivals of American Society of Cataract and Refractive Surgery, American Academy of Opthalmology, and European Society of Cataract and Refractive Surgeries. He has written more than 60 books, which have been published in various languages: English, Spanish, and Polish. He trains doctors from all over the world in his center on phaco, bimanual phaco, LASIK, and retina. He is chairman and managing director of Dr. Agarwal's Group of Eye Hospitals, which has 60 eye hospitals worldwide. He is professor of ophthalmology at Ramachandra Medical College in Chennai, India and can be contacted at dragarwal@vsnl.com. The hospital's website is http://www.dragarwal.com

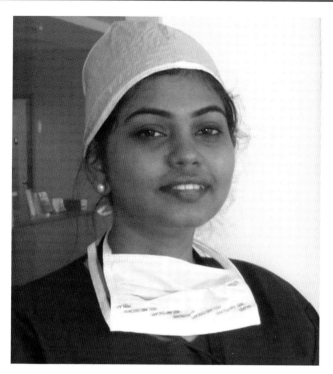

Dr. Dhivya Ashok Kumar, MD, FICO
Consultant Ophthalmologist and Head of R & D
Dr. Agarwal's Group of Eye Hospitals and Eye Research Centre
Chennai, Tamil Nadu
India

Dhivya Ashok Kumar, MD, completed her ophthalmology residency training at the All India Institute of Medical Sciences, New Delhi, India, and has been affiliated with Dr. Agarwal's Eye Hospital and Eye Research Centre, Chennai, India, since 2007. She is now working as consultant in uvea and oculoplasty services in Dr. Agarwal's Eye Hospital. She has an immense passion for research and innovative methods for the evaluation of ocular disorders. Her regions of interest involve anterior-segment imaging, glued intraocular lens (IOL), and ocular inflammation. Dr. Kumar had the opportunity to perform various research studies on glued IOL under the guidance of her mentor, Professor Amar Agarwal. The results of this work have been published in leading peer-reviewed journals, books, and conference presentations. Dr. Kumar has formulated a novel optical coherence tomography (OCT) classification of anterior-chamber cellular reaction for grading uveitis, introduced a new algorithm for IOL tilt determination by OCT, and proposed OCT-guided posterior sub-Tenon triamcinolone injection in patients with uveitis to prevent scleral perforation by using direct visualization of intravenous cannula.

Contributors

Mehreen Adhi, MBBS
Research Fellow
Department of Opthalmology
New England Eye Center
Tufts University School of Medicine
Boston, Massachusetts

Amar Agarwal, MS, FRCS, FRCOphth
Professor and Head
Dr. Agarwal's Group of Eye Hospitals and Eye Research Centre
Chennai, Tamil Nadu
India

Athiya Agarwal, MD
Director and Senior Consultant
Dr. Agarwal's Group of Eye Hospitals and Eye Research Centre
Chennai, Tamil Nadu
India

Ashvin Agarwal, MS, FERC
Director and Consultant - Cornea
Dr. Agarwal's Group of Eye Hospitals and Eye Research Centre
Chennai, Tamil Nadu
India

J. Fernando Arevalo, MD
Chief
Vitreoretinal Division
The King Khaled Eye Specialist Hospital
Riyadh, Kingdom of Saudi Arabia

Fernando A. Arevalo, BS
Surgeon
Clinica Oftalmologica Centro Caracas
San Bernadino, Caracas
Venezuela

Amin Ashrafzadeh, MD
Cornea and Refractive Surgeon
Modesto Eye Center
Modesto, California

Sanjay Asrani, MD
Professor of Ophthalmology
Duke University
Duke Eye Center
Durham, North Carolina

Georges Baikoff, MD
Ophthalmologist
Clinique Floutialli
Marseille, France

Rekha S. Bainchincholemath, DOMS, DNB, FMRF
Retina Consultant
Dr. Agarwal's Group of Eye Hospitals and Eye Research Centre
Chennai, Tamil Nadu
India

Vincent Borderie, MD, PhD
National Eye Institute
Paris, France

Jason Philip Brinton, MD
Partner
Hunter Vision
Clinical Assistant Professor of Opthalmology
University of Kansas Medical Center
Kansas City, Kansas

Jay S. Duker, MD
Director
New England Eye Center
Professor and Chairman of Opthalmology
Tufts Medical Center
Tufts University School of Medicine
Boston, Massachusetts

Jeff Fingler, PhD
Senior Research Scientist
University of Southern California
Los Angeles, California

Scott E. Fraser, PhD
Director of Science Initiatives
Provost Professor of Biological Sciences & Biomedical Engineering
University of Southern California
Los Angeles, California

Anat Galor, MD
MSPH Staff Physician
Miami Veterans Affairs Medical Center
Associate Professor of Clinical Ophthalmology
Bascom Palmer Eye Institute
University of Miami Miller School of Medicine
Miami, Florida

Susan Garcia, BA, COT
Research Coordinator
Davis Eye Center
University of California
Sacramento, California

Santosh G. Honavar, MD, FACS
Director
Ophthalmic Plastic Surgery and Ocular Oncology
Centre for Sight Eye Hospital
Banjara Hills, Hyderabad
India

Soosan Jacob, MS, FRCS, DNB
Dr. Agarwal's Group of Eye Hospitals and Eye Research Centre
Chennai, Tamil Nadu
India

Vishal Jhanji, MD
Assistant Professor
Department of Ophthalmology and Visual Sciences
The Chinese University of Hong Kong
Kowloon, Hong Kong SAR

Carol L. Karp, MD
Professor of Opthalmology
Bascom Palmer Eye Institute
University of Miami Miller School of Medicine
Miami, Florida

Dae Yu Kim, PhD
Assistant Research Professor
Beckman Laser Institute Korea
Dankook University
Cheonan-si, Chungnam
Korea

Ronald R. Krueger, MD
Medical Director
Department of Refractive Surgery
Cleveland Clinic
Cole Eye Institute
Cleveland, Ohio

Dhivya Ashok Kumar, MD, FICO
Consultant Ophthalmologist and Head of R & D
Dr. Agarwal's Group of Eye Hospitals and Eye Research Centre
Chennai, Tamil Nadu
India

Mandeep Lamba, MD
Dr. Agarwal's Group of Eye Hospitals and Eye Research Centre
Chennai, Tamil Nadu
India

Laurent Laroche, MD, PhD
Surgeon
National Eye Institute
Paris, France

Andres F. Lasave, MD
Vitreoretinal Specialist
The Retina and Vitreous Service
Clinica Privada de Ojos
Mar del Plata, Argentina

Scott M. McClintic, MD
Vitreoretinal Surgery Fellow
Casey Eye Institute
Oregon Health and Science University
Portland, Oregon

Yuri McKee, MD
Corneal and Refractive Surgeon
Price Vision Group
Indianapolis, Indiana

Lawrence S. Morse, MD, PhD
Professor of Ophthalmology
Department of Ophthalmology
University of California Davis
Sacramento, California

Juan C. Murillo, MD
Research Fellow
Bascom Palmer Eye Institute
University of Miami Miller School of Medicine
Miami, Florida

Richard Packard, MD, DO, FRCS, FRCOphth
Consultant
Prince Charles Eye Unit
King Edward VII Hospital
Windsor, England

Susanna S. Park, MD, PhD
Professor
Davis Eye Center
University of California
Sacramento, California

Francis Price, Jr, MD
President
Price Vision Group
Indianapolis, Indiana

Karolinne Maia Rocha, MD, PhD
Assistant Professor
Medical University of South Carolina
Storm Eye Institute
Charleston, South Carolina

Jullia Ann Rosdahl, MD, PhD
Assistant Professor of Ophthalmology
Duke University
Duke Eye Center
Durham, North Carolina

Philip J. Rosenfeld, MD, PhD
Professor of Opthalmology
Bascom Palmer Eye Institute
University of Miami Miller School of Medicine
Miami, Florida

Jason P. Ruggiero, MD
Surgeon
Retina Associates
Winchester, Virginia

Tika Siburt
Opthalmic Photographer
Wills Eye Hospital
Philadelphia, Pennsylvania

Soundari Sivagnanam, DO, DNB, FRCS
Senior Consultant
Dr. Agarwal's Group of Eye Hospitals and Eye Research Centre
Chennai, Tamil Nadu
India

Otman Sandali, MD
Surgeon
National Eye Institute
Paris, France

Kaladevi Satish, MD
Consultant
Dr. Agarwal's Group of Eye Hospitals and Eye Research Centre
Chennai, Tamil Nadu
India

Gabor B. Scharioth, MD
Professor
Aurelios Augenzentrum
Recklinghausen, Germany

Evan D. Schoenberg, MD
Corneal and Refractive Surgeon
George Eye Partners
Atlanta, Georgia

Daniel M. Schwartz, MD
Director of Vitreoretinal Service
Professor of Clinical Ophthalmology
Department of Ophthalmology
University of California
San Francisco, California

Carol L. Shields, MD
Co-Director
Ocular Oncology Service
Wills Eye Hospital
Philadelphia, Pennsylvania

Roger F. Steinert, MD
Professor and Chair
Department of Ophthalmology
Irving H. Leopold
Director
Gavin Herbert Eye Institute
Professor of Biomedical Engineering
University of California Irvine
Irvine, California

Mariana R. Thorell, MD
Post-Doctoral Associate
Bascom Palmer Eye Institute
University of Miami Miller School of Medicine
Miami, Florida

George O. Waring IV, MD FACS
Director of Refractive Surgery
Assistant Professor of Ophthalmology
Medical University of South Carolina
Adjunct Assistant Professor of Bioengineering
College of Engineering and Science at Clemson University
Clemson, South Carolina

John S. Werner, PhD
Surgeon
University of California Davis
Department of Ophthalmology & Vision Science
Department of Neurobiology, Physiology & Behavior
Brown University
Davis, California

Cong Ye, PhD
Department of Ophthalmology and Visual Sciences
The Chinese University of Hong Kong
Kowloon, Hong Kong SAR

Robert J. Zawadzki, MD
Associate Researcher
Department of Ophthalmology & Vision Science
University of California Davis
Sacramento, California

Video Contents

Video 1: Room with a View
Video 2: Corneal Biomechanics: The New Mantra
Video 3: Posterior Chamber Phakic IOL: The Right Way Up
Video 4: Contact Lens Assisted Collagen Crosslinking: New Technique for Crosslinking in Thin Corneas
Video 5: Descemet's Detachment New Classification and management
Video 6: Pre-Descemet's Endothelial Keratoplasty
Video 7: Sub 1mm Cataract Surgery
Video 8: Glued IOL Reloaded
Video 9: What Lies Beneath
Video 10: Stab Incision Glaucoma Surgery

Part 1

Basics

1 History, Principles, and Instrumentation of Optical Coherence Tomography

Dhivya Ashok Kumar and Amar Agarwal

1.1 History

Optical coherence tomography (OCT) is a newer medical investigational modality that has been widely used in ophthalmology. It performs real-time, high-resolution, micrometer-scale, cross-sectional imaging of ocular tissues in less time. Although it has been used in other medical fields, the ophthalmologic specialty has used this application widely for the diagnosis, prognosis, and management of ocular pathologies. OCT uses low-coherence interferometry to produce a two-dimensional image of optical scattering from internal tissue microstructures in a way that is analogous to ultrasonic pulse-echo imaging.

The noninvasive nature and higher resolution compared with other imaging techniques, such as ultrasound, magnetic resonance imaging, and computerized tomography, have made OCT one of the standard diagnostic tests for many ocular disorders. OCT was first used for in vitro imaging in the peripapillary area of the retina and in the coronary artery, two clinically relevant examples that are representative of transparent and turbid media, respectively. In 1991, Huang and associates demonstrated the OCT evaluation of the retina using infrared light of ~ 800-nm wavelength and axial resolution 10 µm.[1] They reported OCT correlation with the histologic appearance of the retina. Their images were displayed as false color scale, depending on the magnitude of the backscattering. OCT was also used in cadaver eyes for ex vivo imaging of the retina and optic nerve head. It was the effort and vision of the physical scientists and ophthalmologists, namely, Doctors David Huang, Joel Schumann, James Fujimoto, Eric Swanson, and Carmen A. Puliafito, that led to the conversion of the interferometry principle to a widely used imaging modality in the eye.[2] OCT gained popularity in ophthalmology as a result of the transparent nature of the ocular media and the ease in evaluation of anterior and posterior segments of the eye.

Initially, OCT was used for the evaluation of retinal structures and the optic nerve head.[3,4,5,6] The wavelength of light used for retinal study was 830 nm; however, this wavelength was not adequate for imaging the anterior ocular structures, such the cornea, anterior-chamber, angles, and lens. OCT imaging of the anterior segment with a longer wavelength of 1310 nm was developed later. Izatt et al first introduced micrometer-scale resolution imaging of the anterior eye with OCT in 1994.[7] It had the advantages of better penetration through sclera as well as real-time imaging at eight frames per second.[8]

Since the introduction of OCT in ophthalmology, this imaging method has been used extensively for the diagnosis of various clinical disorders of the retina. Quantification of macular edema, diagnosis of central serous retinopathy, grading of macular holes, assessment of age-related macular degeneration, and determination of epiretinal membrane are some of the widely applied fields of macular OCT.[9,10,11,12,13] In analysis of the optic nerve head, OCT was initially used for determination of the thickness of the retinal nerve fiber layer, which is an important parameter for glaucoma assessment.[5,14] In 1995, Schuman and associates showed that the thickness of the retinal nerve fiber layer as measured by OCT demonstrated a high degree of correlation with the functional status of the optic nerve as measured by visual field examination.[5] Emergence of OCT in anterior-segment evaluation has opened the new world of using OCT for corneal surgeries, especially refractive surgeries.[15,16,17,18] With the evolution of OCT, new clinical entities have been identified, and innovative OCT-guided surgical techniques are being performed.[19,20,21,22] The last decade saw massive innovative applications of OCT in ophthalmology.[18,19,20,21,22,23,24] High-speed anterior-segment OCT has been applied to visualize anywhere from the cornea to the lens.[24,25,26,27] In 2010, anterior-segment OCT was combined with femtosecond laser for cataract extraction.[28]

1.2 Principle

Interferometry is the basic physical principle used in OCT. The Michelson interferometer causes interference by splitting a beam of light into two parts. Each part is made to travel a different path and brought back together, where they interfere according to their path length difference.[2]

1.2.1 Coherence

Coherent lights are light waves that are "in phase" with one another (▶ Fig. 1.1a). Two waves are coherent if the crests of one wave are aligned with the crests of the other and the troughs of one wave are aligned with the troughs of the other. Otherwise, these light waves are considered incoherent. Light

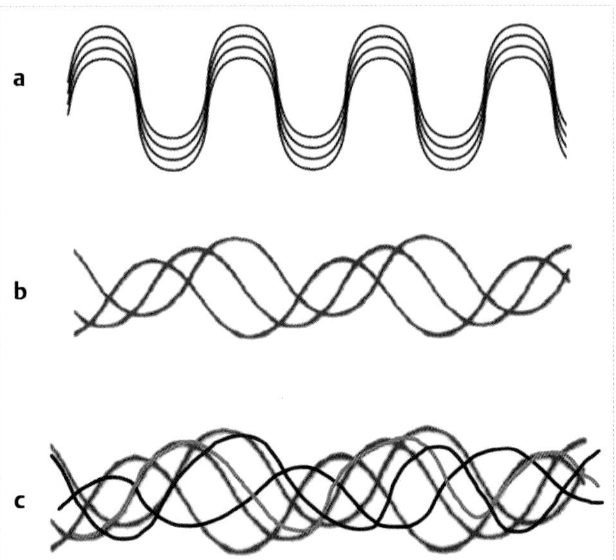

Fig. 1.1 Image of (**a**) coherent and (**b, c**) noncoherent waves. (**b**) Light bulb. (**c**) Sun.

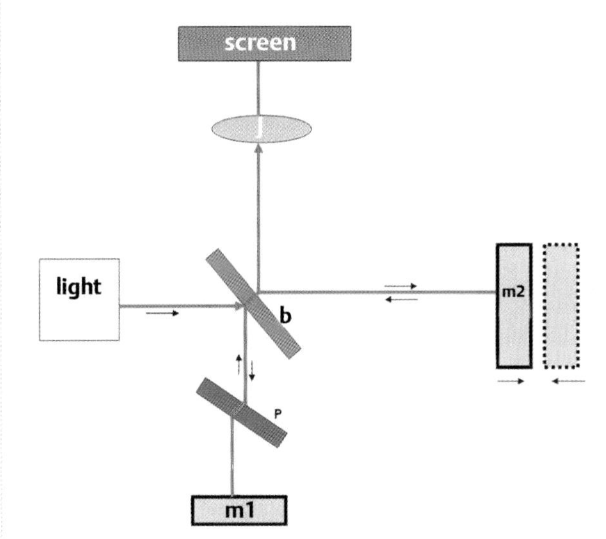

Fig. 1.2 Schematic diagram of interferometry. Light strikes the beam splitter (b), which splits the light into two, one transmitted to mirror m1 and the other to mirror m2. The light rays reflected from mirrors m1 and m2 are received on the screen where the two beams are superposed making it possible to observe the interference. P: compensatory plate, L: Focusing lens

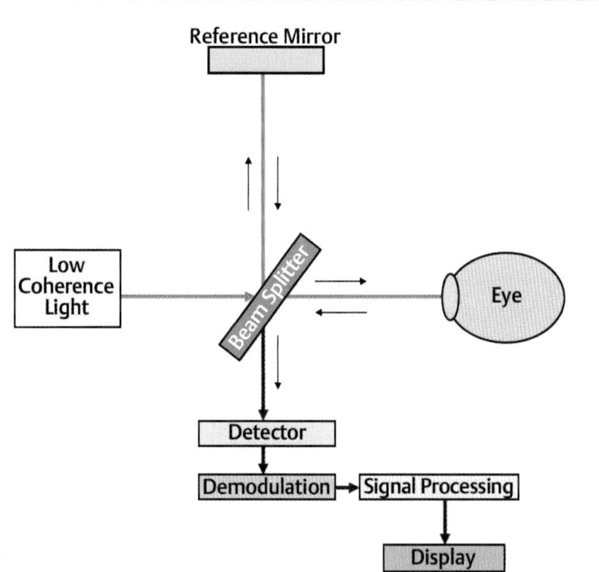

Fig. 1.3 Optics in optical coherence tomography. Near-infrared low-coherence light is directed onto a beam splitter, from which one beam is incident onto the eye; the second beam travels a reference path (reference mirror). The backscattered light from the eye is interfered with the reflected light from the reference arm and detected with a photodetector. It then undergoes demodulation and processing at the output of the interferometer.

produced by lasers is *coherent light*. Light from light bulbs or the sun, however, is *incoherent light* (▶ Fig. 1.1b,c).

1.2.2 Interferometer

Light from the source (▶ Fig. 1.2) strikes the beam splitter (B). The beam splitter allows 50% of the radiation to be transmitted to the translatable mirror M1. The other 50% of the radiation is reflected resected to the fixed mirror M2. The compensator plate P is introduced along this path to make each path have the same optical path length when M1 and M2 are the same distance from the beam splitter. After returning from M1, 50% of the light is reflected toward the frosted glass screen. Likewise, 50% of the light returning from M2 is transmitted to the glass screen. At the screen, the two beams are superposed, and one can observe the interference between them.

1.2.3 Interferometry in OCT

Low coherence was initially described by Sir Issac Newton.[29] This principle of interferometry has been used technically in fiber-optic instrumentation in the last two decades. Distance or spatial information may be determined from the time delay of reflected echoes according to the formula $\Delta T = z/v$, where ΔT is the echo delay, z is the distance that the echo travels, and v is the velocity of the sound wave or light wave.[2] Low-coherence interferometry was first applied in ophthalmology to perform precision measurements of axial eye length and corneal thickness.[29] Light from a source is directed onto a beam splitter, and one of the beams is incident onto the sample to be imaged; the second beam travels a reference path with a variable path length and time delay (▶ Fig. 1.3). The backscattered light from the sample is interfered with reflected light from the reference arm and detected with a photo detector at the output of the interferometer. If the light source is coherent, interference fringes will be observed as the relative path lengths are varied. However, if low-coherence or short-pulse light is used, interference of the light reflected from the sample and reference path can occur only when the two path lengths match to within the coherence length of the light. The echo time delay and intensity of backscattered light from sites within the sample can be measured by detecting and demodulating the interference output of the interferometer while scanning the reference path length.

When light enters the eye, it goes to the interior of the eye, hits the ocular structures, and comes back. Thus, the light is back-reflected from tissue boundaries and backscattered with varying intensities from tissues of different optical properties.[2] The distances and dimensions of the intraocular structures are determined from the amount of light backreflected and backscattered from the biological tissue by quantifying the echo time delay.[30] The echo time delay depends on the distance travelled by the light and its velocity. We know that the velocity of light is faster than that of sound; thus, resolution of an image acquired by OCT is higher.

1.2.4 Comparison with Ultrasound Imaging

The velocity of sound in water is approximately 1500 m/s, whereas the velocity of light is approximately 3×10^8 m/s. The fundamental physical principle underlying diagnostic ultrasound is the generation of sound waves at frequencies above the range of human hearing (greater than 20,000 Hz or 20 kHz) by the vibration of a thin crystal in the tip of the probe that is

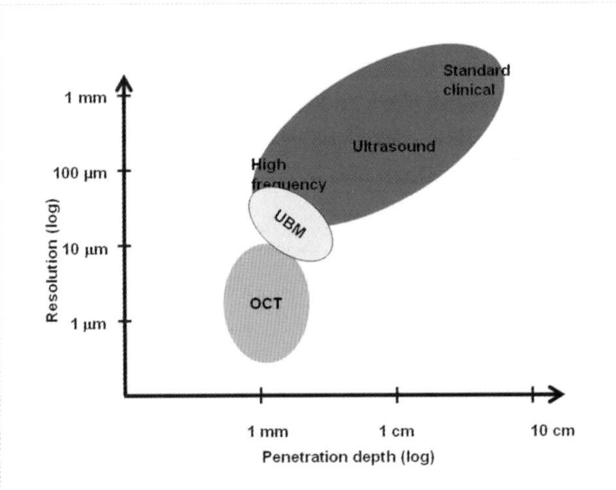

Fig. 1.4 Graphical representation showing the difference in the resolution of optical coherence tomography (OCT) and ultrasound imaging. UBM, ultrasound biomicroscopy.

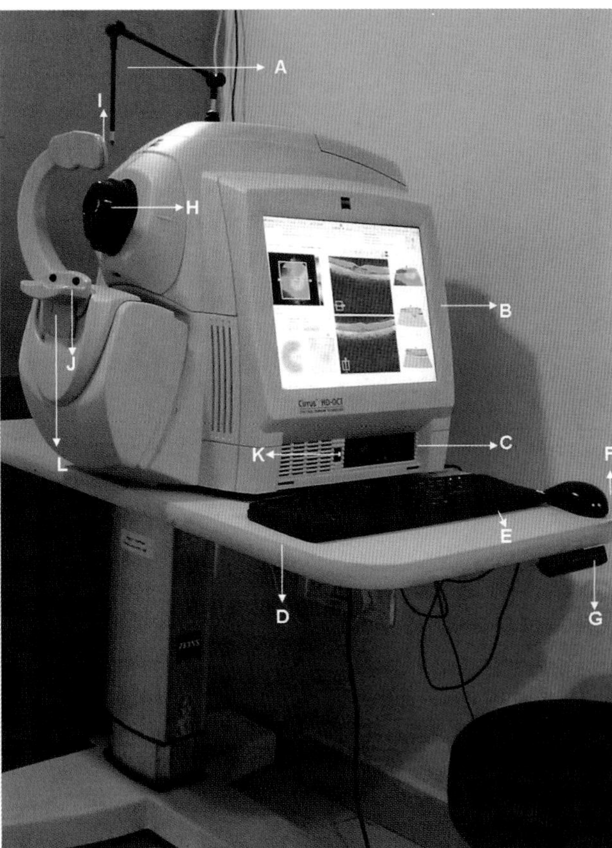

Fig. 1.5 Commercial optical coherence tomography (OCT) machine showing the system hardware in operational setup. External fixator (A). Integrated video monitor (B). CD drive or USB port (C). Power table (D). Keyboard (E). Mouse (F). Table height controls (G). Imaging aperture (H). Patient headrest (I). Chin rest (J). System power switch (K). Three-dimensional motorized patient alignment unit (L).

stimulated by pulses of electric current. The B-scan (brightness amplitude) probe contains a transducer, which sweeps back and forth at an average rate of 25 oscillations per second. It generates sound waves at a frequency of 10 MHz. Higher frequencies of 30 MHz or 50 MHz are used in anterior segment imaging. The conventional ultrasound gives resolution of 150 µm and the high-frequency ultrasound named as ultrasound biomicroscopy gives 50-µm resolution, which is far less than OCT (▶ Fig. 1.4). In ultrasound, there is need for coupling fluid, or viscoelastics, on the eye for image acquisition. Therefore, in post-traumatic cases and eyes with open wounds, ultrasound scan is not performed because of the risk of the transfer of microbes and the induction of globe distortion during the examination. The main advantage of OCT, which is a light-based instrument compared with ultrasound, a sound-based machine, is that it can be applied to all eyes without direct contact onto the biological structure. The limitation of a light-based instrument is the scattering or absorption in the tissues. An important feature of ultrasound imaging is the absence of scattering and ready transmission into deeper structures. Moreover, it can be performed in eyes with opaque media-like dense corneal opacity or vitreous hemorrhage, where an OCT imaging might not be possible.

1.3 OCT Instrumentation

The internal optics of the OCT machine is similar to a fundus camera. The near-infrared light from the superluminescent light-emitting diode source (840 nm) goes through the pupil and reaches the retina. The optical system is built so that the OCT beam pivots about the pupil of the eye when it is scanned. The external structure of the machine includes the patient's side and the examiner's operational side (▶ Fig. 1.5). The patient side has the chin rest, head rest, the imaging aperture, and the fixation target arm; the examiner side of the machine has the viewing integrated video monitor, keyboard, and mouse. The whole OCT system is placed in a power table with height-control buttons.

An objective lens of 78 diopters is used to relay the image of the retina on to the image plane inside the machine.[2] The retinal image is then relayed to the video camera, where the examiner views in real time. The OCT beam is coupled with the optical path of the instrument by the beam splitter and then focused in the image plane by a focusing lens. From there, the OCT beam is relay-imaged onto the retina by another objective lens and the patient's eye.[2] The size of the incident OCT beam at the pupil is approximately 1.4 mm and at the retina (spot size) is 15 to 20 µm. Because the OCT beam pivots around the pupil, there is less possibility of vignette, which causes a reduction in the OCT signal and induces artifacts. Hence, it is necessary that the OCT beam pivots around the pupil and is maintained by placing the patient's eye at the given distance from the objective lens.[2] Vertical and horizontal alignments are adjusted by the chin rest alignment display in the monitor. The mouse scroll wheel works well for fine adjustments (▶ Fig. 1.6).

Once the OCT image is seen in the video screen on the display, the lens can be adjusted for perfect focusing on the retina. Some OCT systems use two additional live-imaging systems simultaneously to facilitate ease of use: a charged coupled device (CCD) video camera monitors the exterior eye and assists with scan alignment, and a line-scanning ophthalmoscope provides a clear image of the retinal area addressed by the scan.

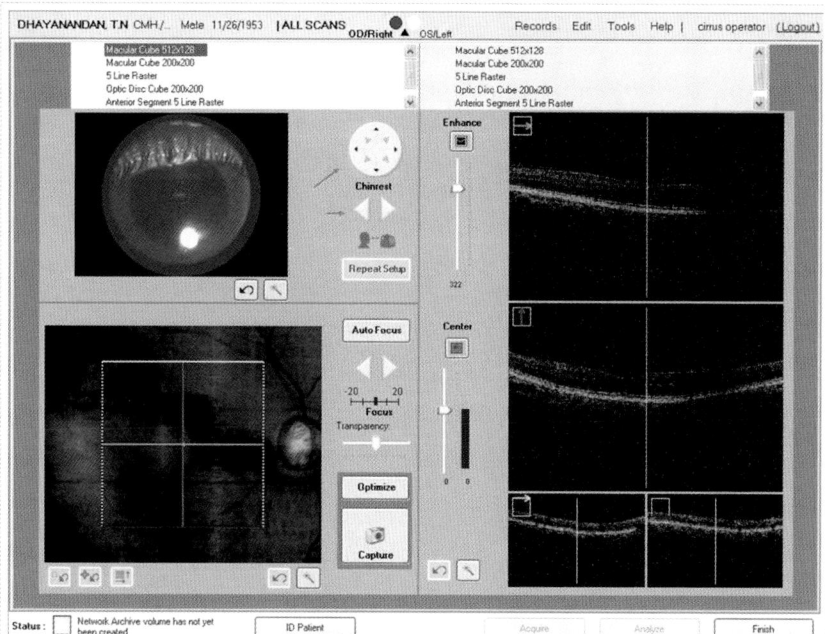

Fig. 1.6 Video monitor showing the fine adjustment options for chin rest and headrest for proper focusing (red arrows).

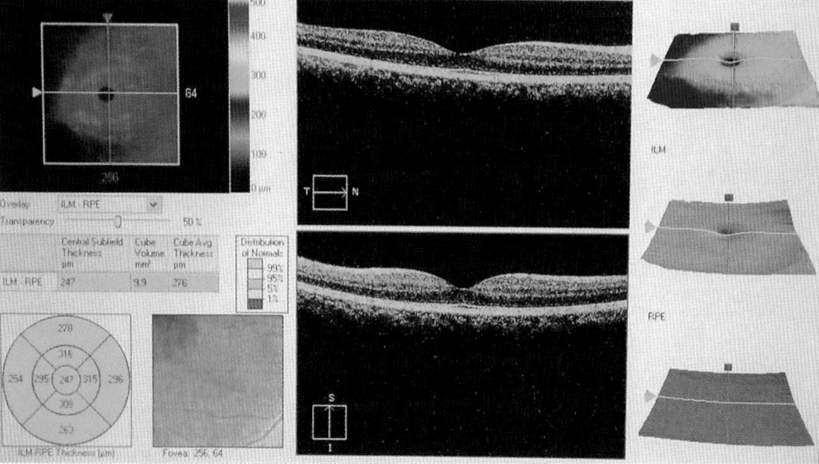

Fig. 1.7 Optical coherence tomography image as seen by macular cube 512 × 128 type scan. ILM, internal limiting membrane; RPE, retinal pigment epithelium.

Tomograms are stored on the computer or on an archive medium and can be quantitatively analyzed. The system can work at about 750 μW because of its high sensitivity. The instrument is intended for use in an environment in which radiated radio frequencies disturbances are controlled.

1.3.1 Type of Scans

Type of scans depends on the commercial OCT instrument used. The following are some of the scan types commonly used for evaluation.

- Posterior-segment (Cirrus OCT; Carl Zeiss Meditec, Dublin, CA, USA) macular cube 512 × 128: Generates a cube of data (▸ Fig. 1.7) through a 6-mm-square grid by acquiring a series of 128 horizontal scan lines, each composed of 512 A-scans.
- Macular cube 200 × 200: Generates a cube of data through a 6-mm-square grid by acquiring a series of 200 horizontal scan lines, each composed of 200 A-scans.
- Five-line raster: Adjustable. Scans through five parallel lines (▸ Fig. 1.8) of equal length; the line length, rotation, and spacing are adjustable. By default, the lines are horizontal, and each line is 6 mm long and separated by 250 μm (0.25 mm) from the next, so that the five lines together cover a 1-mm width. In the custom scan pattern, for line spacing, you can select among the following options, in millimeters: 0 (five lines in same location), 0.01, 0.025, 0.05, 0.075, 0.125, 0.2, 0.25, 0.5, or 1.25. For length, you can select 3, 6, or 9 mm. For rotation, adjust the angle in the ranges of 0 to 90 or 270 to 359 degrees.
- Optic disc cube 200 × 200: Generates a cube (▸ Fig. 1.9) of data through a 6-mm-square grid by acquiring a series of 200 horizontal scan lines, each composed of 200 A-scans.

1.3.2 Interpretation of OCT Output

The OCT image provides a cross-sectional view of the retina with unprecedented resolution and allows detailed structures to be differentiated. Image contrast in OCT depends on the differences in the back-reflection and backscattering of light from different ocular tissues.

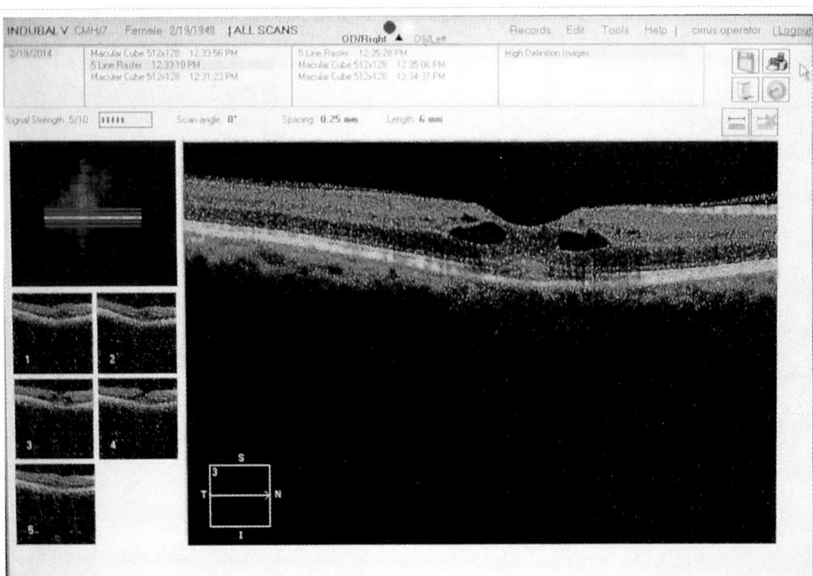

Fig. 1.8 Five-line raster scan (▶ Fig. 1.7) of macula showing cystoid macular edema.

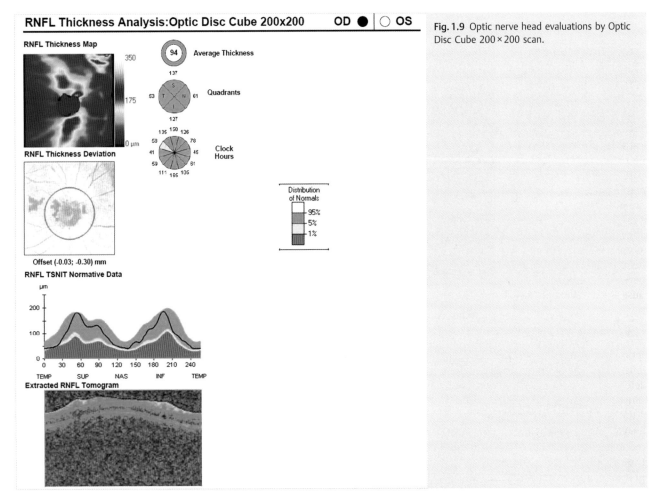

Fig. 1.9 Optic nerve head evaluations by Optic Disc Cube 200 × 200 scan.

1.3.3 Factors Affecting OCT Image

Light Transmission

Transmitted light is the unaffected light, and it goes inside the ocular structures. The better the transmission is, the better the output will be.

Light Absorption

Absorption of light in the biological tissues will reduce the transmitted light. The light is absorbed by the presence of tissue chromophores, which absorb light of a specific wavelength. In the human eye, hemoglobin and melanin are the pigments that cause absorption.

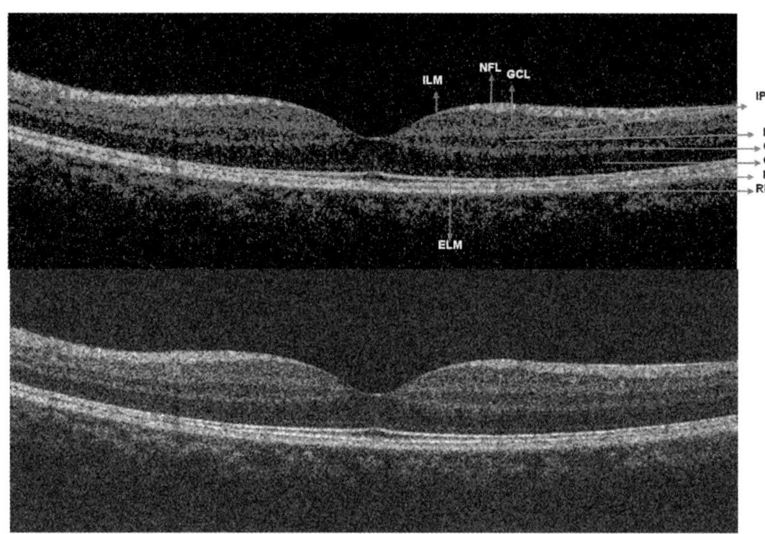

Fig. 1.10 Retinal layers as seen by color-coded optical coherence tomography scan and the corresponding gray scale. CC, choriocapillaries; ELM, external limiting membrane; GCL, ganglion cell layer; ILM, internal limiting membrane; INL, inner nuclear layer; IPL, inner plexiform layer; IS-OS JN, inner segment-outer segment junction; NFL, nerve fiber layer; OPL, outer plexiform layer; ONL, outer nuclear layer; RPE, retinal pigment epithelium.

Reflection

When sharp borders or structures are in the pathway of the light, reflections occur. This happens when different biological tissues of varying refractive indices are present. Reflections are greatest when the light is perpendicular to the structure. In OCT, reflections are usually seen in the fovea.

1.3.4 Scattering

Scattering happens as a result of structural variations within the tissue. Tissues made of heterogeneous proteins where the spatial variations are present produce optical scattering. The internal refractive indices at varying regions of the same structure may show differences. The refractive index variations occur at the intracellular level at the nuclei, cytoplasm, and intracellular organelles. Scattering makes the structure brighter in OCT output. In retinal OCT, the nerve fiber layer, retinal pigment epithelium (RPE), and plexiform layers show more scattering and therefore appear brighter. Excess absorption and scattering can cause light attenuation and shadowing of the deep tissues.

1.3.5 Backscattering

Optical scattering will make the incident light move in all directions. When the scattered light is reversed in direction completely, this is known as backscattered light. OCT output image comprises the backscattered light from the internal structures of the eye. The contrast in the backscattered light depends on the microscopic variations in the specific tissue.

1.3.6 OCT Analysis

The output is obtained in the monitor in false color-coded images (▸ Fig. 1.10) and must be interpreted with respect to histologic variation. For example, in normal retinal OCT, layer differentiation is made with respect to the difference in the histologic characteristics of the individual layers. The nerve-fiber layer (NFL) is the innermost layer and is the first bright line seen in the retinal OCT, in bright red to yellow. The NFL and the two plexiform layers (inner and outer) have axonal structures passing across them, so they are seen as bright green. The inner and outer nuclear layers show weak backscattering and are seen as black. The ganglion cell layer seems to be increasing in the parafoveal region compared with the foveal region, and this can be visualized in OCT by a progressive increase in the green inner layer in the parafoveal region. The thin line seen posterior to the outer nuclear layer represents the external limiting membrane. The layers of photoreceptors are a bright line just anterior to the RPE and choroid. This layer is highly reflecting because of the reflection from the junction of inner and outer segment of the photoreceptors. The outermost layer is the RPE, which has melanin, causing strong backscattering, and it appears as red or bright green.

1.3.7 Artifacts in OCT

Fixation Error

Improper fixation can induce artifact preventing proper evaluation of the structures. Patients with nystagmus and with very low vision can have this problem (▸ Fig. 1.11a).

Focusing Error

Absolute focusing of the retina by fine adjustments made after viewing the retina in the monitor is recommended. The autofocus option can also be used. Ocular media changes like vitreous haze can affect the focusing range during operation (▸ Fig. 1.11b).

Vignette Image

When the OCT beam is not pivoting in the pupil plane, vignetting happens and causes a reduction in the intensity of light entering the eye and, therefore, artifacts. Hence, the patient's eye should remain at the same distance throughout the test.

1.4 Conclusion

Although OCT has been introduced in ocular diagnosis in the last decade, it has revolutionized the imaging field of

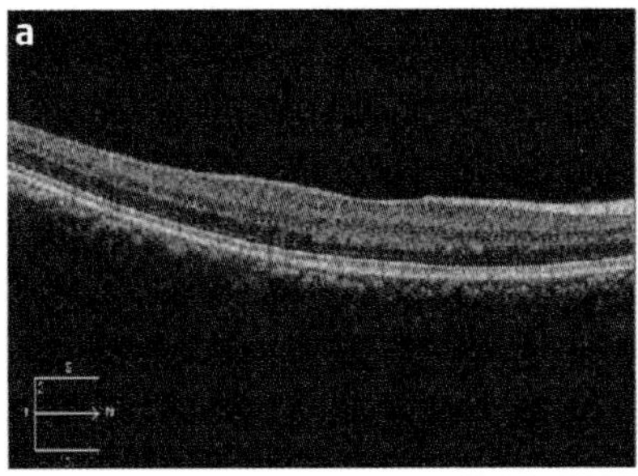
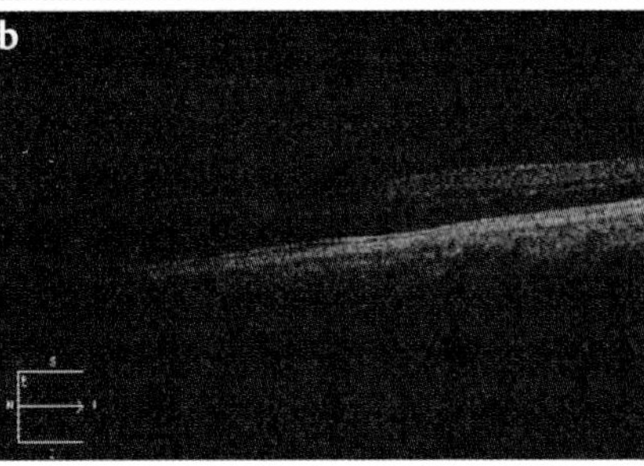

Fig. 1.11 (a) Demonstration of retinal optical coherence tomography scans with fixation error and (b) focusing error.

ophthalmology tremendously during this time, unlike any other investigation so far. In this first chapter, we have gone through a brief history and the basic optical principle and instrumentation of OCT. We have also discussed the basic analysis of OCT output and the optical mechanism behind it and summarized the differences between the ultrasound-based machine and the light-based OCT scan. In subsequent chapters, we detail the different types of OCT mechanisms and the commercially available OCT systems.

References

[1] Huang D, Swanson EA, Lin CP, et al. Optical coherence tomography. Science 1991; 254: 1178–1181

[2] Fujimoto J, Schumann J, Huang D, Duker JS, Carmen A Puliafito ES. Introduction to optical coherence tomography. In: Schumann J, Puliafito CA, Fujimoto J, Duker S III. Optical Coherence Tomography of Ocular Diseases. 3rd ed. Thorofare, NJ: SLACK, Inc.; 2012:3–25

[3] Swanson EA, Izatt JA, Hee MR, et al. In vivo retinal imaging by optical coherence tomography. Opt Lett 1993; 18: 1864–1866

[4] Puliafito CA, Hee MR, Lin CP, et al. Imaging of macular diseases with optical coherence tomography. Ophthalmology 1995; 102: 217–229

[5] Schuman JS, Hee MR, Arya AV, et al. Optical coherence tomography: a new tool for glaucoma diagnosis. Curr Opin Ophthalmol 1995: 89–95 Review

[6] Schuman JS, Hee MR, Puliafito CA, et al. Quantification of nerve fiber layer thickness in normal and glaucomatous eyes using optical coherence tomography. Arch Ophthalmol 1995; 113: 586–596

[7] Izatt JA, Hee MR, Swanson EA, et al. Micrometer-scale resolution imaging of the anterior eye in vivo with optical coherence tomography. Arch Ophthalmol 1994; 112: 1584–1589

[8] Radhakrishnan S, Rollins AM, Roth JE, et al. Real-time optical coherence tomography of the anterior segment at 1310 nm. Arch Ophthalmol 2001; 119: 1179–1185

[9] Hee MR, Puliafito CA, Wong C, et al. Quantitative assessment of macular edema with optical coherence tomography. Arch Ophthalmol 1995; 113: 1019–1029

[10] Hee MR, Puliafito CA, Wong C, et al. Optical coherence tomography of central serous chorioretinopathy. Am J Ophthalmol 1995; 120: 65–74

[11] Hee MR, Puliafito CA, Wong C, et al. Optical coherence tomography of macular holes. Ophthalmology 1995; 102: 748–756

[12] Coker JG, Duker JS. Macular disease and optical coherence tomography. Curr Opin Ophthalmol 1996: 33–38 Review

[13] Wilkins JR, Puliafito CA, Hee MR, et al. Characterization of epiretinal membranes using optical coherence tomography. Ophthalmology 1996; 103: 2142–2151

[14] Burk RO, Völcker HE. Current imaging of the optic disk and retinal nerve fiber layer [Review]. Curr Opin Ophthalmol 1996: 99–108

[15] Maldonado MJ, Ruiz-Oblitas L, Munuera JM, Aliseda D, García-Layana A, Moreno-Montañés J. Optical coherence tomography evaluation of the corneal cap and stromal bed features after laser in situ keratomileusis for high myopia and astigmatism. Ophthalmology 2000; 107: 81–88

[16] Ustundag C, Bahcecioglu H, Ozdamar A, Aras C, Yildirim R, Ozkan S. Optical coherence tomography for evaluation of anatomical changes in the cornea after laser in situ keratomileusis. J Cataract Refract Surg 2000; 26: 1458–1462

[17] Wirbelauer C, Scholz C, Hoerauf H, Engelhardt R, Birngruber R, Laqua H. Corneal optical coherence tomography before and immediately after excimer laser photorefractive keratectomy. Am J Ophthalmol 2000; 130: 693–699

[18] Hirano K, Ito Y, Suzuki T, Kojima T, Kachi S, Miyake Y. Optical coherence tomography for the noninvasive evaluation of the cornea. Cornea 2001; 20: 281–289

[19] Margolis R, Spaide RF. A pilot study of enhanced depth imaging optical coherence tomography of the choroid in normal eyes. Am J Ophthalmol 2009; 147: 811–815

[20] Vajpayee RB, Maharana PK, Kaweri L, Sharma N, Jhanji V. Intrastromal fluid drainage with air tamponade: anterior segment optical coherence tomography guided technique for the management of acute corneal hydrops. Br J Ophthalmol 2013; 97: 834–836

[21] Shah SP, Manjunath V, Rogers AH, Baumal CR, Reichel E, Duker JS. Optical coherence tomography-guided facedown positioning for macular hole surgery. Retina 2013; 33: 356–362

[22] Rush SW, Han DY, Rush RB. Optical coherence tomography-guided transepithelial phototherapeutic keratectomy for the treatment of anterior corneal scarring. Am J Ophthalmol 2013; 156: 1088–1094

[23] Bianciotto C, Shields CL, Guzman JM, et al. Assessment of anterior segment tumors with ultrasound biomicroscopy versus anterior segment optical coherence tomography in 200 cases. Ophthalmology 2011; 118: 1297–1302

[24] Bakri SJ, Singh AD, Lowder CY, et al. Imaging of iris lesions with high-speed optical coherence tomography. Ophthalmic Surg Lasers Imaging 2007; 38: 27–34

[25] Cabot F, Kankariya VP, Ruggeri M, et al. High-resolution optical coherence tomography-guided donor tissue preparation for descemet membrane endothelial keratoplasty using the reverse big bubble technique. Cornea 2014; 33: 428–431

[26] Agarwal A, Ashokkumar D, Jacob S, Agarwal A, Saravanan Y. High-speed optical coherence tomography for imaging anterior chamber inflammatory reaction in uveitis: clinical correlation and grading. Am J Ophthalmol 2009; 147: 413–416, e3

[27] Kumar DA, Agarwal A, Prakash G, Jacob S, Saravanan Y, Agarwal A. Evaluation of intraocular lens tilt with anterior segment optical coherence tomography. Am J Ophthalmol 2011; 151: 406–412, e2

[28] Palanker DV, Blumenkranz MS, Andersen D, et al. Femtosecond laser-assisted cataract surgery with integrated optical coherence tomography. Sci Transl Med 2010: 58ra85

[29] Born M, Wolf E, Bhatia AB. Principles of Optics: Electromagnetic Theory of Propagation, Interference and Diffraction of Light. 7th expanded ed. Cambridge, UK: Cambridge University Press, 1999

[30] Fercher AF, Mengedoht K, Werner W. Eye-length measurement by interferometry with partially coherent light. Opt Lett 1988; 13: 186–188

2 Time-Domain and Fourier-Domain Optical Coherence Tomography

Dhivya Ashok Kumar and Amar Agarwal

Optical coherence tomography (OCT) has revolutionized the investigative field of ophthalmology in the last two decades. Huang et al established OCT evaluation of the retina using infrared light wavelength in 1991.[1] Time-domain (TD) OCT was the first model of in vivo evaluation of the human retina and optic nerve until 1995, when Fourier- or frequency-domain (FD) OCT was introduced for ocular imaging.[2] The mechanisms by which the TD and FD OCT functions have been studied widely since then and have been used accordingly for various clinical conditions. The popularity of the method lies in its ability to delineate micrometer differences or variations in the clinical tissues like macula or cornea. Although TD and FD OCT were introduced in the early 1990s, FD OCT has been applied widely only after 2000. Wojtkowski et al were among the earliest to report an experimental study showing the superior sensitivity of FD over TD OCT.[2]

This chapter presents the basic optical differences between the TD and FD OCT systems. We also mention various studies that have demonstrated the sensitivity differences between the methods.[3,4,5,6] The advantages and limitations of the individual methods are also addressed. appropriately.

2.1 Optics: How They Differ

In a conventional TD system, the source light passes through the beam splitter, which splits the light beam into *sample* and *reference*. The sample arm is directed to the sample or tissue end and the other to the moving reference mirror (▶ Fig. 2.1).

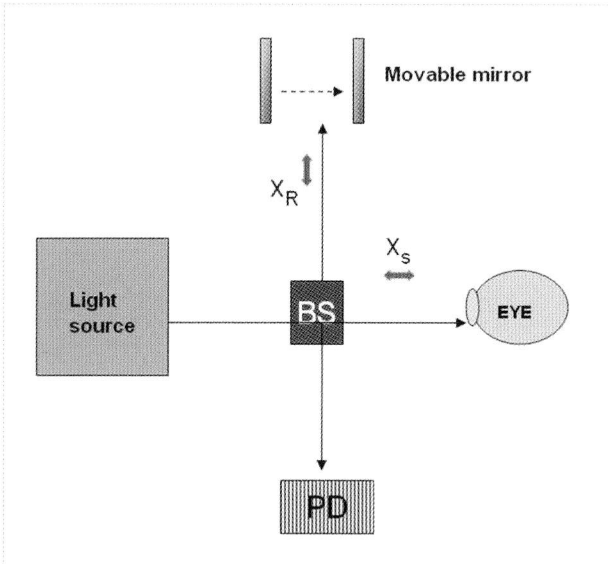

Fig. 2.1 Schematic diagram showing the optical principle of time-domain optical coherence tomography. BS, beam splitter; PD, photodetector; X_R, reference arm interface signal; X_S, sample arm interface signal.

The light beams, which are backscattered and back-reflected from the sample and the reference mirror are rechanneled by the beam splitter and detected by the photodetector. Interference can occur only when the two arms are matched in length so that the returning pulses can arrive at the detector at the same time to interfere. Yaqoob et al reported the bio-optical differences between the two domains of OCTs and have shown the theoretical differences.[3]

2.1.1 Time-Domain OCT

In a TD OCT system, the reference arm is typically displaced and scanned over a distance equal to the depth range, x_{depth} that is to be probed for the sample.[3] For a given total scan time duration, T, we can determine that a TD OCT system will spend a duration $(L_C/\ x_{\ depth}) \times T$ of collecting interference signal from any given interface within the sample, where L_C is the coherence length.[3] A determination of the TD OCT sensitivity can be made by calculating the number of useful signal photons within that duration and comparing that with the noise photon count. The total useful interference signal photons that will be collected in this context are given by the following equation:

$$\mathrm{Signal}_{TDOCT} = 2\sqrt{(P_{ref}P_{sig})}\,(L_C \cdot T/x_{depth})\,(\epsilon/hv)$$

where P_{ref} and P_{sig} are the collected reference and sample power at wavelength k, respectively, and ε is the quantum efficiency of the detector and hv is the photon quantum energy.[3] The noise count is given by the square root of the total photons that are detected by the detector during that time duration. As the reference power P_{ref} typically dominates over all other signal in TD OCT, noise is calculated as follows:

$$\mathrm{Noise}_{TDOCT} = \sqrt{\{P_{ref}\,(L_C \cdot T/x_{depth})\,(\epsilon/hv)\}}$$

Although the photodetector is collecting backscattered photons from the interface of interest for the entire duration of the acquisition, T, the detection scheme is actively selecting only those photons for OCT signal construction over a much shorter duration, $L_{C^*}\ T/\ x_{\ depth}$. This necessarily leads to diminished signal sensitivity compared with a scheme that is capable of using those photons for OCT signal construction over the entire duration of the acquisition (example FD OCT).

2.1.2 Fourier-Domain OCT

In an FD system, the source light passes through the beam splitter, which splits the light beam into sample and reference. The sample arm is directed to the sample or tissue end and the other to the stationary reference mirror (▶ Fig. 2.2). The light beams that are backscattered and back-reflected from the sample and the reference mirror are rechanneled by the beam splitter and detected by the spectrometer. There is an immobile

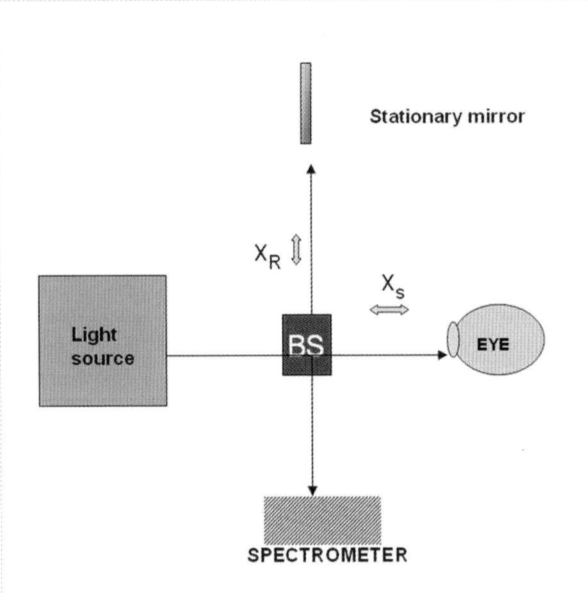

Fig. 2.2 Schematic diagram showing the optical principle of Fourier-domain optical coherence tomography. BS, beam splitter; X_R, reference arm interface signal; X_S, sample arm interface signal.

reference mirror, and instead of a photodetector as in TD OCT, there is a spectrometer (▶ Fig. 2.2). In FD OCT, the spectral variation in the detected signal is analyzed by the low-loss spectrometer. An interface that gives a smaller value (X_R–X_S) will produce a slower sinusoidal spectral oscillation than will an interface with a larger value (X_R–X_S). Therefore, a Fourier transform of the spectral measurement will produce a line-scan profile similar to that obtained from TD OCT. It should be noted that in FD OCT, signal contribution from two or more interfaces may be collected simultaneously as they contribute to different spectral oscillation components.[3] Here the total useful interference signal photons from a given interface collected in this context are given by the following equation:

$$\text{Signal}_{\text{FDOCT}} = 2\sqrt{((P_{\text{ref}}P_{\text{sig}})(T*\epsilon/hv))}$$

where T is the total signal collection time. The noise count is given by the square root of the total photons that are detected by the entire spectrometer during the entire signal collection duration as follows:

$$\text{Noise}_{\text{FDOCT}} = \sqrt{\{P_{\text{ref}}T(\epsilon/hv)\}}$$

The scan depth, x_{depth}, which is achievable with scan-depth (SD) OCT, is given by the range of spectral oscillation frequency that is detectable by the spectrometer.[3] According to Yaqoob and associates, for a spectrometer with N pixels, the highest spectral oscillation periodicity that is detectable is $N/2$.[3] The SD OCT system is intrinsically more sensitive than a TD OCT system by a factor of $N/2$. This improvement is attributable to the fact that SD OCT is capable of collecting signals from all depths of the sample during the entire acquisition time. SD OCT has a scheme that is capable of using photons for OCT signal construction over the entire duration of the acquisition, unlike the TD OCT detection scheme, which actively selects those photons for OCT signal construction over a much shorter duration.

2.1.3 Different Methods of Fourier-Domain OCT

Spectrometer Method

A low-loss spectrometer is used for collection, Fourier transformation, and spectrum detection of the backscattered and back-reflected waves. The grating-based spectrometer measures the interference signal as a function of wavelength, λ. The spectral data are then rescaled and resampled evenly in k-space, before being Fourier transformed to obtain the sample depth profile or A-scan.[3]

Swept-Source Method

In swept-source OCT, the source is a narrowband laser. Chapter 5 gives further details of swept-source OCT.

2.2 Signal-to-Noise Ratio

The sensitivity figure used for assessing OCT performance is the signal-to-noise ratio (SNR) quantity (decibels),[3] which is given by the following equation:

$$\text{SNR}_{\text{OCT}} = 10\log\{\text{Signal}_{\text{OCT}}/\text{Noise}_{\text{OCT}}\}^2$$

The typical SNR of an OCT system can vary depending on the scan parameters of interest, but an SNR of 80 or greater is generally accepted as the minimum required for imaging biological targets.

2.3 Comparison of Time-Domain Versus Fourier-Domain OCT in Clinical Applications

The FD OCT systems may be used to perform OCT imaging at higher speed and (or) scan depth.[7] FD or spectral-domain OCT provides higher resolution and fast image acquisition compared with TD OCT. The commercially available spectral-domain OCT system gives improved image resolution, imaging speed, and sensitivity. ▶ Table 2.1 and ▶ Table 2.2 show the comparison between the differences in commercially available OCT systems for anterior- and posterior-segment evaluation.

2.3.1 Macular Thickness

Compared with TD OCT, FD OCT has shown better repeatability in macular evaluation, especially in thickened macula.[8,9] The foveal and total macular thicknesses measured by FD OCT were significantly greater than those measured by TD OCT (both with $P < 0.001$).[9] Forooghian et al reported that the absolute measures of macular thickness and volume in patients with diabetic macular edema (DME) differed significantly in magnitude between the Stratus OCT and Cirrus HD-OCT systems.[10]

However, both OCT systems demonstrated high intrasession repeatability. Although the two systems cannot be used interchangeably, they appear equally reliable in generating macular measurements for clinical practice and research. The agreement between the two OCTs is low and varies in each macular subfield.[8,11] All reported studies have shown that the OCT system cannot be used interchangeably. Hence, for prognostic evaluation, the same OCT (either the TD or FD) should be compared before and after treatment. FD OCT gives good-quality scans for macular pathologies like macular hole, epiretinal membrane, edema (▶ Fig. 2.3), and pseudohole (▶ Fig. 2.4).

Table 2.1 The difference in time- and Fourier-domain posterior-segment optical coherence tomography

	Time Domain	Fourier Domain
Wavelength	820 µm	840 µm
Axial resolution	10 microns	5 microns
Reference mirror	Moves	Stationary
Interference	Time delay detected	Split spectrally
Spectrometer	Absent	Present
Fourier transform	Does not happen	Happens
Signal loss	Present, affects signal noise ratio	Less
Viewing area	Same	Same
Example	Stratus OCT (Carl Ziess)	Cirrus OCT (Carl Zeiss)

OCT = Ocular Coherence Tomography

Table 2.2 The difference in time- and Fourier-domain anterior-segment optical coherence tomography

	Time Domain	Fourier Domain
Wavelength	1310 µm	840 µm
Axial resolution	18 microns	5 microns
Reference mirror	Moves	Stationary
Interference	Time delay detected	Split spectrally
Spectrometer	Absent	Present
Fourier transform	Does not happen	Happens
Signal loss	Present, affects signal noise ratio	Less
Viewing area	10 mm	3–6 mm
Example	Visante OCT (Carl Ziess)	Rtvue (Optivue), Cirrus OCT (Carl Zeiss)

OCT = Ocular Coherence Tomography

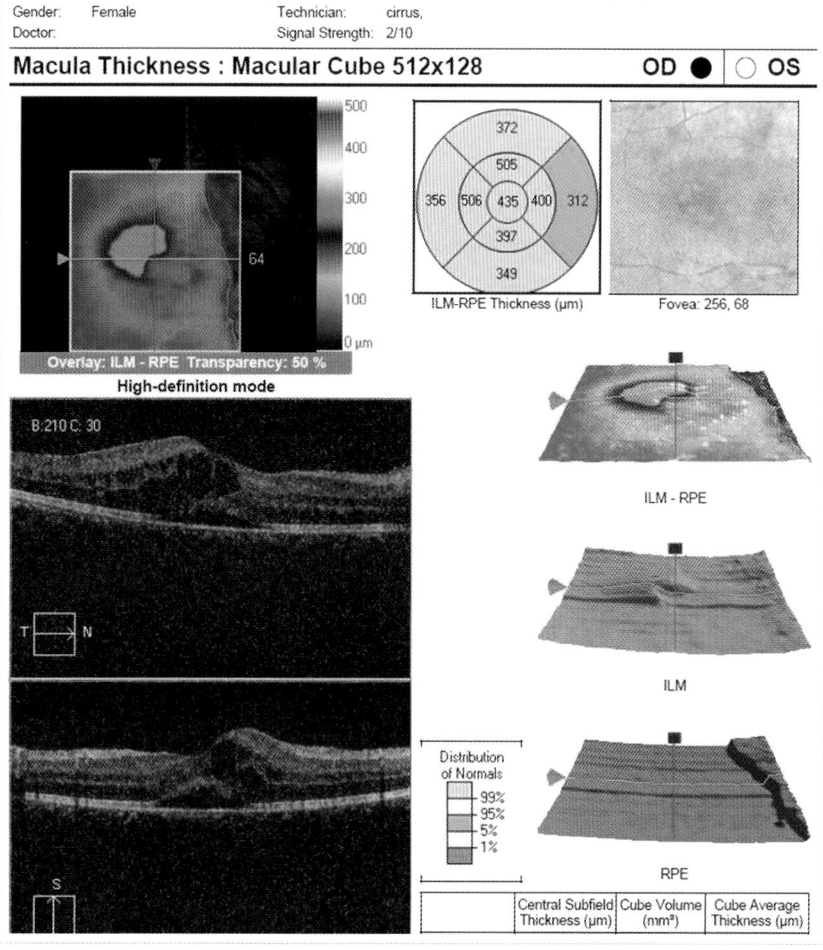

Fig. 2.3 Fourier-domain optical coherence tomography showing macular edema in chronic uveitis. ILM, internal limiting membrane; RPE, retinal pigment epithelium.

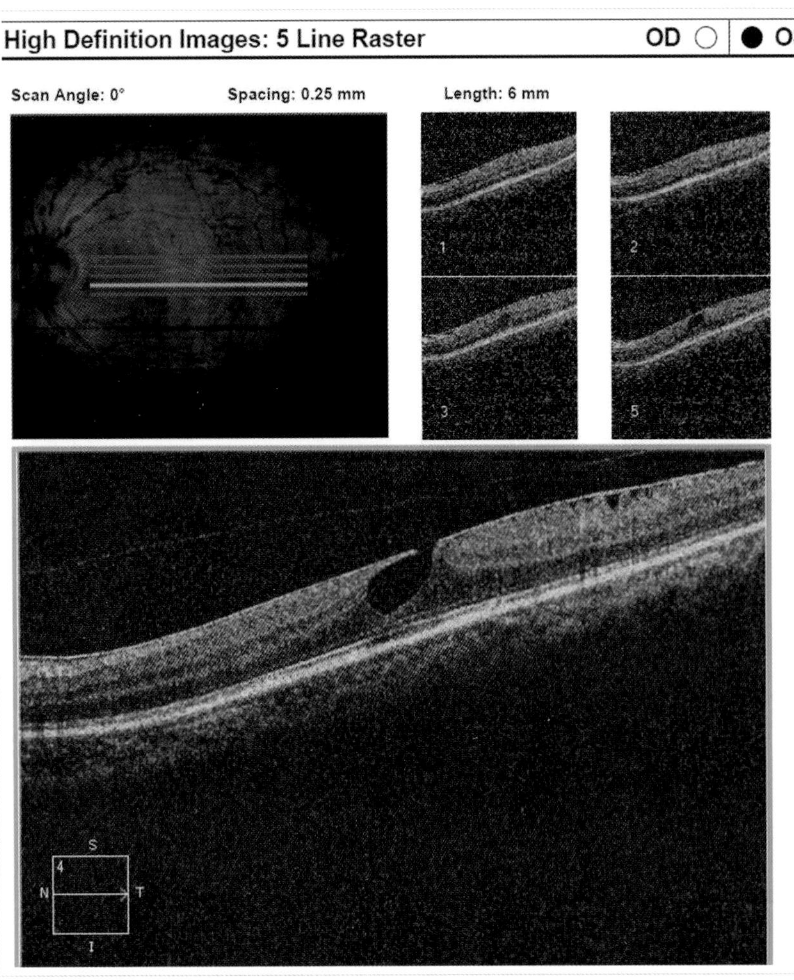

Fig. 2.4 Fourier-domain optical coherence tomography showing macular pseudohole with epiretinal membrane. 5 scans taken at different levels in macula are shown by 5 lines in the left image.

2.3.2 Nerve-Fiber Layer

Optical coherence tomography is a valuable tool in evaluating the peripapillary retinal nerve fiber layer (RNFL) in both glaucomatous and nonglaucomatous optic neuropathies. According to Leung et al, the diagnostic performance and the strength of the structure-function association were comparable between Cirrus (FD OCT) and Stratus (TD OCT) RNFL measurements.[12] FD OCT demonstrated lower measurement variability compared with TD OCT, with significant differences at 1, 3, 4, and 8 to 11 o'clock. Sung et al reported that the average RNFL thickness as determined by the two OCT machines was correlated ($r = 0.94$; $P < 0.001$) but significantly different (Stratus, 98.0 µm, standard deviation [SD] 18.0; Cirrus, 85.6 µm, SD 14.6; $P < 0.001$).[13] The FD OCT classified a significantly higher percentage of eyes as abnormal (Stratus, 12.9%; Cirrus, 23.3%; $P < 0.001$) in average RNFL thickness. FD OCT demonstrated higher sensitivity and specificity (63.6% and 100%) than did TD OCT (40.0% and 96.7%) in normative classification of average RNFL thickness.[13] Scan quality has been known to be better with FD OCT than with the TD OCT system; global RNFL thickness measurements appeared to be in perfect agreement between the two systems.[14]

2.3.3 Cornea and Anterior Segment

Corneal-flap thickness after refractive surgery is one of the main indications for OCT evaluation. Hall et al compared observer variation between the FD and TD OCT systems and noted that the FD OCT had closer agreement between observers and between-instrument measurements than TD OCT and provided more consistent measurements of post-LASIK (laser-assisted in situ keratomileusis) flap thickness.[15] In a study on corneal pachymetry in our center, we noted that the corneal thickness measurements between TD OCT and FD OCT were highly correlated but not similar. Conversion equations may be used for central and paracentral, but not for minimum, corneal thickness (▶ Fig. 2.5). Even though both the OCT instruments had good reliability, FD OCT was better.[16] The scan area examined by the FD OCT is always less than that seen in TD OCT (▶ Fig. 2.6). Hence, we need multiple-region analysis in FD OCT, unlike in TD OCT, where a single image can give you a view of the entire anterior segment. FD OCT acquires scans at a much faster speed than TD-OCT, thereby leading to minimized effects of the patient's eye movements. This could be the reason for the better repeatability for FD OCT found in our study. Wylegała et al compared TD and FD OCT systems in anterior-segment evaluation and observed that FD OCT provided accurate anterior-eye-segment measurements that agreed with those obtained with TD OCT.[17] Although no significant difference between mean values was found, and they were highly correlated, the FD OCT provided precise information in small areas of the anterior chamber.[17] Conditions like epithelial thickness, anterior stromal changes (▶ Fig. 2.7), and endothelial features can be more

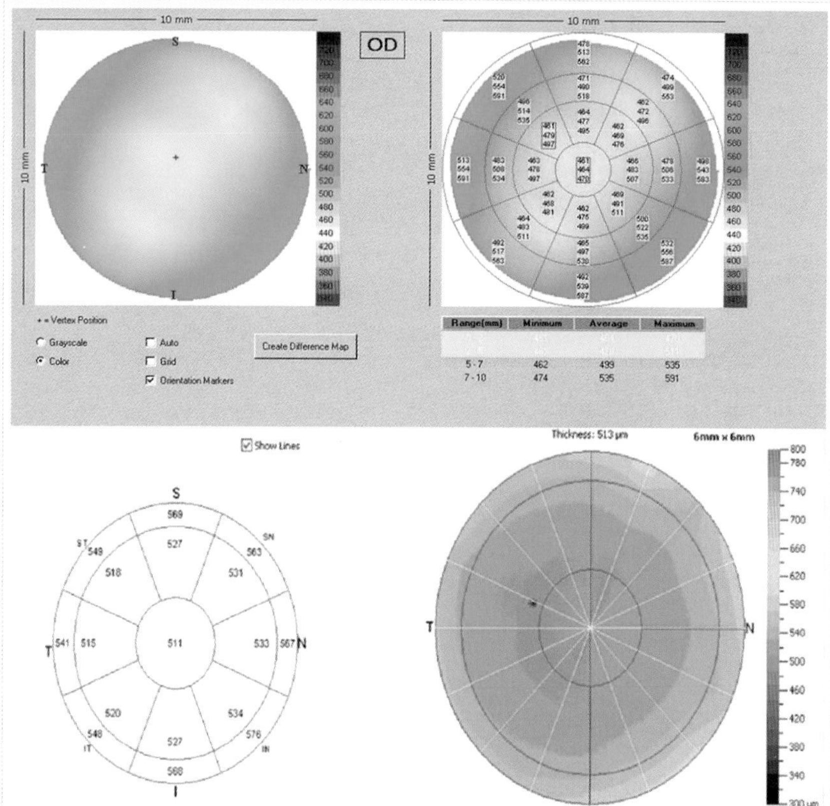

Fig. 2.5 Corneal pachymetry map as seen in time-domain (above) and Fourier-domain (below) optical coherence tomography. OD, right eye.

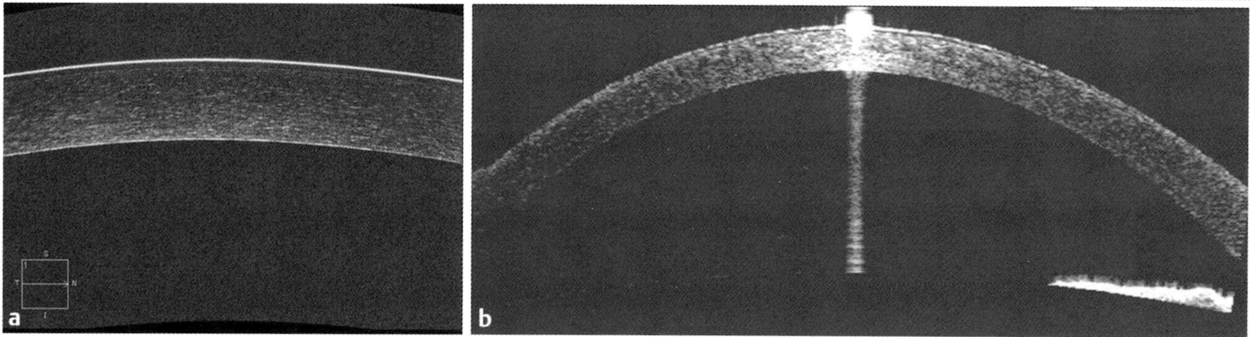

Fig. 2.6 (a) Anterior segment as seen by Fourier-domain and (b) time-domain optical coherence tomography in the same eye.

clearly seen with FD OCT compared with TD OCT. FD OCT has shown superior use in postendothelial keratoplasty (▶ Fig. 2.8) patients, where the micrometer level changes in the endothelial monolayer can be delineated.

2.3.4 En Face OCT

Few spectral domain OCT systems have En-face OCT technology for visualization. It is a newer modality that compiles many transversal priority scans to create frontal images that are compatible with conventional fundus images. It scans the retinal layers and choroid on a coronal plane at 90° from cross-section. It can provide additional information on the clinical conditions. In the en face OCT, the transversal scanner produces the fast lines in the image. OCT C-scans (Type of mode) are represented as two-dimensional transversal slices at any given depth through the retina, thereby enabling visualization of the lateral extent of structures. Internal limiting membrane or ILM is one of the layers of retinal which can be better seen with this technique.[18]

2.4 Future Trends

As the newer-generation OCT machines continue to evolve, there is always the potential for enhanced imaging facilities in the near future. High resolution, speed, precision, image quality, and sensitivity are the common factors that will help ophthalmologists decide on the type of OCT they prefer. Nevertheless, in the current scenario, both OCT systems have widely been used for various clinical applications with excellent prognostic values.

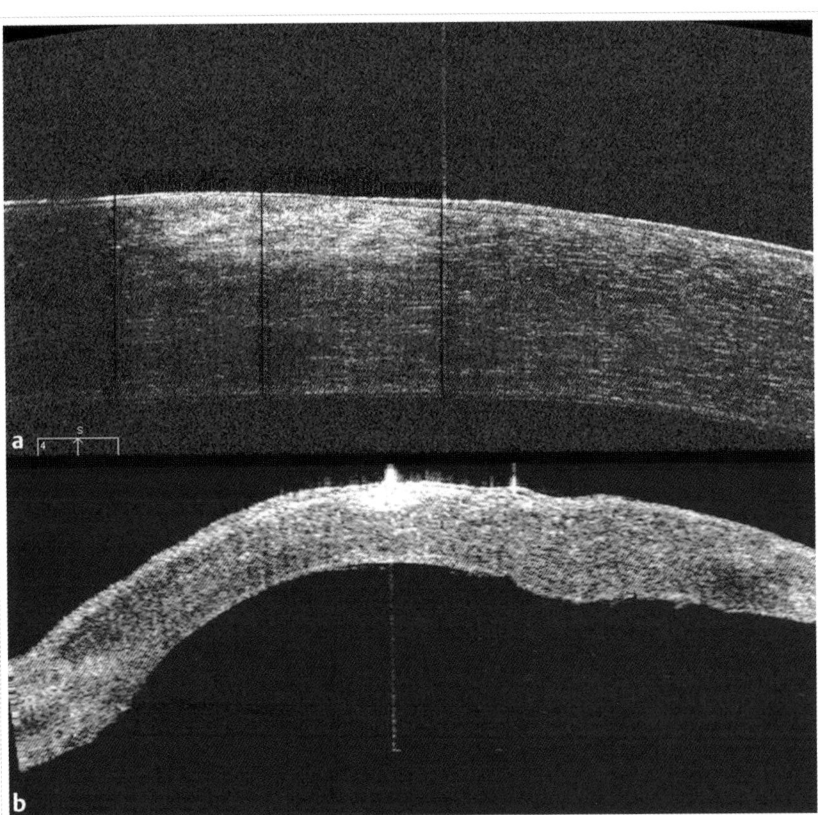

Fig. 2.7 Anterior stromal opacity as seen by Fourier-domain **(a)** and time-domain **(b)** optical coherence tomography.

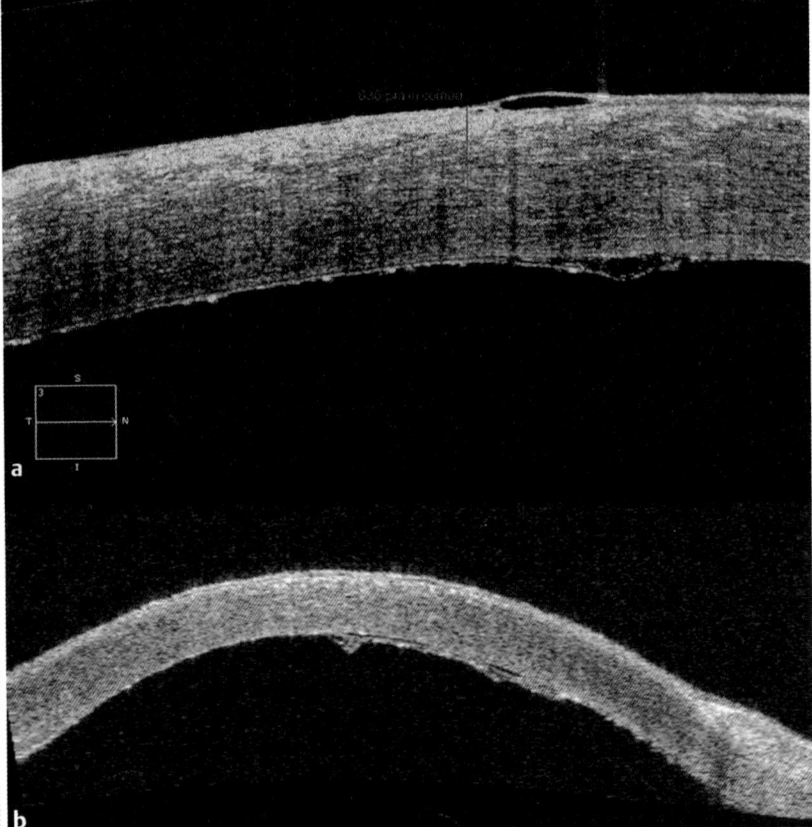

Fig. 2.8 Post-Descemet membrane endothelial keratoplasty with graft detachment is seen in Fourier-domain **(a)** and time-domain **(b)** optical coherence tomography.

References

[1] Huang D, Swanson EA, Lin CP, et al. Optical coherence tomography. Science 1991; 254: 1178–1181

[2] Wojtkowski M, Leitgeb R, Kowalczyk A, Bajraszewski T, Fercher AF. In vivo human retinal imaging by Fourier domain optical coherence tomography. J Biomed Opt 2002; 7: 457–463

[3] Yaqoob Z, Wu J, Yang C. Spectral domain optical coherence tomography: a better OCT imaging strategy. Biotechniques 2005; 39 Suppl: S6–S13

[4] Leitgeb R, Hitzenberger C, Fercher A. Performance of fourier domain vs. time domain optical coherence tomography. Opt Express 2003; 11: 889–894

[5] Choma M, Sarunic M, Yang C, Izatt J. Sensitivity advantage of swept source and Fourier domain optical coherence tomography. Opt Express 2003; 11: 2183–2189

[6] de Boer JF, Cense B, Park BH, Pierce MC, Tearney GJ, Bouma BE. Improved signal-to-noise ratio in spectral-domain compared with time-domain optical coherence tomography. Opt Lett 2003; 28: 2067–2069

[7] Wojtkowski M, Srinivasan V, Ko T, Fujimoto J, Kowalczyk A, Duker J. Ultrahigh-resolution, high-speed, Fourier domain optical coherence tomography and methods for dispersion compensation. Opt Express 2004; 12: 2404–2422

[8] Giammaria D, Ioni A, Bartoli B, Cofini V, Pellegrini G, Giannotti B. Comparison of macular thickness measurements between time-domain and spectral-domain optical coherence tomographies in eyes with and without macular abnormalities. Retina 2011; 31: 707–716

[9] Leung CK, Cheung CY, Weinreb RN, et al. Comparison of macular thickness measurements between time domain and spectral domain optical coherence tomography. Invest Ophthalmol Vis Sci 2008; 49: 4893–4897

[10] Forooghian F, Cukras C, Meyerle CB, Chew EY, Wong WT. Evaluation of time domain and spectral domain optical coherence tomography in the measurement of diabetic macular edema. Invest Ophthalmol Vis Sci 2008; 49: 4290–4296

[11] Patel N, Chowdhury H, Leung R, Sivaprasad S. Sensitivity and specificity of time-domain versus spectral-domain optical coherence tomography in diabetic macular edema. Indian J Ophthalmol 2013; 61: 208–212

[12] Leung CK, Cheung CY, Weinreb RN, et al. Retinal nerve fiber layer imaging with spectral-domain optical coherence tomography: a variability and diagnostic performance study. Ophthalmology 2009; 116: 1257–1263, e1–e2

[13] Sung KR, Kim DY, Park SB, Kook MS. Comparison of retinal nerve fiber layer thickness measured by Cirrus HD and Stratus optical coherence tomography. Ophthalmology 2009; 116: 1264–1270, e1

[14] Moreno-Montañés J, Olmo N, Alvarez A, García N, Zarranz-Ventura J. Cirrus high-definition optical coherence tomography compared with Stratus optical coherence tomography in glaucoma diagnosis. Invest Ophthalmol Vis Sci 2010; 51: 335–343

[15] Hall RC, Mohamed FK, Htoon HM, Tan DT, Mehta JS. Laser in situ keratomileusis flap measurements: comparison between observers and between spectral-domain and time-domain anterior segment optical coherence tomography. J Cataract Refract Surg 2011; 37: 544–551

[16] Prakash G, Agarwal A, Jacob S, Kumar DA, Agarwal A, Banerjee R. Comparison of fourier-domain and time-domain optical coherence tomography for assessment of corneal thickness and intersession repeatability. Am J Ophthalmol 2009; 148: 282–290, e2

[17] Wylegała E, Teper S, Nowińska AK, Milka M, Dobrowolski D. Anterior segment imaging: Fourier-domain optical coherence tomography versus time-domain optical coherence tomography. J Cataract Refract Surg 2009; 35: 1410–1414

[18] Alkabes M, Salinas C, Vitale L, Bures-Jelstrup A, Nucci P, Mateo C. En face optical coherence tomography of inner retinal defects after internal limiting membrane peeling for idiopathic macular hole. Invest Ophthalmol Vis Sci 2011; 52: 8349–55

3 Ultrahigh-Resolution Optical Coherence Tomography for Imaging of Ocular Surface Tumors

Juan C. Murillo, Anat Galor, and Carol L. Karp

Optical coherence tomography (OCT) is a powerful imaging modality that has revolutionized the field of ophthalmology by providing real-time, in vivo, cross-sectional images of ocular tissues. The eye is an optically accessible organ, and OCT technique permits high-resolution (HR) images of normal tissues and pathology. Since its development in 1991, OCT has been used for several clinical applications,[1,2] and even though it was initially conceived as a means of imaging the eye posterior segment, it was later used for the anterior segment (AS).

Early OCT systems detected light echoes using what is known as time-domain (TD) detection. This technology provided resolution of about 15 to 18 µm.[3] These early devices provided some information regarding the AS anatomy but not the fine details of ocular surface lesions. It was not until the development of spectral-domain OCT (SD OCT) devices, capable of HR OCT imaging—down to 5 µm—and ultrahigh-resolution (UHR OCT) devices—less than 5 µm—that the ocular surface was able to be imaged to a degree that structural details of the corneal epithelium, corneal stroma, and conjunctiva were elucidated.[4,5,6,7,8] These newer devices with improved axial resolution and imaging speed made possible the visualization of not only AS dystrophies and degenerations[9] but also of other several ocular surface conditions, disclosing reliable images with high correlation to pathology specimens.[10]

Ultrahigh-resolution OCT has provided a noninvasive method to evaluate ocular surface lesions. Ocular surface squamous neoplasia (OSSN), conjunctival melanoma (CMM), and conjunctival lymphoma are conditions that require biopsy for a definitive diagnosis. However, UHR OCT can provide adjuvant information to a clinical diagnosis before excision, thus allowing early differentiation and management of suspicious lesions.[10,11,12]

As OCT technology improves, it has the potential to revolutionize the management of the ocular surface. The purpose of this chapter is to illustrate the evolution and utilization of AS HR and UHR OCT imaging and its clinical applications, specifically in the diagnosis, differentiation, and management of ocular surface tumors.

3.1 Optical Coherence Tomography: The Evolution to Ultrahigh-Resolution OCT

The first demonstration of OCT imaging was reported by Huang et al,[1] showing a TD OCT ex vivo scan of the human retina and its corresponding histology. The image had an axial resolution of around 15 µm, which was almost 10 times finer than conventional clinical imaging modalities such as ultrasound. The most important advance in OCT technology was the transition from TD OCT to SD OCT because the latter is much more efficient than the serial scanning performed by the TD OCT, discussed in detail later in this chapter.

Imaging with OCT technology is based on the use of an optical device known as the Michelson interferometer. The technology compares or correlates one optical beam of light or light wave (reference) with another as the light waves return from the variably reflective tissue layers of the eye.[4] The device creates an interference pattern by gathering reflected light beams from the target tissue and from the reference. Several interference patterns are created in this fashion.[5]

In early generation TD OCT machines, multiple readings are produced as a reference mirror physically moves in a linear fashion over the target, creating individual A-scans that indicate a specific measure of the depth and reflectivity of the underlying tissue. These A-scans are then combined to form a composite, cross-sectional image (B-scan).[5] Conventional clinical imaging technologies such as ultrasound, magnetic resonance, or computed tomography have poorer resolution compared with that achieved with this novel technology.

In 1994, AS OCT was reported for the first time by Izatt et al.[3] Later, several TD OCT machines were designed and made commercially available for imaging of the AS. Likewise posterior-segment OCT machines, such as the Stratus OCT (Carl Zeiss Meditec, Dublin, CA), were also used for this purpose.[4] Devices using TD detection technology were capable of achieving satisfactory resolution to image the cornea, anterior chamber, and angle.[13,14] Nonetheless, this technology was limited compared with current-generation devices: first, A-scans were limited in number—from 200 to little more than 2000/s—because the reference mirror was required to physically travel as it processed serial A-scans.[15,16] Consequently, image resolution was compromised by relatively fewer A-scans and longer times to capture them, making this early technology state susceptible to patient compliance and vulnerable to motion artifacts.[4] The Zeiss OCT1 (Carl Zeiss Meditec, Dublin, CA) was one of the first available devices; it provided an axial resolution of 15 µm with only 100 A-scans per second.[17] Improvements continued with the Zeiss OCT2 (Carl Zeiss Meditec).[18] Later Stratus OCT (Carl Zeiss Meditec) machines were capable of an axial resolution of 10 µm and 512 A-scans in 1.3 seconds.[19]

The search for quality images of the AS using TD technology continued, and two AS OCT devices were introduced to the market in 2001: the Slit-Lamp OCT (Heidelberg Engineering, Heidelberg, Germany) and the Visante OCT (Carl Zeiss Meditec). Both were capable of up to 2048 A-scans per second,[20] which granted a significant improvement in terms of image quality, with greater penetrance to a depth of approximately 6 to 7 mm while reducing signal scattering.[19] Additionally, both machines improved scan width (compared with earlier devices) to 15 to 16 mm, which could easily cover all AS structures. These devices still had limited resolution of 25 µm for the slit-lamp OCT and 18 µm for the Visante OCT, respectively.[19,20,21]

The evolution from TD OCT to SD OCT technology, which uses a broadband light source, ultimately brought remarkable improvements to image resolution.[4] Replacement of the reference mirror (TD OCT) with systems that depend on a spectrometer and a high-speed camera to capture and decode (at the same time) the multiple spectra across the whole scan is the key to this dramatic progress.[19] This information is then translated into depth images using Joseph Fourier's equations. Therefore, this technology is also known as Fourier-domain OCT.[20]

The SD OCT imaging acquisition technique was then free from the mechanical limitations of a moving reference mirror and therefore capable of collecting as many as 50,000 or more A-scans per second.[20] Signal-to-noise ratio was considerably increased, and much more detailed images were reached. This innovation was then in most commercially available devices in combination with movement-tracking software products to reduce motion artifacts.[20] OCT imaging of the AS still required use of adapted lenses or the development of new software products. Remember that the initial aim of this novel technology was to image the posterior segment. A few examples of devices that were used for the imaging of the AS are the following: the Spectralis (Heidelberg Engineering), the Cirrus device (Carl Zeiss Meditec), a handheld Bioptigen model (Bioptigen Inc., Research Triangle Park, NC), and three-dimensional OCT (Topcon Medical Systems, Oakland, NJ).[22,23,24,25] These devices were able to obtain axial resolutions from 4 to 7 µm,[20,22] making it possible to distinguish epithelium from stroma.[23]

All things considered, SD OCTs were able to generate detailed, HR images of the AS; nevertheless, they presented marked limitations in width and scan depth. Their horizontal scan width was limited to 3 to 6 mm, making scanning of wider structures extremely difficult.[4,23] A new technology that was slightly different from the SD-OCT, called swept-source OCT, was developed (found in devices such as the SS-1000 CASIA [Tomey, Agoya, Japan]). It utilizes a light source with a 1310-nm wavelength and obtains images with a 16-mm horizontal scan width; nonetheless, its axial resolution was only 10 µm.[23]

It was a matter of time for the development of the UHR OCT technology; images with an axial resolution of 1 to 4 µm were then possible.[4] Drexler et al, in 2001, reported UHR OCT imaging for the first time.[26] They used a TD OCT machine with resolution of up to 2 to 3 µm to image and demonstrate the Bowman layer. Later, in 2004,[27] they described in vitro corneal OCT with the ability to obtain images with an axial resolution of 1 µm.

The UHR OCT images were accomplished by using a light source with a broad bandwidth of more than 100 nm, as well as a specifically designed spectrometer that detected the fringes collected from both reference and sample arms.[4] Clinically, this allowed for the detailed imaging of the tear film,[28,29] tear meniscus,[29] contact lens[28,29,30,31,32,33] interfaces, and individual corneal layers.[31,33,34,35,36] Most of the available literature is based on the use of custom-built UHR OCT devices; a few machines are commercially available.[28,29,30,31,32,33,34,35,36]

At our institution, we have available a custom-built UHR OCT machine that has changed our practice regarding the management of ocular surface lesions (▶ Fig. 3.1). This UHR OCT device is capable of UHR imaging with an axial resolution of approximately 2 to 3 µm,[4,10] and it uses a three-module superluminescent diode light source (Broadlighter, T840-HP, Superlumdiodes Ltd., Moscow, Russia) with a center wavelength of 840 nm.[4,9,10,11,12] This low-coherence light is passed through a pigtailed isolator and then coupled into a fiber-based Michelson interferometer, generating up to 24,000 A-scans per second.[4,9,10,11,12]

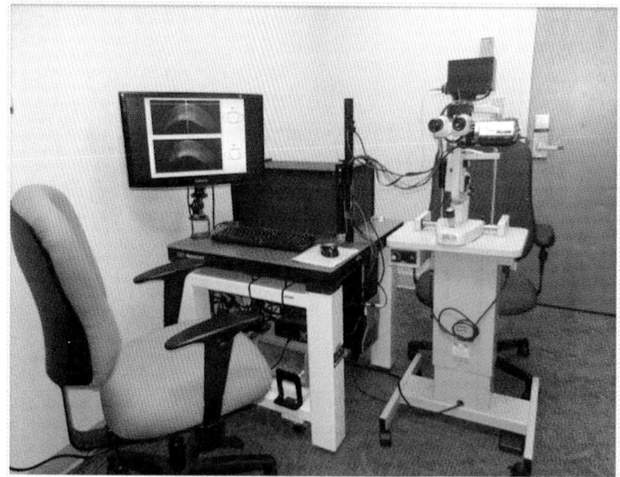

Fig. 3.1 Custom-built ultrahigh-resolution optical coherence tomography device (UHR-OCT) available at our institution. (Developed by Jianhua Wang, MD, PhD).

Based on our previously published experience, certain scan parameters can be recommended: a raster scan with 512 (A-scan) × 2014 (depth) × 128 (frame) pixels with a field of view 8 × 8 mm.[4] These dimensions will allow coverage of the lesion in most cases, although the scan dimension can be increased if necessary. For the generated two-dimensional images, a scan of 2048 (A-scan) × 2048 (depth) pixels provides high-definition of sufficient size to differentiate normal from abnormal tissue and corroborate clinical suspected diagnoses.[37]

The use of HR and UHR OCT has become routine care in our ocular surface clinic. We have been able to capture normal and abnormal structures with extraordinary detail and as a result increased our understanding of numerous AS diseases, which has been especially helpful for ocular surface tumors (▶ Table 3.1).

3.2 Ocular Surface Tumors

3.2.1 Ocular Surface Squamous Neoplasia

Ocular surface squamous neoplasia is a term that encompasses a broad spectrum of neoplastic squamous epithelial abnormalities, including squamous dysplasia, squamous cell carcinoma in situ (also known as conjunctival intraepithelial neoplasia), and invasive squamous cell carcinoma of the cornea or conjunctiva.[38] Clinically, OSSN lesions are elevated, gelatinous, papilliform or leukoplakic and have certain characteristic features that include blood vessel abnormalities and an ameboid and frosted growth pattern when involving the cornea.[39] Whereas most OSSN lesions are clinically obvious to diagnose, some cases are not as straightforward, especially in patients with concomitant complex ocular surface conditions.[37]

Excisional biopsy and histopathologic examination have been the gold standard for diagnosis.[38] As we might expect, the role of several noninvasive diagnostic imaging techniques have been studied to help detect OSSN. Confocal microscopy,[40] HR anterior segment ultrasound biomicroscopy (UBM),[41] and OCT,[10,11,12] have all shown to be beneficial as adjuvant diagnostic techniques; each, however, has its own advantages and disadvantages. For example, UBM and some confocal microscopy devices require eye contact, which increases the level of expertise needed for imaging and also the length of the scan time. Although UBM shows greater depth of penetrance, its resolution is lower than that of other technologies (50 µm).[41] Confocal microscopy can provide optical images at the level of an individual cell, but it can image only a limited area.[10,40,42] Whereas OCT has the advantage of imaging a larger area in a noncontact fashion, not all images can be fully characterized as thick, and leukoplakic lesions often display image shadowing.[43]

Table 3.1 Ultrahigh-resolution optical coherence tomography (UHR OCT) optical signs of ocular surface lesions

Conjunctival lesion	UHR OCT findings
Ocular surface squamous neoplasia	Severely thickened, hyperreflective epithelium Abrupt transition between normal and abnormal epithelium
Conjunctival melanoma	Normal to mildly thickened epithelium Epithelial cleavage indicates some involvement with atypical melanocytes Well-circumscribed subepithelial lesion
Primary acquired melanosis	Normal thickness epithelium with strong hyperreflectivity of the basal layer No involvement of subepithelial layers
Nevus	Normal thickness epithelium Well-circumscribed, highly hyperreflective subepithelial lesion within the substantia propria for subepithelial nevi Epithelial and substantia propria lesions seen in compound nevus Cysts within subepithelial tissue
Conjunctival lymphoma	Normal-thickness epithelium Homogeneous hyporeflective subepithelial lesion

The first OSSN series using UHR OCT was published by Abou Shousha et al in 2011; images of OSSN lesions of seven patients were obtained by UHR OCT and compared with their subsequent histologic appearance.[10] Substantial correlation was detected, and the authors found that a thickened hyperreflective epithelial layer and abrupt transition from normal to abnormal epithelium on UHR OCT were considered classic in OSSN. At times, a distinct plane between the lesion and underlying tissue could be noted in thinner tumors.[10] Not all features, however, were detected to the same extent in all scans (several images per lesion were taken, with 32 frames generated per scan), necessitating looking at multiple scans to evaluate for these characteristics. These abnormal UHR OCT features normalized with successful medical therapy.[10,12] These characteristic OSSN findings have been repeatedly described in our subsequent publications.[12,37](▶ Fig. 3.2)

Shortly thereafter, Vajzovic et al, in 2011, described a case series of UHR OCT images in various AS dystrophies and degenerations.[9] Images revealed various deposits within particular layers of the cornea, creating a specific pattern for such diseases as Salzmann nodular degeneration and also demonstrating the previously listed classic features of OSSN. In a subsequent study, UHR OCT was used to evaluate whether OSSN could be differentiated from pterygium. Kieval et al, in 2012, reported UHR OCT findings in a series of 34 patients with AS lesions suspicious for OSSN or pterygum.[11] The authors reported that UHR OCT could reliably distinguish pterygia from OSSN. Pterygia disclosed a

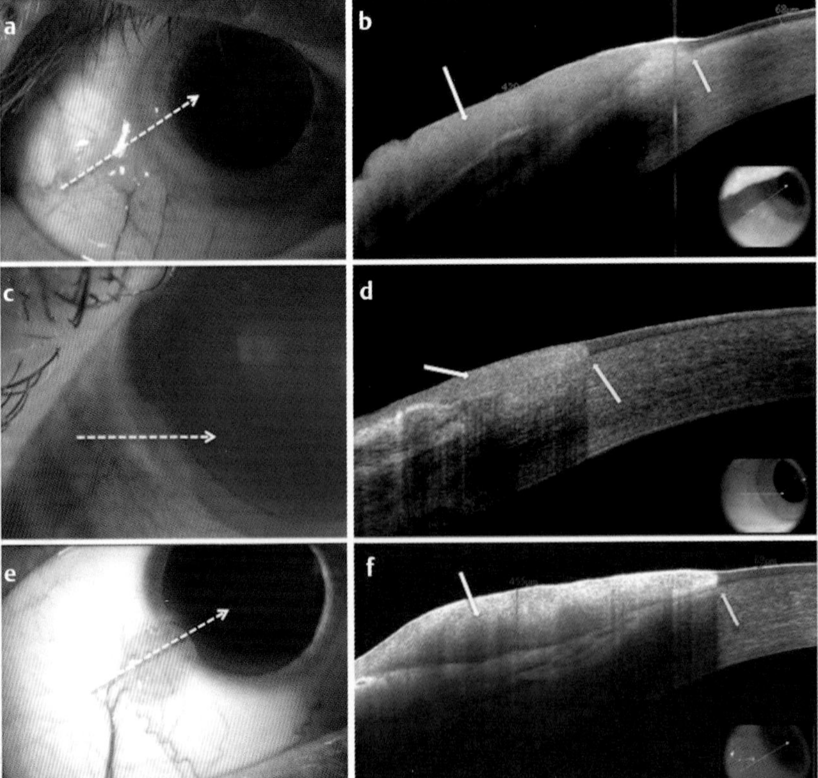

Fig. 3.2 Clinical photographs and ultrahigh-resolution optical coherence tomography (UHR OCT) scans of ocular surface squamous neoplasia (OSSN). **(a-c)** Clinical images of limbal lesions suspicious for OSSN. White dotted arrows represent UHR-OCT-imaged area. **(d-f)** Corresponding UHR OCT images demonstrating thickened hyperreflective epithelial layer (white arrows) and an abrupt transition from normal to hyperreflective epithelium (yellow arrows).

thin, dark epithelium layer with the presence of subepithelial hyperreflective tissue, whereas OSSN showed the previously mentioned features of a thickened and hyperreflective epithelium, usually with distinct transition zones. These findings were particularly useful in cases where the clinical differentiation between the two entities was not clear. Both groups correlated with the histopathology of resected specimens.[11] In ▶ Fig. 3.3, we illustrate several pterygium cases that have been followed up in our institution and have shown consistency with these findings. Additional publications evidenced that UHR OCT could be used to diagnose OSSN in patients with concomitant ocular surface diseases.[9] For example, in Salzmann nodular degeneration, the UHR OCT of the Salzmann nodules revealed a thin, normal epithelium and a subepithelial lesion, and the area of OSSN revealed a hyperreflective, thickened epithelium with distinct transition zones.[9] Furthermore, Thomas et al described how UHR OCT was effective in detecting focal neoplastic disease in a patient with complex ocular surface disease.[37] Future studies will be necessary to more fully evaluate the role of this technology.

Surgical excision with wide surgical margins has been the traditional therapy for OSSN, often with adjunctive cryotherapy.[44] Topical chemotherapeutics agents such as mitomycin-C,[45] 5-fluorouracil,[46] and interferon α-2b[47] have also been found to be effective in the management of OSSN. Consequently, as we move forward into the direction of treating OSSN medically, the importance of this noninvasive adjuvant technique gains more significance. It might help physicians to avoid unnecessary corneal or conjunctival scarring or even limbal stem cell deficiency caused from multiple biopsies or extensive surgical excisions.[48,49]

As we recently reported,[37] we use UHR OCT for regular monitoring of the ocular surface of patients diagnosed with and treated—surgically or medically—for OSSN. UHR OCT imaging often plays a confirmatory role, affirming the lesion resolution seen on clinical examination.[10,37] However, it is important to mention that we have encountered patients who were noted to have disparities between clinical and OCT resolution of the tumor (i.e., patients who had a normal slit-lamp examination but evidenced residual disease by UHR OCT). Further studies are necessary to assess the frequency of these findings. In our experience, a few guidelines exist to help direct the use of UHR OCT in the treatment of OSSN: we follow up with patients who are on medical therapy every 6 to 8 weeks with serial UHR OCT scans; this is frequent enough to monitor improvement and prevent prolonged and unncessary use of medications. After lesion resolution, we follow up with such patients with serial scans every 3 to 4 months. After a year of normal examinations, follow-up visits are scheduled every 6 to 12 months.[37] We examine and supervise closely all of our OSSN patients with UHR OCT. The main goal is to ensure that every lesion has been fully resolved and also to remain vigilant for early recurrences with the assistant of this novel technology.

3.2.2 Pigmented Conjunctival Lesions

The routine use of our custom-built UHR OCT device for imaging pigmented conjunctival lesions has added an extra step in confirming our clinical suspicion before performing surgical excision and definitive diagnosis by histopathologic analysis. UHR OCT has been able to delineate the morphologic/microscopic location and the extent of several pigmented conjunctival

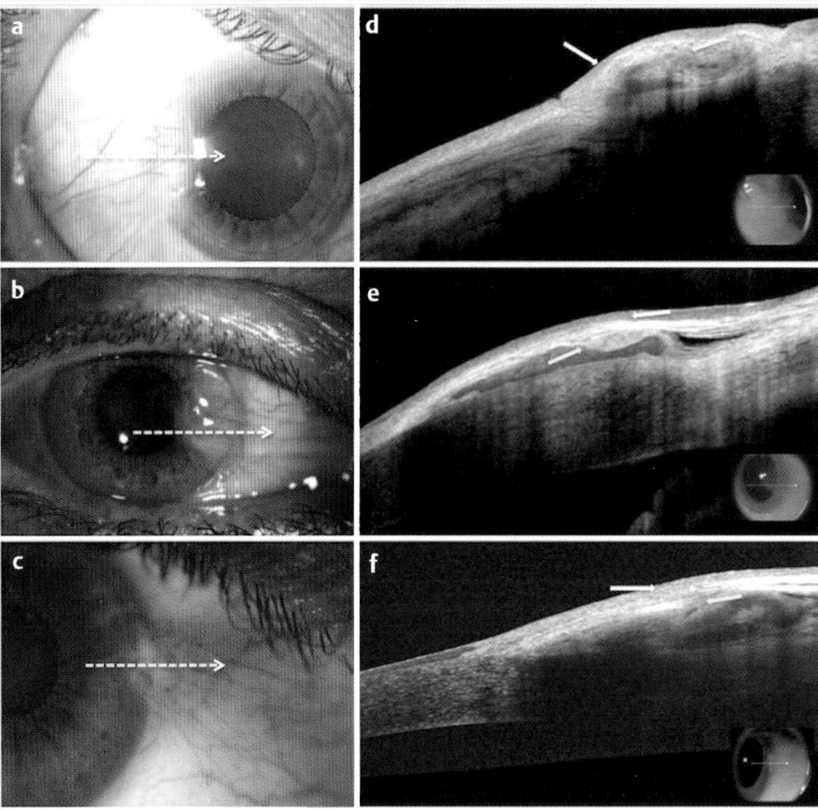

Fig. 3.3 Clinical photographs and ultrahigh-resolution optical coherence tomography (UHR OCT) scans of pterygia. **(a-c)** Raised growths of bulbar conjunctiva invading the cornea. White dotted arrows represent UHR-OCT-imaged area. **(d-f)** UHR-OCT of corresponding images demonstrating a thin, mostly dark epithelium layer (white arrows) with the presence of a subepithelial hyperreflective tissue (yellow arrows).

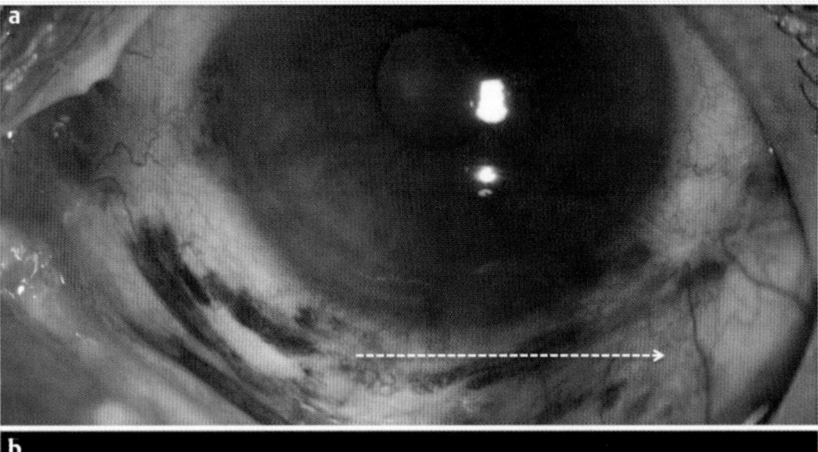

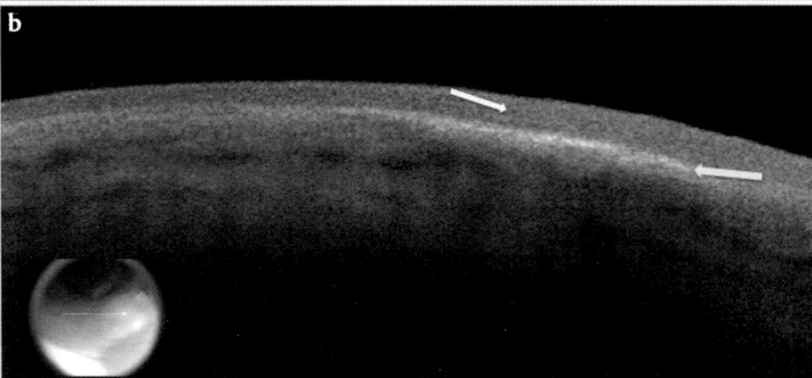

Fig. 3.4 Clinical photographs and ultrahigh-resolution optical coherence tomography (UHR OCT) scan of primary acquired melanosis. **(a)** Diffuse pigmented conjunctiva. White dotted arrow represents UHR OCT-imaged area. **(b)** UHR OCT image showing epithelium of normal thickness (white arrow) with strong hyperreflectivity of the basal epithelium (yellow arrow).

lesions (i.e., primary acquired melanosis [PAM], CMM, and nevi).

3.2.3 Primary Acquired Melanosis

The clinical features of PAM have been fully described: nonhomogeneous, unilateral pigmentations with waxing and waning over time. The appearance is mottled or dusted pigment that can cover quite large aspects of the conjunctiva.[50,51] Although clinical diagnosis might be straightforward, PAM has malignant potential and can develop into CMM[51]; therefore, close follow-up with clinical photos are necessary. UHR OCT may also provide crucial information for the detection of CMM foci, given that specific features for both these conditions have been fully described.[12]

Abou Shousha et al, in 2013,[12] performed UHR OCT scans in eight patients with a preliminary clinical diagnosis of PAM. Images demonstrated epithelium of normal thickness that was moderately hyperreflective (whitish) with strong hyperreflectivity of the basal epithelium. This hyperreflectivity seemed to be regular and pronounced in the basal layer of the epithelium with no invasion toward the subepithelial layers. These findings highly correlated with subsequent histopathologic diagnosis, given that the conjunctiva contained melanocytes located within the basal epithelium with no invasion of the underlying tissue. In ▶ Fig. 3.4, we illustrate a case of PAM that has been monitored in our clinic in which we have found consistency with the previously described features of PAM. Future studies with larger samples will be necessary to compare and assess the reliability of this diagnostic tool for the detection of CMM in the setting of PAM.

The potential of PAM to become CMM is particularly high in cases of PAM with atypia.[52] Clinically, lesions with or without atypia are indistinguishable, and although this is exceptionally important for the selection of further treatment, differentiation between the two was not possible by UHR OCT technology.[12] Consequently, histopathologic analysis is always necessary for differentiation between the two variables of this entity.

3.2.4 Conjunctival Melanoma

With an increase in incidence of 295% over a 27-year period in the United States,[53] CCM can arise de novo, from PAM or from nevus. In a series of 382 cases from Shields et al,[54] melanoma most commonly originated from PAM (74%), followed by de novo (21%), and nevus (4%). In general, these lesions are elevated, immobile, and manifest with vascularity. Interestingly, in 59% of CMMs, the lesion is pigmented, but it can also be nonpigmented or amelanotic.[54] The latter category is of special interest, because on clinical examination, amelanotic melanomas can be quite difficult to differentiate from OSSN. UHR OCT has shown to be particularly helpful in this setting, and the establishment of this diagnostic difference early in management is crucial. OSSN usually follows a benign course, whereas CMM has an aggressive behavior with high mortality rates.

In the series by Abou Shousha and colleagues,[12] five patients who were referred for evaluation for OSSN were imaged with UHR OCT and found instead to have CMM. Clinically, these lesions were gelatinous and nonpigmented, consistent clinically with OSSN. UHR OCT images, however, revealed a normal or mildly thickened epithelial layer with a subepithelial lesion, ruling out the diagnosis of OSSN. In these cases, histopathology

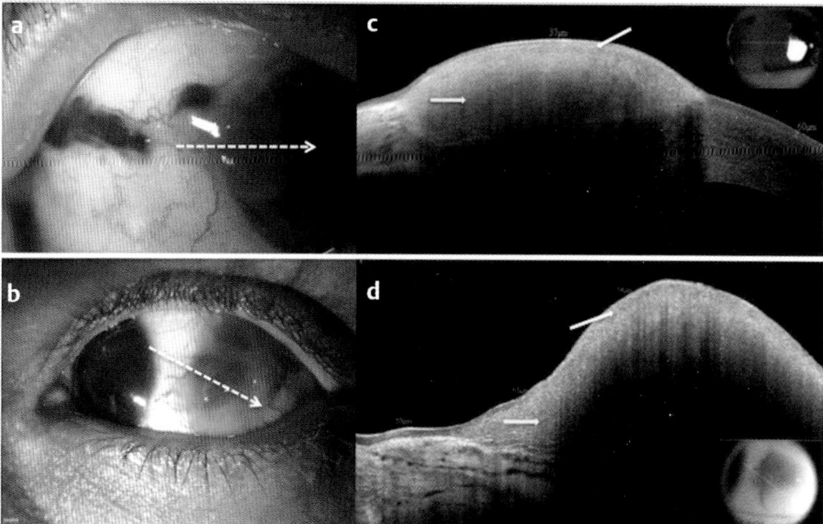

Fig. 3.5 Clinical photographs and ultrahigh-resolution optical coherence tomography (UHR OCT) scans of conjunctival melanomas. **(a,b)** Raised, mostly pigmented, conjunctival lesions. White dotted arrows represent UHR-OCT imaged area. **(c,d)** Corresponding UHR-OCT images with subepithelial lesions (black arrows) beneath a normal to mildly thickened epithelium (yellow arrows).

confirmed the diagnosis of CMM. This UHR OCT diagnosis prompted immediate surgical resection and avoided incisional biopsy (generally not recommended in CMM) or treatment with ineffective topical medications. In recently unpublished data from our group, we evaluated 108 patients (101 OSSNs and 7 CMMs) with UHR OCT. Differences in the measured epithelial thickness on UHR OCT between the two entities were statistically significant ($P = 0.01$). (▸ Fig. 3.5) In this way, the morphologic features displayed by the UHR OCT can be an important adjunct in evaluating OSSN and melanoma.

3.2.5 Nevus

Nevus is the most common pigmented conjunctival tumor, representing 52% of all melanocytic tumors.[55] Clinical features include focality of the lesion, unilaterality, long-term presence, and cysts.[50,56] Nevi are pigmented in 51% of cases, partially pigmented in 28%, and nonpigmented or amelanotic in 21%, giving in this way a broad phenotypic spectrum in its clinical manifestation.[55] With several overlapping features between nevi, PAM, and CMM, the presence of cysts is most suggestive of nevus. Cysts are visible on slit-lamp examination in 57 to 65% of cases[55,57]; however UHR OCT imaging may be of great assistance in their detection, particularly in the group of lesions that are not easily perceived on biomicroscopic examination. This technology can be extremely useful in nonpigmented cases, when clinical characteristics such as gelatinous or translucent appearance and presence of feeder vessels make clinical diagnosis a challenge. (▸ Fig. 3.6)

Shields et al,[58] in 2011, reported the evaluation of conjunctival nevi using a commercially available TD OCT machine. Images disclosed that the deep margin of a nevus can be visualized in 100% of cases, the posterior margin in 82%, and the lateral margin in 86%. The nevi were optically dense in all cases, and cysts could be visualized in 77% (with a sensitivity of 80% and specificity of 100% compared with histopathology). Additionally, two cases were later reported with the use of UHR OCT[12] for nevi. UHR OCT images seemed to demonstrate which tissue layers were involved by nevus cells (i.e., epithelium and substantia propria in the compound nevus and only epithelium in the junctional nevus). Lesions were highly hyperreflective, usually well circumscribed, and cysts were noted within the subepithelial tissue. These findings correlated with the histopathology which disclosed nests of nevus cells within the conjunctival tissue with epithelial-lined cysts. Both studies conclude that the main drawback of the OCT was optical shadowing of deeper structures from pigment within the nevi.[12,58] Furthermore, the presence of a cyst does not provide absolute assurance that the lesion is benign. CMM can develop from nevi. It is exceptionally important to differentiate nevus from CMM, given that nevus has low to no risk of malignant transformation,[55,57,59] whereas CMM is malignant. UHR OCT cannot differentiate between the two lesions with certainty.

3.2.6 Conjunctival Lymphoma

Conjunctival lymphoma is an ocular surface tumor that is clinically described as a salmon-pink, "fleshy" patch, with a generally smooth surface that usually occurs in the superior or inferior conjunctival quadrants.[60,61] It can also have a multinodular appearance and even manifest as follicular conjunctivitis.[62] When the manifestation is not classic, the UHR OCT may provide additional information.

Six cases of lymphoma imaged with UHR OCT have been reported in the literature.[12] UHR OCT disclosed homogeneous dark images lesions in the substantia propria, with a normal overlying epithelium. The lesion was hyporeflective and appeared to be formed of stippled hyperreflective dots suggestive of homogeneous cell population; some shadows were cast by the masses on the underlying tissues.[12] Even though this adjunctive diagnostic technology effectively discloses the presence of subepithelial lesions (▸ Fig. 3.7), differentiation between lymphoid hyperplasia and malignant lymphoid tumors is not possible; therefore, histopathologic evaluation and immunohistochemical studies are always needed.

In addition, UHR OCT has been shown to be effective in demonstrating resolution of conjunctival lymphoma after external-beam radiotherapy,[12] which (30–36 Gy) is the mainstay of treatment for localized disease.[63] This novel imaging technique may be helpful in detecting tumor resolution after treatment and may prove an effective noninvasive approach of monitoring efficacy and perhaps reveal residual disease or recurrences.

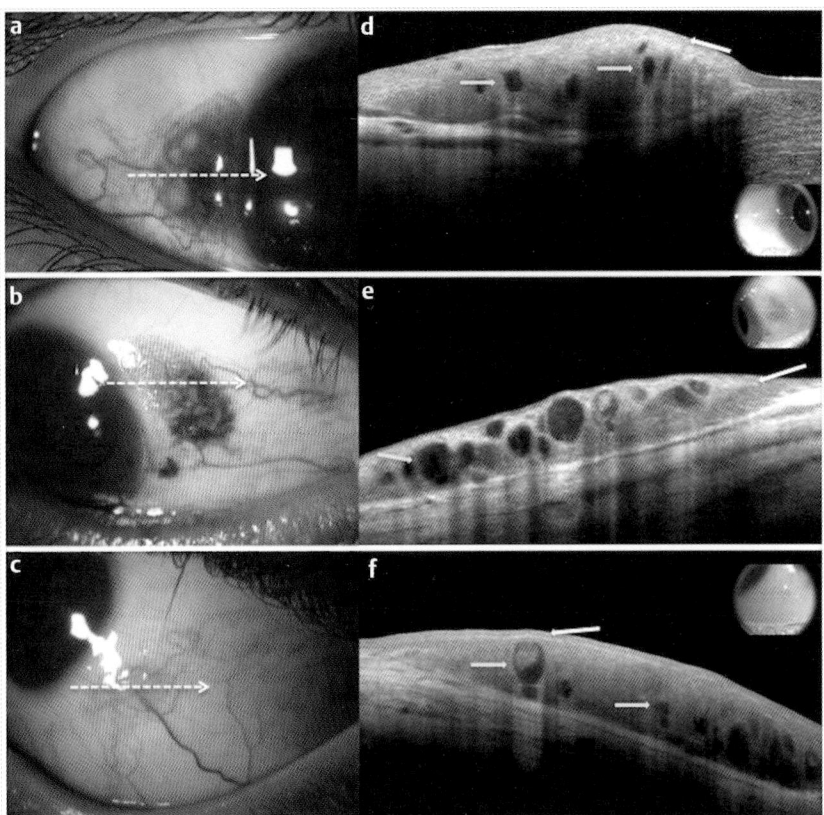

Fig. 3.6 Clinical photographs and ultrahigh-resolution optical coherence tomography (UHR OCT) scans of nevi. **(a,b)** Two localized limbal, pigmented lesions with multiple cysts. **(c)** Localized, limbal, nonpigmeted (amelanotic) lesion. White dotted arrows represent UHR OCT-imaged area. White dotted arrows represent UHR OCT-imaged area. **(d-f)** UHR OCT images with thickened epithelium (white arrows) and well circumscribed hyperreflective subepithelial lesions with multiple cysts (yellow arrows).

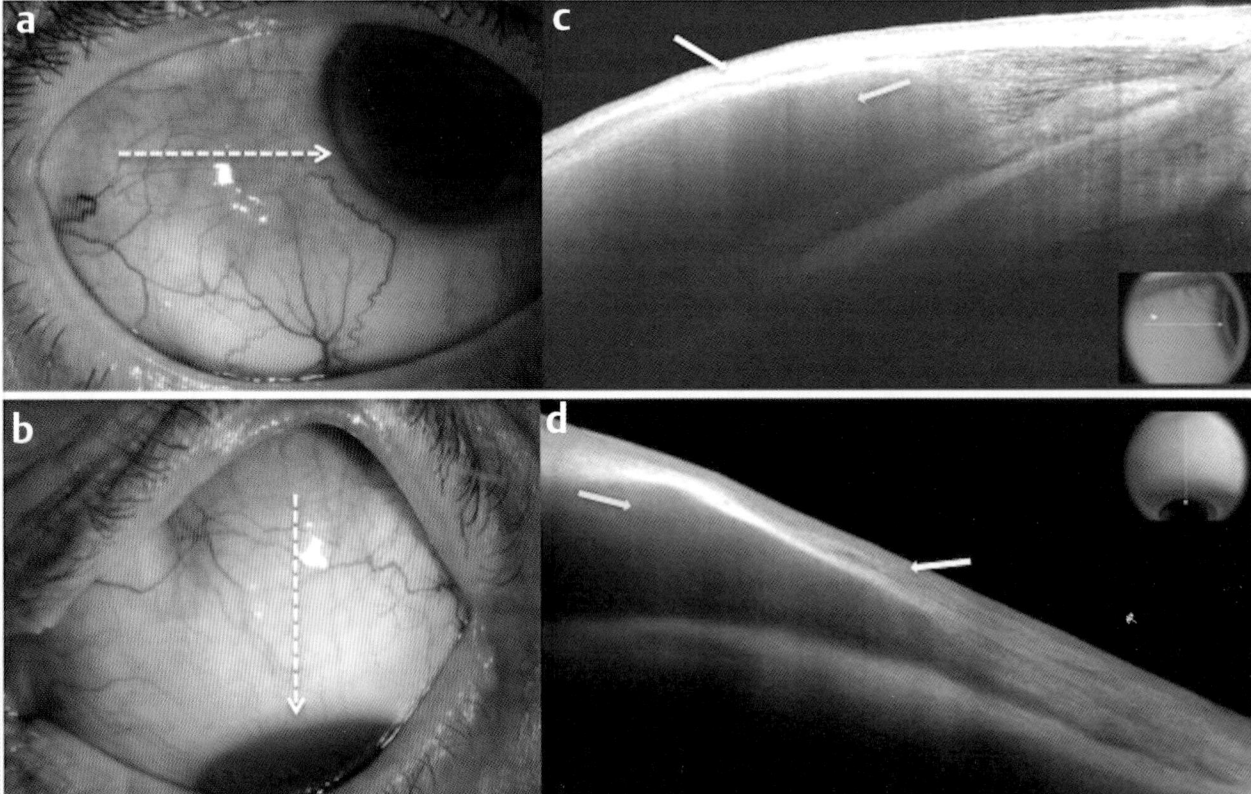

Fig. 3.7 Clinical photographs and ultrahigh-resolution optical coherence tomography (UHR OCT) scans of conjunctival lymphoma. **(a,b)** Salmon-colored lesions of the conjunctiva. White dotted arrows represent UHR-OCT imaged area. **(c,d)** UHR OCT images with homogeneous hyporeflective (dark) subepithelial lesions, with subtle stippled hyperreflective dots within the substantia propria (black arrows). A normal overlying epithelium is also noted (yellow arrows).

3.3 Conclusions

This chapter presents a summary of the history of anterior-segment OCT as well as an overview of how OCT technology works, including TD OCT, SD OCT, and the evolution to HR and UHR OCT devices. This novel, noninvasive adjuvant diagnostic technique has shown to be helpful for the management of several ocular surface pathologies. In particular, it seems most helpful with the management of OSSN. Biopsy with histopathologic analysis remains the "gold standard" for diagnosing ocular surface lesions, but as this technology continues, the OCT is becoming an "optical biopsy." As with any other imaging technique, UHR OCT images should always be evaluated within the proper clinical context, and several scans should be reviewed.

The distinctive characteristics of OSSN in UHR OCT have proven this technology to be valuable in detecting and ruling out OSSN, especially in the setting of subtle or clinically indeterminate lesions. During the medical treatment of OSSN monitoring disease resolution and detecting residual subclinical disease are important features accomplished by the UHR OCT.

Melanocytic lesions, such as CMM, PAM, and nevus, have several overlapping clinical features. UHR OCT may show clues to suggest a diagnosis, but at this point it cannot diagnose. Its main strength is the ability to differentiate nonpigmented (amelanotic) melanomas from OSSNs. UHR OCT was also found to have characteristic features in conjunctival lymphoma and can be used to monitor treatment efficacy.

In the future, newer-generation machines will likely have improved penetrance and scan width, allowing UHR OCT to be used for anterior-segment disease beyond the conjunctival and corneal epithelium, and even higher resolution could perhaps allow imaging to the level of individual cells.

In conclusion, the imaging modality of UHR OCT continues to refine our ability to diagnose ocular surface lesions more accurately, and it also allows for monitoring during and after different treatment modalities. As additional studies become available, clinical applications of this novel technology will continue to expand as a noninvasive, in vivo optical biopsy. Further studies are needed, however, to evaluate how well this technology can be incorporated into different ophthalmology practices.

References

[1] Huang D, Swanson EA, Lin CP, et al. Optical coherence tomography. Science 1991; 254: 1178–1181

[2] Fujimoto J, Drexler W. Introduction to optical coherence tomography. In: Drexler W, Fujimoto J, eds. Optical Coherence Tomography, 2008, Berlin Heidelberg: Springer; 2008:1–45

[3] Izatt JA, Hee MR, Swanson EA, et al. Micrometer-scale resolution imaging of the anterior eye in vivo with optical coherence tomography. Arch Ophthalmol 1994; 112: 1584–1589

[4] Wang J, Shousha MA, Perez VL, Karp CL, et al. Ultra-high resolution optical coherence tomography for imaging the anterior segment of the eye. Ophthalmic Surg Lasers Imaging 2011; 42 Suppl: S15–S27

[5] Ramos JL, Li Y, Huang D. Clinical and research applications of anterior segment optical coherence tomography: a review. Clin Experiment Ophthalmol 2009; 37: 81–89

[6] Grieve K, Paques M, Dubois A, Sahel J, Boccara C, Le Gargasson JF. Ocular tissue imaging using ultrahigh-resolution, full-field optical coherence tomography. Invest Ophthalmol Vis Sci 2004; 45: 4126–4131

[7] Simpson T, Fonn D. Optical coherence tomography of the anterior segment. Ocul Surf 2008: 117–127

[8] Feng Y, Simpson TL. Corneal, limbal, and conjunctival epithelial thickness from optical coherence tomography. Optom Vis Sci 2008; 85: E880–E883

[9] Vajzovic LM, Karp CL, Haft P, et al. Ultra high-resolution anterior segment optical coherence tomography in the evaluation of anterior corneal dystrophies and degenerations. Ophthalmology 2011; 118: 1291–1296

[10] Shousha MA, Karp CL, Perez VL, et al. Diagnosis and management of conjunctival and corneal intraepithelial neoplasia using ultra high-resolution optical coherence tomography. Ophthalmology 2011; 118: 1531–1537

[11] Kieval JZ, Karp CL, Abou Shousha M, et al. Ultra-high resolution optical coherence tomography for differentiation of ocular surface squamous neoplasia and pterygia. Ophthalmology 2012; 119: 481–486

[12] Shousha MA, Karp CL, Canto AP, et al. Diagnosis of ocular surface lesions using ultra-high-resolution optical coherence tomography. Ophthalmology 2013; 120: 883–891

[13] Baikoff G, Lutun E, Ferraz C, Wei J. Static and dynamic analysis of the anterior segment with optical coherence tomography. J Cataract Refract Surg 2004; 30: 1843–1850

[14] Radhakrishnan S, Rollins AM, Roth JE, et al. Real-time optical coherence tomography of the anterior segment at 1310 nm. Arch Ophthalmol 2001; 119: 1179–1185

[15] Stanga PE, Bird AC. Optical coherence tomography (OCT): principles of operation, technology, indications in vitreoretinal imaging and interpretation of results. Int Ophthalmol 2001; 23: 191–197

[16] Li Y, Tang M, Zhang X, Salaroli CH, Ramos JL, Huang D. Pachymetric mapping with Fourier-domain optical coherence tomography. J Cataract Refract Surg 2010; 36: 826–831

[17] Pierre-Kahn V, Tadayoni R, Haouchine B, Massin P, Gaudric A. Comparison of optical coherence tomography models OCT1 and Stratus OCT for macular retinal thickness measurement. Br J Ophthalmol 2005; 89: 1581–1585

[18] Bitton E, Keech A, Simpson T, Jones L. Variability of the analysis of the tear meniscus height by optical coherence tomography. Optom Vis Sci 2007; 84: 903–908

[19] Jancevski M, Foster CS. Anterior segment optical coherence tomography. Semin Ophthalmol 2010; 25: 317–323

[20] Kiernan DF, Mieler WF, Hariprasad SM. Spectral-domain optical coherence tomography: a comparison of modern high-resolution retinal imaging systems. Am J Ophthalmol 2010; 149: 18–31

[21] Hurmeric V, Yoo SH, Mutlu FM. Optical coherence tomography in cornea and refractive surgery. Expert Rev Ophthalmol 2012; 7: 241–250

[22] Maeda N. Optical coherence tomography for corneal diseases. Eye Contact Lens 2010; 36: 254–259

[23] Leite MT, Rao HL, Zangwill LM, Weinreb RN, Medeiros FA. Comparison of the diagnostic accuracies of the Spectralis, Cirrus, and RTVue optical coherence tomography devices in glaucoma. Ophthalmology 2011; 118: 1334–1339

[24] Shetty R, Malhotra C, D'Souza S, Wadia K. WaveLight FS200 vs Hansatome LASIK: intraoperative determination of flap characteristics and predictability by hand-held bioptigen spectral domain ophthalmic imaging system. J Refract Surg 2012; 28 Suppl: S815–S820

[25] Matonti F, Hoffart L, Alessi G, et al. [Spectral-domain optical coherence tomography in anterior segment imaging: the 3rd dimension] J Fr Ophtalmol 2009; 32: 727–734

[26] Drexler W, Morgner U, Ghanta RK, Kärtner FX, Schuman JS, Fujimoto JG. Ultrahigh-resolution ophthalmic optical coherence tomography. Nat Med 2001; 7: 502–507

[27] Drexler W. Ultrahigh-resolution optical coherence tomography. J Biomed Opt 2004: 47–74

[28] Wang J, Jiao S, Ruggeri M, Shousha MA, Chen Q. In situ visualization of tears on contact lens using ultra high resolution optical coherence tomography. Eye Contact Lens 2009; 35: 44–49

[29] Chen Q, Wang J, Tao A, Shen M, Jiao S, Lu F. Ultrahigh-resolution measurement by optical coherence tomography of dynamic tear film changes on contact lenses. Invest Ophthalmol Vis Sci 2010; 51: 1988–1993

[30] Gonzalez-Meijome JM, Cerviño A, Carracedo G, Queiros A, Garcia-Lázaro S, Ferrer-Blasco T. High-resolution spectral domain optical coherence tomography technology for the visualization of contact lens to cornea relationships. Cornea 2010; 29: 1359–1367

[31] Shousha MA, Perez VL, Wang J, et al. Use of ultra-high-resolution optical coherence tomography to detect in vivo characteristics of Descemet's membrane in Fuchs' dystrophy. Ophthalmology 2010; 117: 1220–1227

[32] Kaluzny BJ, Fojt W, Szkulmowska A, Bajraszewski T, Wojtkowski M, Kowalczyk A. Spectral optical coherence tomography in video-rate and 3D imaging of contact lens wear. Optom Vis Sci 2007; 84: 1104–1109

[33] Kałuzny BJ, Kaluzny JJ, Szkulmowska A, et al. Spectral optical coherence tomography: a new imaging technique in contact lens practice. Ophthalmic Physiol Opt 2006; 26: 127–132

[34] Suh LH, Shousha MA, Ventura RU, et al. Epithelial ingrowth after Descemet stripping automated endothelial keratoplasty: description of cases and assessment with anterior segment optical coherence tomography. Cornea 2011; 30: 528–534

[35] Hurmeric V, Yoo SH, Karp CL, et al. In vivo morphologic characteristics of Salzmann nodular degeneration with ultra-high-resolution optical coherence tomography. Am J Ophthalmol 2011; 151: 248–256, e2

[36] Hurmeric V, Yoo SH, Fishler J, Chang VS, Wang J, Culbertson WW. In vivo structural characteristics of the femtosecond LASIK-induced opaque Bubble Layers with ultrahigh-resolution SD-OCT. Ophthalmic Surg Lasers Imaging 2010; 41: S109–S113

[37] Thomas BJ, Galor A, Nanji AA, et al. Ultra high-resolution anterior segment optical coherence tomography in the diagnosis and management of ocular surface squamous neoplasia. Ocul Surf 2014; 12: 46–58

[38] Shields CL, Demirci H, Karatza E, Shields JA. Clinical survey of 1643 melanocytic and nonmelanocytic conjunctival tumors. Ophthalmology 2004; 111: 1747–1754

[39] Sanders N, Bedotto C. Recurrent carcinoma in situ of the conjunctiva and cornea (Bowen's disease). Am J Ophthalmol 1972; 74: 688–693

[40] Xu Y, Zhou Z, Xu Y, et al. The clinical value of in vivo confocal microscopy for diagnosis of ocular surface squamous neoplasia. Eye (Lond) 2012; 26: 781–787

[41] Finger PT, Tran HV, Turbin RE, et al. High-frequency ultrasonographic evaluation of conjunctival intraepithelial neoplasia and squamous cell carcinoma. Arch Ophthalmol 2003; 121: 168–172

[42] Balestrazzi A, Martone G, Pichierri P, Tosi GM, Caporossi A. Corneal invasion of ocular surface squamous neoplasia after clear corneal phacoemulsification: in vivo confocal microscopy analysis. J Cataract Refract Surg 2008; 34: 1038–1043

[43] Dada T, Sihota R, Gadia R, Aggarwal A, Mandal S, Gupta V. Comparison of anterior segment optical coherence tomography and ultrasound biomicroscopy for assessment of the anterior segment. J Cataract Refract Surg 2007; 33: 837–840

[44] Fraunfelder FT, Wingfield D. Therapy of intraepithelial epitheliomas and squamous cell carcinoma of the limbus. Trans Am Ophthalmol Soc 1980; 78: 290–300

[45] Frucht-Pery J, Sugar J, Baum J, et al. Mitomycin C treatment for conjunctival-corneal intraepithelial neoplasia: a multicenter experience. Ophthalmology 1997; 104: 2085–2093

[46] Parrozzani R, Lazzarini D, Alemany-Rubio E, Urban F, Midena E. Topical 1% 5-fluorouracil in ocular surface squamous neoplasia: a long-term safety study. Br J Ophthalmol 2011; 95: 355–359

[47] Galor A, Karp CL, Chhabra S, Barnes S, Alfonso EC. Topical interferon alpha 2b eye-drops for treatment of ocular surface squamous neoplasia: a dose comparison study. Br J Ophthalmol 2010; 94: 551–554

[48] Schwartz GS, Holland EJ. Iatrogenic limbal stem cell deficiency. Cornea 1998; 17: 31–37

[49] Hatch KM, Dana R. The structure and function of the limbal stem cell and the disease states associated with limbal stem cell deficiency. Int Ophthalmol Clin 2009; 49: 43–52

[50] Oellers P, Karp CL. Management of pigmented conjunctival lesions. Ocul Surf 2012; 10: 251–263

[51] Shields JA, Shields CL, Mashayekhi A, et al. Primary acquired melanosis of the conjunctiva: experience with 311 eyes. Trans Am Ophthalmol Soc 2007; 105: 61–72

[52] Jakobiec FA, Folberg R, Iwamoto T. Clinicopathologic characteristics of premalignant and malignant melanocytic lesions of the conjunctiva. Ophthalmology 1989; 96: 147–166

[53] Yu GP, Hu DN, McCormick S, Finger PT. Conjunctival melanoma: is it increasing in the United States? Am J Ophthalmol 2003; 135: 800–806

[54] Shields CL, Markowitz JS, Belinsky I, et al. Conjunctival melanoma: outcomes based on tumor origin in 382 consecutive cases. Ophthalmology 2011; 118: 389–395, e1–e2

[55] Shields CL, Fasiuddin AF, Mashayekhi A, Shields JA. Conjunctival nevi: clinical features and natural course in 410 consecutive patients. Arch Ophthalmol 2004; 122: 167–175

[56] Folberg R, Jakobiec FA, Bernardino VB, Iwamoto T. Benign conjunctival melanocytic lesions: clinicopathologic features. Ophthalmology 1989; 96: 436–461

[57] Levecq L, De Potter P, Jamart J. Conjunctival nevi clinical features and therapeutic outcomes. Ophthalmology 2010; 117: 35–40

[58] Shields CL, Belinsky I, Romanelli-Gobbi M, et al. Anterior segment optical coherence tomography of conjunctival nevus. Ophthalmology 2011; 118: 915–919

[59] Shields CL, Shields JA. Tumors of the conjunctiva and cornea. Surv Ophthalmol 2004; 49: 3–24

[60] Bardenstein DS. Ocular adnexal lymphoma: classification, clinical disease, and molecular biology. Ophthalmol Clin North Am 2005; 18: 187–197

[61] Shields CL, Shields JA, Carvalho C, Rundle P, Smith AF. Conjunctival lymphoid tumors: clinical analysis of 117 cases and relationship to systemic lymphoma. Ophthalmology 2001; 108: 979–984

[62] Stefanovic A, Lossos IS. Extranodal marginal zone lymphoma of the ocular adnexa. Blood 2009; 114: 501–510

[63] Tsai PS, Colby KA. Treatment of conjunctival lymphomas. Semin Ophthalmol 2005; 20: 239–246

4 Phase-Variance Optical Coherence Tomography

Scott M. McClintic, Dae Yu Kim, Jeff Fingler, Susan Garcia, Robert J. Zawadzki, Lawrence S. Morse, Susanna S. Park, Scott E. Fraser, John S. Werner, Jason P. Ruggiero, and Daniel M. Schwartz

Angiography of the retinal and choroidal vasculature is a valuable diagnostic tool and is essential to the evaluation of many vision-threatening diseases, including age-related macular degeneration (AMD), cystoid macular edema, diabetic retinopathy, posterior uveitis, and retinal vascular occlusion. Fluorescein angiography (FA) is the gold-standard modality for imaging of the retinal circulation, whereas indocyanine green angiography (ICGA) is used primarily for its visualization of the choroidal vasculature.[1] However, each of these modalities requires intravenous dye infusion, is time-consuming, requires significant operator skill, and carries the risk of both minor and major adverse events.[2,3]

Dye-based angiography is also limited in its imaging capabilities. Leakage of dye from the vessels can obscure vascular detail, particularly when imaging the fenestrated vessels of the choriocapillaris. Compared with fluorescein, indocyanine green dye is more protein-bound and has higher absorption (~ 805 nm) and emission (~ 835 nm) wavelengths.[1] These properties reduce dye extravasation from intact choroidal vessels and improve signal penetration, both of which enable enhanced visualization of the choroidal vasculature. However, its ability to resolve the microvasculature, particularly the choriocapillaris, remains limited.[4,5]

As an alternative to dye-based modalities, optical coherence tomography (OCT) provides highly detailed, noninvasive imaging of the retinal architecture, and recent developments have enabled the production of uniquely informative data. Machines capable of performing both scanning laser ophthalmoscopy and OCT permit the combined use of microperimetry and OCT to assess precisely the relationship between visual function and retinal structures.[6] The application of adaptive optics uses wavefront analysis to facilitate correction of higher-order optical aberrations and increase scan resolution.[7] The development of faster and more sensitive imaging techniques (e.g., Fourier-domain systems, such as spectral-domain (SD) and swept-source OCT), along with progress in OCT data processing, has enhanced the ability of OCT to create retinovascular angiograms.[8,9,10,11,12,13,14,15,16,17,18,19,20,21,22,23,24,25,26,27,28,29,30] Multiple approaches, each with certain advantages and limitations, have been developed for this purpose. Phase-variance OCT (pvOCT) is a noninvasive technique that creates three-dimensional representations of the retinal and choroidal vasculature by analyzing motion-related changes in OCT signal phase over time that occur between consecutive B-scans.[24,25,26,27,28,29,30]

4.1 Basic Principles

Optical coherence tomography of the eye relies on the principles of optical interferometry.[31] A beam of low-coherence, near-infrared light is split into two arms: a *reference signal* that is projected toward a reference mirror and a *sample signal* of equal optical path length that is projected onto the sample tissue. As the sample signal passes through tissue, some portion of it is scattered, and the portion that is backscattered is combined with the reflected reference signal. In Fourier-domain OCT systems, the resulting spectral interference pattern is Fourier-transformed to produce a depth-resolved scattering profile that is then used to generate a structural image of the sample tissue.

Although OCT can produce images of the retinal and choroidal blood vessels, standard visualization of the B-scan (intensity of back-scattered light) is unable to highlight flow through the retinal structures; however, the reconstructed OCT B-scan contains phase information that can be analyzed to detect motion. When the sample beam is reflected by medium that is moving, the resulting phase value varies over time.[32] Phase-variance OCT is a technique that interprets phase shifts between series of consecutive B-scans to detect areas of motion.[24,25,26]

An A-scan is a one-dimensional depth-scattering profile taken at a single location, and a B-scan is a two-dimensional cross-section composed of multiple, consecutive A-scans taken over a range of transverse locations. In the most common pvOCT technique, multiple successive OCT B-scans (BM-scan) are acquired consecutively at the same location, and this process is repeated over a spatial region of the retina to obtain a volumetric scan.[24] Interpretation of the statistical variance of the phase shifts occurring between the B-scans can be used to identify areas of mobility (i.e., blood flow) that contrast with the relatively static retinal tissue.[24,25,26] The ability to determine the phase contrast between successive B-scans is dependent on the image acquisition speed of the OCT system, and improvements in acquisition speed should reduce motion artifact and increase the potential imaging size.[25]

An alternative method for visualizing motion is Doppler OCT. Doppler-based methods identify motion by detecting changes in the signal occurring in the axial direction of the imaging beam; pvOCT is able to characterize flow occurring in both axial and transverse planes.[25] Furthermore, because Doppler-based methods rely on detecting signal scattering that occurs on successive A-scans, increasing the image acquisition speed allows less time for scatter changes to occur and the ability to detect slow flow is reduced.[33,34,35] In contrast, pvOCT can identify motion over a wide dynamic range of flow rates and, as stated previously, benefits from improved acquisition speed.[25]

4.2 Technique

4.2.1 Equipment

A primary advantage of pvOCT over other methods of OCT-based angiography is the ability to use conventional SD OCT machines to acquire the data required for phase-variance imaging. The pvOCT technique relies on analysis of phase-specific data that are normally collected, but not used, during standard SD OCT imaging; however, although no hardware modifications are necessary, specialized software-based imaging protocols must be applied to capture the entire raw data set and perform BM-scans in the appropriate fashion. Average volumetric scan times are less than 5 seconds, and irradiance levels conform to

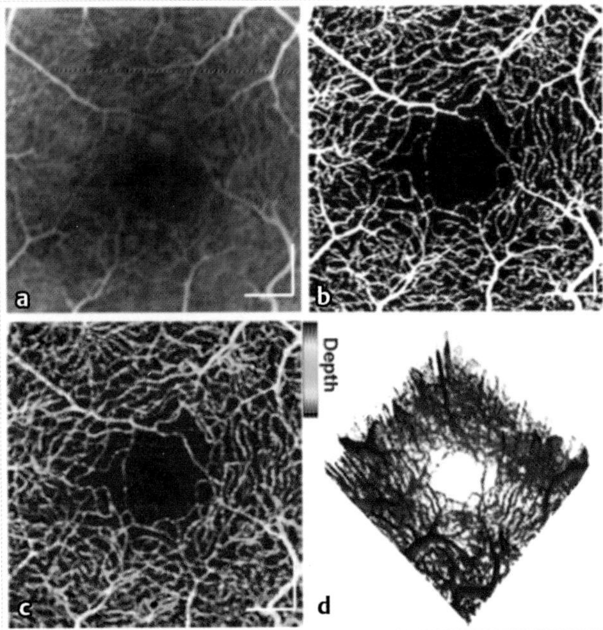

Fig. 4.1 Retinal perfusion images of the parafoveal region measuring 1.5 × 1.5 mm. (a) Fluorescein angiography. (b) En face phase-variance optical coherence tomography (pvOCT) image. (c) Pseudocolor-coded depth representation of image. (d) Three-dimensional depth color-coded pvOCT image. Scale bar, 250 µm. Colors in depth: Superficial layer, red; intermediate layer, green; deep layer, blue. (From Kim DY, Fingler J, Zawadzki RJ, et al. Noninvasive imaging of the foveal avascular zone with high-speed, phase-variance optical coherence tomography. Invest Ophthalmol Vis Sci 2012;53:85–92. Used with permission.)

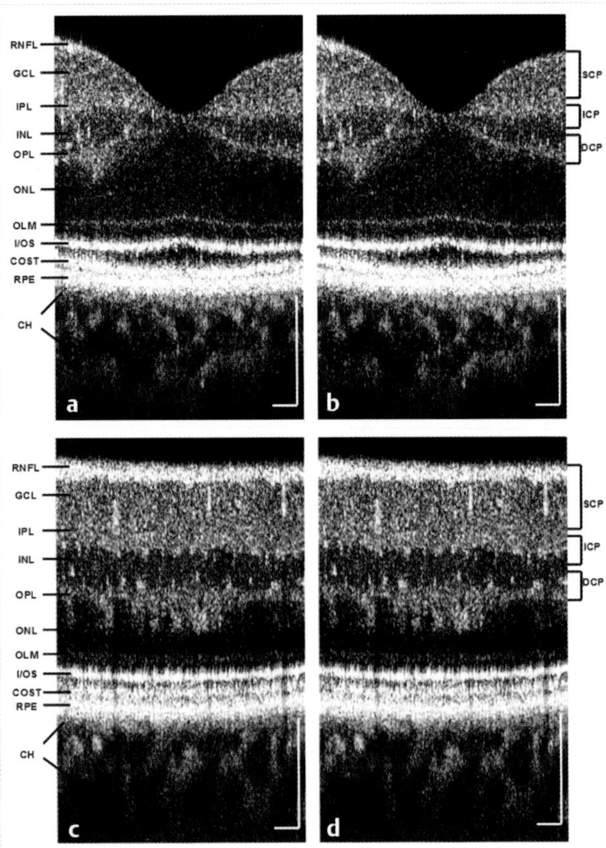

Fig. 4.2 Spectral-domain optical coherence tomography (SD OCT) and phase-variance OCT (pvOCT) retinal images from a 59-year-old healthy man. (a) Averaged SD OCT intensity images from two sequential multiple successive (BM) scans (three B-scans each) at the fovea. (b) Composite image of the SD OCT intensity (gray) and the pv-OCT image (red). (c) An averaged SD OCT image near the foveal center. (d) Composite image of the SD OCT intensity (gray) and the pv-OCT image (red). CH, choriocapillaris and choroid; COST, cone outer segment tip; DCP, deep capillary plexus; GCL, ganglion cell layer; ICP, intermediate capillary plexus; INL, inner nuclear layer; I/OS, inner/outer segment junction; IPL, inner plexiform layer; OLM, outer limiting membrane; ONL, outer nuclear layer; OPL, outer plexiform layer; RPE, retinal pigment; SCP, superficial capillary plexus. Scale bar, 150 µm. (From Kim DY, Fingler J, Zawadzki RJ, et al. Noninvasive imaging of the foveal avascular zone with high-speed, phase-variance optical coherence tomography. Invest Ophthalmol Vis Sci 2012;53:85–92. Used with permission.)

the established American National Standards Institute (ANSI) standards.[27,28] The generation of images comparable to those produced on custom OCT machines has been demonstrated using a commercial SD OCT platform. With existing technology, the approximate axial resolution ranges from 3 to 4.5 µm, and lateral resolution ranges from 10 to 15 µm.[30]

4.2.2 Image Processing

Once raw scan data are collected, phase information must be extracted and analyzed. Acquired OCT data are initially processed using standard procedures, and bulk axial motion is calculated and corrected for each location to separate vascular flow from gross eye motion.[26,27] Intensity thresholding reduces signal noise, and the phase differences between sequential B-scans are extracted for phase-variance calculations.[28] This process is repeated over the entire scan area to yield a three-dimensional image. Volumetric data are segmented according to depth, and pseudocolor depth coding may be applied to highlight depth position of vascular networks.[28,30]

4.2.3 Image Format

Phase-variance OCT images may be viewed as standard two-dimensional tomograms or as en face projections.[28] An en face projection may represent a single depth layer of the retina or choroid, or multiple depth layers may be overlaid, each with an assigned pseudocolor (▶ Fig. 4.1). Images of specific depth layers may be produced to evaluate a particular vascular network (e.g., the Sattler versus the Haller layer of the choroid). Color-coded pvOCT B-scans may also be displayed over standard OCT tomograms to produce composite B-scan images in which color indicates areas of flow (▶ Fig. 4.2).

4.3 Applications

The ability of pvOCT to produce high-resolution, three-dimensional angiographic images of the retinal and choroidal circulation makes it well suited for a variety of clinical applications. These features also provide a noninvasive alternative to conventional dye-based angiography that may easily be repeated on sequential office visits. Because the fine retinal

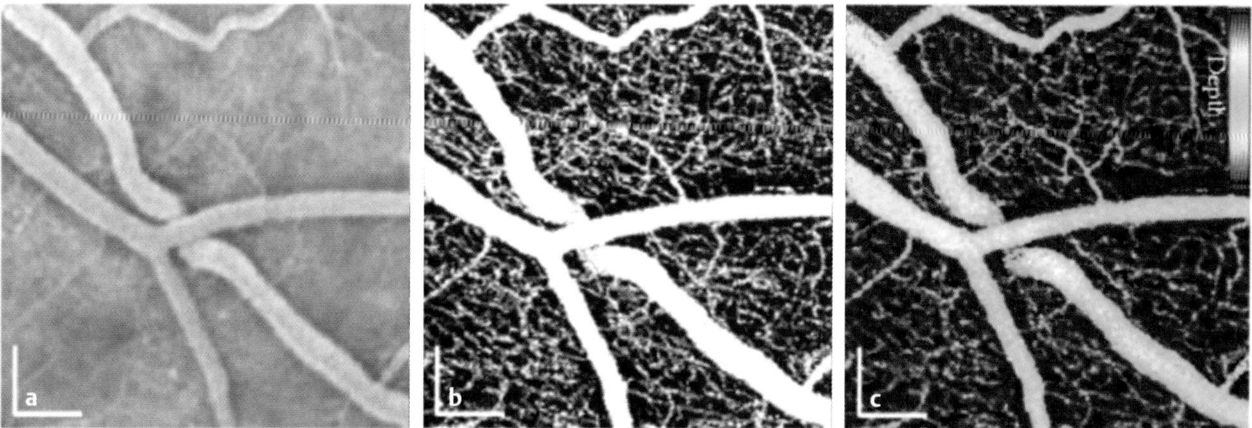

Fig. 4.3 Fine detail of in vivo retinal microcapillary network. Image size 1.5 × 1.5 mm. **(a)** Fluorescein angiography. **(b)** En face phase-variance optical coherence tomography (pvOCT) image. **(c)** Three-dimensional depth color-coded pvOCT image. Upper right shows depth scale bar: superficial layer, red; intermediate layer, green; deep layer, blue. Scale bar, 250 µm. (From Kim DY, Fingler J, Werner JS, et al. In vivo volumetric imaging of human retinal circulation with phase-variance optical coherence tomography. Biomed Opt Express [serial online] 2011;2:1504–1513. Used with permission.)

microvasculature is often obscured by background choroidal fluorescence in FA, the resolution of pvOCT is often superior (▶ Fig. 4.3). This level of detail extends posteriorly into the choroid, enabling visualization of the choriocapillaris and deeper choroidal vascular beds (▶ Fig. 4.4).

4.3.1 Age-Related Macular Degeneration

Angiographic evaluation in AMD is important for establishing the diagnosis, detecting the presence of exudative disease, characterizing choroidal neovascularization, and monitoring response to treatment. Because management of neovascular AMD has become focused predominantly on intravitreal anti-vascular endothelial growth factor therapy, clinicians have relied on OCT to guide treatment decisions. OCT has become the standard of care to study the morphologic changes associated with active exudative AMD, such as macular edema or subretinal exudation.[36] It can also be used to detect subretinal fibrosis, which has been shown to correlate closely in size and location with choroidal neovascularization visualized by FA.[37] However, conventional OCT cannot differentiate active neovascularization from avascular subretinal fibrosis because it does not provide flow information within the neovascular complex. It also provides limited resolution of the choriocapillaris, the loss of which may be critical to the development of geographic atrophy and/or choroidal neovascularization.[38]

Like conventional OCT, pvOCT is able to be repeated at sequential office visits and therefore may be used to inform routine treatment decisions. While extravasated dye limits visualization of neovascular membranes in FA, pvOCT is able to provide high-resolution views and three-dimensional localization of neovascular vessels (▶ Fig. 4.5). The improved localization and visualization of the neovascular membrane may result in a more accurate and sensitive diagnosis of retinal angiomatous proliferation or occult choroidal neovascularization associated with exudative AMD. This potential advantage of using OCT has been reported with high-resolution OCT instrumentation, although it lacks the flow information provided by pvOCT.[37,39] This degree of detail also provides a means of monitoring disease progression and response to therapy. Color-coded composite tomograms can be used to evaluate the presence of vascular flow, which may aid in the early detection of vascularization in pigment epithelial detachments (▶ Fig. 4.6). Furthermore, pvOCT may provide an alternative to ICGA for detection of vascular networks and polyps associated with polypoidal choroidal vasculopathy.

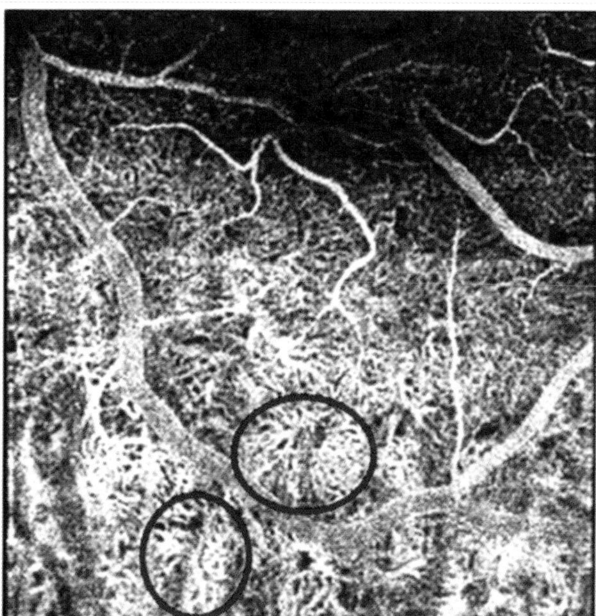

Fig. 4.4 En face phase-variance optical coherence tomography image of the retinal and choroidal vasculature. Putative choroidal lobules are circled in red. (From Schwartz DM, Fingler J, Kim DY, et al. Phase-variance optical coherence tomography: a technique for noninvasive angiography. Ophthalmology 2014;121:180–187. Used with permission.)

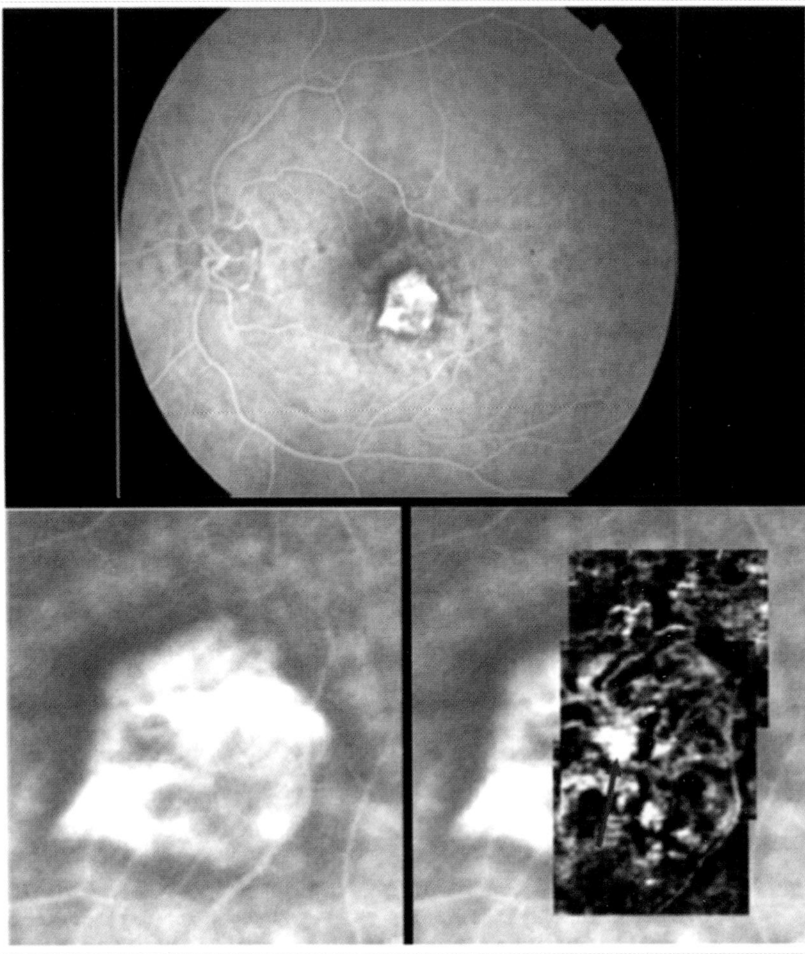

Fig. 4.5 Wet age-related macular degeneration with subfoveal choroidal neovascularization (CNV). Top shows early laminar flow transit fluorescein angiography (FA) of subfoveal classic CNV. Lower left shows magnification of FA, zoomed into region of CNV. Lower right shows a phase-variance optical coherence tomography montage (1 × 1-mm scans) of the subfoveal CNV, overlaid onto the FA. Note the cartwheel shape of multiple vascular spokes emanating from a probable central feeder vessel (red arrow). (From Schwartz DM, Fingler J, Kim DY, et al. Phase-variance optical coherence tomography: a technique for noninvasive angiography. Ophthalmology 2014;121:180–187. Used with permission.)

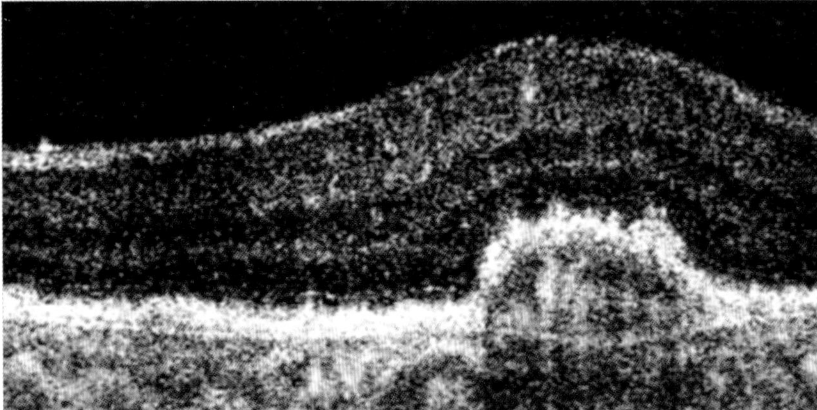

Fig. 4.6 Composite spectral-domain optical coherence tomography (OCT) and phase-variance OCT tomogram demonstrating a flow signal beneath the elevated retinal pigment epithelium and likely representing a vascularized pigment epithelial detachment.

4.3.2 Diabetic Retinopathy

In patients with diabetes, FA may be used to assess the severity of retinopathy by demonstrating the presence and extent of capillary nonperfusion, microaneurysms, intraretinal microvascular abnormalities, macular edema, and neovascularization (▶ Fig. 4.7). It can also assess the size of the foveal avascular zone, which may be predictive of visual potential.[40,41,42] These features are central to the standardized grading system used for diabetic retinopathy and are used to guide follow-up intervals and treatment decisions, including the timing of pan-retinal photocoagulation. However, because of the cost and inconvenience, patients typically receive an FA only when the fundus appearance first suggests advanced disease or to evaluate subsequent significant events (e.g., unexplained visual loss or a vitreous hemorrhage in the absence of clinically detectable neovascularization). Identification of areas of nonperfusion on pvOCT images is comparable to FA; however, microaneurysms may be more visible on FA. Whereas all depth layers are overlaid and are viewed simultaneously with FA, the creation of a three-dimensional pvOCT image requires the combination of data taken at multiple depth layers, and microaneurysms

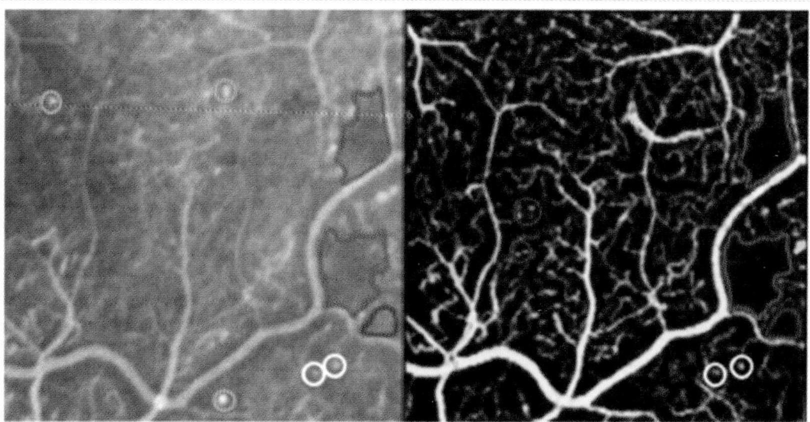

Fig. 4.7 View of temporal retina in subject with proliferative diabetic retinopathy. Fluorescein angiography (FA) on the left shows multiple microaneurysms and regions of capillary nonperfusion are outlined in red. A 3 × 3-mm phase-variance optical coherence tomography (pvOCT) image on the right shows similarly shaped regions of capillary nonperfusion outlined in red. Although some microaneurysms are shown by FA and pvOCT (white circles), others are only shown in the FA image (blue circles) or pvOCT (red circles). (From Schwartz DM, Fingler J, Kim DY, et al. Phase-variance optical coherence tomography: a technique for noninvasive angiography. Ophthalmology 2014;121:180–187. Used with permission.)

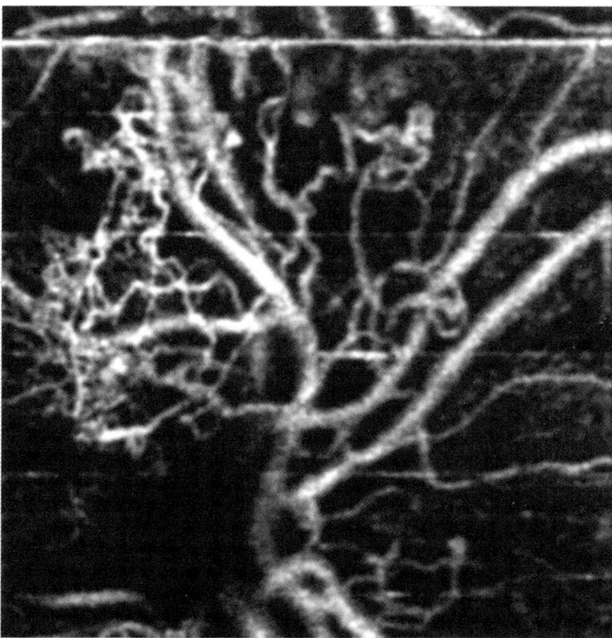

Fig. 4.8 En face phase-variance optical coherence tomography image of retinal neovascularization of the optic disc in a patient with proliferative diabetic retinopathy.

located in the intervening layers may not be captured.[30] Also, while associated dye leakage is often used to detect retinal neovascularization on FA, on pvOCT these vessels are located by identification of the actual neovascular structures (▶ Fig. 4.8).

4.4 Advantages

Phase-variance OCT offers many advantages over dye-based methods of fundus angiography and also provides several novel capabilities. Because it is noninvasive, side effects of FA and ICGA are avoided, including difficult needle sticks, local tissue damage from dye extravasation, and systemic side effects including, rarely, severe allergic reactions.[2,3] Retinovascular imaging with pvOCT can be performed with the same commercial instruments used in SD OCT, and exposure levels fall within established ANSI standards.

Scans can be quickly obtained in the office using existing OCT equipment, and operators require no additional skills aside from familiarity with the software interface and perhaps an increased attention to patient movement and positioning. Compared with dye-based angiography, it is faster, cheaper, more easily repeatable, and does not require the assistance of skilled nurses and technicians.

The resulting high-resolution, three-dimensional representations of the retinal and choroidal vasculature have the potential to be clinically useful. The microvascular detail is comparable to, and may exceed, that provided by FA and ICGA.[27,29,30] The exact size and position of features may be determined and monitored over time using sequential scans. Also, because scans produce both conventional OCT and pvOCT images, the two can be overlaid to provide a single composite image, which may provide information about vascularization in relation to other structural changes, including pigment epithelial detachment, macular edema, or subretinal fibrosis. Furthermore, the ability to assess sequential changes in the choriocapillaris could improve our understanding of the pathogenesis of inflammatory diseases of the retina and choroid.

4.5 Limitations

The phase-variance technique is subject to several important limitations. Because it relies on the detection of motion-related phase shifts, pvOCT is particularly sensitive to motion artifact. Obtaining a high-quality scan may be difficult with frail or elderly patients who struggle to maintain the proper position. Stabilization devices such as forehead rests and fixation lights may reduce patient movement and postscan image processing is used to reduce bulk motion signals. Eye-tracking devices are also currently being developed.

Also, the need to perform sequential B-scans at multiple locations requires the handling of large amounts of data. Depending on the capabilities of the OCT machine, maintaining a relatively small image frame may be necessary to prevent data overload. Raw OCT scan data must then be processed and analyzed to yield an image. At present, data are extracted from the OCT machine and transferred to a separate computer for manual processing. Automation of this process, with the ability to quickly create and view images on the OCT machine, is a subject of current investigation.

Because dynamic dye extravasation does not occur in pvOCT, the identification of sites of leakage (e.g., central serous chorioretinopathy and choroiditis) may be difficult. Identification of retinal neovascularization may also be more difficult using pvOCT. In these cases, dye-based angiography may remain the preferred imaging modality.

Lastly, whereas a primary advantage of pvOCT is the ability to detect flow occurring both in the perpendicular and transverse imaging planes, the analysis that allows for this ability makes it difficult to determine quantitative flow data (e.g., volume, velocity).[25] Once a three-dimensional map of the vasculature has been created, other flow methods, including Doppler-based techniques, may be used to quantify flow within these structures.[25]

4.6 Future

Because pvOCT is a software-based technique, it has the potential to be quickly integrated into clinical practice. This integration will be aided by the development of automated image processing so that physicians can review the scans immediately after acquisition. Features that reduce the effect of motion artifact may also improve image quality and make the process easier for both patients and technicians.

In many cases, pvOCT may be a preferred alternative to FA and ICGA. The ability to obtain sequential scans may increase the information available to clinicians in the ongoing treatment of chronic retinal and choroidal diseases. The enhanced visualization of the choriocapillaris compared with dye-based angiography is also a novel capability that may improve our understanding of disease behavior and pathogenesis. Further research will be required to determine how best to apply these features to practice.

References

[1] Owens SL. Indocyanine green angiography. Br J Ophthalmol 1996; 80: 263–266

[2] Lipson BK, Yannuzzi LA. Complications of intravenous fluorescein injections. Int Ophthalmol Clin 1989; 29: 200–205

[3] Kwan AS, Barry C, McAllister IL, Constable I. Fluorescein angiography and adverse drug reactions revisited: the Lions Eye experience. Clin Experiment Ophthalmol 2006; 34: 33–38

[4] Pauleikhoff D, Spital G, Radermacher M, Brumm GA, Lommatzsch A, Bird AC. A fluorescein and indocyanine green angiographic study of choriocapillaris in age-related macular disease. Arch Ophthalmol 1999; 117: 1353–1358

[5] Flower RW, Fryczkowski AW, McLeod DS. Variability in choriocapillaris blood flow distribution. Invest Ophthalmol Vis Sci 1995; 36: 1247–1258

[6] Landa G, Rosen RB, Garcia PM, Seiple WH. Combined three-dimensional spectral OCT/SLO topography and microperimetry: steps toward achieving functional spectral OCT/SLO. Ophthalmic Res 2010; 43: 92–98

[7] Deák GG, Schmidt-Erfurth U. Imaging of the parafoveal capillary network in diabetes. Curr Diab Rep 2013; 13: 469–475

[8] White B, Pierce M, Nassif N, et al. In vivo dynamic human retinal blood flow imaging using ultra-high-speed spectral domain optical coherence tomography. Opt Express 2003; 11: 3490–3497[serial online]

[9] Leitgeb RA, Schmetterer L, Hitzenberger CK, et al. Real-time measurement of in vitro flow by Fourier-domain color Doppler optical coherence tomography. Opt Lett 2004; 29: 171–173

[10] Makita S, Hong Y, Yamanari M, Yatagai T, Yasuno Y. Optical coherence angiography. Opt Express 2006; 14: 78217840 [serial online]

[11] Tao YK, Kennedy KM, Izatt JA. Velocity-resolved 3D retinal microvessel imaging using single-pass flow imaging spectral domain optical coherence tomography. Opt Express 2009; 17: 4177–4188[serial online]

[12] Grulkowski I, Gorczynska I, Szkulmowski M, et al. Scanning protocols dedicated to smart velocity ranging in spectral OCT. Opt Express 2009; 17: 23736–23754[serial online]

[13] Zotter S, Pircher M, Torzicky T, et al. Visualization of microvasculature by dual-beam phase-resolved Doppler optical coherence tomography. Opt Express 2011; 19: 1217–1227[serial online]

[14] Makita S, Jaillon F, Yamanari M, Miura M, Yasuno Y. Comprehensive in vivo micro-vascular imaging of the human eye by dual-beam-scan Doppler optical coherence angiography. Opt Express 2011; 19: 1271–1283 [serial online]

[15] Wang RK, Jacques SL, Ma Z, Hurst S, Hanson SR, Gruber A. Three dimensional optical angiography. Opt Express 2007; 15: 4083–4097[serial online]

[16] Braaf B, Vermeer KA, Vienola KV, de Boer JF. Angiography of the retina and the choroid with phase-resolved OCT using interval-optimized backstitched B-scans. Opt Express 2012; 20: 20516–20534[serial online]

[17] Kurokawa K, Sasaki K, Makita S, Hong YJ, Yasuno Y. Three-dimensional retinal and choroidal capillary imaging by power Doppler optical coherence angiography with adaptive optics. Opt Express 2012; 20: 2279622812 [serial online]

[18] Braaf B, Vienola KV, Sheehy CK, et al. Real-time eye motion correction in phase-resolved OCT angiography with tracking SLO. Biomed Opt Express 2013; 4: 51–65[serial online]

[19] Schmoll T, Singh AS, Blatter C, et al. Imaging of the parafoveal capillary network and its integrity analysis using fractal dimension. Biomed Opt Express 2011; 2: 1159–1168[serial online]

[20] Mariampillai A, Leung MK, Jarvi M, et al. Optimized speckle variance OCT imaging of microvasculature. Opt Lett 2010; 35: 1257–1259

[21] Motaghiannezam R, Fraser S. Logarithmic intensity and speckle-based motion contrast methods for human retinal vasculature visualization using swept source optical coherence tomography. Biomed Opt Express 2012: 503–521 [serial online]

[22] Jia Y, Tan O, Tokayer J, et al. Split-spectrum amplitude-decorrelation angiography with optical coherence tomography. Opt Express 2012; 20: 4710–4725 [serial online]

[23] Liu G, Chou L, Jia W, Qi W, Choi B, Chen Z. Intensity-based modified Doppler variance algorithm: application to phase instable and phase stable optical coherence tomography systems. Opt Express 2011; 19: 11429–11440[serial online]

[24] Fingler J, Schwartz D, Yang C, Fraser SE. Mobility and transverse flow visualization using phase variance contrast with spectral domain optical coherence tomography. Opt Express 2007; 15: 12636–12653[serial online]

[25] Fingler J, Readhead C, Schwartz DM, Fraser SE. Phase-contrast OCT imaging of transverse flows in the mouse retina and choroid. Invest Ophthalmol Vis Sci 2008; 49: 5055–5059

[26] Fingler J, Zawadzki RJ, Werner JS, Schwartz D, Fraser SE. Volumetric microvascular imaging of human retina using optical coherence tomography with a novel motion contrast technique. Opt Express 2009; 17: 22190–22200[serial online]

[27] Kim DY, Fingler J, Werner JS, Schwartz DM, Fraser SE, Zawadzki RJ. In vivo volumetric imaging of human retinal circulation with phase-variance optical coherence tomography. Biomed Opt Express 2011; 2: 1504–1513[serial online]

[28] Kim DY, Fingler J, Zawadzki RJ, et al. Noninvasive imaging of the foveal avascular zone with high-speed, phase-variance optical coherence tomography. Invest Ophthalmol Vis Sci 2012; 53: 85–92

[29] Kim DY, Fingler J, Zawadzki RJ, et al. Optical imaging of the chorioretinal vasculature in the living human eye. Proc Natl Acad Sci U S A 2013; 110: 14354–14359

[30] Schwartz DM, Fingler J, Kim DY, et al. Phase-variance optical coherence tomography: a technique for noninvasive angiography. Ophthalmology 2014; 121: 180–187

[31] Hee MR, Izatt JA, Swanson EA, et al. Optical coherence tomography of the human retina. Arch Ophthalmol 1995; 113: 325–332

[32] Zhao Y, Chen Z, Saxer C, Xiang S, de Boer JF, Nelson JS. Phase-resolved optical coherence tomography and optical Doppler tomography for imaging blood flow in human skin with fast scanning speed and high velocity sensitivity. Opt Lett 2000; 25: 114–116

[33] Park B, Pierce MC, Cense B, et al. Real-time fiber-based multi-functional spectral-domain optical coherence tomography at 1.3 microm. Opt Express 2005; 13: 3931–3944

[34] Yazdanfar S, Yang C, Sarunic M, Izatt J. Frequency estimation precision in Doppler optical coherence tomography using the Cramer-Rao lower bound. Opt Express 2005; 13: 410–416

[35] Vakoc B, Yun S, de Boer J, Tearney G, Bouma B. Phase-resolved optical frequency domain imaging. Opt Express 2005; 13: 5483–5493

[36] Fung AE, Lalwani GA, Rosenfeld PJ, et al. An optical coherence tomography-guided, variable dosing regimen with intravitreal ranibizumab (Lucentis) for neovascular age-related macular degeneration. Am J Ophthalmol 2007; 143: 566–583

[37] Park SS, Truong SN, Zawadzki RJ, et al. High resolution Fourier-domain optical coherence tomography of choroidal neovascular membranes associate with age-related macular degeneration. Invest Ophthalmol Vis Sci 2010; 51: 4200–4206

[38] Bhutto I, Lutty G. Understanding age-related macular degeneration (AMD): relationships between the photoreceptor/retinal pigment epithelium/Bruch's membrane/choriocapillaris complex. Mol Aspects Med 2012; 33: 295–317

[39] Truong SN, Alam S, Zawadzki RJ, et al. High resolution Fourier-domain optical coherence tomography of retinal angiomatous proliferation. Retina 2007; 27: 915–925

[40] Arend O, Wolf S, Harris A, Reim M. The relationship of macular microcirculation to visual acuity in diabetic patients. Arch Ophthalmol 1995; 113: 610–614

[41] Arend O, Remky A, Evans D, Stüber R, Harris A. Contrast sensitivity loss is coupled with capillary dropout in patients with diabetes. Invest Ophthalmol Vis Sci 1997; 38: 1819–1824

[42] Sim DA, Keane PA, Zarranz-Ventura J, et al. The effects of macular ischemia on visual acuity in diabetic retinopathy. Invest Ophthalmol Vis Sci 2013; 54: 2353–2360

5 Swept-Source Optical Coherence Tomography

Cong Ye and Vishal Jhanji

5.1 Background

Optical coherence tomography (OCT) was first applied in ophthalmology by Huang et al in 1991 to image the retinal layers.[1] Since then, OCT technology has been advanced from time domain (TD) to Fourier domain (FD), providing a noninvasive imaging method with high scanning speed and high resolution to visualize the structures inside the eye. The unique cross-sectional view of the eye enables not only morphologic but also quantitative assessment of the structure, which facilitates the diagnosis and monitoring of eye diseases. This chapter summarizes the applications of the latest generation of OCT, swept-source optical coherence tomography (SS OCT) for assessment of both the anterior and posterior segments of the eye.

5.2 Optical Coherence Tomography: From Time-Domain to Swept-Source

Low-coherence interferometry, the fundamental principle of OCT, detects and analyses the interference signals generated by superimposing backscattered light from the tissue of interest and that from a reference path to obtain optical intensity and depth information. The information is then translated into a color-coded or gray-scaled image to reveal the internal structures of the tissue. In TD OCT, a mobile reference arm mirror is used to ensure that the path lengths of both sample and reference arms are the same or nearly the same to allow interference between light reflected from the two arms, so that optical intensities of structures with varied depths can be sequentially documented while the reference mirror goes through the whole depth of the tissue. Because of the mobile reference mirror, the image acquisition time is rather long, which limits the image sampling density and makes TD OCT prone to motion artifacts. Additionally, the power of the light source of TD OCT is restricted by the inherited long image acquisition time and safety standards of total light exposure to the eye. Therefore, image resolution of TD OCT is also limited.

With the advent of FD technology, including spectral-domain OCT (SD OCT) and later the SS OCT, the axial image resolution and image acquisition speed of OCT have been significantly improved over the TD method. In SD OCT, the depth information is acquired without mechanical movement of the reference mirror, which significantly increases the scan speed.[2,3,4] Although the stationary reference mirror causes mismatch of path lengths, the light reflected from the structures with different depths will still interfere with the light from reference arm, generating interference signals coded with different beat frequencies. The beat frequency will be higher if the path lengths have a greater mismatch and vice versa. Then the interference signals with different beat frequencies will be dispersed by a spectrometer. After Fourier transformation of the separated interference signals, the optical intensity and depth information within the whole tissue will be determined simultaneously. This method increases the scan speed up to 100 times compared with TD OCT. However, the grating and detecting systems of SD OCT sample signals with higher frequencies in a nonlinear manner, so the higher frequency signals cannot be separated to the same extent as lower-frequency signals can, which restricts the ability of SD OCT to visualize deeper structures. Despite methods such as enhanced depth imaging and image averaging having been combined with SD OCT for better resolution of imaging deeper structures, SD OCT can produce high-resolution images of the structures only at either the proximal or the distal limit of the tissue, but not both at the same time.

Swept-source OCT uses a short cavity-swept laser as light source, which has a narrow bandwidth and is tunable to emitted light with different frequencies. When the tissue is scanned by the laser across a range of frequencies in an orderly and rapid fashion, the spectral interference patterns are generated and then detected by a photodiode in almost real time. With such a process, the interference signals from different depths are coded by time rather than by frequency. Afterward, the spectral interference pattern will be Fourier-transformed to give a depth profile of the sample's reflectance, which is similar to what happens in SD OCT. By using a more complicated light source and simple detection system, SS OCT gains additional advantages over TD OCT, including better sensitivity with imaging depth, higher imaging resolution, longer imaging range, and even shorter imaging acquisition time. All the advantages allow us to see into the eye in a better and deeper way, providing better understanding of the eye diseases we are currently treating.

5.3 Applications of Swept-Source OCT

5.3.1 Glaucoma

Since the first commercially available model, OCT has been adopted for the detection of glaucomatous damage and progression. Now, with SS OCT, more information can be readily obtained.

Glaucoma, a chronic degenerative optic neuropathy, is characterized by progressive loss of retinal ganglion cells and remodeling of the optic nerve head (ONH). Therefore, quantitative assessment of the peripapillary retinal nerve fiber layer (RNFL) and displacement of lamina cribrosa (LC) is of great interest to glaucoma specialists. SD OCT is capable of measuring RNFL thickness around the ONH region with low test-retest variability; however, the wider imaging range provided by SS OCT can cover a larger retinal area to avoid missing subtle RNFL defects, which could be located away from the optic disc margin and even close to the macular region. This capability not only indicates involvement of the macular region in glaucoma development, but it also offers an opportunity to understand the natural history of glaucomatous damage to the RNFL from an early disease stage.

Visualization of the LC is feasible with SS OCT.[5,6] Lopilly Park et al reported that the lamina thickness measured with SS OCT

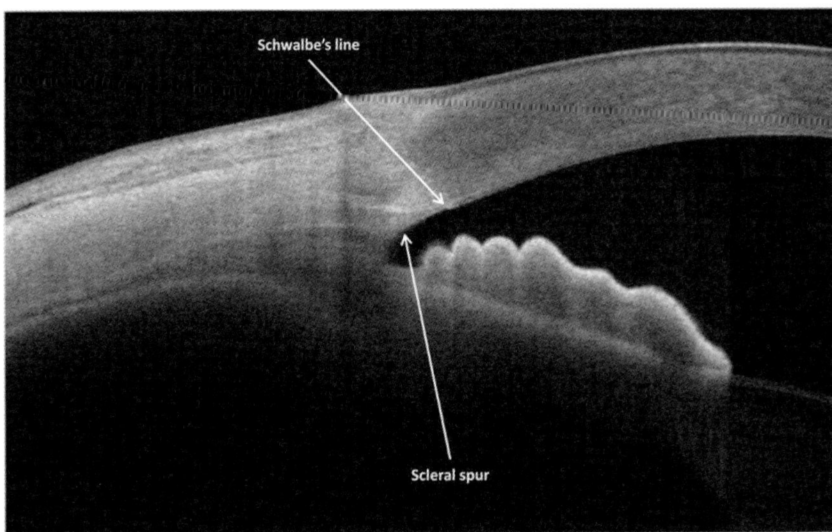

Fig. 5.1 Swept-source optical coherence tomography image of the anterior-chamber angle showing the scleral spur and Schwalbe line.

in primary open-angle glaucoma and normal-tension glaucoma eyes was significantly decreased compared with normal controls.[7] Yoshikawa et al studied the change of displacement of LC using SS OCT in glaucoma patients after surgical reduction of intraocular pressure (IOP) and concluded that changes in LC may correlate with the IOP level and disease severity.[8] In contrast to SD OCT, SS OCT permits simultaneous imaging of the retina, choroid, and LC with high sensitivity in one scan, so that landmarks, like the Bruch's membrane opening, and delineation of lamina will be determined reliably to generate quantitative data over time for further understanding of the process of ONH remodeling and its significance in glaucoma progression.

In addition, SS OCT has been used to image the choroid and sclera to study their roles in glaucoma. Usui et al measured choroidal thickness in highly myopic eyes with and without normal tension glaucoma using SS OCT and reported that choroidal thickness was significantly thinner in highly myopic eyes with normal-tension glaucoma compared with age- and refractive error–matched controls.[9] After measuring the subfoveal sclera using an SS OCT system, Lopilly Park et al found that subfoveal scleral thickness in normal-tension glaucoma eyes was thinner than in primary open-angle glaucoma eyes.[7]

Application of SS OCT in glaucoma is not limited to the posterior part of the eye. Anterior-segment imaging has also been improved by enabling three-dimensional imaging and increasing sampling density. Identification of scleral spur is crucial for quantification of angle status (▶ Fig. 5.1). A study by McKee et al assessed the visibility of scleral spur in SS OCT images of the anterior-chamber angle. Using high-density raster scan (64 A-scan/mm), visibility ranged from 95 to 100% for the superior, inferior, nasal, and temporal quadrants.[10] Although currently the scleral spur needs to be determined manually, measurement reproducibility was found to be high by Liu et al.[11] Compared with gonioscopy, SS OCT provides the feasibility to examine the angle in different lighting conditions and the possibility of quantification of the extent of angle closure. Additionally, the contribution of the iris to angle closure has been studied using SS OCT. Mak et al measured the iris and anterior chamber volume in open-angle and angle-closure eyes before and after dilation and found that the iris volume decreased after pupil dilation and the degree of reduction was less in eyes with a smaller anterior-chamber volume.[12] Therefore, both iris volume and anterior chamber volume contribute to angle closure. Lai et al also used SS OCT to visualize and measure the area and degree of peripheral anterior synechia.[13]The authors concluded from the low measurement variability that SS OCT would be useful to detect peripheral anterior synechia progression in relation to IOP increase and glaucoma progression (▶ Fig. 5.2).

5.3.2 Swept-Source OCT in the Cornea

Along with the development of refractive surgery, precise and detailed assessment of the cornea is becoming increasingly important as one of the determinants of surgical outcome. Studies have shown the applicability of SS OCT in morphologic, biometric, and topographic assessments of the cornea. Fukuda et al used an SS OCT device to measure the central corneal thickness (CCT) and corneal volume within a diameter of 10 mm at the center.[14] Comparisons were made with various devices, including ultrasonic pachymetry, Scheimpflug camera, and specular microscopy, and they reported that the CCT measured by SS OCT was comparable with those measured with the Scheimpflug camera and specular microscopy but thinner than ultrasonic CCT measurement. The corneal volume measurements agreed between those from SS OCT and the Scheimpflug camera. Karnowski et al presented corneal topographic analysis based on SS OCT in patients with keratoconus, postinfectious scar, and penetrating keratoplasty.[15] The quantitative corneal topographic analysis by SS OCT agreed well with other widely used commercial devices, but SS OCT took a shorter time for the topographic measurement and provided better tomographic images of the cornea, which were of value for morphologic evaluation of the cornea. The SS OCT corneal biometric and topographic measurements have also been assessed. Intrarater and interrater variability of the CCT, anterior chamber depth, and anterior chamber width measurements using SS OCT have been studied by Fukuda et al.[16] Both repeatability and reproducibility of all the measurements were found to be high. Neri et al also reported the excellent repeatability of CCT

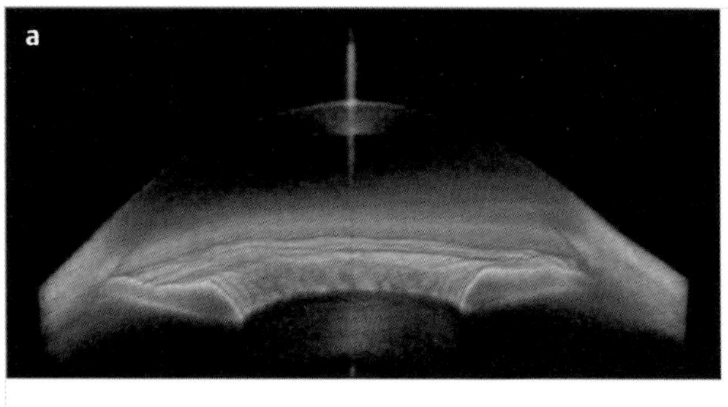

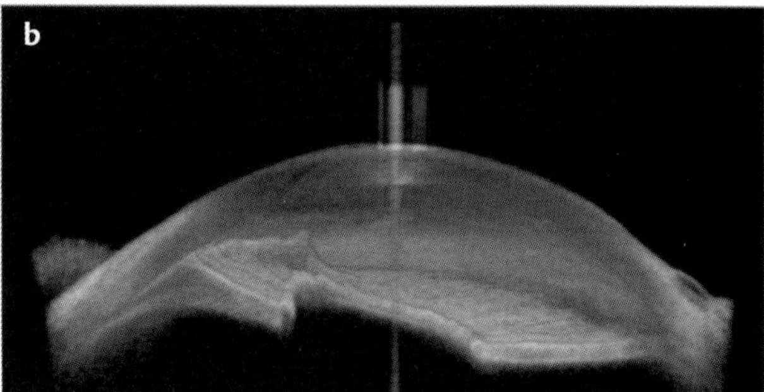

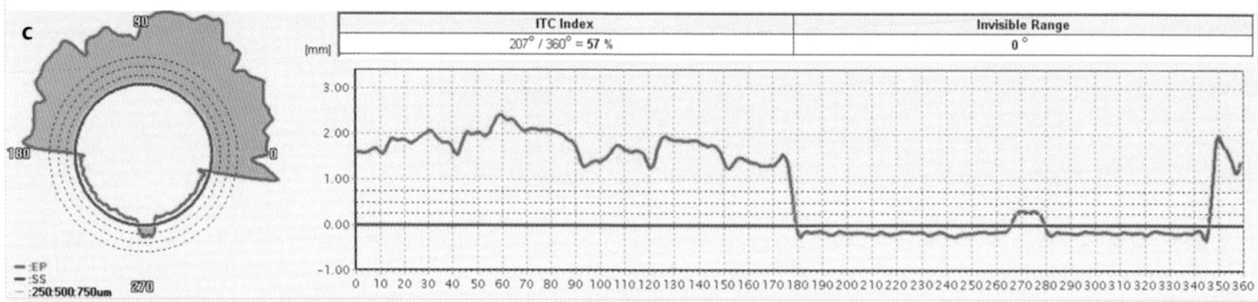

Fig. 5.2 **(a)** Three-dimensional reconstruction of the swept-source optical coherence tomography (SS OCT) images provides the gonioscopic view of the anterior chamber of a normal eye and **(b)** an eye with peripheral anterior synechia. **(c)** By identification of the location of scleral spur (red line) and anterior tip of the irido-angle adhesion (green line) in each SS OCT image, quantification of the extent of peripheral anterior synechia is enabled as the iris-trabecular contact (ITC) index.

measurement obtained by SS OCT.[17] Jhanji et al compared corneal thickness and corneal elevation measurements using SS OCT and slit-scanning topography in both normal and keratoconic eyes and reported that corneal thickness and elevation measurements were significantly different between SS OCT and slit-scanning topography.[18] With lower measurement variability, OCT may provide a reliable alternative for measurement of corneal parameters. Nakagawa et al also studied the corneal topographic analysis in patients with keratoconus using SS OCT[19] and found that SS OCT, compared with the Scheimpflug camera, performed better for imaging the opacified cornea and had a higher success rate of correctly delineating the corneal surfaces in keratoconic eyes.

The precise corneal measurement also extends the use of SS OCT in laser-assisted in-situ keratomileusis (LASIK) to assess the corneal structures created during the procedure, such as LASIK flap and stromal bed, to ensure a safe and satisfactory surgical outcome (▶ Fig. 5.3). From our unpublished data, stromal bed thickness measured intraoperatively using an SS OCT instrument was highly repeatable, and agreement was excellent with the readings acquired with another SD OCT device; however, we also found that OCT tends to underestimate the stromal bed thickness, taking ultrasonic pachymetry as the gold standard, which may be due to the different imaging and segmentation methods used by the two instruments. It is important to understand that the SS OCT corneal measurement could not be used interchangeably with those taken by other technologies. Because the safety requirements on minimal corneal thickness and residual stromal thickness of the LASIK procedure were determined using measurements obtained by ultrasonic pachymetry, caution should be exercised when using SS OCT for perioperative assessment of the cornea. With its advantages over conventional devices, SS OCT will be eventually accepted as an alternative for cornea evaluation to accommodate the increasing demand for precision.

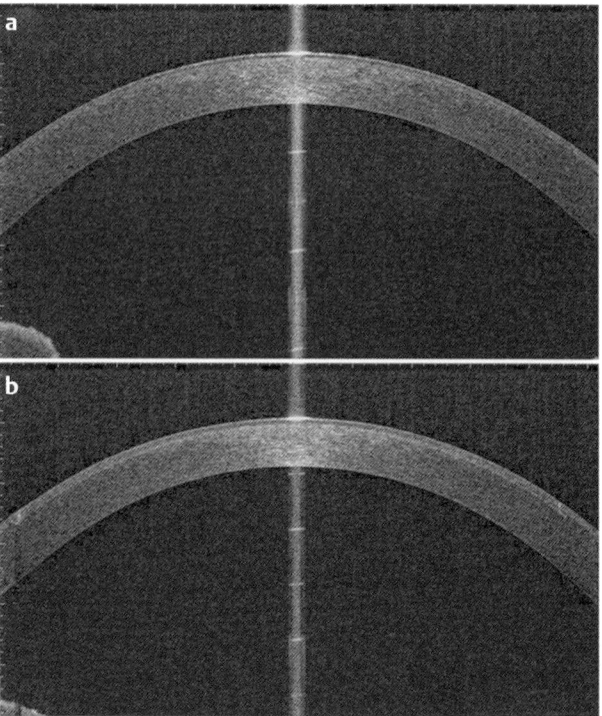

Fig. 5.3 **(a)** Swept-source optical coherence tomography images of the cornea before and **(b)** 1 month after laser-assisted in-situ keratomileusis (LASIK) for perioperative assessment.

5.3.3 Posterior Segment

The deep penetration capability of SS OCT makes it a promising method in visualizing the ophthalmic structures in the posterior part of the eye. Ferrara et al evaluated the use of SS OCT in chronic central serous chorioretinopathy.[20] SS OCT was able to reveal pathological changes in the retinal pigment epithelium and choroid that could not be shown by SD OCT. The en face SS OCT image provided additional information on the choroidal vasculature with different depths without the use of angiography. The curvature and thickness of sclera in highly myopic eyes were evaluated by Ohno-Matsui et al using SS OCT.[21] Whereas the sclera was thinner in highly myopic eyes, the irregular scleral curvature was associated with higher frequency of myopia-related retinochoroidal lesions. The same group also investigated vasculature within and posterior to the sclera in pathological myopia.[22] With identification of intrascleral and retrobulbar blood vessels in the macular area, quantitative analysis of the entry, distribution pattern, and displacement of the blood vessels could be established. Longitudinal studies will determine the relationship between alterations of the intrascleral and retrobulbar blood vessels and the development of complications of pathological myopia. Ohno-Matsui et al found that the retrobulbar subarachnoid space around optic nerve could be visualized in more than 90% patients with a high degree of myopia.[23] The optic subarachnoid space appeared to be expanded, which may contribute at least partially to staphyloma formation and development of glaucoma. With the ability to visualize the "invisibles" of the past, SS OCT has shown its tremendous potential for providing insights on variable ocular diseases of the posterior segment.

5.3.4 Future Directions

With further maturation of SS OCT technology and in combination with other imaging methods and postimaging processing algorithms, applications for SS OCT in ophthalmology will be greatly enhanced. Real-time SS OCT imaging has been demonstrated by Alonso-Caneiro et al to reveal the dynamic change in the cornea after deformation by an air puff.[24] The SS OCT imaging in video rate will play an important role in assisting surgical procedures intraoperatively for a better delineation of tissue margins and also in understanding the biomechanics of the eyeball. Fujimoto's group has integrated the ability of detecting Doppler shift[25] and polarizing property[26] into the SS OCT system. Doppler SS OCT can measure the total retinal blood flow, and polarization-sensitive SS OCT is able to analyze tissue integrity based on birefringence and provides additional information for structure segmentation. Another impactful method, adaptive-optics OCT, improves the imaging resolution to nearly cellular resolution by correcting the high-order aberration of the eye. Zawadzki et al has presented images captured with adaptive-optics OCT showing the inner and outer segments of an individual cone photoreceptor.[27] In summary, the emerging SS OCT technology will continue to offer new approaches to expand significantly our knowledge of various eye diseases. Understanding of the technology, including the principles, advantages, and disadvantages, will facilitate optimal applications of these methods.

References

[1] Huang D, Swanson EA, Lin CP, et al. Optical coherence tomography. Science 1991; 254: 1178–1181

[2] Wojtkowski M, Leitgeb R, Kowalczyk A, Bajraszewski T, Fercher AF. In vivo human retinal imaging by Fourier domain optical coherence tomography. J Biomed Opt 2002; 7: 457–463

[3] Nassif N, Cense B, Park BH, et al. In vivo human retinal imaging by ultrahigh-speed spectral domain optical coherence tomography. Opt Lett 2004; 29: 480–482

[4] Wojtkowski M, Srinivasan V, Fujimoto JG, et al. Three-dimensional retinal imaging with high-speed ultrahigh-resolution optical coherence tomography. Ophthalmology 2005; 112: 1734–1746

[5] Srinivasan VJ, Adler DC, Chen Y, et al. Ultrahigh-speed optical coherence tomography for three-dimensional and en face imaging of the retina and optic nerve head. Invest Ophthalmol Vis Sci 2008; 49: 5103–5110

[6] Takayama K, Hangai M, Kimura Y, et al. Three-dimensional imaging of lamina cribrosa defects in glaucoma using swept-source optical coherence tomography. Invest Ophthalmol Vis Sci 2013; 54: 4798–4807

[7] Lopilly Park HY, Lee NY, Choi JA, Park CK. Measurement of scleral thickness using swept-source optical coherence tomography in patients with open-angle glaucoma and myopia. Am J Ophthalmol 2014; 157: 876–884

[8] Yoshikawa M, Akagi T, Hangai M, et al. Alterations in the neural and connective tissue components of glaucomatous cupping after glaucoma surgery using swept-source optical coherence tomography. Invest Ophthalmol Vis Sci 2014; 55: 477–484

[9] Usui S, Ikuno Y, Miki A, Matsushita K, Yasuno Y, Nishida K. Evaluation of the choroidal thickness using high-penetration optical coherence tomography with long wavelength in highly myopic normal-tension glaucoma. Am J Ophthalmol 2012; 153: 10–16

[10] McKee H, Ye C, Yu M, Liu S, Lam DS, Leung CK. Anterior chamber angle imaging with swept-source optical coherence tomography: detecting the scleral spur, Schwalbe's line, and Schlemm's canal. J Glaucoma 2013; 22: 468–472

[11] Liu S, Yu M, Ye C, Lam DS, Leung CK. Anterior chamber angle imaging with swept-source optical coherence tomography: an investigation on variability of angle measurement. Invest Ophthalmol Vis Sci 2011; 52: 8598–8603

[12] Mak H, Xu G, Leung CK. Imaging the iris with swept-source optical coherence tomography: relationship between iris volume and primary angle closure. Ophthalmology 2013; 120: 2517–2524

[13] Lai I, Mak H, Lai G, Yu M, Lam DS, Leung CK. Anterior chamber angle imaging with swept-source optical coherence tomography: measuring peripheral anterior synechia in glaucoma. Ophthalmology 2013; 120: 1144–1149

[14] Fukuda R, Usui T, Miyai T, Mori Y, Miyata K, Amano S. Corneal thickness and volume measurements by swept source anterior segment optical coherence tomography in normal subjects. Curr Eye Res 2013; 38: 531–536

[15] Karnowski K, Kaluzny BJ, Szkulmowski M, Gora M, Wojtkowski M. Corneal topography with high-speed swept source OCT in clinical examination. Biomed Opt Express 2011; 2: 2709–2720

[16] Fukuda S, Kawana K, Yasuno Y, Oshika T. Repeatability and reproducibility of anterior ocular biometric measurements with 2-dimensional and 3-dimensional optical coherence tomography. J Cataract Refract Surg 2010; 36: 1867–1873

[17] Neri A, Malori M, Scaroni P, Leaci R, Delfini E, Macaluso C. Corneal thickness mapping by 3D swept-source anterior segment optical coherence tomography. Acta Ophthalmol (Copenh) 2012; 90: e452–e457

[18] Jhanji V, Yang B, Yu M, Ye C, Leung CK. Corneal thickness and elevation measurements using swept-source optical coherence tomography and slit scanning topography in normal and keratoconic eyes. Clin Experiment Ophthalmol 2013; 41: 735–745

[19] Nakagawa T, Maeda N, Higashiura R, Hori Y, Inoue T, Nishida K. Corneal topographic analysis in patients with keratoconus using 3-dimensional anterior segment optical coherence tomography. J Cataract Refract Surg 2011; 37: 1871–1878

[20] Ferrara D, Mohler KJ, Waheed N, et al. En face enhanced-depth swept-source optical coherence tomography features of chronic central serous chorioretinopathy. Ophthalmology 2014; 121: 719–726

[21] Ohno-Matsui K, Akiba M, Modegi T, et al. Association between shape of sclera and myopic retinochoroidal lesions in patients with pathologic myopia. Invest Ophthalmol Vis Sci 2012; 53: 6046–6061

[22] Ohno-Matsui K, Akiba M, Ishibashi T, Moriyama M. Observations of vascular structures within and posterior to sclera in eyes with pathologic myopia by

swept-source optical coherence tomography. Invest Ophthalmol Vis Sci 2012; 53: 7290–7298

[23] Ohno-Matsui K, Akiba M, Moriyama M, Ishibashi T, Tokoro T, Spaide RF. Imaging retrobulbar subarachnoid space around optic nerve by swept-source optical coherence tomography in eyes with pathologic myopia. Invest Ophthalmol Vis Sci 2011; 52: 9644–9650

[24] Alonso-Caneiro D, Karnowski K, Kaluzny BJ, Kowalczyk A, Wojtkowski M. Assessment of corneal dynamics with high-speed swept source optical coherence tomography combined with an air puff system. Opt Express 2011; 19: 14188–14199

[25] Baumann B, Potsaid B, Kraus MF, et al. Total retinal blood flow measurement with ultrahigh speed swept source/Fourier domain OCT. Biomed Opt Express 2011: 1539–1552

[26] Baumann B, Choi W, Potsaid B, Huang D, Duker JS, Fujimoto JG. Swept source/ Fourier domain polarization sensitive optical coherence tomography with a passive polarization delay unit. Opt Express 2012; 20: 10229–10241

[27] Zawadzki RJ, Cense B, Zhang Y, Choi SS, Miller DT, Werner JS. Ultrahigh-resolution optical coherence tomography with monochromatic and chromatic aberration correction. Opt Express 2008; 16: 8126–8143

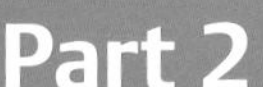

Part 2

Anterior-Segment Optical Coherence Tomography

6 Visante Anterior-Segment Optical Coherence Tomography in Evaluation of Patients for Refractive Surgery

Amin Ashrafzadeh and Roger F. Steinert

Optical coherence tomography (OCT) is a technique that uses light to create a two-dimensional cross-section image of the eye.[1] This technique allows imaging of either the anterior segment or the posterior segment of the eye. Decision making for refractive surgery is aided by evaluations in either the preoperative or postoperative stages. The main focus of this chapter is to discuss the Visante anterior-segment OCT, its properties, capabilities, and functions in evaluation of patients being considered for excimer laser treatment and phakic intraocular lens (IOL) implantation. Although one of the most common refractive surgery procedures is cataract extraction, that topic is outside the scope of this chapter.

6.1 Visante Anterior-Segment OCT

Optical coherence tomography is a noncontact, real-time technique that uses low-energy infrared laser energy to image structures. The most commonly used retinal OCT uses 820-nm light, which allows excellent tissue penetration to the level of the retina. The Visante anterior-segment OCT (Carl Zeiss Meditec, Dublin, CA) uses 1310-nm light, which has greater absorption, resulting in limited penetration, allowing increased intensity of the light as decreased amounts reach the retina. As such, in the Visante, the light is 20 times more intense, giving a much greater signal-to-noise ratio. This increased intensity allows imaging speed to be increased by 20 while retaining signal-to-noise ratio levels similar to those with retinal OCT but with resultant decreased motion artifact. Additionally, the 1310-nm light has reduced scattering and therefore better penetration through opaque tissue, such as an opaque cornea and sclera, thereby resulting in better evaluation of the anterior segment and visualization of the angle and, to a lesser degree, the ciliary body.

The Visante OCT has two modes: standard-resolution imaging and high-resolution imaging. Standard-resolution imaging provides a broader view of the anterior segment with a 16-mm-width and 6-mm-depth image, providing a full overview of the anterior segment, including the cornea, anterior chamber, iris, and both angles. The high-resolution imaging mode ("high-res mode") provides a more detailed image with dimensions of 10-mm width and 3-mm depth. High-res mode is more appropriate for imaging of the cornea and any segment in need of detailed evaluation.

In the standard-resolution mode, the Visante performs 256 scans assessing the 16 × 6-mm area in 0.125 seconds. In high-res mode, the Visante performs 512 scans to assess the 10 × 3-mm area in 0.250 seconds. The resolution of the Visante images is limited by the spacing between the scans performed. The resolution of the Visante reaches 18 µm axially and 60 µm transversally.

In addition to a single scan, the operator has the option of selecting automatic dual or quad scans. The dual-scan mode performs two scans, one at a selected orientation between 20 and 200 degrees, the second scan between 160 and 340 degrees. The quad-scan mode performs four scans between axes of 0 to 180, 45 to 225, 90 to 270, and 135 to 315 degrees. All scans in all modes can be rotated manually to any of the 180 axis lines at the discretion of the operator performing the imaging.

The corneal pachymetry mapping ("pachy map") module in the standard software performs eight modified high-resolution scans of the cornea in preset radial axis lines starting at 0-degree axis and rising at 22.5-degree intervals. The high-res mode allows for the pachy map to be performed in 0.5 seconds with little artifactual distortion. It produces a 10 × 10-mm pachymetry map of the cornea, revealing the corneal thickness in all locations. The preset grid separates the cornea into the central 0- to 2-mm area along with eight radial regions at 2 to 5 mm, 5 to 7 mm, and 7 to 10 mm concentric to the central region. All areas produce three numbers: the thinnest area, noted as the top number; the average, noted as the middle number; and the thickest area, noted as the bottom number. The global pachy map in the Visante 2.0 software performs 16 modified high-resolution scans of the cornea in 1.0 second. The preset radial axis lines start at 0 degrees and rise at 11.25-degree intervals. The global pachy map is able to provide twice as many data points and therefore a more detailed evaluation. The repeatability of the Visante pachy map in the standard mode was noted at 7-µm standard deviation in the center and 14 µm standard deviation in the periphery.

The Visante is also equipped with an optometer capable of changing focus from a + 20 to −35 diopters. As the optometer changes focus, accommodation can be induced; and, as such, dynamic changes of the anterior segment can be quantitatively measured.

In the Visante 2.0 software, there is an additional enhanced mode for anterior-segment mode scan and the high-res mode scan. In the enhanced mode, four consecutive scans are performed and compressed into a single image to produce a higher-density, higher-contrast image. Additionally, new software tools to produce a phakic IOL template and measurement tools for endothelial clearance and lens vault distance, along with more sophisticated angle measurement tools, are among the few enrichments that have been devised.

Visante anterior-segment OCT images can be used in evaluating the refractive patient both preoperatively and postoperatively. It is capable of providing broad overview images of the anterior segment and more detailed high resolutions of specific areas. Pachymetry mapping, angle evaluations, corneal flap evaluations, and phakic IOL templates are some of the useful features that are demonstrated in examples in the remainder of this chapter.

6.2 LASIK Patients

In the evaluation of a patient for LASIK (laser-assisted in-situ keratomileusis) eye surgery, the Visante is able to provide

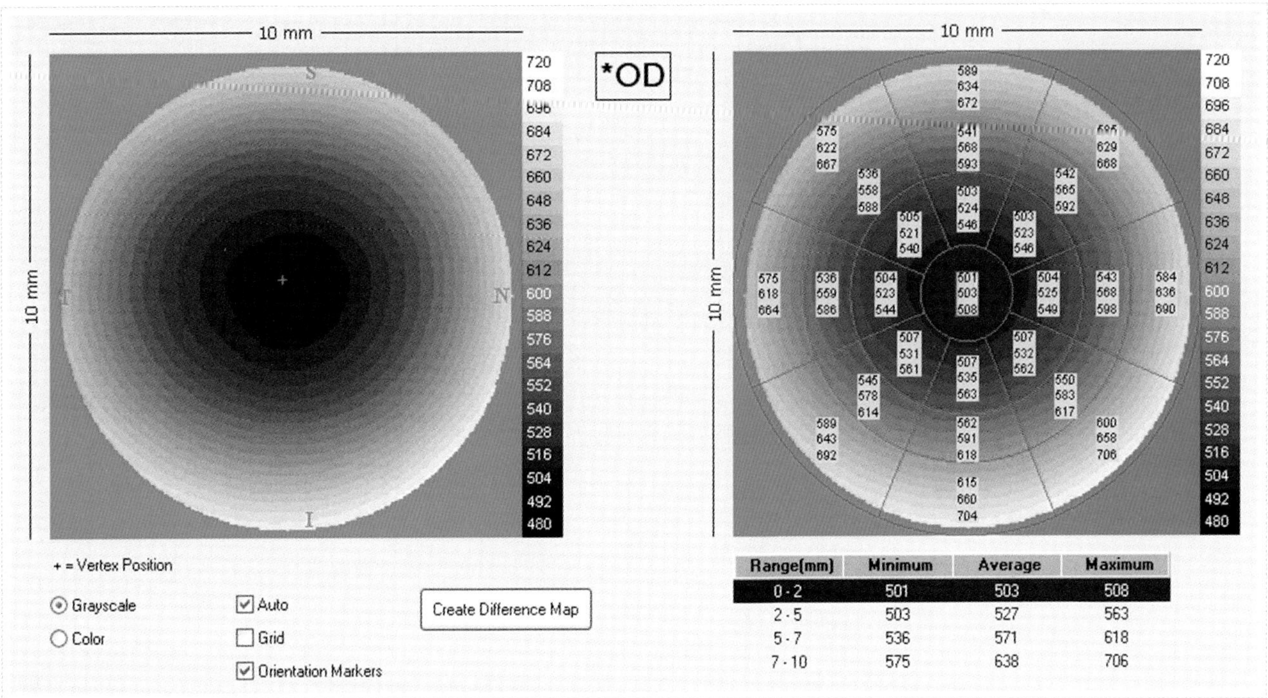

Range(mm)	Minimum	Average	Maximum
0 - 2	501	503	508
2 - 5	503	527	563
5 - 7	536	571	618
7 - 10	575	638	706

Fig. 6.1 Normal pachymetric map of the cornea demonstrating the thinnest area in the center with concentric thickening of the tissue toward the periphery. OD, right eye.

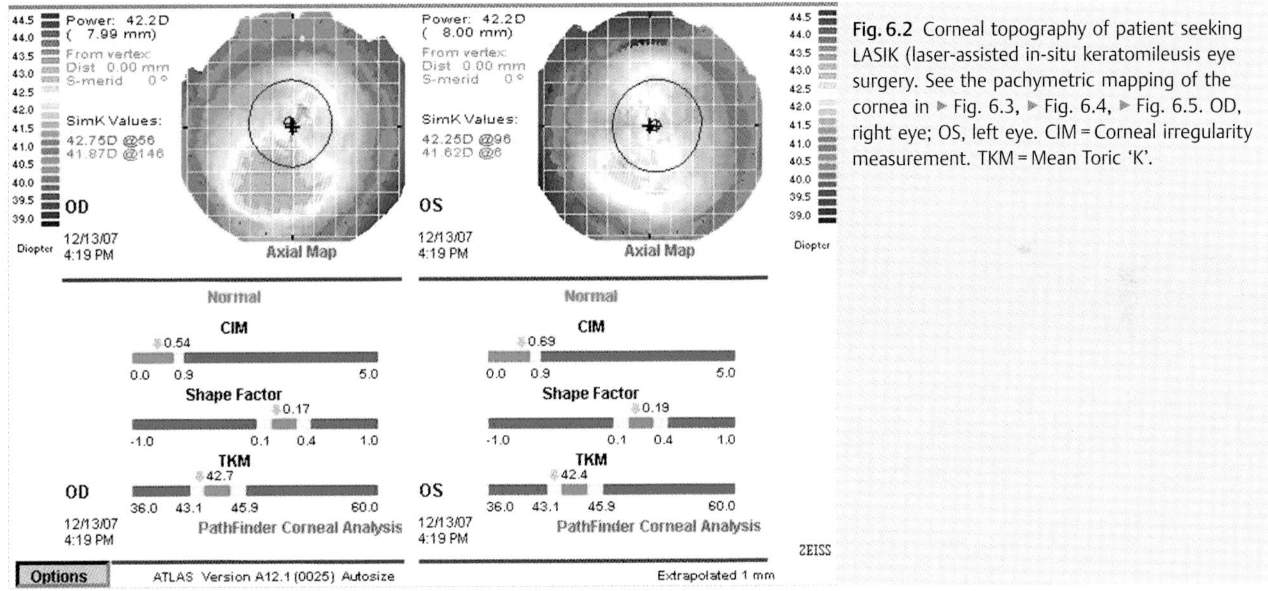

Fig. 6.2 Corneal topography of patient seeking LASIK (laser-assisted in-situ keratomileusis eye surgery. See the pachymetric mapping of the cornea in ▶ Fig. 6.3, ▶ Fig. 6.4, ▶ Fig. 6.5. OD, right eye; OS, left eye. CIM = Corneal irregularity measurement. TKM = Mean Toric 'K'.

preoperative pachymetry mapping of the cornea, evaluation of the angles, and any corneal pathology that is present. In evaluation of post-LASIK surgery patients, detailed anatomical data may be obtained to further guide in clinical decision making.

6.2.1 Pachymetry Mapping

Pachymetry mapping of the cornea, combined with the corneal topographic map, provides a powerful set of information, which may be especially important in cases where possibility of corneal ectasia is raised. A normal pachymetry map of the cornea (▶ Fig. 6.1) has the thinnest portion in the center with concentrically thicker tissue as it approaches the periphery.

A 19-year-old man was being considered for LASIK eye surgery; he had refractions of −1.75–0.25 × 111 in the right eye and −2.00 sphere in the left eye, with best-corrected vision a weak 20/20−. His corneal topographies (▶ Fig. 6.2) were interpreted by the computer software as normal (PathFinder Corneal Analysis Software, Atlas Topographer, Carl Zeiss Meditec, CA). Slight interior steepening of the right eye prompted concerns of possible forme fruste keratoconus. A global pachy map of both eyes (▶ Fig. 6.3, ▶ Fig. 6.4, ▶ Fig. 6.5) revealed an inferotemporal

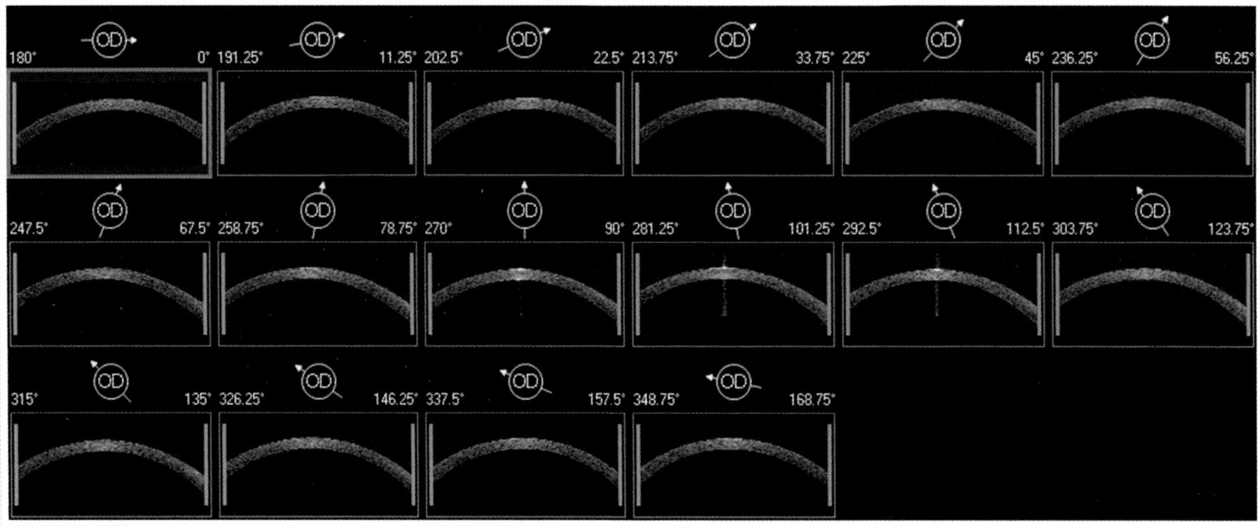

Fig. 6.3 Global pachymetric map is created from 16 modified high-res images as noted in this figure.

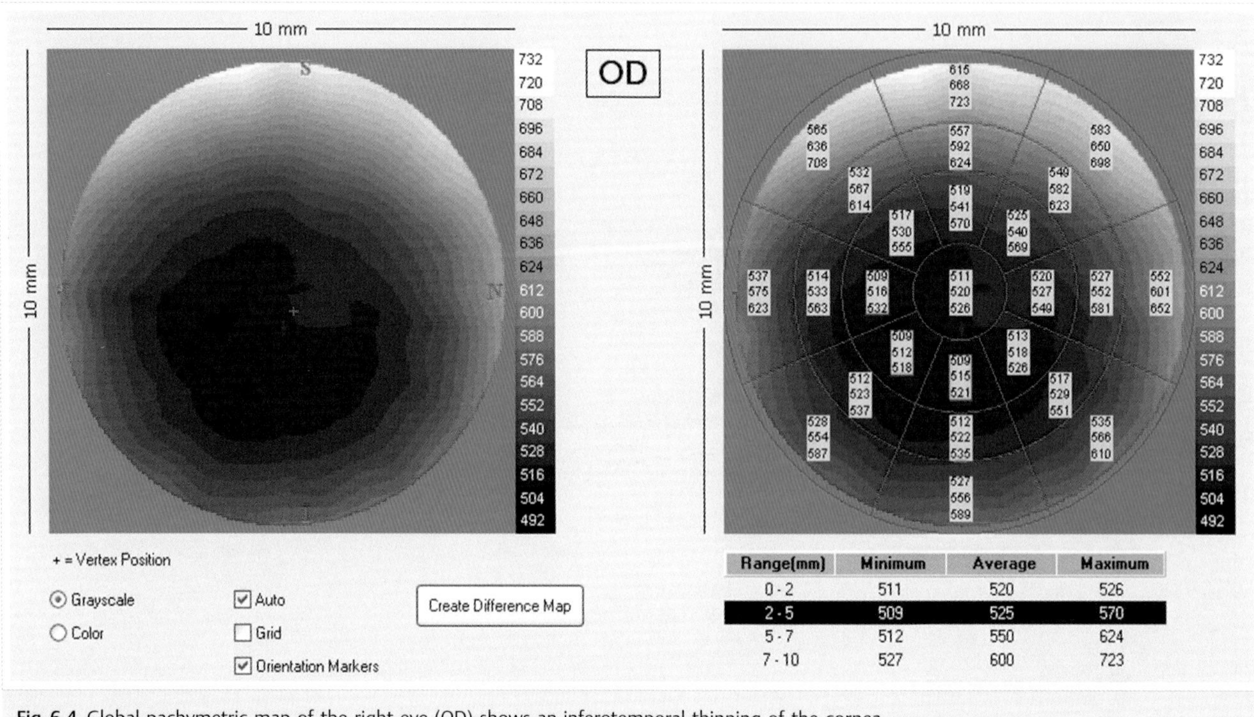

Fig. 6.4 Global pachymetric map of the right eye (OD) shows an inferotemporal thinning of the cornea.

thinning, consistent with bilateral inferotemporal steepening seen on topography. Diagnosis of forme fruste keratoconus was confidently made, and the patient was encouraged to continue with his regular corrective methods and not to consider excimer laser therapy at that time.

To counterbalance the previous example, a 13-year-old adolescent boy with rapidly progressive keratoconus had undergone standard penetrating keratoplasty 11 months earlier in his left eye. In the span of 11 months, the keratometric measurement in his right eye had progressed from a mean of 48 to 58 diopters. His vision had also declined from best-corrected 20/20 to 20/400. In his preoperative evaluation for IntraLase-enabled keratoplasty, the pachy map (▶ Fig. 6.6) revealed a perfectly normal pattern of pachymetric distribution, despite the clearly pathologic cornea. This case demonstrates that one must consider pachymetry mapping only as an augmentation to other information in considering LASIK surgery and that it may appear normal despite such advanced pathology.

6.2.2 Angle Evaluation

In the care of a refractive patient, one must never overlook the ophthalmic care that may be required. A 55-year-old woman with 2.0 diopters of hyperopia planned to undergo LASIK eye

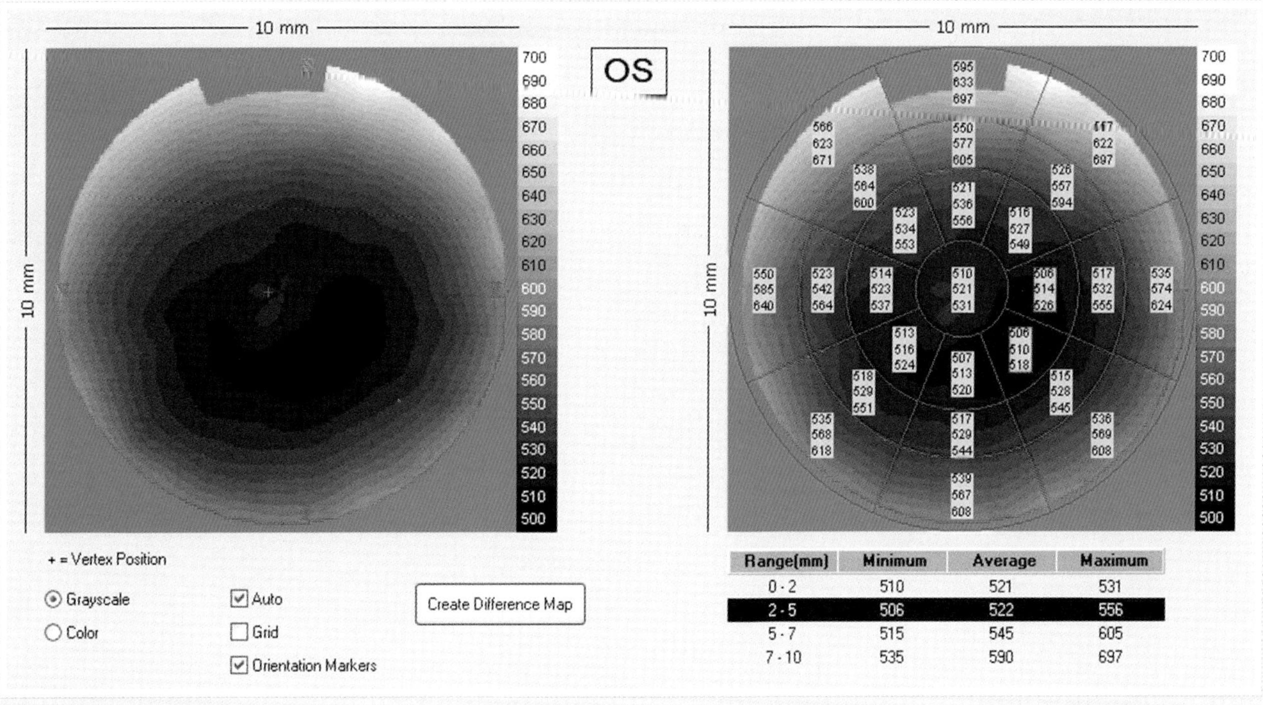

Fig. 6.5 Global pachymetric map of the left eye (OS) showing inferotemporal thinning of the cornea.

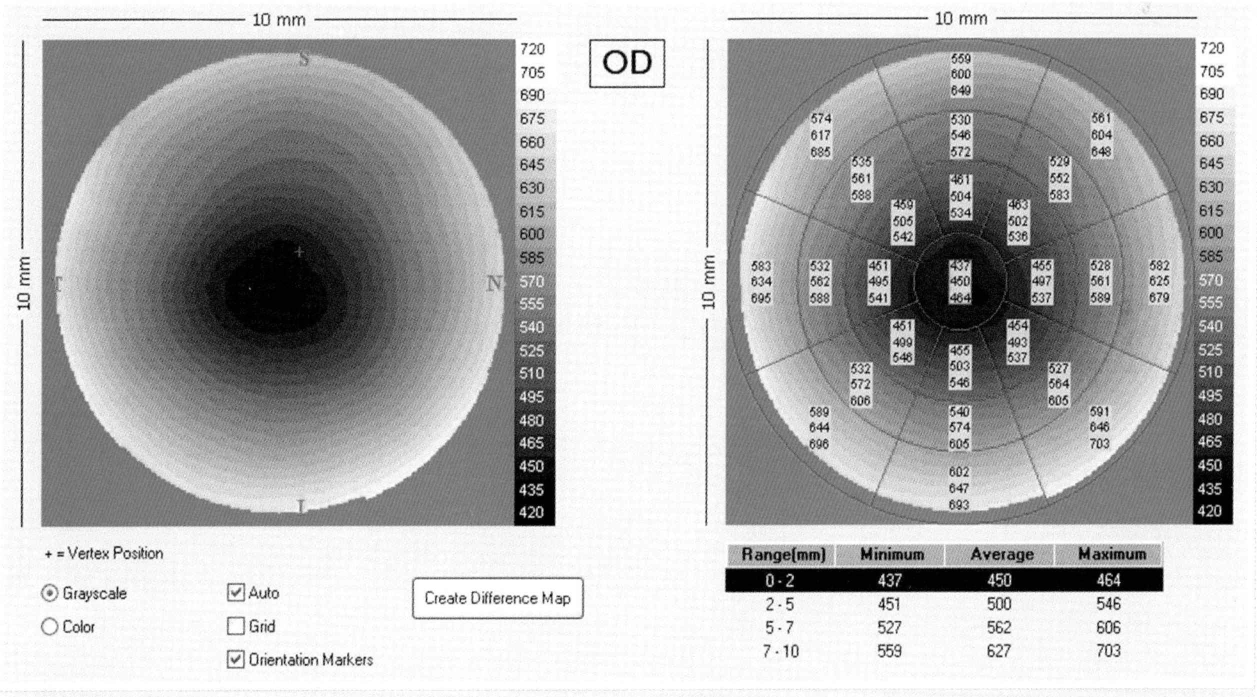

Fig. 6.6 Pre-IntraLase-enabled keratoplasty. Visante pachymetric mapping of patient with advanced keratoconus and central keratometric readings of 58 diopters. OD, right eye.

surgery. Preoperative Visante evaluation (▶ Fig. 6.7) revealed narrow angles of approximately 10 degrees. Moderate anterior bowing of the posterior iris pigmented line was noted. Peripheral iridotomies were performed weeks before her scheduled LASIK eye surgery. After iridotomy (▶ Fig. 6.8), despite the fact that the pupils were larger compared with the preoperative images, the angles were significantly more open at approximately 25 degrees with near complete flattening of the posterior pigmented iris lines. Compared with standard slit-lamp gonioscopic examination of the eye, the angle is identified quantitatively with multiple methods of calculated angle area and distance measurements. Trabecular-iris space area (TISA)

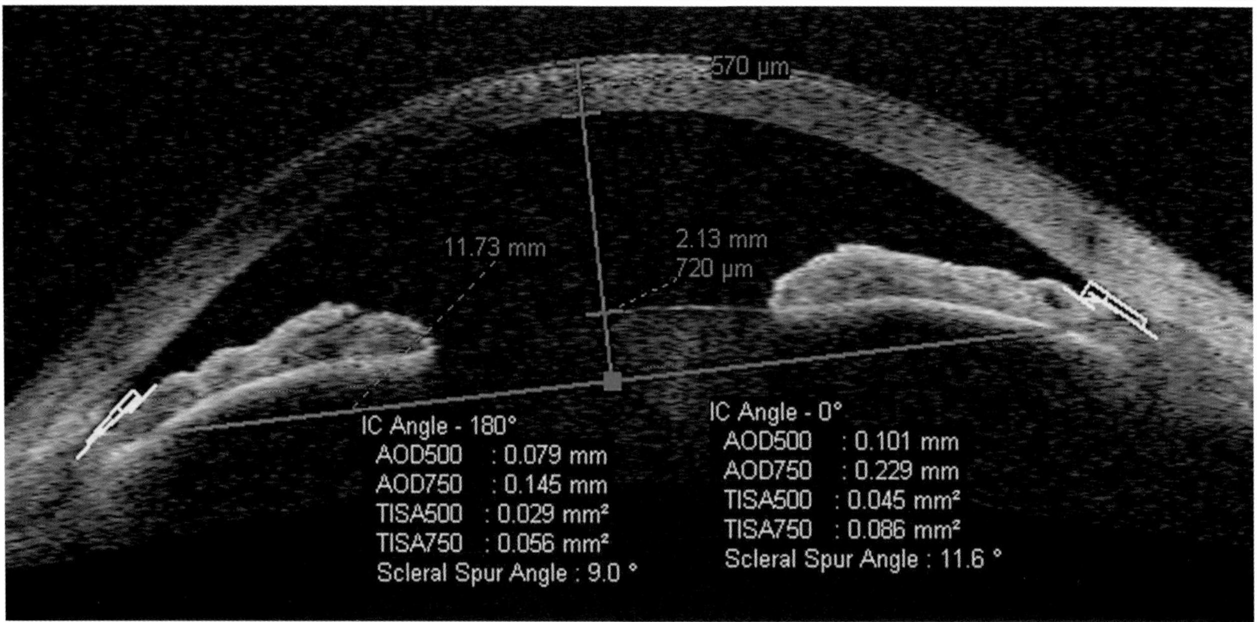

Fig. 6.7 Preoperative evaluation of the anterior segment of a patient with 2 diopters of hyperopia in consideration of LASIK (laser-assisted in situ keratomileusis). IC, iris curvature.

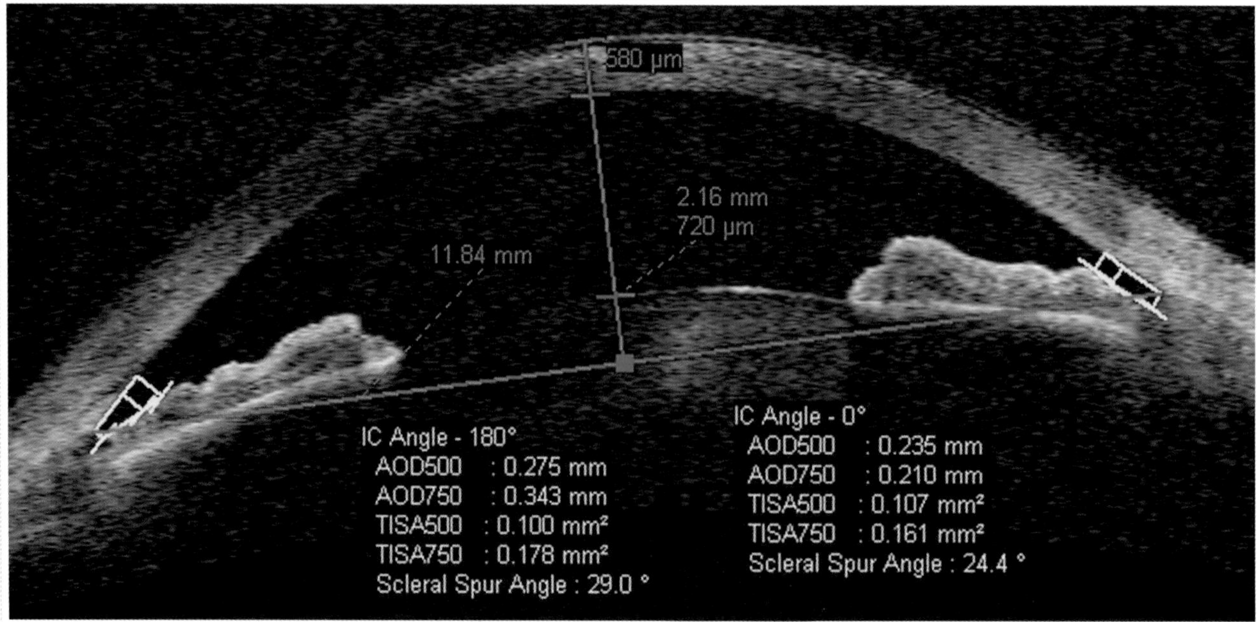

Fig. 6.8 Postiridotomy evaluation of the same patient as ▶ Fig. 6.1 showing greater opening of the angle and flatting of the posterior pigmented iris line. IC, iris curvature.

and angle-opening distance (AOD) are both measured at 500 and 750 µm away from the scleral spur. The AOD is defined as the distance perpendicularly away from the trabecular meshwork/endothelial surface to the surface of the iris. The TISA is a trapezoidal area bordered by the AOD at 500 or 750 µm and a line drawn perpendicularly from the scleral spur to the iris. The ability to acquire and present all this information in real time to a patient represents a major advance in both diagnosis and patient education.

6.2.3 Corneal Pathology

A 44-year-old woman, a contact lens user, had developed a corneal ulcer in her dominant eye 5 years earlier with complete healing and resolution; however, best-corrected visual acuity had been reduced to 20/40. The patient was seeking consultation for LASIK eye surgery. Her cornea had a paracentral scar with concordant flattening on the topographic map (▶ Fig. 6.9). Her preoperative refraction was −4.00–1.50 × 110, leading to

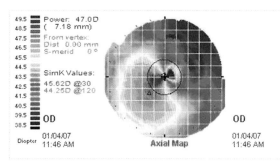

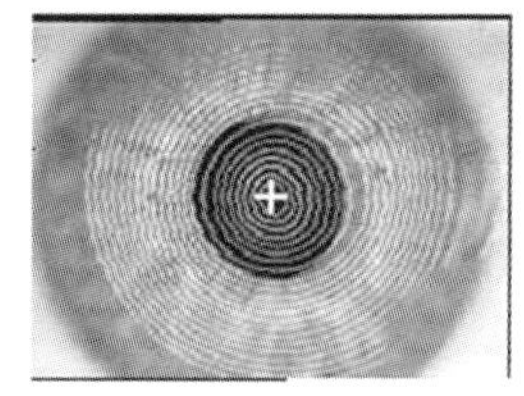

Fig. 6.9 Corneal topography before photoreactive keratectomy showing area of flattening associated with corneal scar at the 2 o'clock paracentral position. OD, right eye.

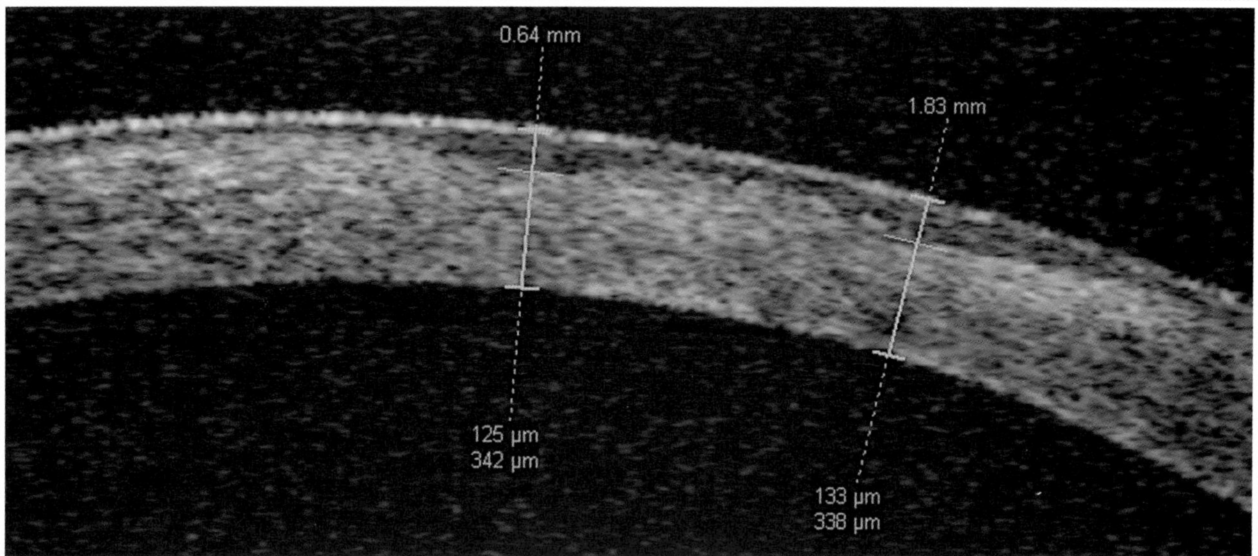

Fig. 6.10 Corneal scar of the same patient as ▶ Fig. 6.9 showing loss of corneal tissue and filling with epithelium.

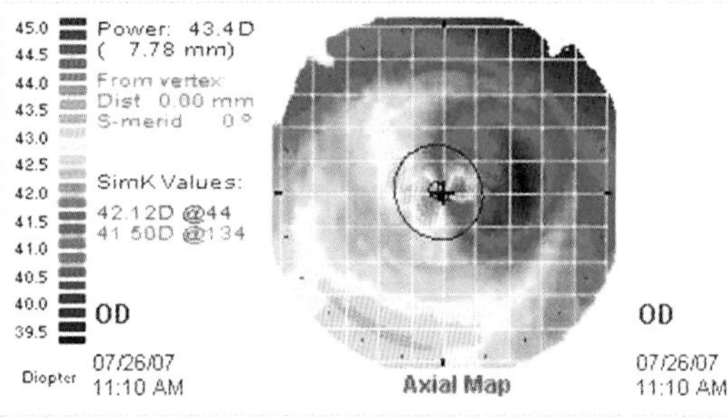

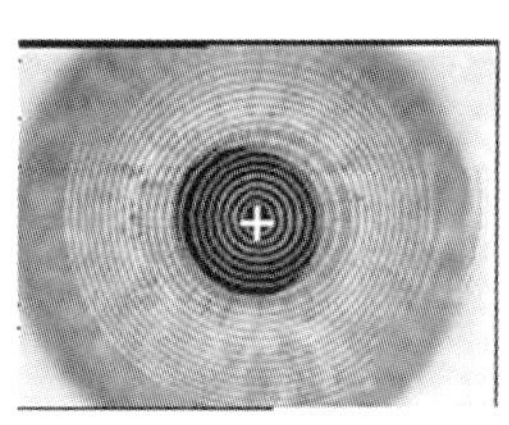

Fig. 6.11 Corneal topography of the same patient as ▶ Fig. 6.9 after photoreactive keratectomy. OD, right eye.

20/40 vision. The Visante was used to measure the depth of tissue loss, epithelial filing, and the corneal scar (▶ Fig. 6.10). A decision was made to correct this eye conservatively using a stepwise approach; such treatment of only −2.25–1.50 × 110 was delivered via photorefractive keratectomy (PRK). Six months after PRK, the patient had 20/25 + uncorrected visual acuity, correctable to 20/20 with plano −0.75 × 135. The corneal topography (▶ Fig. 6.11) had improved mire rings. The corneal scar, although not obliterated by the excimer laser, was reduced in thickness and opacity intensity (▶ Fig. 6.12). Additionally, the epithelial pooling over the depressed scar was noted to be significantly less. It was also noted that the Bowman membrane, seen as a black line under the white epithelium in ▶ Fig. 6.10, was obliterated and nonexistent in ▶ Fig. 6.12 after PRK.

6.2.4 Flap Evaluation

In the evaluation of postoperative LASIK patients who may be considering enhancement, the Visante can provide detailed information that would be essential to the safety of the procedure. The Visante can provide details of corneal flap shape and regularity. The LASIK flaps are created using either a mechanical microkeratome or a femtosecond laser microkeratome. An example of a mechanical microkeratome flap created using the Amadeus II (Ziemer Ophthalmic Group AG, Switzerland) (▶ Fig. 6.13) can be noted to have a tapered edge with a thicker peripheral flap and a thinner central flap. This configuration is referred to as the *meniscus flap*. An example of a femtosecond laser microkeratome flap created using the IntraLase (Advanced

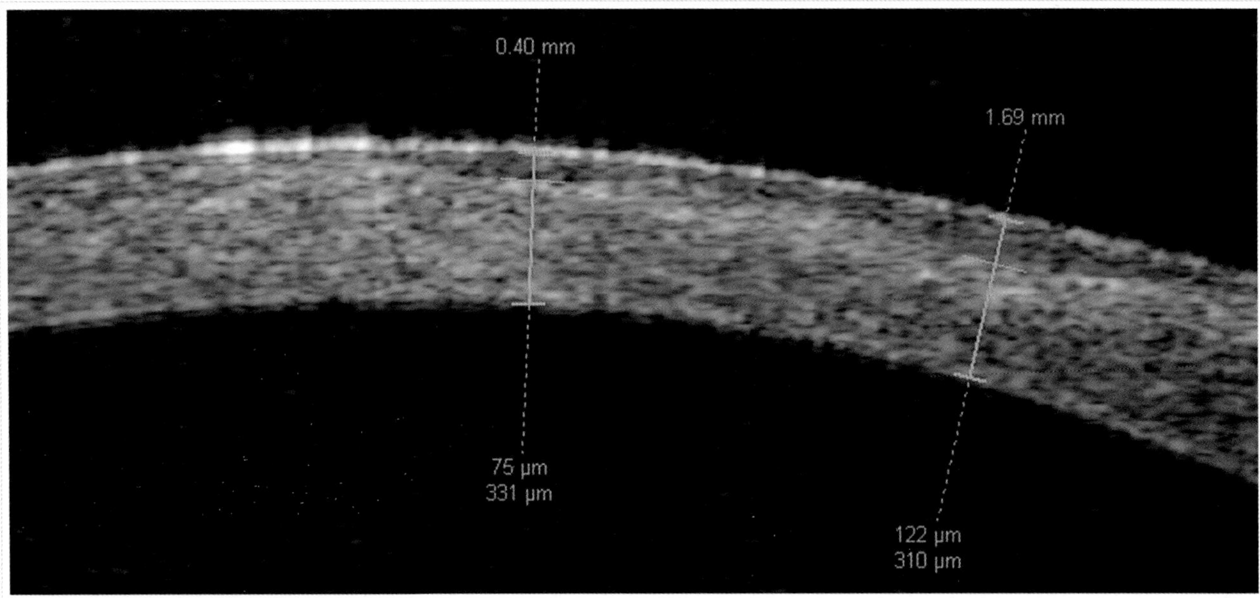

Fig. 6.12 Corneal scar of the same patient as ▶ Fig. 6.9 after photoreactive keratectomy.

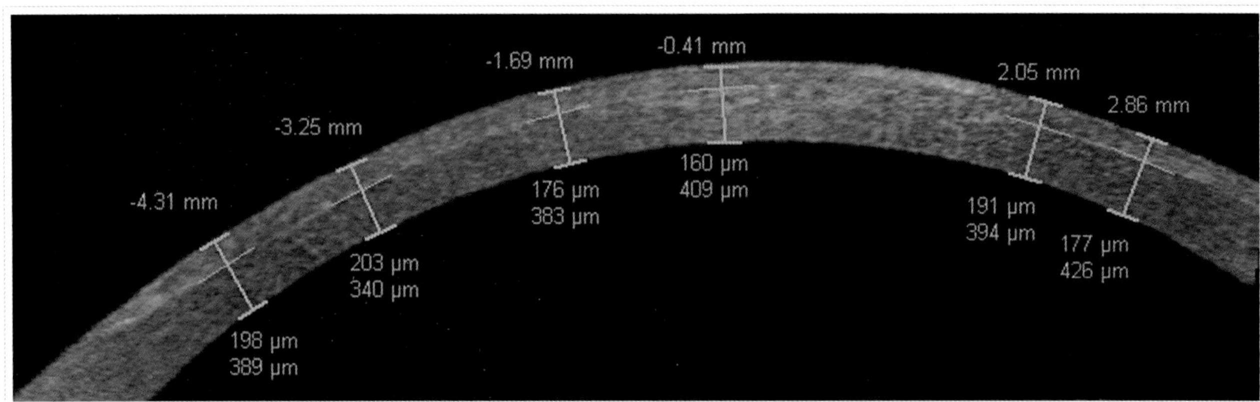

Fig. 6.13 Amadeus II microkeratome created flap showing the tapered flap edge and meniscus flap configuration.

Medical Optics, Inc., Santa Ana, CA) shows a sharp 70-degree flap edge and an evenly thick flap throughout (▶ Fig. 6.14). This flap configuration is referred to as the *linear flap*.

A 35-year-old man had undergone LASIK eye surgery 5 years previously elsewhere, and no records were available. A LASIK flap with jagged edge was noted peripherally. The Visante was able to demonstrate the presence of a very thin LASIK flap (▶ Fig. 6.15). A decision was made to perform a surface ablation rather than try to lift the previous LASIK flap. The patient obtained 20/15 vision postoperatively.

A 35-year-old woman with a refraction of −8.00–2.75 × 020 with central corneal thickness of 515 µm had CustomVue IntraLase LASIK eye surgery with iris registration (iLASIK) (Advanced Medical Optics, Inc., Santa Ana, CA). As shown in ▶ Fig. 6.16, the central residual stromal bed remaining after the initial iLASIK was in the range of only 280 µm. Postoperative refraction stable over 6 months is −0.25–1.75 × 010. Many opinions and options regarding the safety of LASIK and its enhancements might have been possible in this patient because residual microns were left, but the data provided allowed the individual patient and surgeon to discuss the plan and practice the art of medicine in this case. In this LASIK case, one notes the 70-degree flap edge on the left side of the image and the linear flap thickness created by the IntraLase femtosecond laser. Although the range of the flap thickness is measured from 107 to 118 µm, one must also note the limitation in the gradation of the flap tool in the Visante software that may be stepwise and in accordance with the resolution limits of the hardware. Specifically, the axial resolution of the Visante is 18 µm and has a repeatability of ± 7 µm in measurement of the flap and ± 11 µm in the measurement of the stromal tissue. It should also be noted that flap visibility is diminished over time. The sensitivity at 1 day is 99% and 95% at 6 months.

6.2.5 Complication Evaluation

A 38-year-old man had undergone LASIK eye surgery 8 years previously elsewhere, with no records available, and he planned

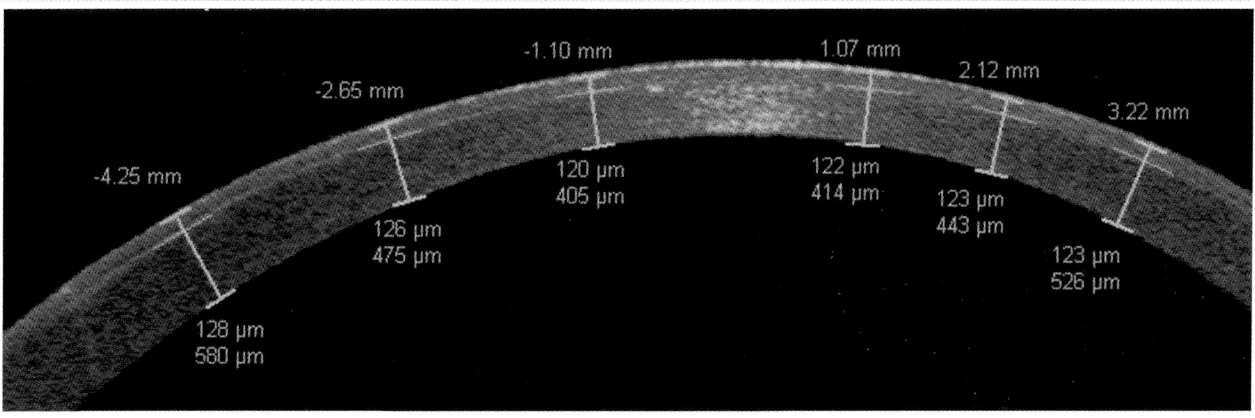

Fig. 6.14 IntraLase-created LASIK (laser-assisted in situ keratomileusis) flap with vertical edge and linear flap configuration.

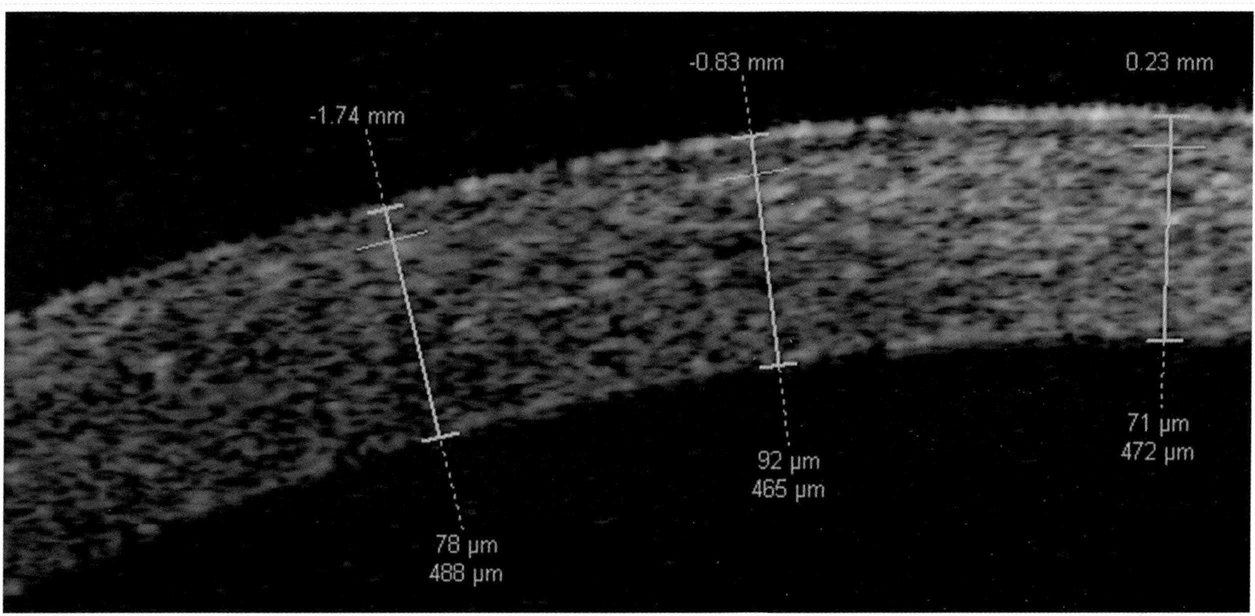

Fig. 6.15 Patient asking for enhancement 5 years after initial LASIK (laser-assisted in-situ keratomileusis) surgery.

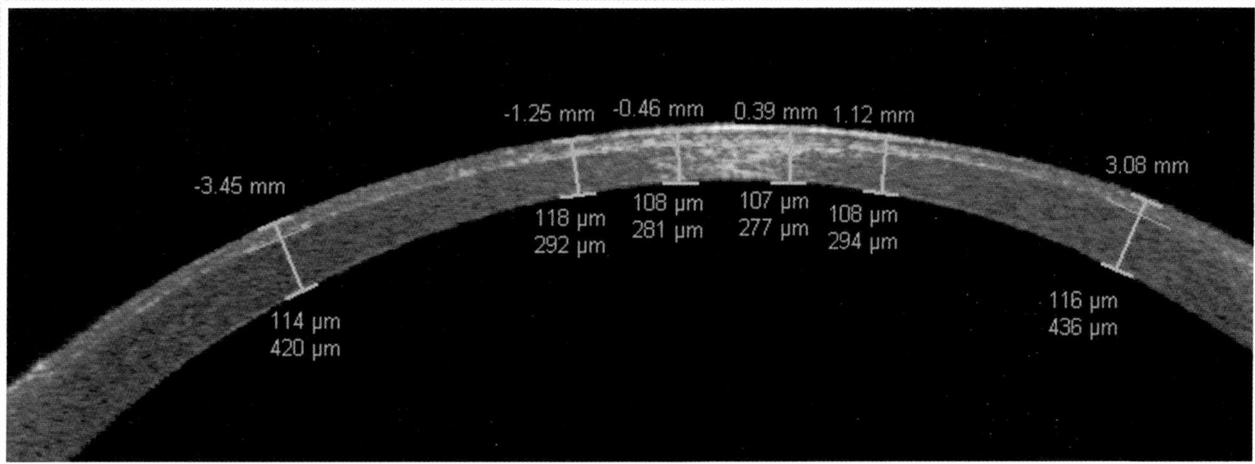

Fig. 6.16 Highly myopic patient after iLASIK (laser-assisted in-situ keratomileusis with iris registration) in need of minor enhancement.

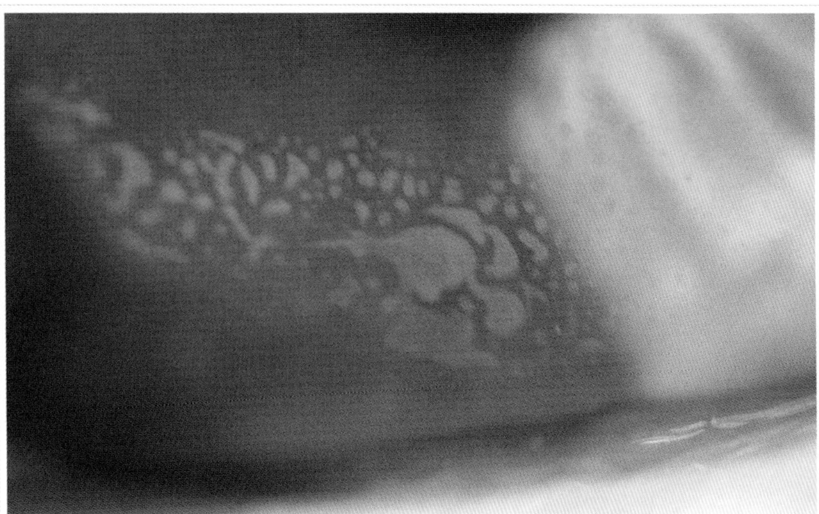

Fig. 6.17 Epithelial ingrowth after LASIK (laser-assisted in-situ keratomileusis) enhancement.

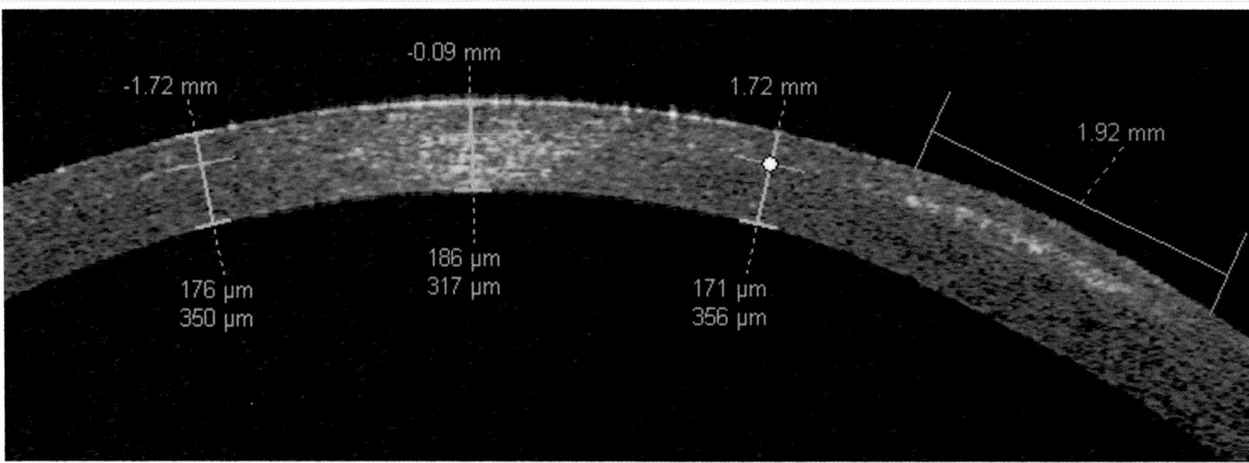

Fig. 6.18 Visante (standard high-resolution mode) 2 months after LASIK (laser-assisted in-situ keratomileusis) enhancement.

to have LASIK enhancement. The Visante was able to demonstrate clearly the flap and residual stromal bed thickness. The patient was assured that LASIK enhancement via lifting of the flap could be performed. The patient, however, developed epithelial ingrowth postenhancement. The patient, with uncorrected 20/15 vision after the enhancement, chose not to have any intervention. The Visante is able to identify the leading edge of the epithelial ingrowth and allow precise monitoring overtime. The clinical appearance of the epithelial ingrowth at 2 months can be noted in ▶ Fig. 6.17. The Visante image (▶ Fig. 6.18), in regular high-res mode in a rainbow color scheme, performed 2 months after the LASIK enhancement, demonstrated the leading edge of the epithelial ingrowth from the flap edge. At follow-up 6 months later (8 months postoperatively), the clinical appearance was unchanged. The Visante image (▶ Fig. 6.19), however, was acquired in the enhanced high-res mode. In this enhanced format, four high-resolution images are composited together to provide an enhanced view with reduced graininess and increased contrast within the image. Please note that the epithelial ingrowth on the Visante has remained identical.

A 63-year-old man, 1 year post-LASIK, acquired a pet kitten. The kitten, with her sharp, narrow claws, punctured the LASIK flap and seeded the interstromal space with a small infiltrate, forming an ulcer (▶ Fig. 6.20), which was treated conservatively with close evaluation intervals, without lifting the flap, with combined aminoglycoside (tobramycin) and fluoroquinolone (moxifloxacin) for complete resolution without any loss of visual acuity.

A 56-year-old man with a history of initial refractive errors of −0.50–3.00 × 050 right eye and −0.75–2.25 × 115 left eye with pre-LASIK corneal topographies, as noted in ▶ Fig. 6.21, underwent LASK eye surgery elsewhere. The patient later underwent two enhancement procedures for correction of residual refraction in the right eye and one enhancement procedure in the left eye. The patient sought a second opinion in regard to his progressively declining vision. The Visante (▶ Fig. 6.22) demonstrated that despite the residual stromal tissue of at least 300 µm, ectasia of the cornea was clearly notable. The patient underwent corneal transplant surgery for the right eye and was fitted with hard contact lens in the left eye.

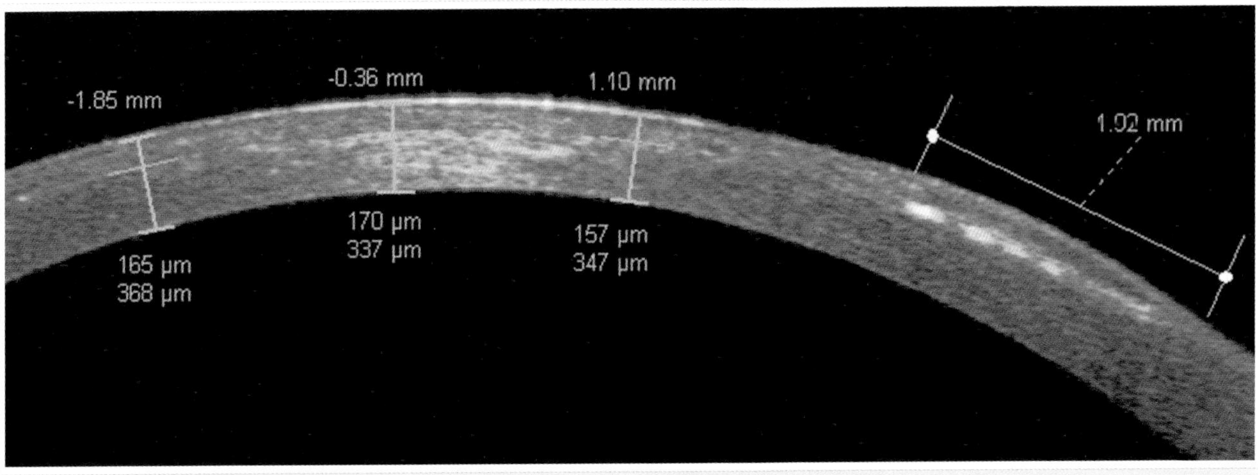

Fig. 6.19 Visante (enhanced high-resolution mode) 8 months after LASIK (laser-assisted in-situ keratomileusis) enhancement.

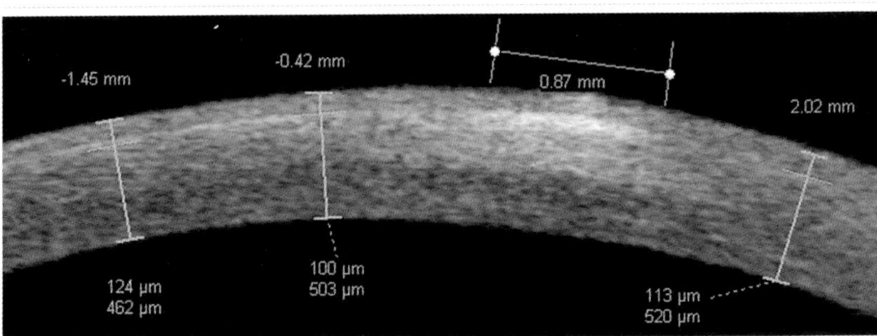

Fig. 6.20 Visante image of interflap space ulcer.

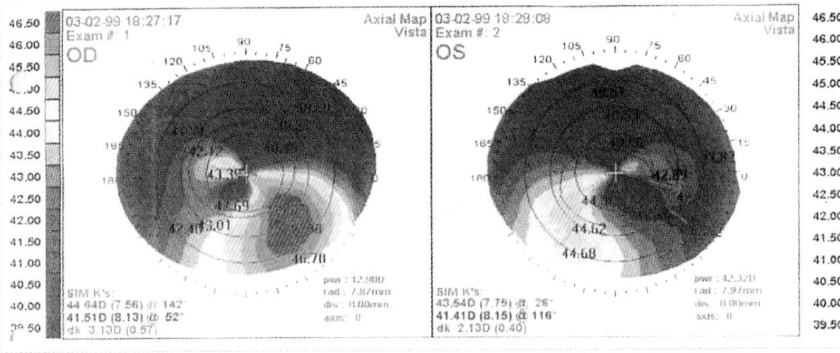

Fig. 6.21 Pre-LASIK (laser-assisted in-situ keratomileusis) topography of patient in ▶ Fig. 6.22. OD, right eye; OS, left eye.

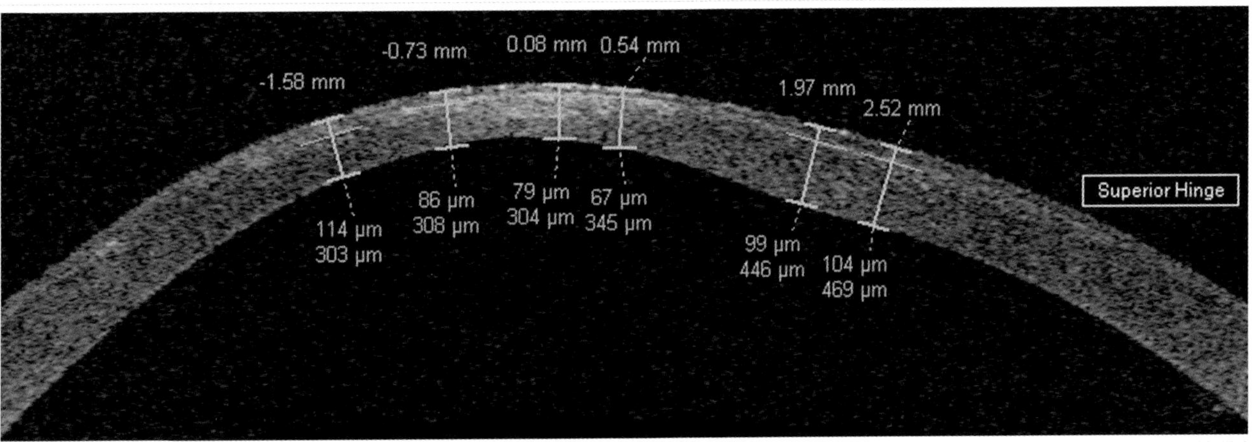

Fig. 6.22 Corneal ectasia after LASIK (laser-assisted in-situ keratomileusis).

As demonstrated in these cases, the Visante anterior-segment OCT is useful in preoperative evaluation of LASIK patients, for example, in evaluation of the corneal pachymetric map as an adjunct to the corneal topographic map and quantitative assessment of the angles. Postoperative care is also enhanced in evaluating patients for enhancement and also for the management of complications.

6.3 Phakic Intraocular Lenses

Phakic IOLs are relatively new to the U.S. market, but they have had much greater acceptance and use internationally. As of January 2008, only two phakic IOLs have been approved by the U.S. Food and Drug Administration: the Verisyse (Advanced Medical Optics, Inc.) and the Visian intracorneal lens (ICL; Staar Surgical, Inc., Monrovia, CA). Both phakic IOLs are approved only for the correction of myopia in the United States. The Verisyse is an anterior chamber lens that has undergone enclavation to the iris (▶ Fig. 6.23). The Visian ICL is a posterior chamber lens that rests in the sulcus space anterior to the crystalline lens. Many other lenses are available in the international markets and also in clinical trials in the United States.

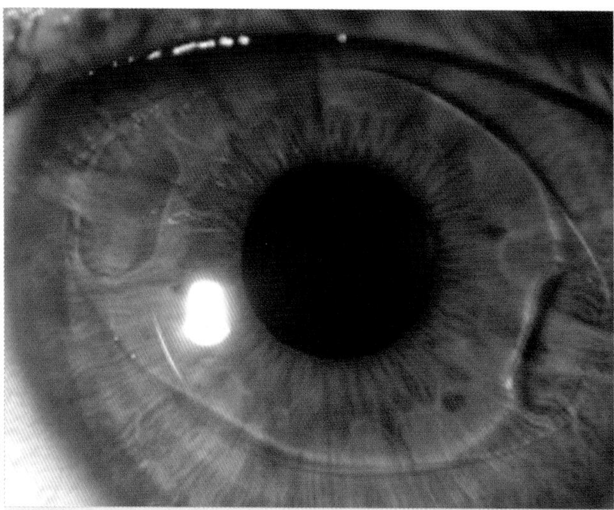

Fig. 6.23 Image of an eye implanted with Verisyse.

6.3.1 Endothelial Clearance

The inner lining of the cornea is populated by the corneal endothelium cells. With placement of the phakic IOLs, there is always concern of the lifetime consequences that placement of these prostheses may pose on the population of these cells. Two of the risk factors noted and emphasized by Advanced Medical Optics (AMO, Abbott laboratories Inc, Illinois, USA) are the 1.5-mm minimal clearance of the anterior aspect of the prosthesis to the corneal endothelium and the minimum anterior chamber depth of 3.2 mm. Advanced Medical Optics has a computer software program called the VeriCalc, which requires the patient's prescription in sphere and cylinder, along with anterior-chamber depth and the corneal keratometric measurements. Although the VeriCalc is helpful, the Visante, with its new phakic IOL module, may provide a much more accurate assessment of acceptable implantation requirements.

The next case is of a patient who had Verisyse implantation before the Visante and its phakic IOL module became available. A 28-year-old woman with a prescription of right eye –15.00 – 1.50 × 165 and left eye –14.25–1.25 × 175, with the VeriCalc was estimated to have a postoperative minimal endothelial clearance of 1.56 and 1.65 in the right and left eye, respectively. However, on postoperative evaluation (▶ Fig. 6.24, ▶ Fig. 6.25), the patient was noted to have significantly less endothelial Verisyse clearance, ranging from 1.22 to 1.66 mm in the right eye,

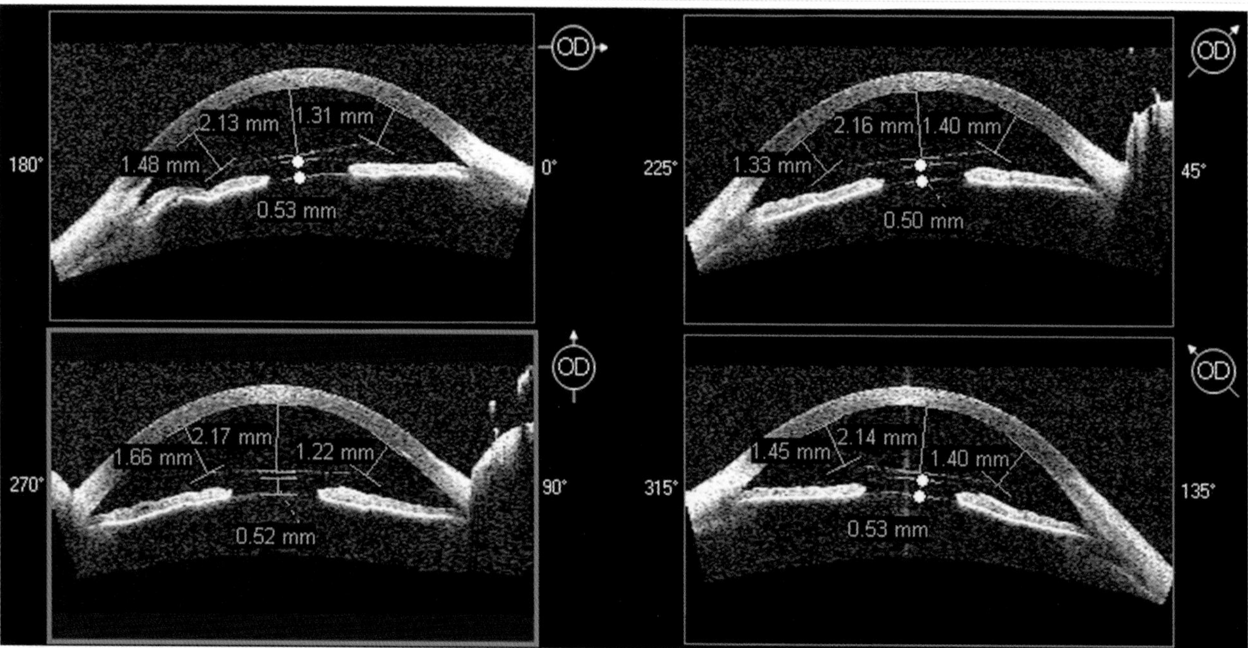

Fig. 6.24 Visante images (quad scan) of the right eye (OD) implanted with Verisyse.

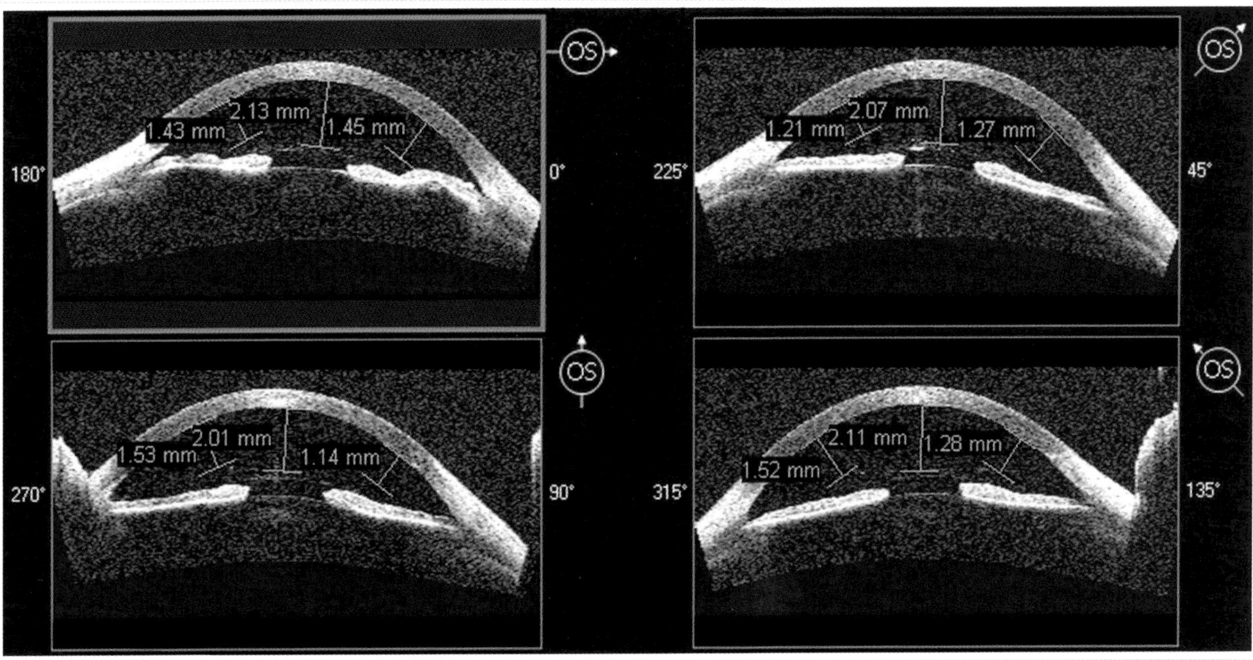

Fig. 6.25 Visante images (quad scan) of the left eye (OS) implanted with Verisyse.

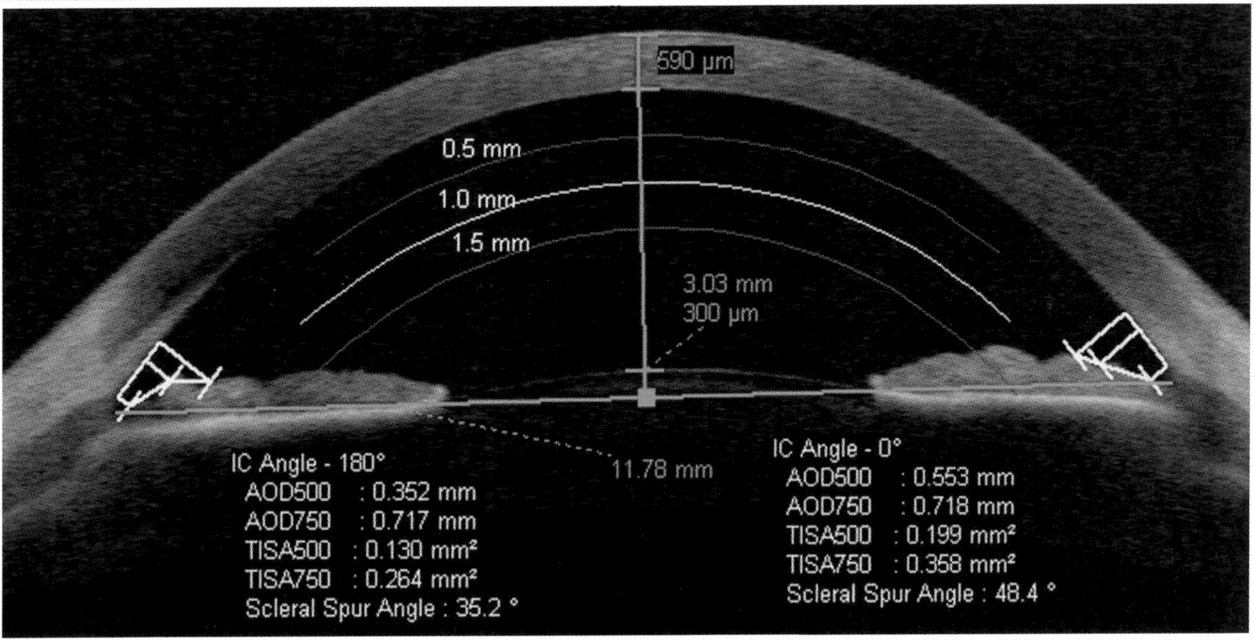

Fig. 6.26 Preoperative evaluation of eye for Verisyse. Evaluations of the angles, crystalline lens rise, anterior chamber depth, and safety endothelial distance clearance are noted. IC, iris curvature.

with average of 1.41 mm, and ranging from 1.14 to 1.53 mm in the left eye, with an average of 1.35 mm.

6.3.2 Crystalline Lens Rise

In the following case, however, the patient was evaluated using the new Phakic IOL module available with the Visante 2.0 software. A 20-year-old man with right eye refraction of −14.25 −2.75 × 115 leading to 20/40 vision, with slight amblyopia, was evaluated for the Verisyse implantation. In ▶ Fig. 6.26, one can evaluate the angles, anterior chamber, and the gross endothelial clearance, using the "rainbow" module. The anterior chamber depth (ACD) in this case equals to the anterior lens surface to endothelial distance (3.03 mm) plus the corneal thickness (590 μm = 0.59 mm). Therefore, the ACD would equal 3.03 mm + 0.59 mm = 3.62 mm. Baikoff described the crystalline lens rise (CLR) as measurement of lens rise above or below the horizontal line across the deepest portion of the angles.[2] Note that

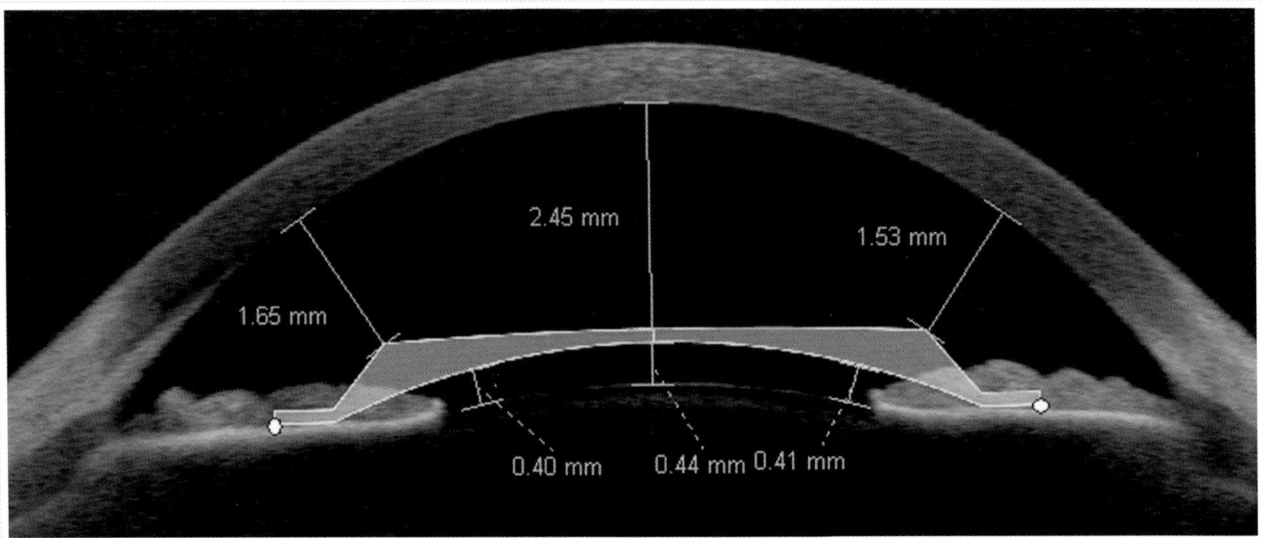

Fig. 6.27 Preoperative Verisyse model placement using the Visante. The Verisyse model and power are programmed and placed properly. The lens-endothelial clearance and the vault distances are measured preoperatively.

although the angle measurements are done from the scleral spur, these measurements are done from the deepest angle positions. In this case the CLR is found to be 300 µm. Baikoff describes a form of pigment dispersion syndrome (PDS) in nine patients, eight of whom had a CLR greater than 600 µm. This form of PDS is a direct result of iris pigment liberation from traumatized iris tissue between the phakic IOL and the crystalline lens. As an example, the patient (▶ Fig. 6.27) had a CLR of 720 µm and would have sufficient clearance of neither the ACD nor the CLR and would not be a candidate for Verisyse.

6.3.3 Preoperative Phakic Intraocular Lens Model

After the initial quick evaluation (▶ Fig. 6.27), one may proceed to a much more in-depth evaluation with the Verisyse model number and power. Once the model is aligned just anterior to the posterior iris pigmented epithelium and centered, the measurement via the safety lines and the lens vault can be placed. The safety lines are to evaluate for the anterior surface of the phakic IOL to the posterior aspect of the cornea. The vault caliper is used to evaluate the distance from posterior aspect of the phakic IOL to the anterior crystalline lens distance.

This patient did subsequently undergo Verisyse implantation and was evaluated by the Visante (▶ Fig. 6.28). The VeriCalc calculated the minimum endothelial clearance as 1.92 mm. The Visante model calculated an average of 1.59-mm phakic IOL to endothelium clearance and a vault distance of 41.67 µm. The actual postoperative data revealed a 1.64-mm phakic IOL to endothelial clearance and a vault distance of 38.67 µm.

6.3.4 Dynamic Changes of the Anterior Chamber with Accommodation

Verisyse, as currently available in the United States, is a solid polymethylmethacrylate lens available in 6.0-mm or 5.0-mm optics and must be inserted through a similar-size wound. Artiflex is a foldable version of the same that may be inserted through a smaller wound. Guell and colleagues published a study in which they implanted Verisyse in one eye and Artiflex in the second eye.[3] They then did an accommodative dynamic study on each eye of the 11 patients in their study. Using the optometer, accommodation was induced in the patient's eye, 1 diopter at a time, up to 7 diopters. Their conclusion was that there were no clinical differences in how these phakic IOLs behaved relative to each other; however, with accommodation, there was a total anterior movement of the iris-lens diaphragm of up to a maximal 250 µm at the center of the phakic IOL to the endothelial distance. It must be noted that the distance of the phakic IOL edge to the endothelium is much less than the center and may prove to be more significant than the measurement of the center of the lens. Additionally, a maximal 1.5-mm pupillary constriction with accommodation was noted. Accommodation did not cause significant change in the vault distance between the crystalline lens and the posterior aspect of the phakic IOL.

In another study, Kiovula and Kugelberg studied the phakic refractive lens (PRL; Medennium, Inc., Irvine, CA), which is not currently approved by the FDA in United States.[4] The PRL is a posterior-chamber lens that floats in the posterior chamber, rests on the zonules, and freely rotates. In their study, in the hyperopic group, there were no contacts between the crystalline lens and the PRL at baseline; however, with accommodation, contact was noted in three cases (27%), and a decrease in the distance noted in another six cases (55%). In the myopic group, with the lens model PRL 100, there was one case of contact (10%) at baseline, two crystalline lenses had contact with the PRL with accommodation (20%), and three cases (30%) had a decrease in the distance between the PRL and the crystalline lens. With the myopic PRL 101, two patients (6%) had baseline PRL-crystalline lens contact at baseline, and another lens came in contact with accommodation (10%); in 21 cases (68%) there was a decrease in the PRL-crystalline lens distance without

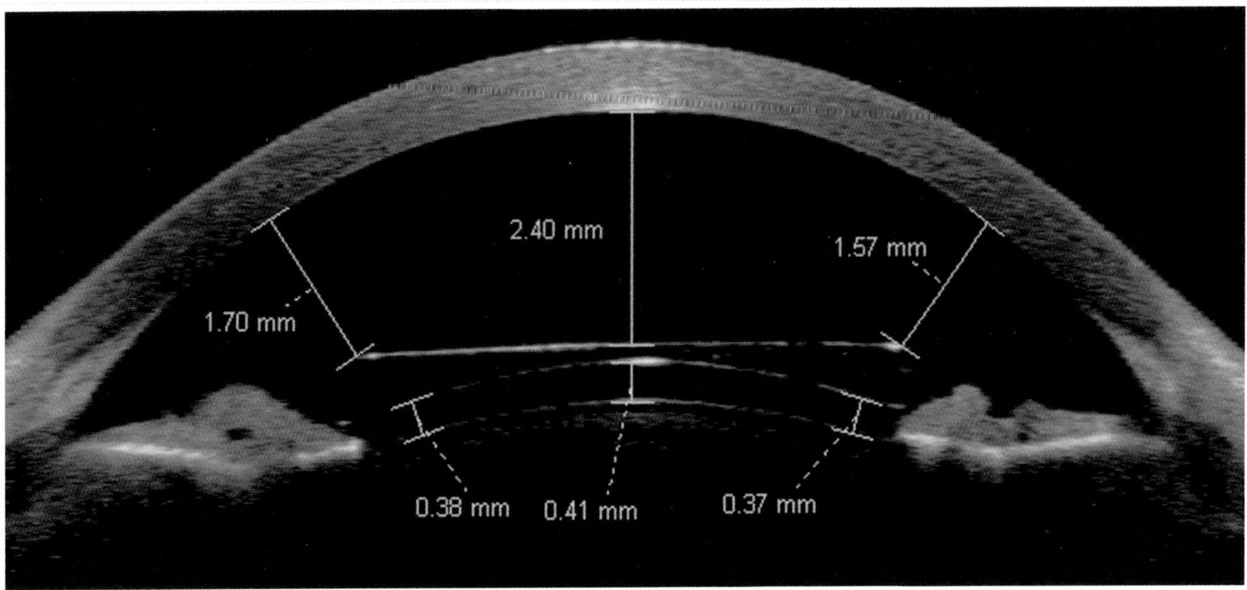

Fig. 6.28 Postoperative actual Visante scan of eye implanted with Verisyse. Endothelial clearance and vault distances are measured. The iris claw hooks are noted as black spots in the iris tissue.

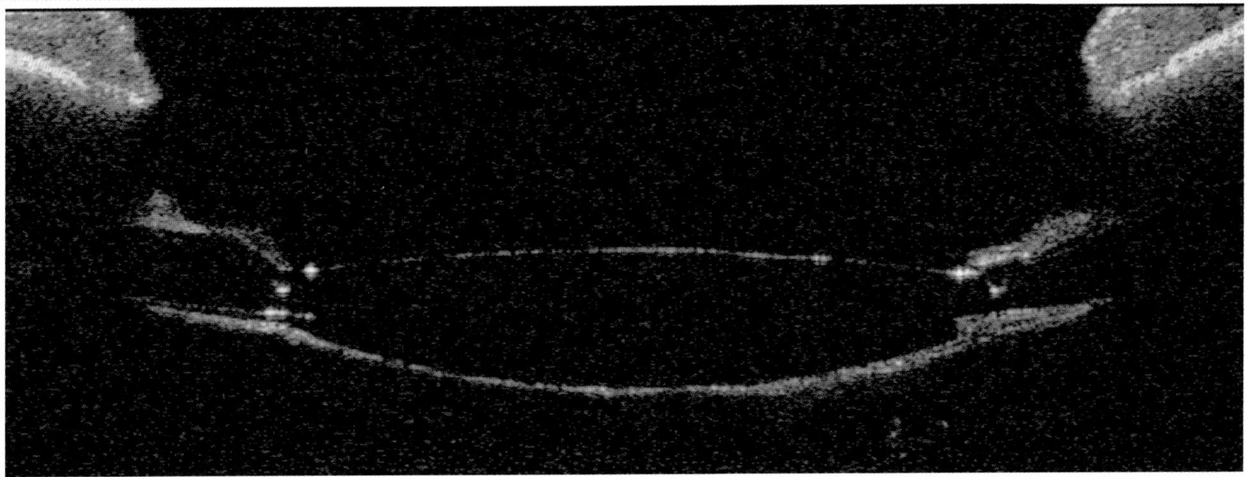

Fig. 6.29 CrytaLens implanted in the eye. The optic and the hinges are clearly noted.

contact. A mean reduction of 84 µm in the PRL-crystalline lens distance in the PRL models 101 and 200 was noted; however, there was no reduction in the PRL model 100. The authors suggest that the smaller size of this model prevents the reduction in the PRL-crystalline lens caused by pupillary constriction and the anterior lens movement. They also suggest that despite greater prosthesis-crystalline touch, the reason for fewer cataract complications of this lens compared with the sulcus fixated posterior-chamber Visian ICL phakic IOL is that the lens rotation allows for aqueous exchange.

In evaluation of the phakic IOL candidate, the Visante anterior-segment OCT plays a crucial role in safely evaluating the anterior-chamber depth, the crystalline lens rise, the endothelial-phakic IOL distance, the phakic IOL-crystalline lens vault, and the dynamic accommodative changes of the anterior segment.

6.3.5 Conclusion

In one of the most commonly performed refractive surgeries, namely, cataract surgery or clear lens extraction, there is also a significant role for the Visante anterior-segment OCT in those cases as well. With increasing emphasis on the premium IOL, including the accommodative lenses, the Visante becomes invaluable in demonstrating the efficacy of the lenses and can also be used to induce accommodation using the built-in optometer as noted under the *Phakic Intraocular Lens* section of this chapter. An example of CrystaLens implanted in a patient is presented, although no measurable movement in the lens could be noted (▶ Fig. 6.29).

As demonstrated through the case presentations, the Visante anterior-segment OCT is a powerful noncontact, real-time imaging system of the eye that shows excellent accuracy. In the care of excimer laser patients, from the preoperative stages, the patient's candidacy may be enhanced with additional information, such as pachymetric mapping of the cornea. The health of the eye may be assessed beyond its refraction, such as the quantitative measurement of the angle, as opposed to the qualitative capabilities of the standard slit-lamp gonioscope. Corneal pathologies, such as scars, infections, flap configurations, and irregularities, are quantitatively noted and are only some of the examples of the usefulness of the Visante in the care of a past, present, and future refractive patient.

6.4 Reference

[1] Roger F Steinert DH. Anterior Segment Optical Coherence Tomography. Thorofare, NJ: Slack; 2008

[2] Baïkoff G. Anterior segment OCT and phakic intraocular lenses: a perspective. J Cataract Refract Surg 2006 Nov; 32: 1827–35

[3] Guell JL, Morral M, Gris O, Gaytan J, Sisquella M, Manero F. Evaluation of Verisyse and Artiflex phakic intraocular lenses during accommodation using Visante optical coherence tomography. J Cataract Refract Surg 2007 Aug; 33: 1398–404

[4] Koivula A, Kugelberg M. Optical coherence tomography of the anterior segment in eyes with phakic refractive lenses. Ophthalmology 2007 Nov; 114: 2031–7

7 Anterior-Segment Exploration with Optical Coherence Tomography

Georges Baikoff

Until recently, most efforts in ocular imaging concerned posterior-segment exploration. One of the most important events was the commercialization of the Carl Zeiss Meditec Stratus optical coherence tomography (OCT 3–820 nm wavelength), which made it possible to visualize different layers of the retina with a great deal of precision (resolution 3–4 µm). Efforts are under way to develop increasingly precise scanning of the neurosensorial layers using three-dimensional visualization (Carmen Puliafito Innovators Lecture, American Society of Cataract and Refractive Surgery, Washington, 2005).

Because it is possible to observe the anterior segment directly using the slit lamp, extensive research has not been a priority. In daily practice, ultrasonic evaluations of corneal pachymetry and anterior-chamber depth along the optical axis of the eye have been considered sufficient. With the development of sophisticated surgical techniques, however, it became essential to obtain elaborate static and dynamic measurements of the anterior segment to meet modern safety requirements. Here one can briefly refer to X-ray imaging of the eye (conventional X-ray, MRI (Magnetic Resonance Imaging), TDM (computer tomography)) because its use in daily practice is unlikely to undergo further development. The choice now lies between optical and ultrasonic exploration of the anterior segment. Slit-lamp images are simply frontal images with a subjective estimation of a few external measurements of the eye. Development of the Scheimpflug technique with oblique images resulted in a new capability to evaluate the distances in the eye's anterior segment along different optical sections. The major drawbacks of this technology are a difficult mathematical reconstruction and scleral overexposure when taking photographs. In particular, the whole of the angle area is masked by this overexposure, and the fine structures are indiscernible (i.e., the scleral spur, iridocorneal sinus).

The idea of using infrared wavelengths in optical coherence is expanding rapidly (IOLMaster, Visant OCT; Carl Zeiss Meditec).[1,2] About 10 years ago, Izatt and colleagues[3] suggested using the OCT for anterior-segment imaging. Reflection of the infrared light rays is captured and analyzed by an optical sensor, and appropriate software readjusts the dimensions of the images by erasing distortion errors attributable to different corneal optical transmission differences. Measuring software capable of evaluating the distance between two points, the curvature radius and angles, is also integrated.

Ultrasonic exploration of the anterior segment appears to have reached its limits, whether in ultrasound biomicroscopy or ultrahigh-frequency ultrasound equipment (Artemis; Ultralink, LLC). Today, resolution is identical to 1310-nm wavelength anterior segment OCT, which is available on the market (15–20 µm for axial resolution, 50–100 µm for transverse resolution). Manipulation is fairly complex, and even if some ultrasonic measurements are used as references to calibrate a certain number of instruments, there is no certainty of exact in vivo or ultrasonic measurements. However, the error can be considered relative as long as the reference scale remains constant with each device and technology.

7.1 Anterior-Segment Exploration

7.1.1 Time-Domain Anterior-Segment OCT

The anterior-segment time-domain OCT (Visante, Carl Zeiss Meditec) is on the verge of being commercialized, and we have been fortunate to be able to use it for 2 years as a prototype.[4,5,6,7,8,9,10,11,12,13,14,15,16] The equipment uses a 1310-nm wavelength, but in its present form, the infrared light is blocked by pigments; however, the nonpigmented opaque structures are permeable, and images can be obtained through a cloudy or white cornea, through the conjunctiva, and through the sclera. Axial resolution is 18 µm and transverse resolution 50 µm. The procedure is noncontact and quite easy; therefore, a technician can be rapidly trained to carry out the examinations. It is possible to choose the axis to be explored or carry out an automatic 360-degree exploration along the four meridians.

An optical target can be focused or defocused with positive or negative lenses. Natural accommodation can be stimulated, and anterior-segment modifications during accommodation can be explored in vivo. Image reconstruction software has been criticized, but in our experience, we have been able to show that the sections obtained were reproducible. We believe this notion of reproducibility is quite important. A few errors regarding the precision of the readings may be important, but as long as the reference scale remains constant and the areas explored can easily be found during successive examinations, these errors can be considered relative (▶ Fig. 7.1,▶ Fig. 7.2).

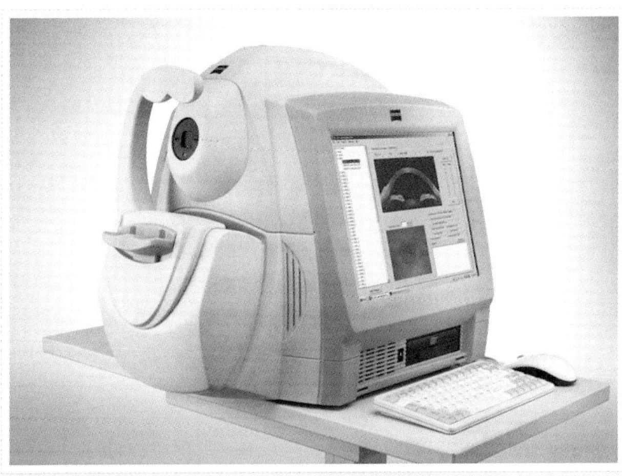

Fig. 7.1 Visante optical coherence tomograph.

7.1.2 Static Measurement of the Anterior Segment (▶ Fig. 7.3)

With the Visante OCT prototype at our disposal, we were able to explore hundreds of eyes and to evaluate the different measurements of the anterior segment. We were able to show a new notion: in most cases, the anterior chamber was not a circle. We were able to prove in vivo that in 75% of cases, the internal vertical diameter of the anterior chamber was larger than the internal horizontal diameter by at least 100 µm. Using the Artemis instrument (ultra high-frequency ultrasound) on cadaver eyes, this notion had already been put forward by Liliana Werner. This discovery has essential implications when an anterior chamber phakic or pseudophakic angle-supported implant is scheduled. The measurement obtained with the Visante OCT is much more precise than the white-to-white evaluation that was previously used, and it is more precise and much easier to acquire than the anterior-segment images obtained using the classic B-scan instruments, even the most recent ones.

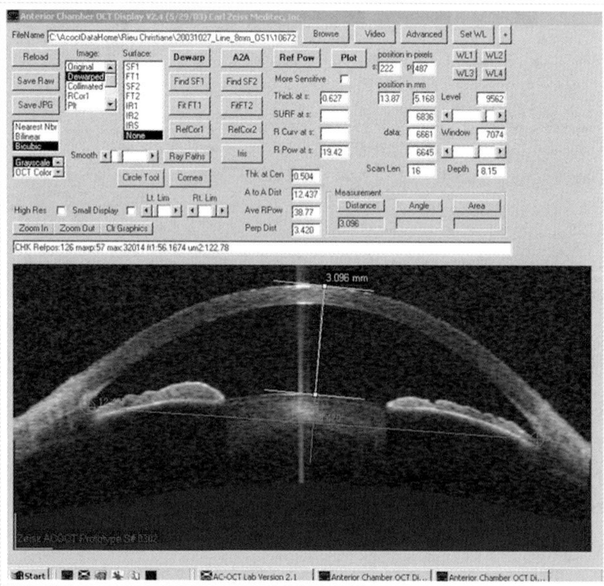

Fig. 7.2 Prototype of the image exploitation software.

Furthermore, with ultrasonic scanning devices, the water bath placed before the patient's cornea makes the examination difficult, and because there is no fixation point, it is not possible to visualize the optical axis. The optical axis, which is a fixed reference point, allows one to know with certainty the position of the examined optical section. Thus, with the Artemis, there is lack of reproducibility.

7.1.3 Dynamic Evaluation of the Anterior Segment

▶ Fig. 7.4 comprises images of the eye of a 10-year-old child with 10 diopters of accommodation; the images speak for themselves. Distortion of the anterior surface of the crystalline lens, myosis, and modifications to the anterior chamber depth during accommodation can be observed. This shows that in young subjects the anterior segment of the eye is quite dynamic; for 1-diopter accommodation, there is approximately a 30-µm forward thrust of the crystalline lens' anterior pole. Therefore, it is usual to observe a 100- to 200-µm variation of the anterior chamber in a young subject (a candidate for a phakic implant).

With aging, crystalline lens flexibility reduces and fewer modifications to the anterior segment occur during accommodation; however, the anterior chamber becomes flatter as the crystalline lens' anterior pole moves forward by about 20 µm per year. Specific software could perhaps be used to simulate the aging of the anterior segment and thus help to explain that as the crystalline lens thickens with time, contact between the crystalline lens and all models of phakic implants is probable, regardless of their type of fixation in the anterior segment.

7.1.4 Evaluation of the Crystalline Lens with the Anterior Chamber OCT

- ▶ Fig. 7.5a shows that by focusing behind the iris, it is possible to observe the entire thickness of the crystalline lens.
- ▶ Fig. 7.5b shows the image of a 2-year-old child with Peter syndrome and lens-cornea adherence; the different layers of the crystalline lens are perfectly visible.

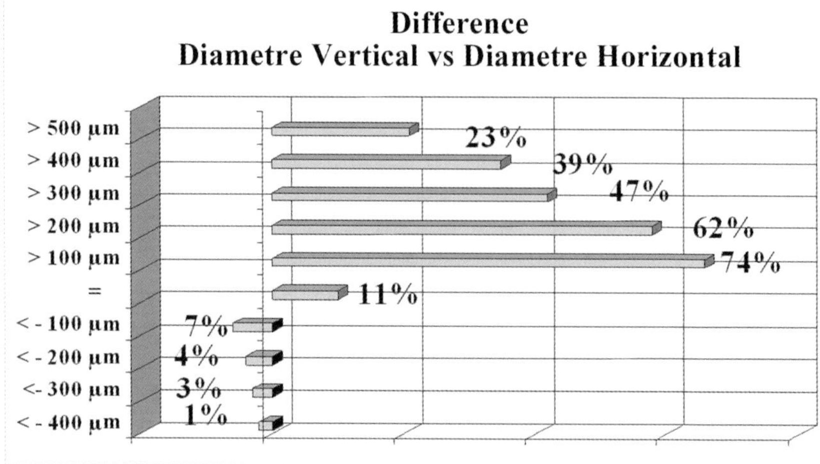

Fig. 7.3 In vivo statistical evaluation of the vertical internal diameter versus the horizontal internal diameter of the anterior chamber of the human eye. In 74% of cases, the anterior chamber's vertical internal diameter was larger than the horizontal internal diameter by 100 µm. The vertical and horizontal diameters were equal in only 11% of cases. The horizontal diameter was larger in 15% of cases.

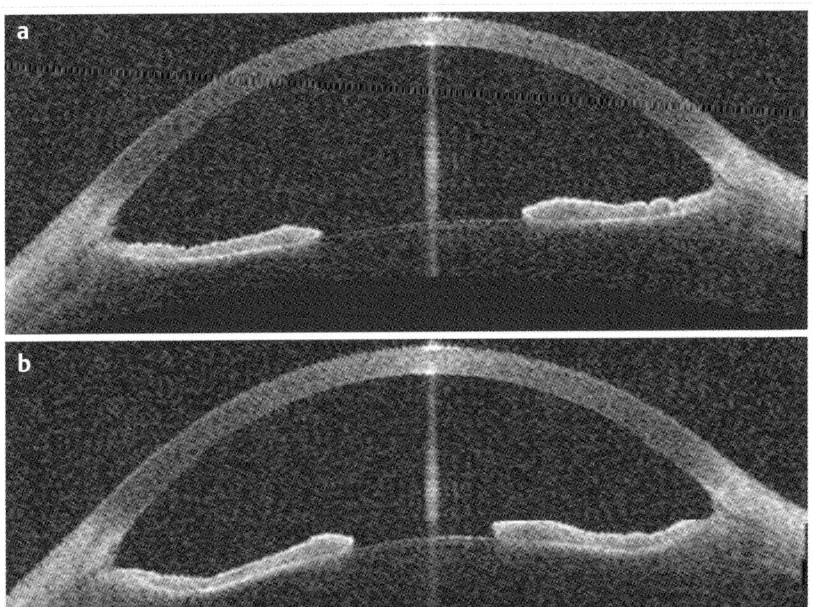

Fig. 7.4 (a,b) Dynamic image of accommodation of the anterior segment in a 10 year-old child (10-diopter accommodation).

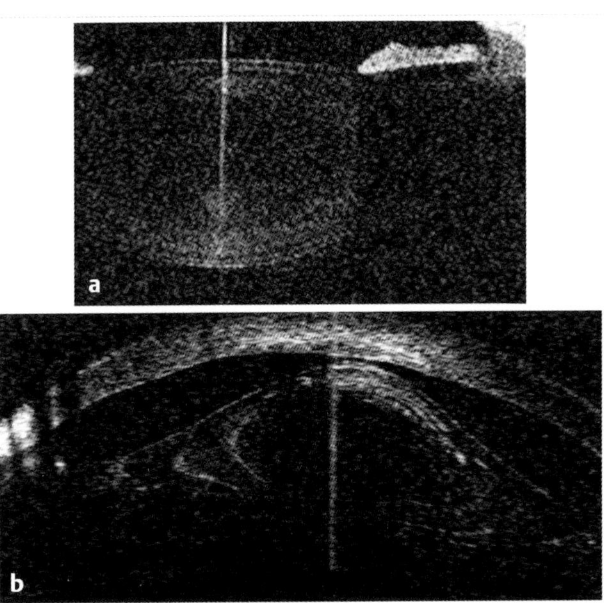

Fig. 7.5 (a) View of natural crystalline lens' entire thickness. (b) View of different layers of a pathological crystalline lens with Peters syndrome (in a 2-year-old child).

With current equipment, densitometric evaluation of the crystalline lens is not possible, but it is hoped that with ongoing studies, such analysis will be possible shortly.

7.1.5 Pseudophakic Artificial Crystalline Lens

▶ Fig. 7.6 shows two examples of a piggyback implant, and ▶ Fig. 7.6a shows perfectly well-adapted piggyback intraocular lens with the main lens behind and the secondary lens in front. The interface between the two lenses is virtual but perfectly

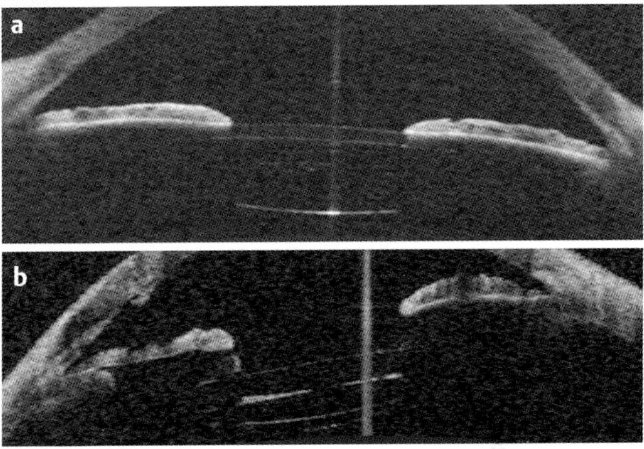

Fig. 7.6 Piggyback intraoperative lenses. (a) Perfect aspect and interface's optical void. (b) Aspect of an interlenticular proliferation.

visible on the images. In this case, there was no proliferation of unwanted deposits on the interface. In ▶ Fig. 7.6b, perforating keratoplasty was carried out on a corneal pseudophakic edema. Using the slit-lamp, an after-cataract was diagnosed postoperatively. In fact, after an examination with the OCT, we noticed a proliferation of newly formed tissues between the two piggyback implants. We changed our diagnosis of after-cataract to intralenticular proliferation.

7.1.6 Phakic Implants

Inserting a phakic implant (Artisan, Verysise), a method that has obtained Food and Drug Administration approval in the United States, should not be done without a thorough preoperative evaluation and postoperative follow-up. Until recently, measuring the depth of the anterior chamber and checking the endothelium cell count using a specular microscope were considered sufficient. With the development of techniques such as the OCT, surgical indications can be streamlined, and a regular checkup of the anterior chamber after such an intervention is mandatory. ▶ Fig. 7.7a shows a posterior chamber intracorneal lens inserted in a patient over the age of 45 years having developed cataract and severe optical problems. Although the intracorneal lens was been placed in the posterior chamber, on the endothelial safety scale, we note that the edges of the optic are approximately 1 mm from the endothelium. This distance is considered insufficient because it has been demonstrated that a minimum safety distance of 1.5 mm between the edges of the lens' optic and the endothelium is necessary.

In ▶ Fig. 7.7b, a pigment dispersion syndrome was observed after insertion of an Artisan hyperopic implant. Compared with a normal anterior segment, we observed that the iris was unusually thin and that pigment cysts had developed on the pupil between the implant and the patient's anterior capsule. We also demonstrated that a convex iris, which is a contraindication for Artisan implants, can be evaluated in a precise way using the crystalline lens-rise method (distance from the crystalline lens' anterior pole to the internal diameter of the iridocorneal angle).[6,14] When the crystalline lens rise is greater than 600 µm, the risk of developing pigment dispersion syndrome with a drop in visual acuity is probable in 70% of cases.

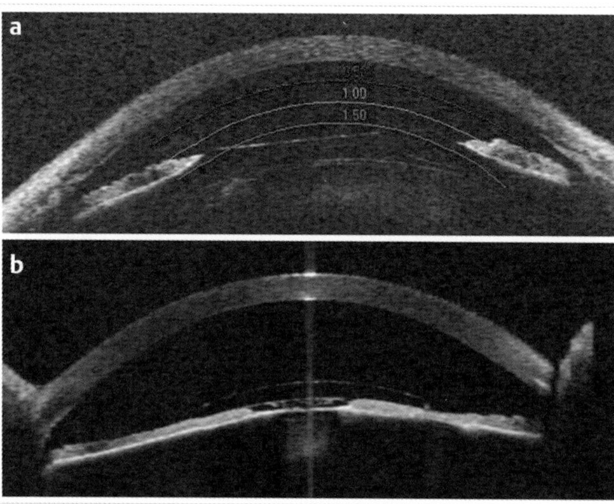

Fig. 7.7 Phakic implants **(a)** Posterior chamber ICL Implant; note that the edges of the optic are inside the 1.5-mm endothelial safety zone. **(b)** Artisan hyperopic implant with pigment dispersion in the pupil area. Note the flattening of the iris and the pigment cysts in the pupil area behind the implant.

7.1.7 Cornea

At present, with the prototype used, corneal imaging is essentially qualitative. Although resolution is not sufficient enough to determine intracorneal disorders or specify different types of dystrophies (▶ Fig. 7.8), three obvious pathologies were visible: in ▶ Fig. 7.8a, Terrien degeneration with peripheral thinning; in ▶ Fig. 7.8b, an old central descemetocele; and in ▶ Fig. 7.8c, keratoglobus with considerable thinning of the entire cornea. In ▶ Fig. 7.9, we were able to show the presence and the position of intracorneal rings used to treat myopia, and in ▶ Fig. 7.10 a lasik flap is perfectly visible with a nylon suture (marked by the arrow) to secure a "free cap."

Today, the anterior segment can be explored behind a cloudy and edematous cornea. ▶ Fig. 7.11 shows excellent examples of the performance of the Visante OCT. ▶ Fig. 7.11a represents a

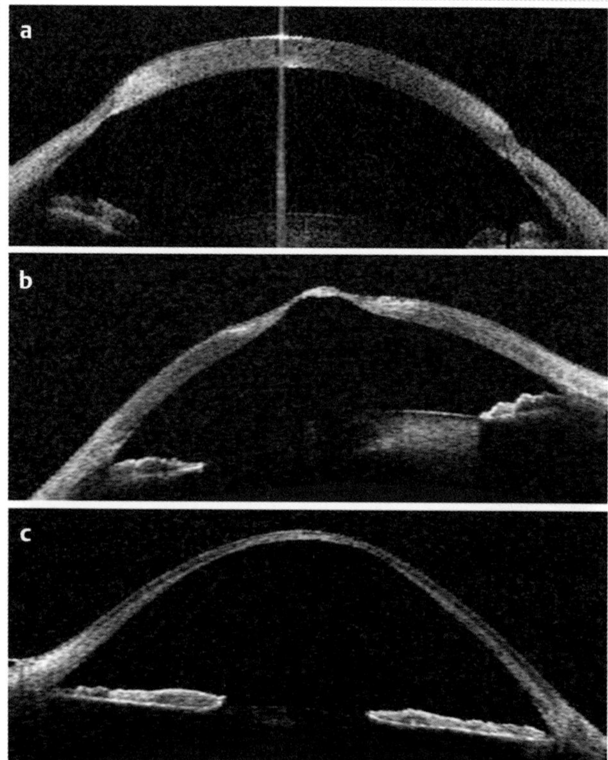

Fig. 7.8 Different aspects of corneal pathologies. **(a)** Terrien degeneration. **(b)** Descemetocele. **(c)** Keratoglobus.

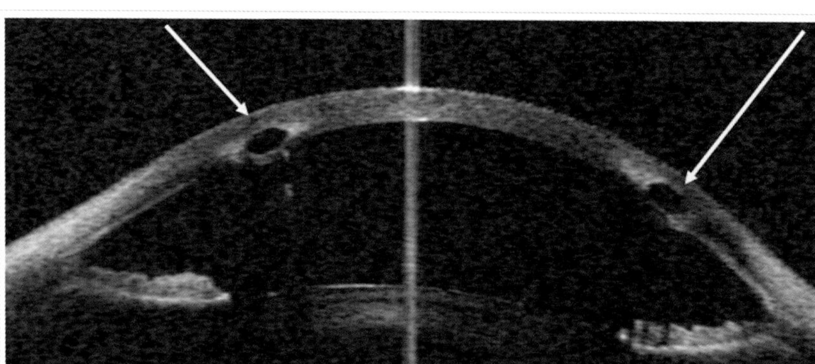

Fig. 7.9 Intracorneal rings to treat myopia (white arrow).

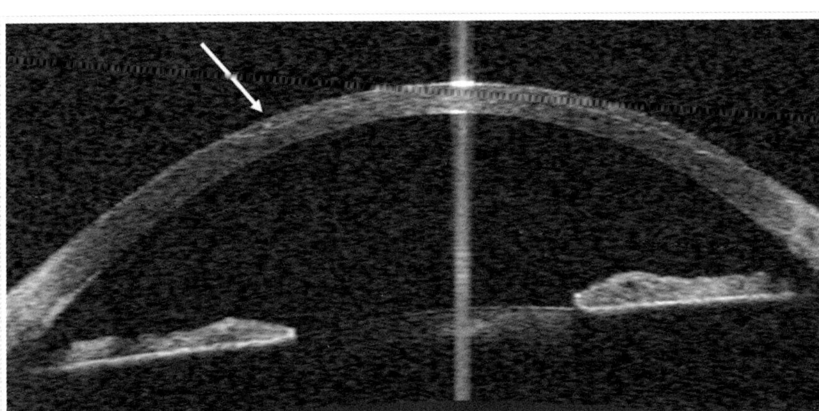

Fig. 7.10 Aspect of a LASIK freecap (white arrow). View of a 10.0 nylon suture.

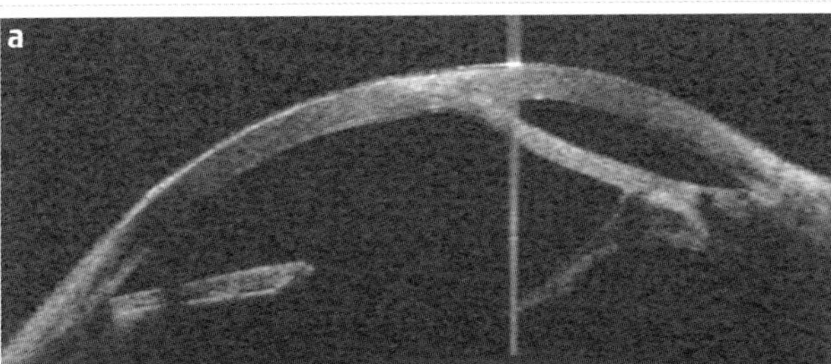

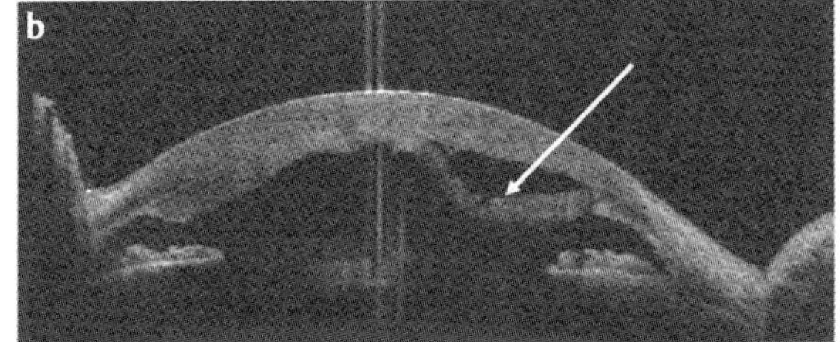

Fig. 7.11 Different aspects of the anterior segment behind a corneal edema. **(a)** Vitreous strands and anterior synechiae. **(b)** Failed descemetic graft. White arrow shows detached graft.

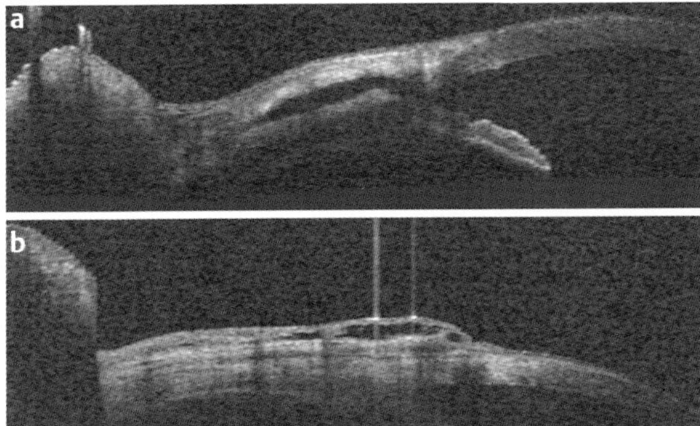

Fig. 7.12 Postoperative trabeculectomy. **(a)** Excessive scleral filtration with hypotonia. **(b)** Conjunctival filtration after scleral flap enhancement.

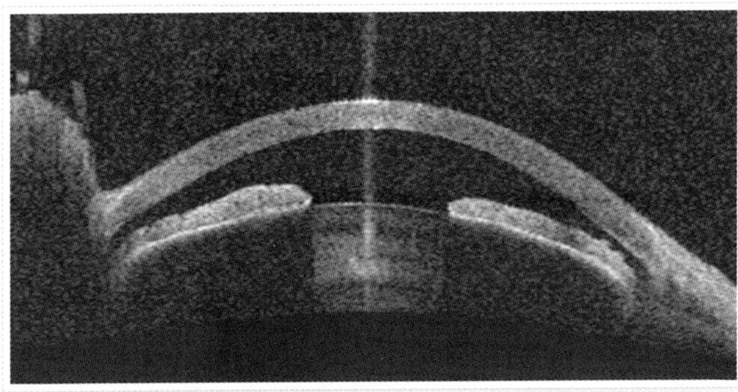

Fig. 7.13 Aspect of angle-closure glaucoma.

postaphakic corneal dystrophy clearly showing anterior synechiae with vitreous strands around the iris. As the eye is aphakic, it is easy for the surgeon to know what type of surgery is needed. ▶ Fig. 7.11b shows a corneal edema after an endothelial graft. It was not possible to explain, using a slit-lamp examination, why the cornea remained cloudy after surgery; however, using OCT during a simple postoperative visit, we were able to observe two corneal stromas without adherence. In this case, the endotheliodescemetic graft was a failure because the initial corneal edema not only remained but worsened. A normal penetrating keratoplasty was carried out later with satisfactory results.

7.1.8 Angle

Visualizing angle structures, as well as exploring the sclera and conjunctiva, is possible with anterior segment OCT. ▶ Fig. 7.12a shows excessive scleral filtration with persistent hypotonia after surgery. Intraocular pressure was brought back to normal by scleral flap enhancement and resulted in subconjunctival filtration (▶ Fig. 7.12b). The risk of angle closure (▶ Fig. 7.13) is easy to evaluate and can be objectively and precisely measured.

7.2 Conclusions and the Future

This general overview should give the reader an idea of the importance of this imaging technique. The main thing to remember is how simple this equipment is to use. Once the patient has fixed the target, manipulation is as easy as a corneal topography. There is no contact, the images are taken quickly, and the technician decides which axis he or she wishes to explore. Resolution is similar to the ultrahigh-frequency scanner, but the zones explored are easier to find because the fixation point is on the optical axis. The iridocorneal angle is perfectly visible, and to evaluate the measurements or check the evolution of an anterior segment, either the iridocorneal angle sinus or the scleral spur area can be used as a reference point because both remain constants of the anterior chamber anatomy during its dynamic or senile modifications. Because it is possible to measure multiple meridians, three-dimensioinal reconstruction of the anterior segment could perhaps be the next step. A 10-mm-diameter pachymetric mapping of the cornea is already possible (▶ Fig. 7.14). Another objective for the near future would be to estimate the quality of a LASIK (laser-assisted in-situ keratomileusis) flap over a certain length of time. (▶ Fig. 7.15).

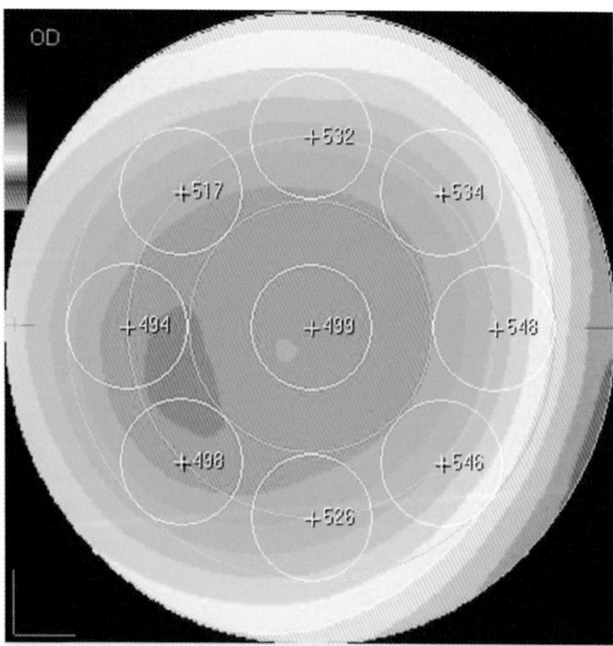

Fig. 7.14 Pachymetry map. OD, right eye.

Finally, in the laboratory, with a more appropriate wavelength or a modification of the power of the light ray, it has been possible to obtain images close to histology. On pseudophakic cadaver eyes, Linnola and colleagues[17] were able to show cell proliferation on the posterior capsule. The images obtain using high-resolution OCT are similar to a pathological study done on these same eyes.

The technological evolution of the Visante OCT for exploring the anterior segment is something to look forward to and anticipate. ▶ Fig. 7.16, ▶ Fig. 7.17, ▶ Fig. 7.18, ▶ Fig. 7.19, ▶ Fig. 7.20, ▶ Fig. 7.21, ▶ Fig. 7.22, ▶ Fig. 7.23, ▶ Fig. 7.24, ▶ Fig. 7.25, ▶ Fig. 7.26 show cases of various indications where anterior-segment OCT can be used. In the near future, these improvements should be similar to those of OCT for exploring the posterior pole: more precise images, resolution of a few

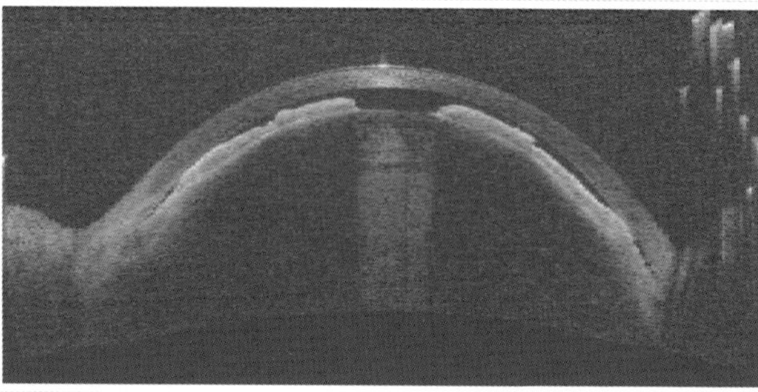

Fig. 7.16 Iridocorneal angle. This figure illustrates an extreme case of nanophthalmos with maximum shallowing of the anterior chamber and narrowing of the iridocorneal angle. The small diameter of the cornea and the very steep curvature and the maximum forward protrusion of the crystalline lens must be noted. Treating eyes like this is a delicate task because of the risk of preoperative or postoperative uveal effusion. It is recommended to combine lens extraction with large zones of lamellar sclerectomy to encourage transscleral aqueous outflow.

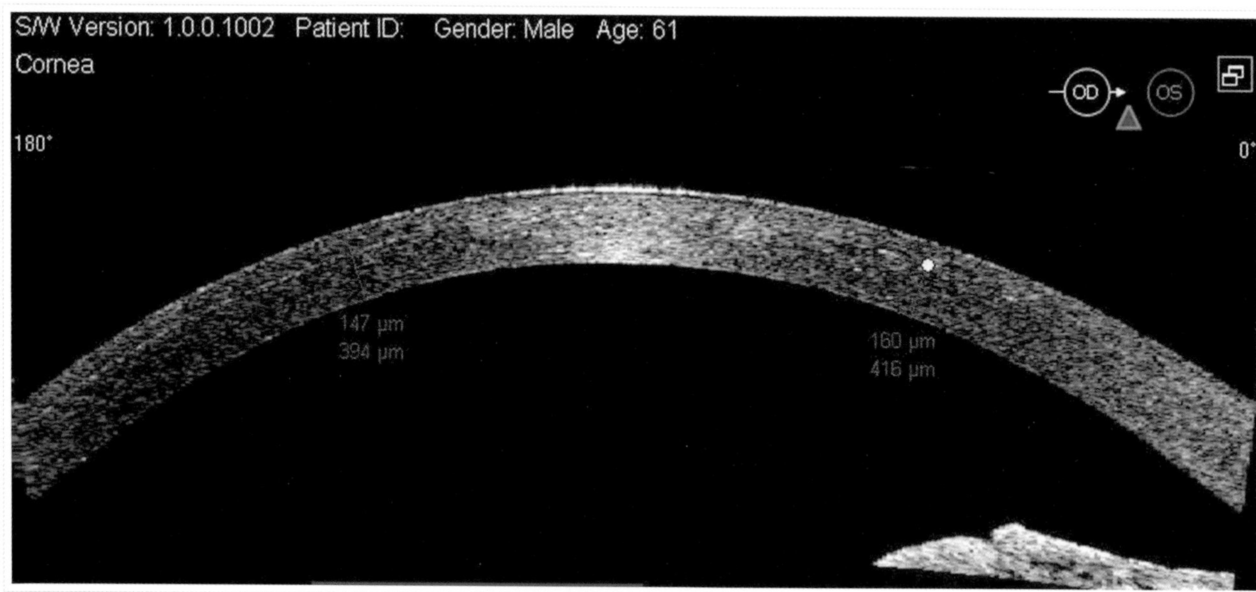

Fig. 7.15 Measurement of LASIK (laser-assisted in-situ keratomileusis) flap thickness with corneal software. OD, right eye; OS, left eye.

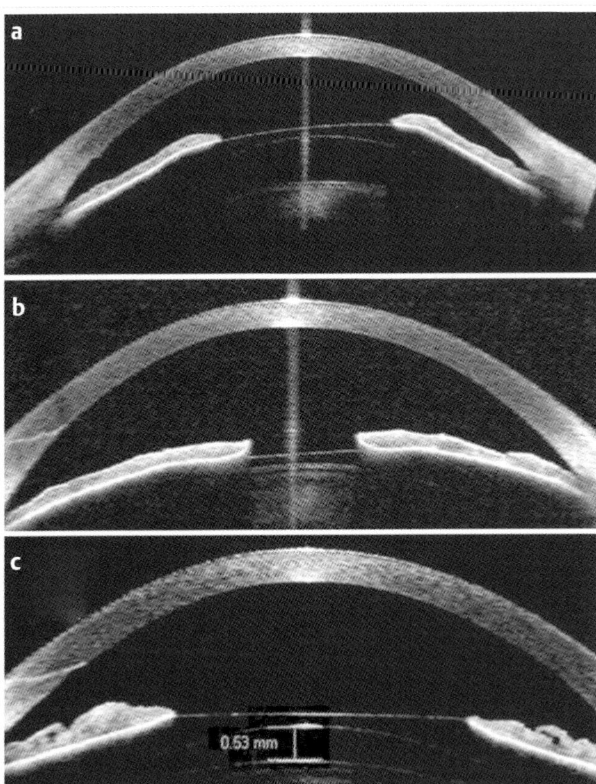

Fig. 7.17 Posterior chamber ICL STAAR phakic implants. This figure illustrates the importance of implant sizing. **(a)** The implant diameter is too large and pushes the iris forward with a risk of angle closure. **(b)** The implant is too small and the posterior surface comes into contact with the crystalline lens. **(c)** The ideal position for the implant with a distance of 530 µm between the anterior surface of the crystalline lens and the posterior surface of the implant. By using optical coherence tomography to calculate a formula, we were able to evaluate preoperatively the correct size of the implant.

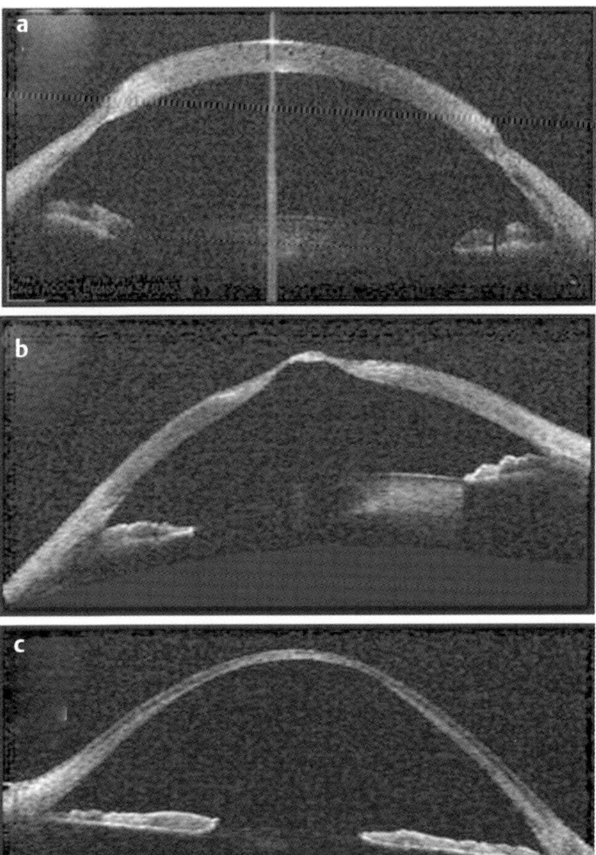

Fig. 7.18 Corneal melting. Different types of corneal melting according to Anglo-Saxon terminology. **(a)** Terrien syndrome shows circular peripheral thinning. **(b)** A descemetocele with substantial central thinning. **(c)** A keratoglobus with an anterior chamber (AC) diameter of about 14 mm and a cornea that is 250 µm thick. Optical coherence tomography enables a rapid diagnosis and the possibility to follow objectively the modifications to all the disorders over the years.

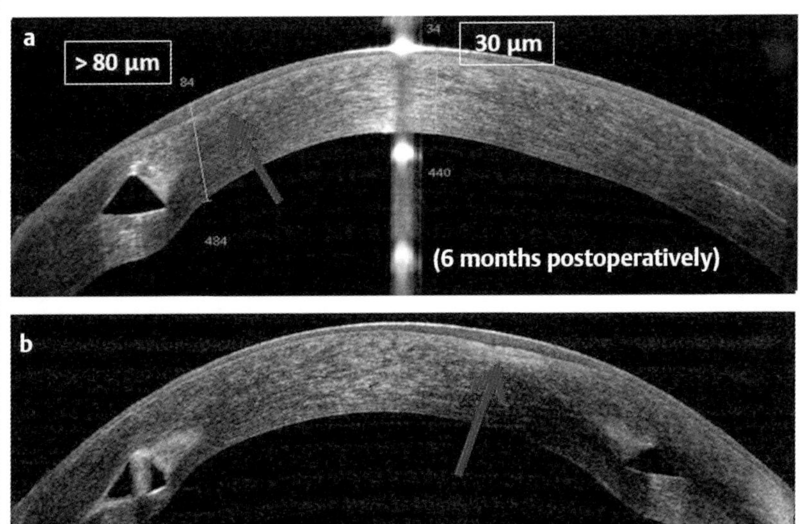

Fig. 7.19 Intracorneal rings. Regarding keratoconus, it is possible to verify the correct (or incorrect) positioning of intracorneal rings. The ring is correctly positioned; stromal distortion induced by the ring is obvious. There is epithelial thickening around the depression close to the ring (red arrows). This epithelial proliferation will smooth the optical surface and slowly contribute to improving the optical results, which continue over the months and years following the insertion of the rings.

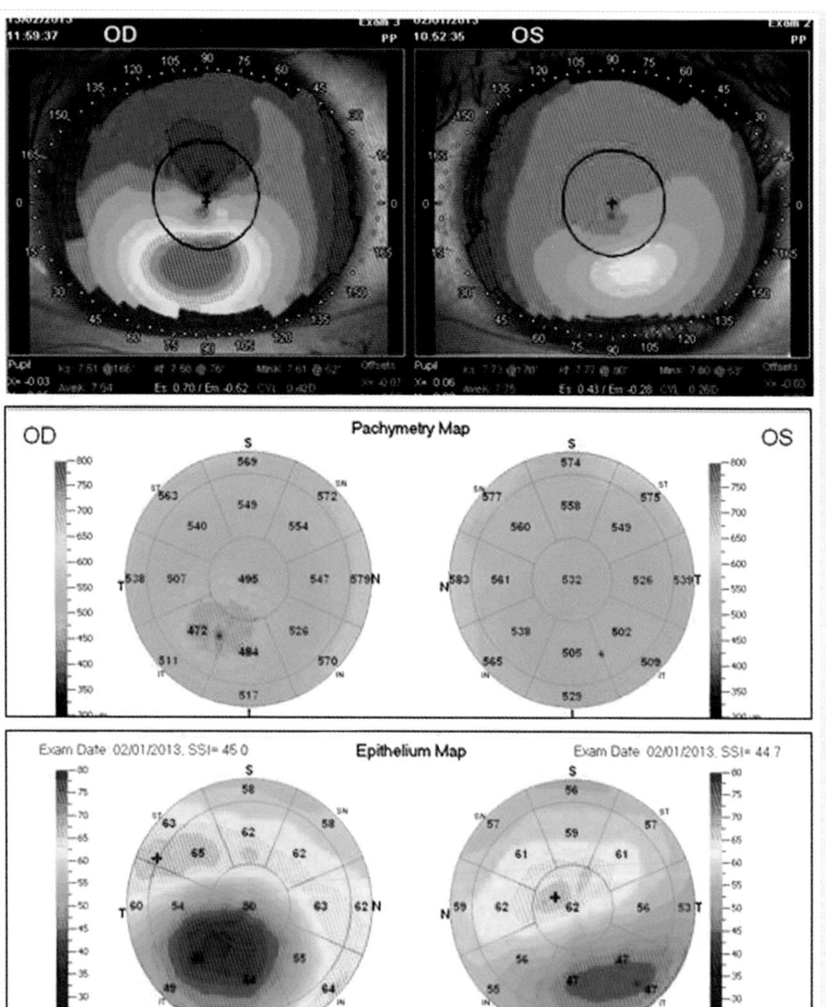

Fig. 7.20 The sequence of topographic, stromal and epithelial pachymetric disorders is illustrated here. In both eyes, epithelial thinning is situated at the apex of the cone, which is itself, the thinnest part of the cornea. The image of the right eye (OD) speaks for itself, as for the left eye (OS), already diagnosed with fruste keratoconus, the disorders are already present.

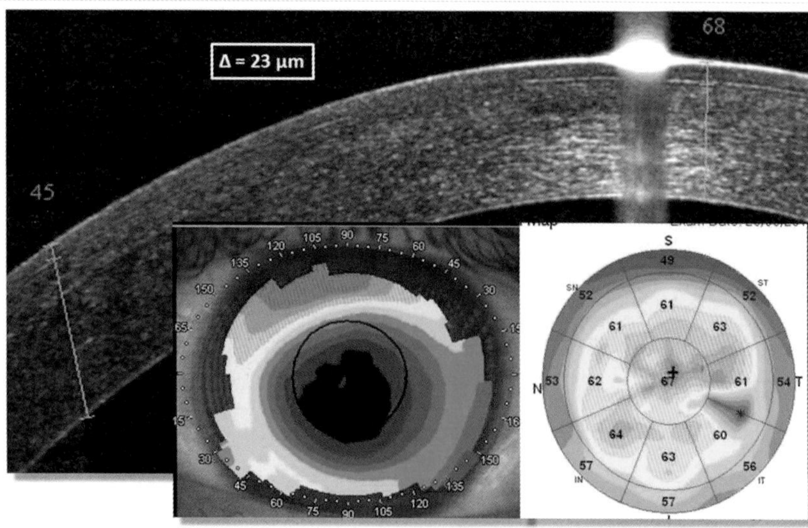

Fig. 7.21 LASIK (laser-assisted in-situ keratomileusis): Myopic laser and corneal epithelium. After LASIK, modifications to the corneal curvature will be accompanied by variations to the epithelial thickness. To summarize, one can say that the epithelium spreads to fill the corneal valleys and thins out at the tip. Epithelial pachymetry Δ can be defined as the difference of epithelial thickness between the center and the periphery.

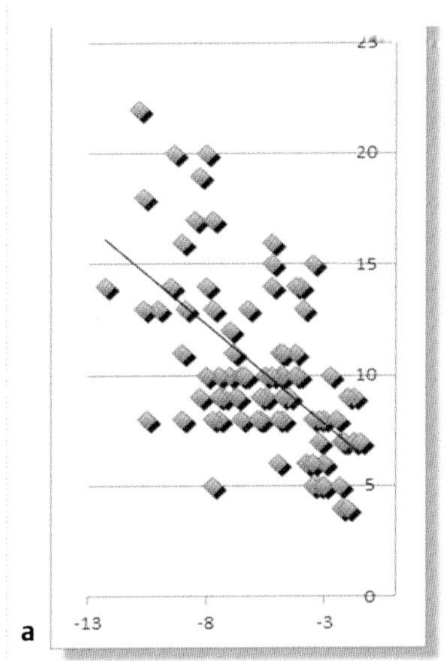

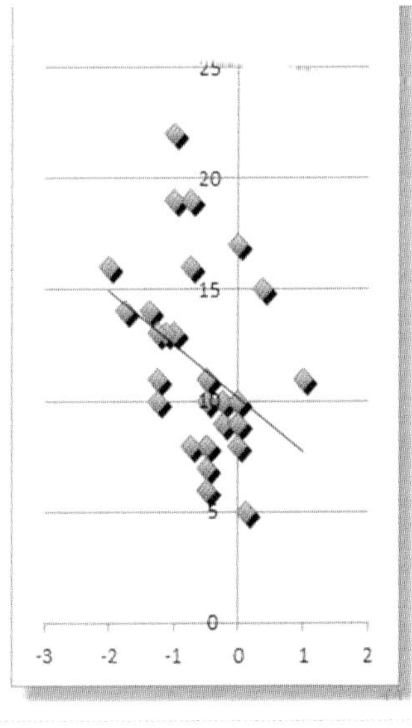

Fig. 7.22 LASIK (laser-assisted in-situ keratomileusis): Myopic laser and corneal epithelium. (a) We were able to establish that the central epithelium thinning is correlated with the value of the preop myopia. **(b)** Likewise, after myopic LASIK, we observed that when there is a regression of the optical effects, the central epithelium thickness increased.

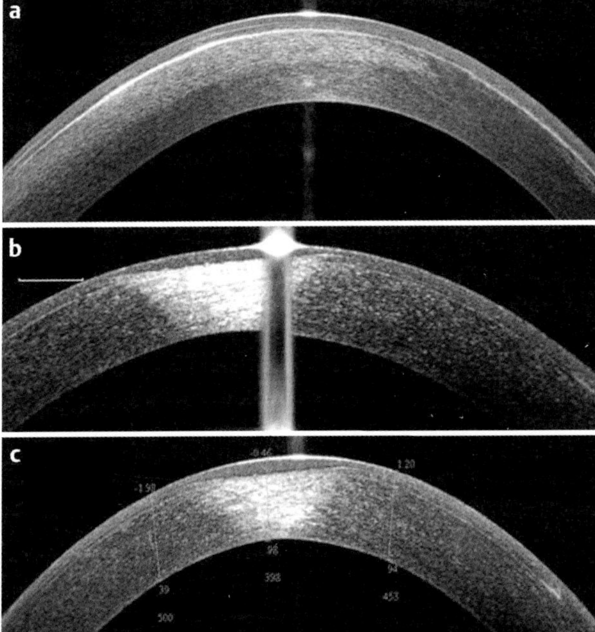

Fig. 7.23 Sands of Sahara (SOS) syndrome. A conclusive example of post-LASIK epithelial modification is depicted showing the evolution of an SOS syndrome after myopic LASIK. The apex inflammation zone **(a)** leads to stromal necrosis **(b, c)**, which is itself the cause of a central flattening that theoretically should lead to considerable hyperopia. In fact, in the present case, there is an apical epithelium proliferation that will more or less reshape a normal central corneal curvature and avoid development toward high hyperopia. In time, the stromal scars will practically clear and visual acuity will improve.

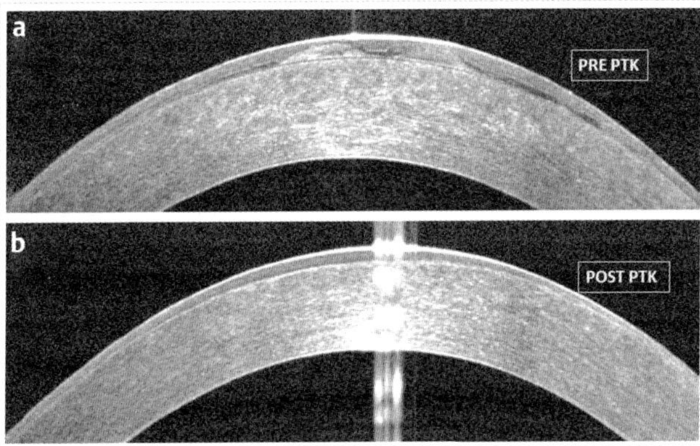

Fig. 7.24 Corneal dystrophies. A Cogan dystrophy before **(a)** and after **(b)** therapeutic photoablation (PTK). In this case, it was possible to evaluate preoperatively the transepithelial ablation depth to avoid following the flaws of the anterior curvature. The cornea was smoothed over and the optical properties restored.

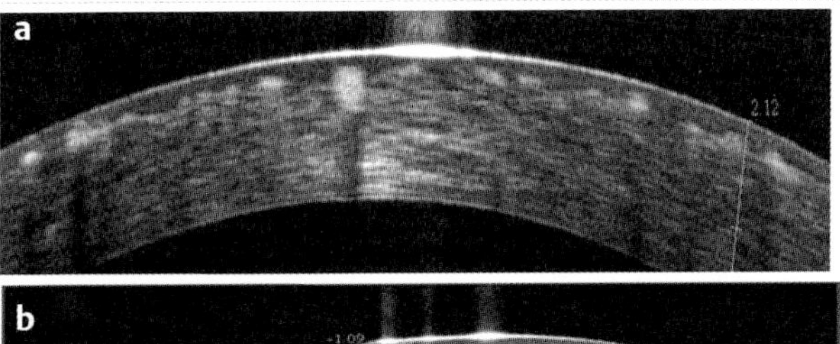

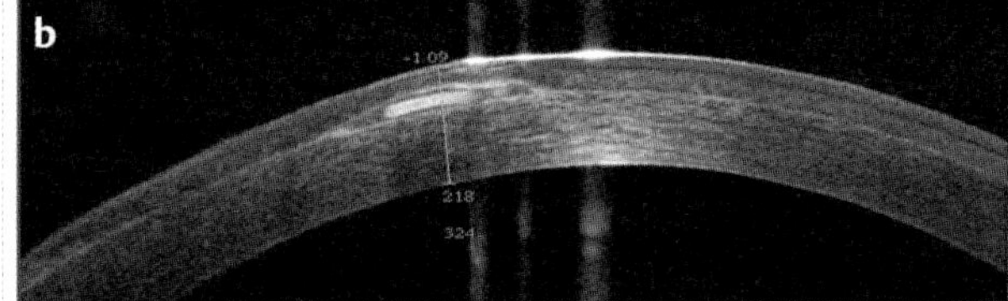

Fig. 7.25 (a) A Groenouw dystrophy with deep opacities that will require a pre-Descemet lamellar graft rather than a surface photoablation, generally limited to 200 µm, and often insufficient. **(b)** A recurring epithelial ingrowth is at the center of the cornea. The inflammatory reaction produced by this epithelial island is obvious as well as the thinning of the corneal flap opposite this lesion.

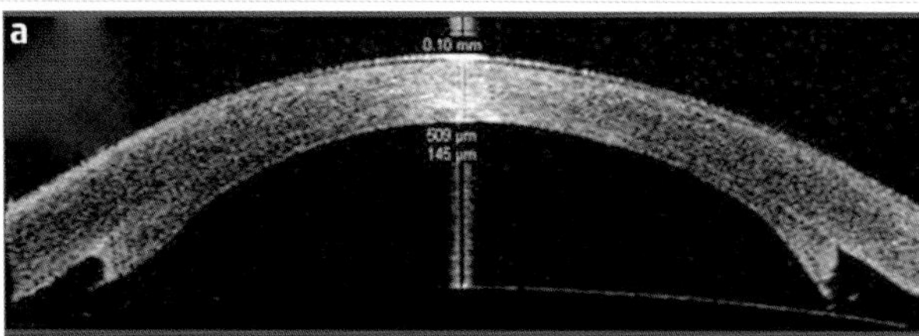
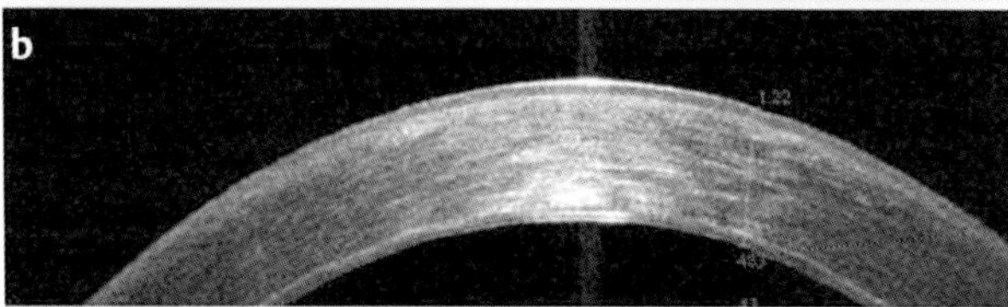
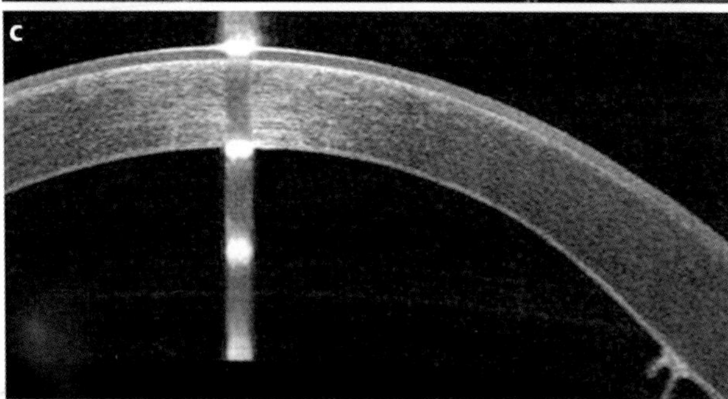

Fig. 7.26 Descemetic pathologies. The evolution of Descemetic grafts. **(a)** In the early days, obtaining donor graft tissue was done mechanically using a microkeratome; the grafts were thick with a meniscus shape (central thickness, 145 µm). **(b)** With the femtosecond laser, it is much easier to obtain very thin graft tissue (thickness, 43 µm). The visual result obtained is between a mechanical DSEK (Descemet Stripping Endothelial Keratoplasty) and a manual Descemet membrane endothelial keratoplasty. **(c)** To improve the results and produce thinner grafts, manual Descemetic dissection is possible but quite delicate. It gives a perfect postoperative anatomical aspect, and recovery is of better quality.

microns, and three-dimensional reconstruction of the structures under study. It is quite certain that this imaging system will, in daily practice, shortly replace ultrasound equipment for anterior segment exploration.

References

[1] Huang D, Swanson EA, Lin CP, et al. Optical coherence tomography. Science 1991; 254: 1178–1181

[2] Puliafito C, Hee MR, Schuman JS, et al. Optical Coherence Tomography of Ocular Diseases. Thorofare, NJ: Slack Inc; 1996

[3] Izatt JA, Hee MR, Swanson EA, et al. Micrometer-scale resolution imaging of the anterior eye in vivo with optical coherence tomography. Arch Ophthalmol 1994; 112: 1584–1589

[4] Baikoff G, Lutun E, Ferraz C, et al. Static and dynamic analysis of the anterior segment with optical coherence tomography. J Cataract Refract Surg 2004; 30: 1843–1850

[5] Baikoff G, Lutun E, Ferraz C, et al. Contact between 3 phakic intraocular lens models and the crystalline lens: an anterior chamber optical coherence tomography study. J Cataract Refract Surg 2004; 30: 2007–2012

[6] Baikoff G, Bourgeon G, Jitsuo Jodai H, et al. Pigment dispersion and Artisan phakic intraocular lenses: crystalline lens rise as a safety criterion. J Cataract Refract Surg 2005; 31: 674–680

[7] Baikoff G, Lutun E, Wei J, Ferraz C. Anterior chamber optical coherence tomography study of human natural accommodation in a 19-year-old albino. J Cataract Refract Surg 2004; 30: 696–701

[8] Baikoff G, Rozot P, Lutun E, Wei J. Assessment of capsular block syndrome with anterior segment optical coherence tomography. J Cataract Refract Surg 2004; 30: 2448–2450

[9] Baikoff G, Jitsuo Jodai H, Bourgeon G. Evaluation of the measurement of the anterior chamber's internal diameter and depth: IOLMaster vs AC OCT. J Cataract Refract Surg 2004; In press

[10] Baikoff G, Lutun E, Wei J, Ferraz C. Contact entre le cristallin naturel et différents modèles d'implants phakes: etude avec l'OCT de chambre antérieure: a propos de trois observations. [Refractive phakic IOLs: three differerent models and contact with the crystalline lens: an AC-OCT study]. J Fr Ophtalmol 2005; 28: 303–308

[11] Rozot P, Baikoff G, Lutun E, Wei J. Evaluation d'un syndrome de blocage capsulaire tardif avec l'OCT de segment antérieure [Evaluation of capsular block syndrome with an anterior segment OCT]. J Fr Ophtalmol 2005; 28: 309–311

[12] Baikoff G, Lutun E, Wei J, Ferraz C. Etude in vivo de l'accommodation naturelle chez un sujet albinos de 19 ans avec un tomographe à cohérence optique: a propos d'un cas [An invivo OCT study of human natural accommodation in a 19-year-old albino]. J Fr Ophtalmol 2005; 28: 514–519

[13] Baikoff G, Lutun E, Ferraz C, Wei J. Analyse du segment antérieur de l'oeil avec un tomographe à cohérence optique. Etude statique et dynamique [Analysis of the eye's interior segment with optical coherence tomography: static and dynamic study]. J Fr Ophtalmol 2005; 28: 343–352

[14] Baikoff G, Bourgeon G, Jodai HJ, Fontaine A, Vieira Lellis F, Trinquet L. Migrations pigmentaires après implant Artisan: importance de la flèche cristallinienne comme critère de sécurité [Pigment dispersion and Artisan implants: crystalline lens rise as a safety criterion]. J Fr Ophtalmol 2005; 28: 590–597

[15] Baikoff G, Jitsuo Jodai H, Bourgeon G. Evaluation de la mesure du diamètre interne et de la profondeur de la chambre antérieure: IOLMaster vs tomographe à cohérence optique de chambre antérieure. J Fr Ophtalmol 2005 (à paraître)

[16] Goldsmith JA, Li Y, Chalita MR, et al. Anterior chamber width measurement by high-speed optical coherence tomography. Ophthalmology 2005; 112: 238–244

[17] Linnola RJ, Findl O, Hermann B, et al. Intraocular lens-capsular bag imaging with ultrahigh-resolution optical coherence tomography Pseudophakic human autopsy eyes. J Cataract Refract Surg 2005; 31: 818–823

8 Corneal Inflammation and Optical Coherence Tomography

Dhivya Ashok Kumar and Amar Agarwal

8.1 Normal Corneal Texture

The normal cornea is seen as a homogeneous structure by optical coherence tomography (OCT). The usual corneal layers seen in conventional time-domain (TD) OCT are the epithelium, the stroma, and the endothelial layer (▶ Fig. 8.1). The epithelial layer is seen highly reflective as a result of the difference in the refractive indices of air and the cornea with overlying tear film. Stroma is seen below the epithelium as a homogeneous structure. The Bowman layer is not routinely seen in conventional TD OCT, although it may be seen in patients with corneal pathologies like ectasia or keratoconus in spectral or Fourier-domain (FD) OCT. The Descemet membrane is seen as highly reflective layer with the underlying endothelium in the posterior cornea. The high reflection is again due to the difference in the refractive indices of aqueous and endothelium.

8.2 Pathology in Corneal Inflammation

Keratitis may be produced by infectious organisms or by noninfectious stimuli. Microbial keratitis is a common, potentially sight-threatening ocular infection that may be caused by bacteria, fungi, virus, or parasites.[1] It is often assessed by the status of epithelium, type of stromal inflammation, and site of stromal inflammation. The intrinsic virulence of an organism relates to its ability to invade tissue, resist host defense mechanisms, and produce tissue damage. Bacterial invasion is facilitated by proteinases that degrade the basement membrane and extracellular matrix and cause cell lysis.[2] The proteases in keratitis cause degradation of the basement membrane, laminin, extracellular matrix, proteoglycan, and collagen. The infective organism may enter the cornea after trauma or surgery (refractive surgery) easily owing to the presence of a break in the epithelium.

8.3 Role of OCT in Keratitis

Anterior-segment OCT provides a range of qualitative and quantitative information for the assessment of microbial keratitis; serial standardized examination allows objective assessment of microbial keratitis and monitoring of the disease course.[3,4,5,6] Depending on the clinical stage, the parameters in the OCT scan change during the course of the disease. Serial scans can be carried out through the same area of the cornea by adhering to a scanning protocol. The common features noted in OCT are stromal thickness, epithelial integrity, infiltration dimensions, endothelial edema, Descemet changes, scar, or fibrosis. Corneal high-resolution mode is routinely used for corneal infiltration quantification. Both TD and FD OCT have been used widely in the recent past for prognosis of corneal infection.[3,4,5,6]

8.3.1 Early Stages of Inflammation

At the initial stages of microbial keratitis, even mild cases have a thickened cornea at the infiltrated area.[3] Inflammatory cells may appear to be hyperreflective in the corneal stroma in superficial and deep keratitis (▶ Fig. 8.2). In infection involving the deeper cornea and anterior chamber, it may be seen as aggregates on the endothelial surface (▶ Fig. 8.3).[7] Corneal ulcer prognosis can be observed by measuring the change in epithelial defect and infiltration thickness (IT) on serial OCT images. Stromal or corneal thickness is observed regularly during the course of treatment, and the decrease in corneal

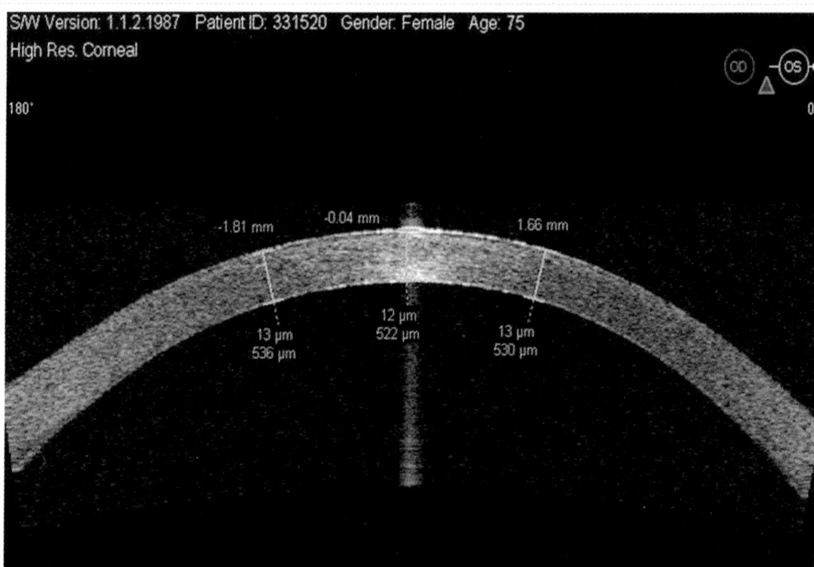

Fig. 8.1 Normal cornea as seen by time domain anterior-segment optical coherence tomography. OD, right eye; OS, left eye.

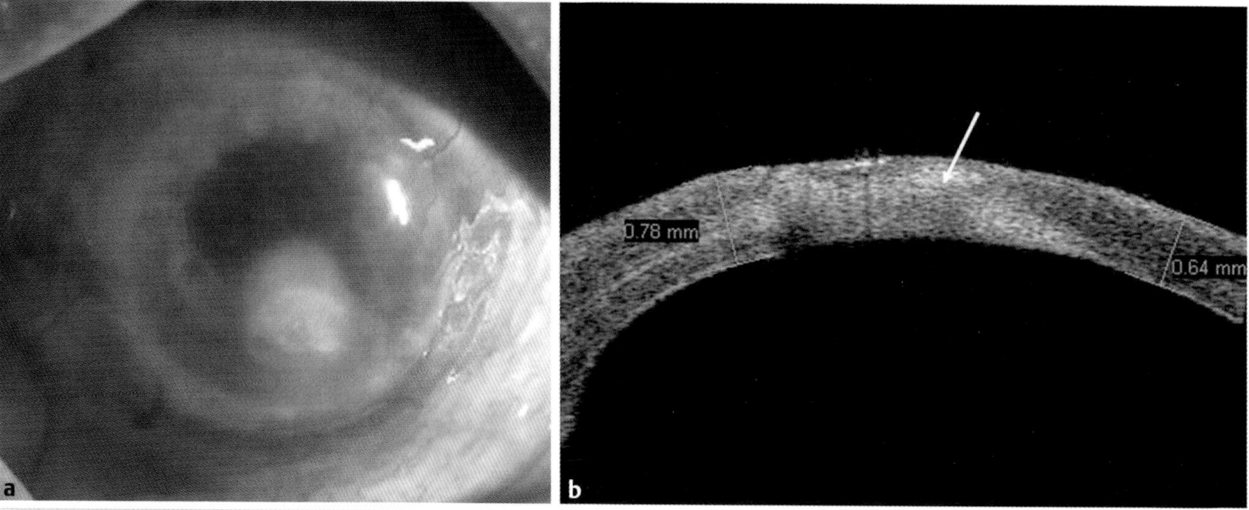

Fig. 8.2 **(a)** Corneal ulcer and **(b)** the corresponding anterior segment optical coherence tomography showing infiltration in stroma (arrow) with increased stromal thickness (0.78 mm).

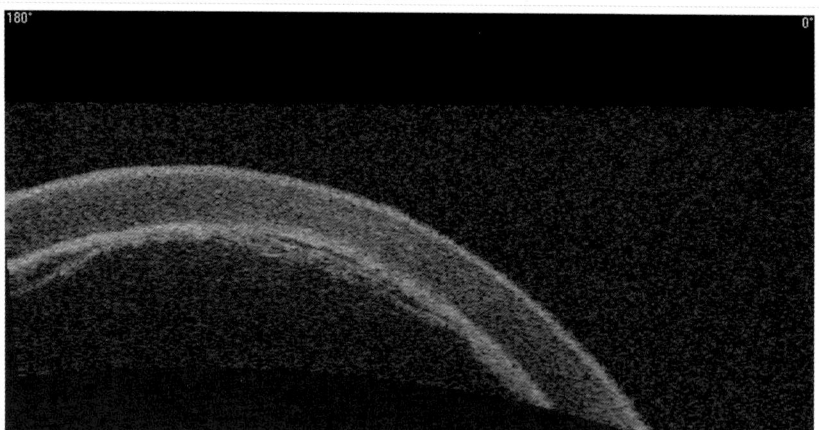

Fig. 8.3 Endothelial inflammation seen as aggregates on the endothelial surface with adjacent fibrinous reaction.

thickness shows response to treatment and resolution of inflammation. Epithelial healing can also be assessed by the absence of "heaped-up" layers and continuous regular reflection from the anterior surface. Anterior-surface OCT also can image and monitor the extent of stromal edema associated with the ulceration. Corneal stromal edema accompanying the ulcer can be visualized as diffuse or local thickening of stroma and increase in the convexity on the posterior surface (▶ Fig. 8.4). Infiltration of microbes and underlying tissue damage is noted as hyperreflective regions in the clear corneal surface (▶ Fig. 8.2). IT is an important parameter that aids in posttreatment monitoring. Descemet folds can be imaged as ruffles in the normally smooth endothelial surface (▶ Fig. 8.5).[3] In early corneal edema, the anterior chamber can be visualized for cellular reaction clearly by OCT, unlike the late stages.[7]

8.3.2 Advanced Inflammation

In advanced lesions, there can be stromal edema, corneal abscess, and diffuse corneal involvement. Severe infection can cause necrosis and liquefaction causing thinning of the affected cornea (▶ Fig. 8.6). Risk of perforation is present in advanced fungal infections (▶ Fig. 8.7). Advanced cases with endothelial inflammatory plaques can be measured using OCT. Measurement of the width of plaque or endothelial abscess (▶ Fig. 8.8) on serial scans allowed objective assessment of the disease course.

8.3.3 Healing Stage

At the later stages of the disease, scar tissue develops and the affected cornea may become thinner than the adjacent healthy tissue. Scar and fibrosis can produce a dense hyperreflective zone in the corneal stroma corresponding to the region of corneal opacity as seen by slit-lamp. Sometimes there can be adherent leukoma (▶ Fig. 8.9) in the chronic stages with synechiae. Long-standing scar can lead to calcareous degeneration or plaque formation. Dense opacification or thick exudates can prevent light from entering the cornea and causes back shadowing. Cornea with blood staining resulting from hyphema may also hinder infrared ray transmission.[7]

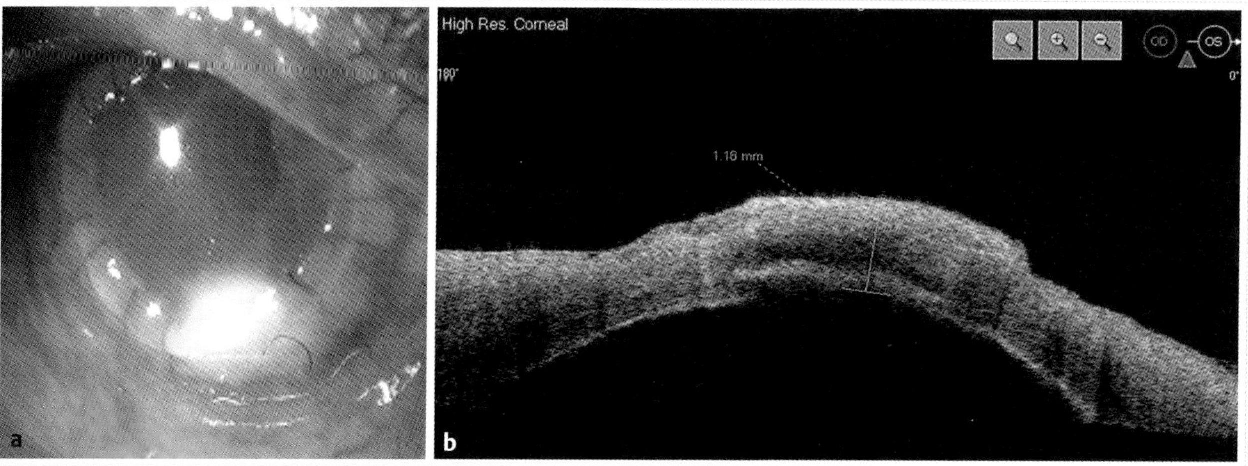

Fig. 8.4 (a) Post-penetrating keratoplasty stromal keratitis and (b) optical coherence tomogram showing deep corneal infiltration with necrosis.

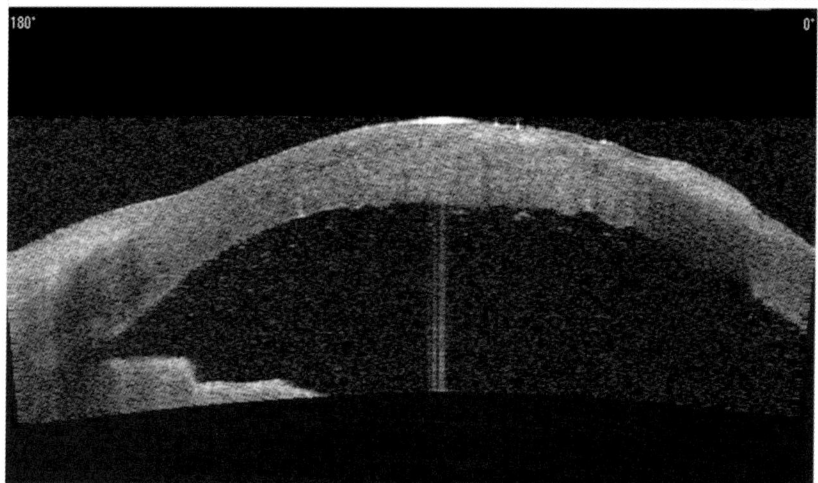

Fig. 8.5 Descemet folds seen on the endothelial surface in microbial keratitis.

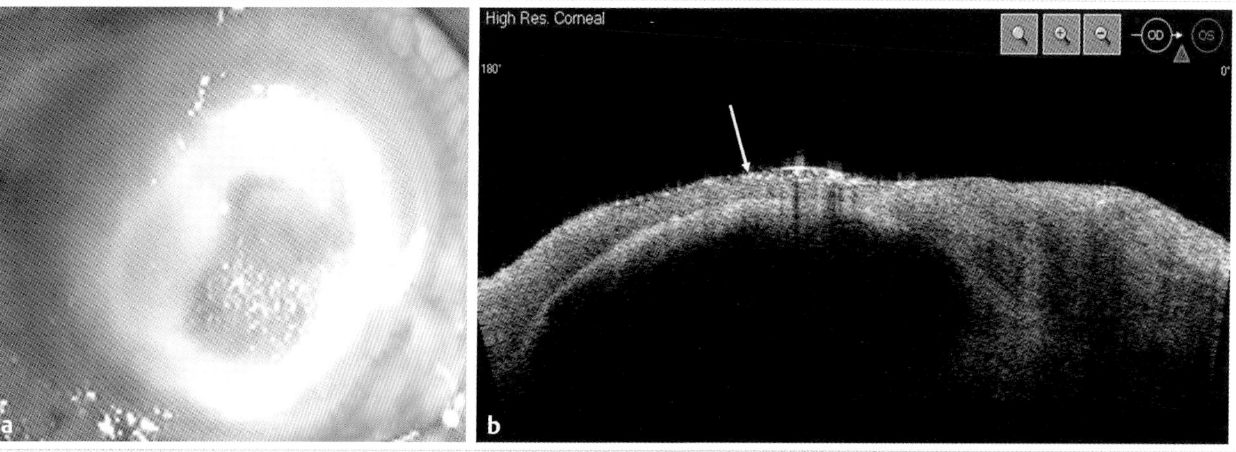

Fig. 8.6 (a) Sclerokeratitis with corneal necrosis in an female patient and (b) the corresponding thinning and stromal changes as seen in the optical coherence tomogram.

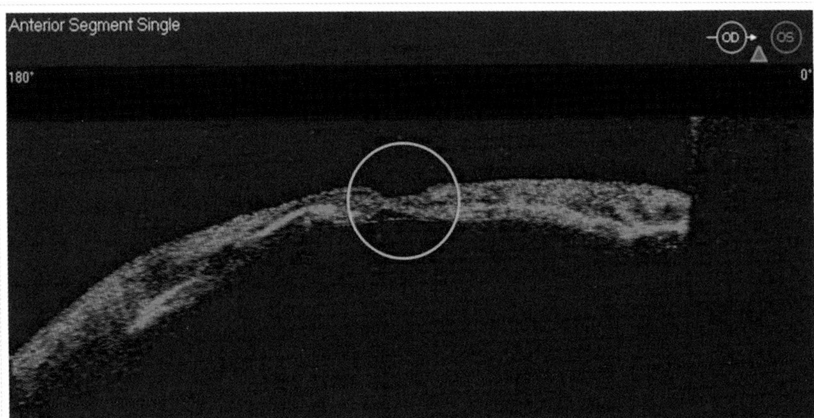

Fig. 8.7 Optical coherence tomogram showing the post-corneal infection perforation with pseudo-cornea formation (circled).

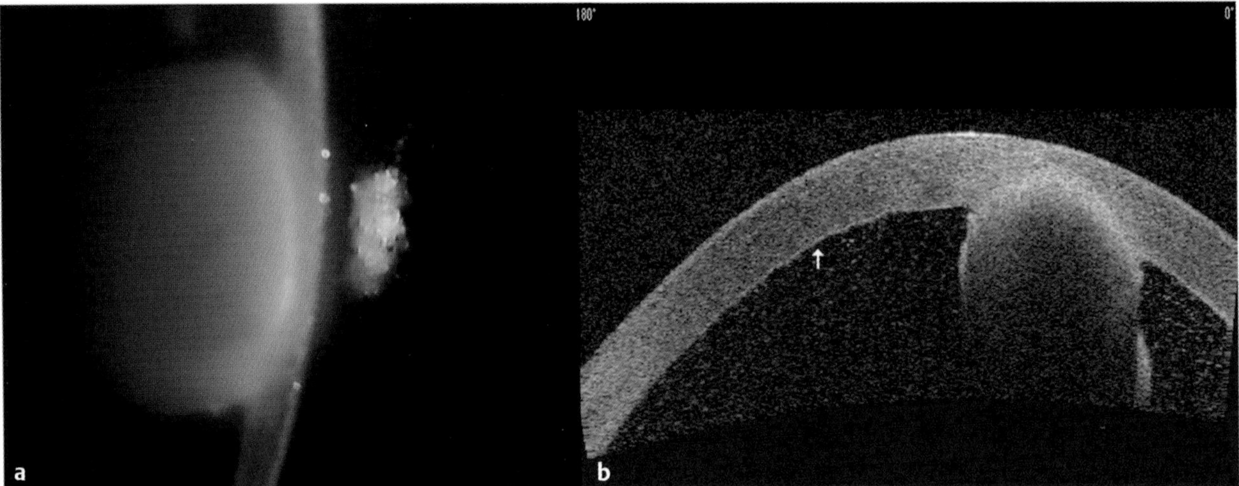

Fig. 8.8 (a) Endothelial abscess in an elderly male and (b) the corresponding OCT scan showing the abscess with infiltration in the posterior cornea and the anterior chamber.

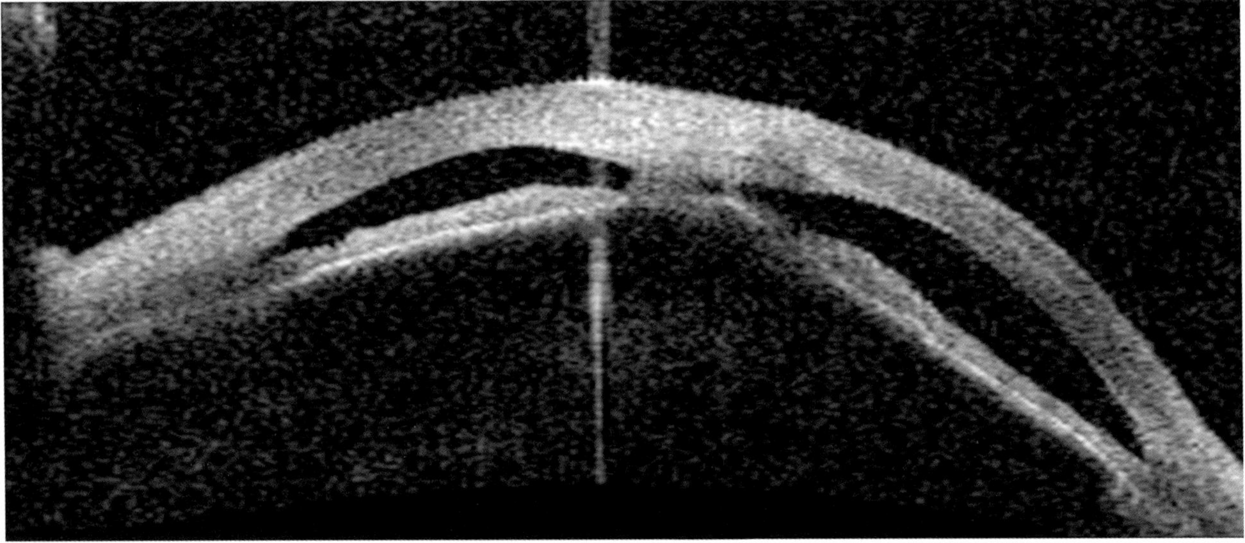

Fig. 8.9 Healed corneal ulcer with adherent leukoma. Note the pulled-up iris to the cornea and shallow anterior chamber.

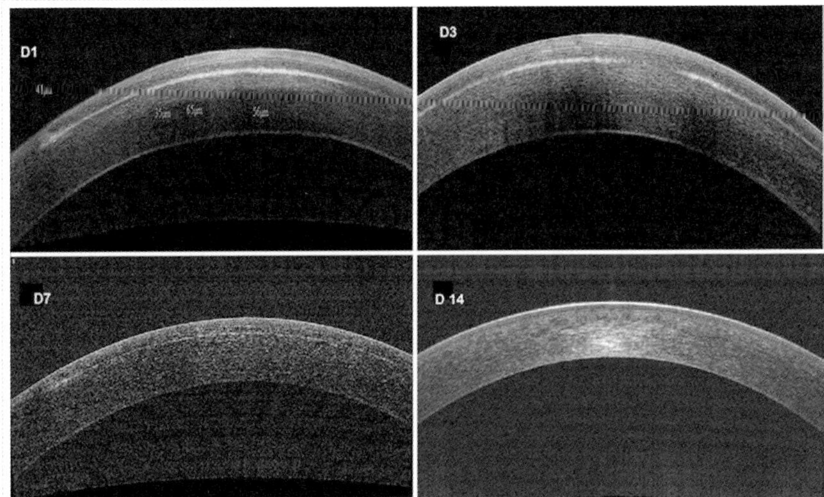

Fig. 8.10 High-resolution Fourier-domain optical coherence tomographic image of the cornea showing the infiltration and interface fluid on day 1 (D1), day 3 (D3), day 7 (D7), and 2 weeks (D14) of treatment.

8.4 Advantage of OCT in Corneal Infiltration

The average sizes of the neutrophils, monocytes, and lymphocytes in inflammation usually range from 10 to 20 mm.[8] Because of the higher resolution of OCT, it may be possible to note even early infiltration. TD OCT has an axial resolution of 18 µm compared with FD, which has a resolution of 5 µm. We have reported on the use of FD OCT in managing post-LASIK (laser-assisted (▶ Fig. 8.10) in-situ keratomileusis) inflammation.[6] The acquisition time of FD OCT is also less than with TD OCT. The number of scans taken by FD OCT is 26,000 A-scan, and TD OCT is 2048 scans; moreover, a three-dimensional image is possible in FD OCT.[6] Therefore, it is possible to document the volume and shape of the lesion in three dimensions. Anterior-segment OCT cannot replace slit-lamp examination, but it does provide information that may aid assessment. Endothelial plaque dimensions and posterior stromal infiltration dimensions can be quantified, even in edematous cornea. Qualitative assessment of the infiltration also is possible because the intensity of hyperreflectivity corresponds to the density of the infiltration on slit-lamp examination.

8.4.1 Anterior-Segment OCT for Prognosis

Instead of a single scan, serial OCT scans are recommended for assessment of response and prognosis after commencing the treatment.[3] OCT software calipers are used for quantification (in microns) of the parameters like infiltration and corneal thicknesses. In the early stages of microbial keratitis, clinical improvement is associated with reduction of IT. Decrease CT is also a necessary OCT parameter which shows the significant response to treatment. Increase in the IT or corneal thickness shows deterioration and no response to antimicrobials. This change may be detected on anterior-segment OCT before deterioration becomes clinically apparent. In postrefractive surgery inflammation, OCT can be used to assess the subflap infiltration thickness and prognosis associated wtih treatment (▶ Fig. 8.10).

8.4.2 Anterior-Segment OCT Assessment for Surgery Plan

In nonresponding microbial keratitis, the depth of involvement of cornea can be measured by OCT, which aids in elective planning for surgery such as corneal debridement or therapeutic penetrating keratoplasty. Corneal abscess, which progressively increases as seen by serial OCT scans, can move into the anterior chamber and therefore requires emergency evacuation with intracameral antibiotics (▶ Fig. 8.8). Eyes with localized postinfective stromal opacity involving the anterior cornea can be assessed by measuring the thickness involved, and anterior lamellar keratoplasty can be planned appropriately. Eyes with localized nonhealing corneal epithelial defect with irregular "heaped-up" margins may require elective amniotic membrane graft. Eyes with corneal edema hindering anterior-chamber evaluation can be seen for the depth of the anterior chamber and iris configuration.

References

[1] O'Brien TP, Green WR. Keratitis. In Mandell GL et al, ed. Principles and Practice of infectious Diseases, 4th ed. New York: Churchill Livingstone; 1995

[2] O'Brien T. Bacterial keratitis. In Krachmer JH, Mannis MJ, Hollane EJ, eds. Cornea, 3rd ed. St. Louis, MO: Mosby; 2011

[3] Konstantopoulos A, Kuo J, Anderson D, Hossain P. Assessment of the use of anterior segment optical coherence tomography in microbial keratitis. Am J Ophthalmol 2008; 146: 534–542

[4] Soliman W, Fathalla AM, El-Sebaity DM, Al-Hussaini AK. Spectral domain anterior segment optical coherence tomography in microbial keratitis. Graefes Arch Clin Exp Ophthalmol 2013; 251: 549–553

[5] Konstantopoulos A, Yadegarfar G, Fievez M, Anderson DF, Hossain P. In vivo quantification of bacterial keratitis with optical coherence tomography. Invest Ophthalmol Vis Sci 2011; 52: 1093–1097

[6] Ashok Kumar D, Prakash G, Agarwal A, Jacob S, Agarwal A. Quantitative assessment of post-LASIK corneal infiltration with frequency domain anterior segment OCT: a case report. Cont Lens Anterior Eye 2009; 32: 296–299

[7] Agarwal A, Ashokkumar D, Jacob S, Agarwal A, Saravanan Y. High-speed optical coherence tomography for imaging anterior chamber inflammatory reaction in uveitis: clinical correlation and grading. Am J Ophthalmol 2009; 147: 413–416, e3

[8] Williams WJ. Clinical evaluation of patient: approach to the patient. In: Williams WJ, Beutler E, Ersler AJ, Litchman MA, eds. Book of Hematology, 3rd ed. New York: McGraw Hill; 1983:11–19

9 Optical Coherence Tomography in Corneal Ectasia

Otman Sandali, Vincent Borderie, and Laurent Laroche

9.1 Keratoconus

Keratoconus is the most common primary ectatic corneal disorder. It is characterized by progressive corneal thinning, irregular astigmatism, and corneal protrusion that may eventually result in scarring and loss of vision. This disease is associated with stromal thinning, a decrease in keratocyte density, various amounts of stromal haze, Bowman layer disruption and splitting in the region of the cone, and epithelial changes.[1] Optical coherence tomography (OCT) provides an accurate assessment of corneal layers changes during keratoconus and should be performed systematically in association with topographic examinations in the evaluation of keratoconus eyes.

9.2 Keratoconus Screening

The diagnosis of moderate to advanced keratoconus is not difficult because of the characteristic topographic patterns. However, identification of forme fruste keratoconus (FFK) in patients with minimum or no clinical signs can be challenging. Preoperative accurate detection of keratoconus among refractive surgery candidates is crucial; FFK is the main cause of postoperative corneal ectasia after LASIK (laser-assisted in-situ keratomileusis) surgery.

Li and colleagues conducted a study using a time-domain OCT system to map pachymetry for keratoconus detection.[2] They determined the criteria for a diagnosis of keratoconus based on the first percentile or 99th percentile cutoff points of the normal range. These criteria include the following:

- Asymmetric parameters: superonasal-inferotemporal (SN-IT) or superior-inferior values greater than 45 µm
- Minimum corneal thickness < 470 µm
- Focal thinning parameter minimum: Maximum value < –100 µm

Early epithelial changes are present in subclinical cases of keratoconus. The epithelium is able to compensate fully for the subsurface cone, which is topographically evident on the back surface, resulting in an apparently normal anterior-surface topography.[3] Analysis of the corneal epithelial thickness profile may aid in the interpretation of corneal topography, improving the detection of FFK. In a recent study of 38 keratoconus cases, we demonstrated that the thinnest epithelial point was located inferiorly compared with the normal cornea and corresponded to the location of the thinnest corneal point on OCT pachymetry and the maximal posterior corneal elevation zone on corneal topography. The epithelial thickness of the thinnest point was thinner in FFK compared with that of normal corneas. A pattern of thin epithelium surrounded by a zone of epithelial thickening ("doughnut pattern") as described by Reinstein et al is suggestive of mild keratoconus (▶ Fig. 9.1).[3]

9.3 Keratoconus Evaluation

Many classifications of keratoconus based on the location of the cone, slit-lamp appearance, and indirect topographic patterns have been proposed in the literature; however, these classifications may have not taken into account direct corneal microstructure and histologic changes occurring during keratoconus

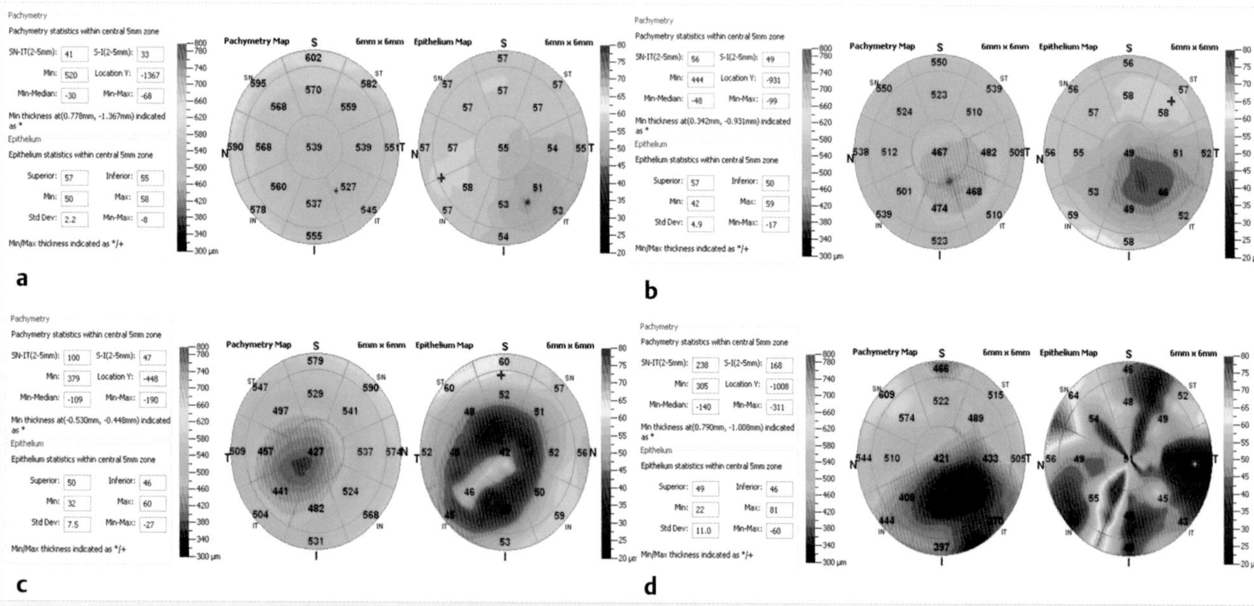

Fig. 9.1 Epithelial thickness map profile of keratoconic patients with various stages of severity. (a) Forme fruste keratoconus. The thinnest epithelial point is located inferiorly and measures 50 µm. **(b)** Pattern of thin epithelium surrounded by a zone of epithelial thickening (doughnut pattern) in mild keratoconus. **(c,d)** Epithelial thickening over the cone in advanced keratoconic eye.

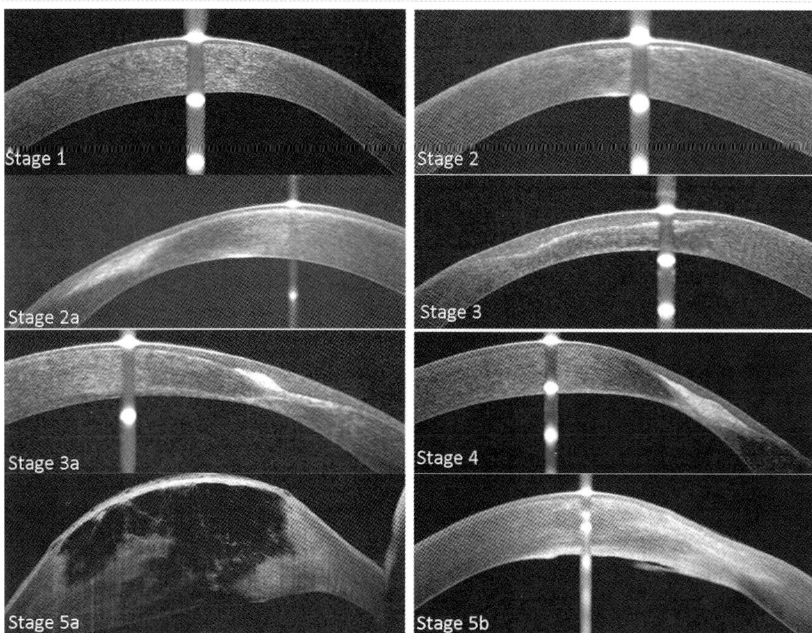

Fig. 9.2 Optical coherence tomography scans of keratoconic patients with various stages of severity and stages.

evolution. Indeed, a microstructural corneal analysis directly reflects abnormalities of corneal layers occurring in keratoconus and is more informative than the corneal topographic changes in the assessment of corneal architecture.

Recently, we established an OCT keratoconus classification based on structural corneal changes occurring at the conus as follows[4] (▶ Fig. 9.2):

- Stage 1: Thinning of epithelial and stromal layers at the conus. Corneal layers have a normal aspect.
- Stage 2: Hyperreflective anomalies occurring at the Bowman layer level (varying from a barely visible hyperreflective line to a hypertrophic scar) and epithelial thickening at the conus (3a, clear stroma; b, stromal opacities)
- Stage 3: Posterior displacement of the hyperreflective structures occurring at the Bowman layer level with increased epithelial thickening and stromal thinning (a, clear stroma; b, stromal opacities)
- Stage 4: Pan-stromal scar. In stage 4, when the residual stroma is thin, it acquires an hourglass-shaped scar with increased epithelial thickening.
- Stage 5. Represents the acute form of keratoconus (hydrops): 5a, acute onset, characterized by the rupture of the Descemet membrane with dilacerations of collagen lamellae, large fluid-filled intrastromal cysts, and the formation of epithelial edema; b, healing stage, pan-stromal scarring with a remaining aspect of Descemet membrane rupture.

Clinical and paraclinical characteristics of keratoconus eyes, including visual acuity, corneal epithelium and stromal thickness changes, corneal topography, biomechanical corneal characteristics, and microstructural changes observed on confocal microscopy were concordant with the OCT classification.

This OCT grading supports the original idea, stated by Chi, Katzin, and Teng, that the earliest ultrastructural changes in keratoconus occur at the epithelial basement membrane and Bowman layer.[1] These changes induce a complex imbalance between proinflammatory and anti-inflammatory cytokines, leading to keratocyte activation and corneal scar formation in advanced cases.

Vogt striaes were predominantly observed in stages 2 and 3. They have the aspect of dark parallel lines running through the stromal thickness between the Descemet and Bowman layers. Their appearance was similar to those observed in confocal microscopy, suggesting that these lines actually represent collagen lamellae under stress rather folds in the Descemet membrane (▶ Fig. 9.3).

9.4 Follow-up of Keratoconus Treatments

9.4.1 Crosslinking

Crosslinking (CXL) is the only treatment available to prevent the progression of keratoconus. This procedure is performed only in progressive keratoconus eyes. Currently, no definitive criteria for progression have been established, but parameters to consider are an increase of diopters in the steepest K-reading and/or the manifest cylinder or an increase of 0.5 diopters in spherical equivalent over 24 months. Contraindications include corneal thickness of less than 400 µm for standard treatment protocols, corneal scarring, a prior herpetic infection, and a history of poor epithelial wound healing, dry eye, and autoimmune disorders.

Thin corneas (< 400 µm) could be treated with modified protocols such as hypo-osmolar riboflavin and transepithelial riboflavin with superficial demarcation line. In this category of patients, OCT is an important tool in the preoperative assessment before CXL, permitting an accurate measurement of epithelial and stromal thicknesses. Epithelium thickening can mask the stromal thinning and compensate the corneal thickness when only total corneal pachymetry is performed. Indeed, we found that epithelium thickness had a negative correlation with stromal thickness in advanced keratoconus cases (▶ Fig. 9.1).

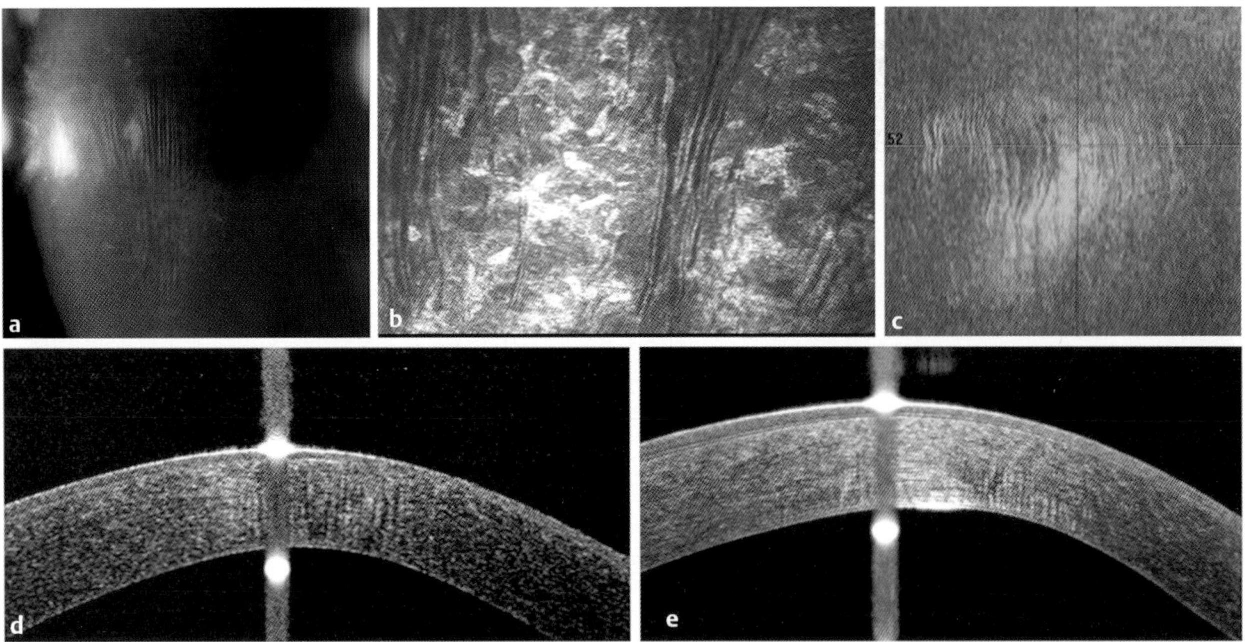

Fig. 9.3 (a) Aspect of Vogt striae in slit-lamp examination. **(b)** Confocal microscopy. **(c)** Optical coherence tomography (OCT): en face or frontal scans. **(d,e)** OCT (axial scans). They have the aspect of dark parallel lines running through the stromal thickness between the Descemet and Bowman layers.

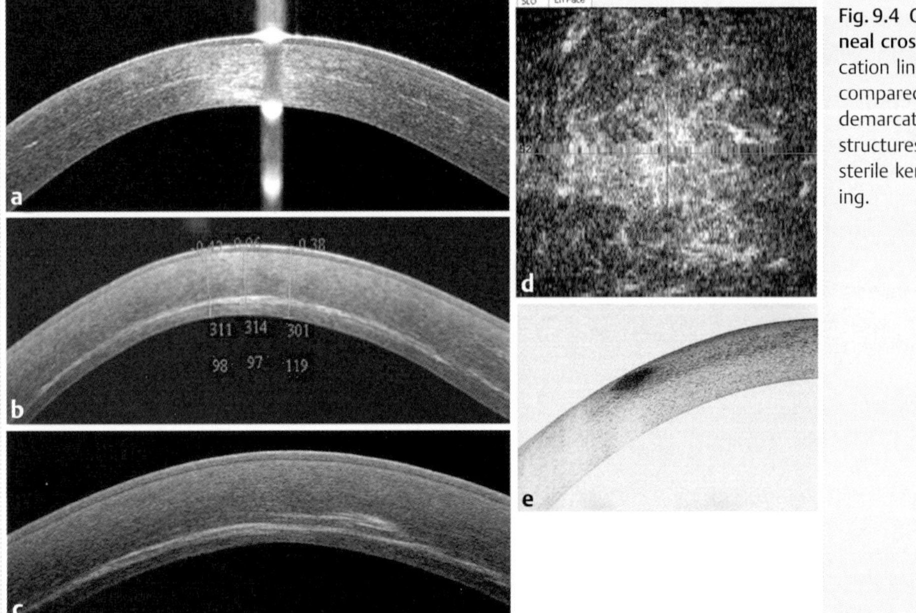

Fig. 9.4 Optical coherence tomography in corneal cross-linking. The corneal stromal demarcation line is deeper in **(b)** and **(c)** cases compared with **(a)**. **(d)** En face aspect of stromal demarcation line demonstrating hyperreflective structures. **(e)** A rare complication of peripheral sterile keratitis occurring after corneal crosslinking.

On OCT images (▶ Fig. 9.4), the corneal stromal demarcation line occurs 1 month after corneal CXL, probably indicating the efficiency of the procedure, and corresponds to the transition zone between the cross-linked anterior corneal stroma and the untreated posterior corneal stroma. Linear hyperreflectivities will be present at the anterior stroma, corresponding to keratocyte activation and synthesis of new collagen fibers.

A temporary anterior stromal haze is frequently seen and decreases between the third and the twelfth postoperative month. Peripheral sterile keratitis will occur rarely after CXL and resolves with topical steroid therapy. Infectious keratitis is associated mainly with CXL protocols with de-epithelialization and postoperative therapeutic contact lens wear.

9.4.2 Intracorneal Ring Implantation

Intracorneal inserts or implants are a minimally invasive surgical option that are used primarily for the treatment of keratoconus. The placement of Intacs corneal implants remodels and reinforces the cornea, thereby eliminating some or all of the

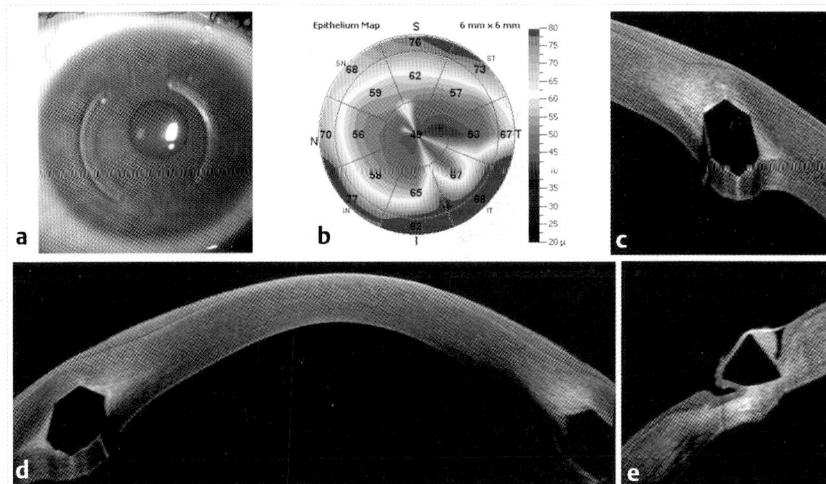

Fig. 9.5 **Intracorneal rings. (a)** Slit-lamp examination. **(b)** Epithelial map showing an epithelial thickening around the ring. **(c,d)** Corneal remodeling after ring implantation on optical coherence tomography. Next to the ring, there is a compression of stromal fibers, and the epithelium compensates the corneal irregularities maintaining the smoothness of corneal surface (epithelial thinning at the stromal protrusion and epithelial thickening around). **(e)** Extrusion of corneal ring segment.

irregularities caused by keratoconus. These implants are indicated in contact lens–intolerant patients who had a keratometry of < 60 diopters and a peripheral corneal thickness of > 450 µm with a clear cornea. The choice of the number of implanted rings (one or two), their diameters, and their thicknesses depends on the corneal topography and the cone location.[5]

The OCT provides more accurate corneal thickness measurements at the peripheral zone of implantation (6–7 mm) compared with topographic pachymetry, improving the results and the safety of the procedure. The best results seem to be obtained when the rings are introduced at 60 to 80% stromal thickness depth. The OCT highlights the anatomical remodeling after ring implantation. The central portion of the cornea becomes flatter. Next to the ring, there is a compression of stromal fibers, and the epithelium compensates for the corneal irregularities, maintaining the smoothness of the corneal surface (epithelial thinning at the stromal protrusion and epithelial thickening around) (▶ Fig. 9.5).

Potential complications of intrastromal ring implantation include accidental penetration through to the anterior chamber when forming the channel, postoperative corneal infection, and migration or extrusion of the segments.

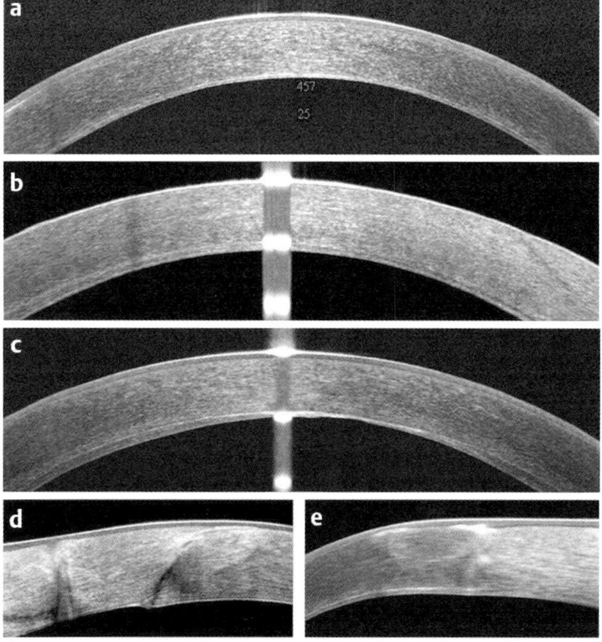

Fig. 9.6 Optical coherence tomography in corneal keratoplasty. (a) DALK (Deep anterior lamellar keratoplasty) (big-bubble technique). **(b)** KLAP (manual dissection with regular stromal interface). **(c)** KLAP (manual dissection with irregular stromal interface). **(d)** Recipient-graft junction in penetrating keratoplasty. **(e)** Better congruency at the recipient-graft junction in KLAP. The endothelium-Descemet membrane complex is continuous at the recipient-graft junction and is discontinuous in penetrating keratoplasty.

9.4.3 Corneal Keratoplasty

In cases of contact lens intolerance or central corneal scars, corneal transplantation is indicated for advanced keratoconus. Deep anterior lamellar keratoplasty (DALK) is currently considered the first-choice operative procedure in patients with severe keratoconus. Removal of the damaged corneal stroma may be achieved by manual dissection with a surgical blade and scissors, microkeratome-assisted lamellar cut, or femtosecond laser–assisted cut. Detachment of the Descemet membrane detachment from the corneal stroma can be achieved by using air injection (the "big-bubble" technique).

Compared with penetrating keratoplasty, long-term, model-predicted graft survival and endothelial densities are higher after DALK than after penetrating keratoplasty (PK). Endothelial immune reactions are prevented in DALK.

Visual recovery depends on postoperative astigmatism, stromal transparency, and the quality of the stromal interface (DALK).The big-bubble technique gives better results than does manual dissection and nearly similar results compared with PK.[6]

Use of OCT enables analysis of the quality of interface and measurement of the residual stroma in DALK (manual dissection) (▶ Fig. 9.6). At the recipient-graft junction, OCT shows an epithelial continuity at the corneal surface in PK (penetrating keratoplasty) and DALK (Deep anterior lamellar keratoplasty). There is a better congruency at the stromal junction in KLAP. The endothelium-Descemet membrane complex is continuous at the recipient-graft junction and is discontinuous in PK.

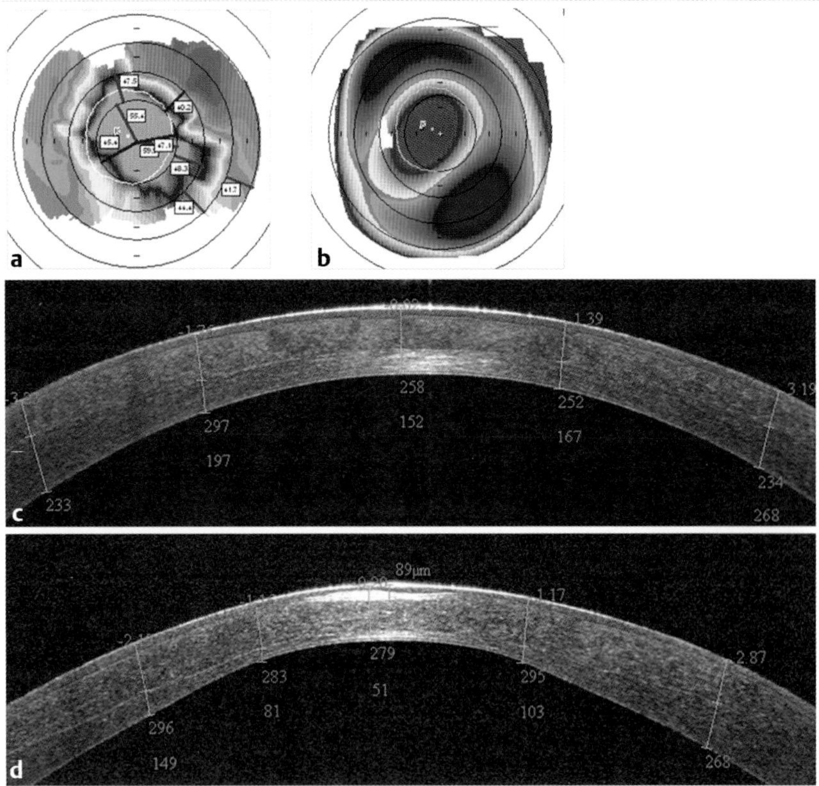

Fig. 9.7 Post-LASIK (laser-assisted in-situ keratomileusis) ectasia. **(a)** Topographic axial power map. **(b)** Posterior elevation map. **(c)** Optical coherence tomography provides accurate measurements corneal flap and residual stromal-bed thicknesses (152 µm). **(d)** Corneal scar at the Bowman layer level and epithelial thickening at the conus in an advanced case of post-LASIK corneal ectasia.

9.5 Other Corneal Ectatic Disorders

9.5.1 Post-LASIK Ectasia

Corneal ectasia is a serious complication of laser in-situ keratomileusis (LASIK). The main risk factors for postoperative corneal ectasia are undiagnosed keratoconus, a family history of keratoconus, preoperative corneal thickness < 500 µm, central keratometry > 47 diopters, age younger than 25 years, correction of myopia > 8 diopters, reverse astigmatism > 2 diopters, and residual posterior stromal bed < 250 µm.[7]

The OCT can accurately measure the corneal flap and the residual stromal bed thicknesses, explaining the cause of ectasia. The presence of Bowman layer anomalies and stromal scars on OCT in advanced cases indicates that the underlying disease is a nondiagnosed keratoconus decompensated by LASIK surgery (▶ Fig. 9.7).

9.5.2 Marginal Pellucid Degeneration

Pellucid marginal degeneration (PMD) is an idiopathic, progressive, noninflammatory ectatic corneal disorder characterized by a peripheral inferior band of corneal thinning in a crescent-shaped pattern (typically 4 o'clock to 8 o'clock). Similarities between PMD and keratoconus have led some ophthalmologists to consider PMD to be a peripheral form of keratoconus.

Distinguishing between the two entities is of potential clinical importance because they differ markedly in prognosis and management. The management of PMD is unique in that PMD is a progressive disease despite the fact that it is encountered in the third to fifth decade of life. Accordingly, corneal CXL should still be one of the treatment options. When intracorneal ring implantation is indicated in the management of PMD, caution should be given to the location of the inferior segment because it passes through the inferior thinned area. Corneal thickness at the thinnest point is more accurate in the pachymetry map provided by the OCT.

In PMD, corneal tomographic analysis reveals a flattening in the vertical meridian, inducing a significant against-the-rule astigmatism and a significant steepening around the area of maximum thinning with a classic aspect of claw pattern. The OCT shows a peripheral and inferior stromal thinning. The central cornea has a normal appearance. The corneal pachymetry map is important to differentiate keratoconus from PMD because PMD shows a lower, more peripheral corneal thinning in PMD (▶ Fig. 9.8).

9.5.3 Keratoglobus

Keratoglobus is a rare corneal disease characterized by limbus-to-limbus corneal thinning, often greatest in the periphery, with globular protrusion of the central cornea. Visual impairment in patients with keratoglobus can be profound owing to severe corneal ectasia, irregular astigmatism, and high myopia, and it may occur secondarily to corneal scarring and rupture.

The natural course of the disease is different from keratoconus. Corneal hydrops are exceptional. However, the evolution is marked by the risk of corneal perforation or rupture.

The OCT topographic map shows a generalized thinning of the cornea (only paracentral in keratoconus). The depth of the anterior chamber is markedly increased. Stromal opacities can occur in advanced cases (▶ Fig. 9.9).

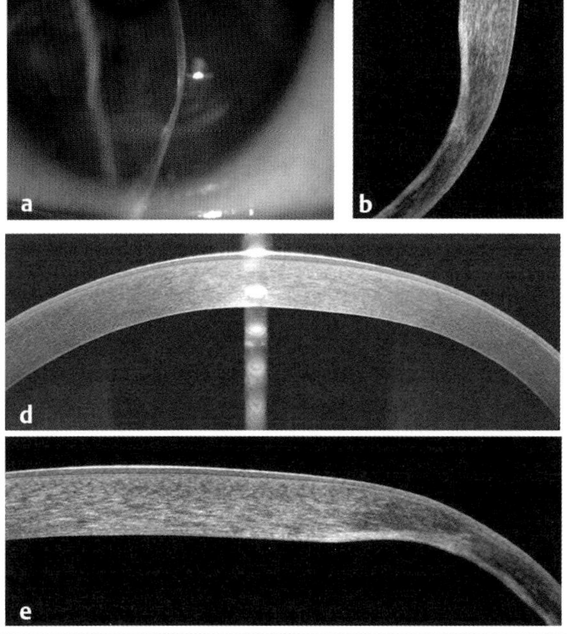

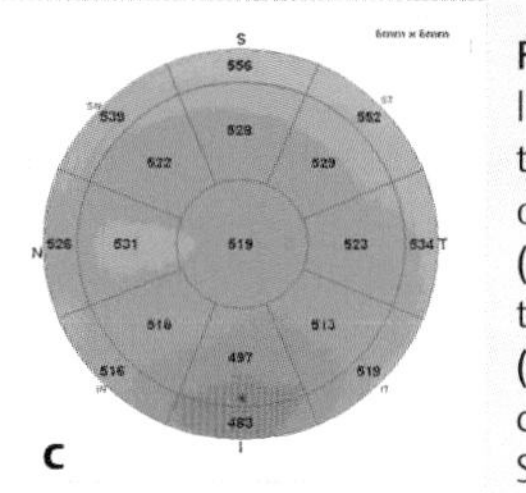

Fig. 9.8 Pellucid marginal degeneration. **(a)** Slit-lamp examination. **(b)** Corneal optical coherence tomography showing a peripheral inferior band of corneal thinning in a crescent-shaped pattern. **(c)** Pachymetry map showing a peripheral corneal thinning in comparison with keratoconus disease. **(d)** In contrast to the peripheral cornea, the central cornea has a normal appearance. **(e)** Stromal opacities in advanced case of pellucid marginal degeneration.

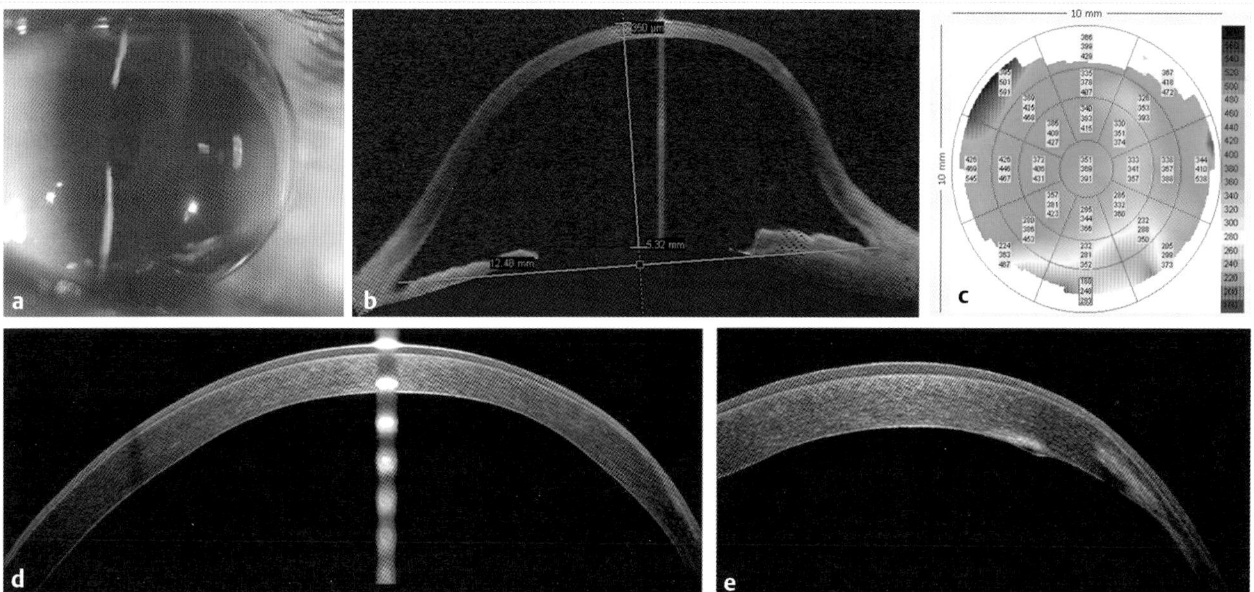

Fig. 9.9 Keratoglobus. **(a)** Slit-lamp examination showing a globular protrusion of the central cornea. **(b)** Anterior chamber is markedly increased on Visante optical coherence tomography (OCT). **(c)** Generalized corneal thinning on Visante OCT map. **(d)** OCT Optovue showing a thinning and protrusion of cornea. **(e)** Stromal and Descemetic lesions in an advanced keratoglobus case.

References

[1] Efron N, Hollingsworth JG. New perspectives on keratoconus as revealed by corneal confocal microscopy. Clin Exp Optom 2008; 91: 34–55

[2] Li Y, Meisler DM, Tang M, et al. Keratoconus diagnosis with optical coherence tomography pachymetry mapping. Ophthalmology 2008; 115: 2159–2166

[3] Reinstein DZ, Archer TJ, Gobbe M. Corneal epithelial thickness profile in the diagnosis of keratoconus. J Refract Surg 2009; 25: 604–610

[4] Sandali O, El Sanharawi M, Temstet C, et al. Fourier-domain optical coherence tomography imaging in keratoconus: a corneal structural classification. Ophthalmology 2013; 120: 2403–2412

[5] Lai MM, Tang M, Andrade EM, et al. Optical coherence tomography to assess intrastromal corneal ring segment depth in keratoconic eyes. J Cataract Refract Surg 2006; 32: 1860–1865

[6] Borderie VM, Sandali O, Bullet J, Gaujoux T, Touzeau O, Laroche L. Long-term results of deep anterior lamellar versus penetrating keratoplasty. Ophthalmology 2012; 119: 249–255

[7] Randleman JB, Woodward M, Lynn MJ, Stulting RD. Risk assessment for ectasia after corneal refractive surgery. Ophthalmology 2008; 115: 37–50

10 Spectral-Domain Anterior-Segment Optical Coherence Tomography in Refractive Surgery

Karolinne Maia Rocha and Ronald R. Krueger

Optical coherence tomography (OCT) is a promising imaging device in refractive surgery because of its real-time, high-speed, and noncontact features. OCT allows for high-resolution, cross-sectional scans and two- and three-dimensional (3-D) reconstructions of the cornea, iris, anterior-chamber angle, and lens as well as 3-D optical biometry.[1,2,3,4,5,6,7,8] OCT images are acquired by measuring the intensity and time delay of wave lights diffracted from anatomical structures passing through an established reference path.[8]

Spectral-domain OCT (SD OCT) systems use a charge coupled device camera to register the diffraction grating of wave lights returning from the eye structures. The time delay and intensity of the wave lights are processed using a mathematical formula (Fourier transformation). The effective acquisition speed is 26,000 axial scans per second, which is up to 100 times faster than the first-generation time-domain (TD) OCT systems. The system operates at 830 nm.[9] Implications of the increased speed and sensitivity offered by SD OCT are images with lower signal-to-noise ratio compared with TD OCT and high axial resolution.[8,9,10,11,12] A wide-angle anterior-segment adaptor (CAM-L mode) for the RTVue-100 OCT (Optovue, Inc., Fremont, CA) provides denser pixel cross-sectional imaging of the cornea and anterior segment with an axial resolution of 5 µm and transverse resolution of 15 µm.[10]

A custom-developed SD OCT system, including full distortion correction (fan and optical), as well as segmentation and merging of the different volumes (cornea, iris, and lens), was built to process and generate high-resolution 3-D images.[1,2,13,14,15,16,17] The main features of this device are its 840-nm (50-nm bandwidth) super luminescent diode (SLD) illuminating source; a spectrometer with a 4096-pixel line CMOS (complementary metal-oxide semiconductor) camera; an axial pixel resolution of 3.4 µm; and a predicted axial resolution of 6.9 µm. As a result, 3-D biometrical quantification of the anterior segment can be generated.

Three-dimensional epithelial and total corneal maps can be generated by interpolating thickness profiles from multiple meridians.[18] In addition, SD OCT-based corneal tomography and visualization of all corneal layers by high-resolution cross-sectional scans are essential tools for evaluating refractive candidates, including screening and risk of ectasia assessment, progression of corneal ectasia, corneal collagen crosslinking, intrastromal corneal rings and inlays, custom ablation profiles, and presbyopic treatments.

10.1 Refractive Surgery Screening and Corneal Ectasia Risk Scoring System

One of the most important screening strategies in refractive surgery is to identify risk factors for corneal ectasia and to minimize its occurrence. Several Placido-based computerized video keratoscopy indices have been described for the diagnosis of keratoconus.[19,20,21] The diagnosis and progression of keratoconus are based on clinical features and anterior corneal curvature data as classically seen with the Amsler-Krumeich classification.[22] Over the last few years, a comprehensive corneal analysis from the anterior and posterior corneal curvature and full pachymetric data has been used for preoperative refractive screening and early detection signs of keratoconus. New corneal tomography parameters using rotating Scheimpflug devices[23,24,25] and slit-scanning elevation topography[26] have shown changes on both the posterior cornea and/or corneal thickness map as earlier indicators of corneal ectasia.

Spectral-domain OCT measures the anterior and posterior cornea curvature in addition to qualitative and quantitative analysis of the relationship of the corneal epithelium and stroma that can be expressed as topographic thickness variations. The Optovue RTVue-CAM (Optovue, Inc., Fremont, CA) pachymetry-corneal power software (Cpwr), with 1024 axial scans and 6-mm diameter scanning, measures the cornea in eight meridians. The high-resolution, cross-sectional scans are repeated five times and averaged to generate the pachymetry maps. The air-tear interface and the epithelial-Bowman layer landmark were identified automatically by a computer algorithm to generate the epithelial thickness maps, as described by Li et al.[27] The corneal pachymetry map and epithelial thickness map are divided into zones by octants and 2-, 5-, and 6-mm annular rings. The map is obtained in 0.32 seconds and comprises eight meridional scans. The average of 6-mm paracentral pachymetry measurements of superior (S), inferior (I), temporal (T), nasal (N), superotemporal (ST), superonasal (SN), inferotemporal (IT), and inferonasal (IN) zones are displayed. The central measurement corresponds to the average pachymetry of the central 2 mm. The pachymetry map also includes minimum corneal thickness and location, anterior and posterior corneal power and curvature radius, and total corneal power (▶ Fig. 10.1). In previous studies, SD OCT pachymetry maps have shown high reproducibility in detecting eccentric and asymmetric corneal thinning in keratoconus.[27] Recently, an SD OCT pachymetry map–based keratoconus risk scoring system was developed based on these pachymetric variables.[28]

Additionally, the cross-sectional high-resolution scans can show localized areas of epithelial compensation overlying areas of stromal thinning in keratoconus (▶ Fig. 10.2). SD OCT high-resolution cross-sectional scans demonstrated significant regional variability in corneal epithelial thickness profiles, as well as greater patterns of thickness deviation in eyes with keratoconus and postoperative corneal ectasia, compared with normal eyes.[28,29,30] ▶ Fig. 10.3 shows two patients with inferior steepening seen on Placido-based corneal topography; SD OCT epithelial thickness map shows localized zone of epithelial thinning surrounded by thickened epithelium over the region of the cone in keratoconus and thickened epithelium, corresponding to the area of inferior steepening seen on topography, in

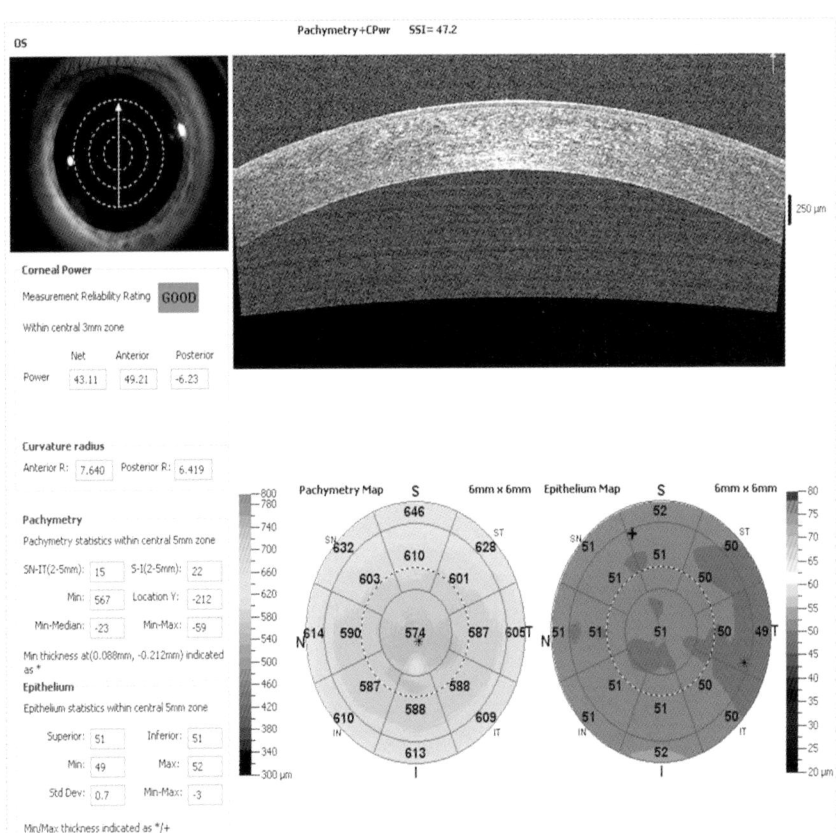

Fig. 10.1 Spectral-domain optical coherence tomography CAM-L raster module scan (6-mm pachymetry + corneal power scans, Optovue RTVue-100) display of a normal cornea, including pachymetry map, epithelial thickness profile map, and corneal power.

corneal warpage. Analysis of the epithelial thickness profile can be used as an adjunctive tool in refractive screening and possible early detection of keratoconus.

10.2 Epithelial Thickness Remodeling in Refractive Surgery

Recently, detailed analysis of the corneal epithelial thickness profile in laser-assisted in-situ keratomileusis (LASIK) using SD OCT has been described.[31,32] The corneal epithelium has a fast turnover, and compensatory changes of the corneal epithelium help to generate a smoother corneal surface in the setting of irregularities of the underlying stroma.[29,30,31,32,33,34,35]

We evaluated epithelial thickness remodeling and changes in the flap architecture after myopic LASIK using high-resolution SD OCT to correlate the anatomical findings to the preoperative spherical equivalent manifest refraction and refractive outcomes.[31] ▶ Fig. 10.4 shows the air-tear film interface and the epithelial-Bowman layer landmark automatic segmentation and reconstruction, as described by Li et al[36]; the distance between the anterior surface of the cornea and the flap-stroma interface were manually detected to generate flap-thickness maps (see *LASIK Flap Mapping by Spectral-Domain OCT* section).

Forty myopic eyes were included in this prospective, randomized, contralateral eye study. The preoperative manifest refraction ranged from −1.00 to −7.25 diopters (mean −3.25 ± 1.9). Flap creation was randomized between eyes by using the IntraLASE FS60 (IL, Abbott Medical Optics, Irvine, CA) in one eye and WaveLight FS200 (FS, Alcon Laboratories Inc., Fort Worth, TX) in the contralateral eye, and all eyes were treated with the ALLEGRETTO Eye-Q excimer laser (Alcon Laboratories Inc.). SD OCT (Optovue RTVue-100, Fremont, CA) was used to evaluate the epithelial and flap thickness profiles and corneal power preoperatively and at 1 week, 1 month, 3 month, and 9 months postoperatively. Statistically significant epithelial thickening was observed in both the IL and FS groups as early as 1 month postoperatively (P = 0.033 and P=0.042), but this thickening stabilized between 3 (P=0.042 and P=0.035) and 9 months postoperatively (P = 0.043 and P=0.041) (▶ Fig. 10.5). The magnitude of epithelial and flap thickness remodeling correlated to the preoperative spherical equivalent refraction. We found a statistically significant correlation between the magnitude of preoperative myopic refraction and the central epithelial thickness at 1, 3, and 9 months (Pearson correlation coefficients 0.485, 0.587, and 0.576) (P=0.0021, 0.0010, and 0.0011), respectively. Additionally, the corneal power change reconstructed from the SD OCT maps showed steepening at 3 and 9 months, in correlation with both the thicker epithelium and a mild myopic shift in manifest and wavefront refraction.

The use of SD OCT in refractive surgery is important to recognize the initial instability seen after LASIK and to characterize the spatial relationship of epithelial remodeling with refractive outcomes. We think the pattern of epithelial remodeling with different ablation profiles should be considered in the future planning of customized excimer laser ablations, including topography-guided, wavefront-guided, and multifocal presbyopic excimer laser treatments.

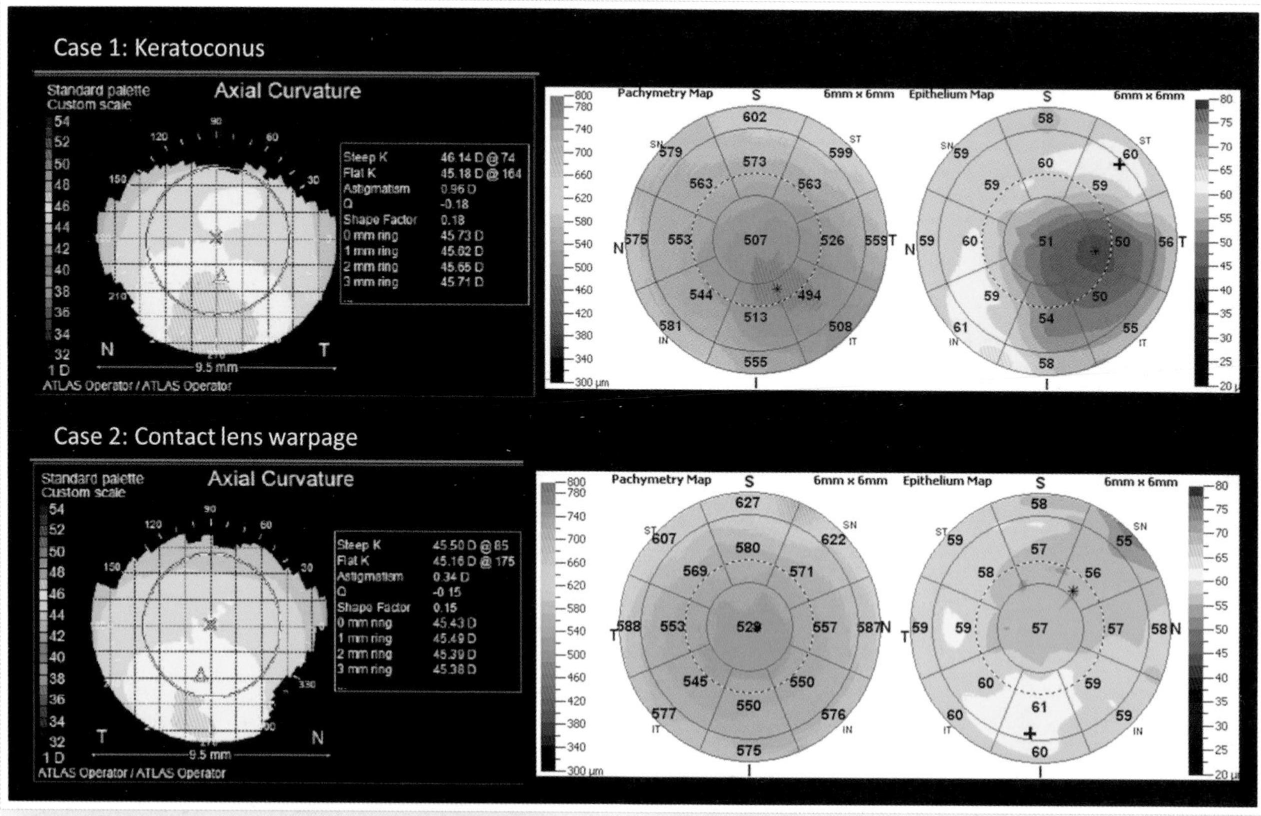

Fig. 10.2 Corneal topography and spectral-domain optical coherence tomography epithelial thickness profile map in corneal warpage and keratoconus. Epithelial thickness map shows localized zone of epithelial thinning over the region of the cone in keratoconus and thickened epithelium corresponding to the area of inferior steepening seen on topography in corneal warpage.

10.3 LASIK Flap Mapping by Spectral-Domain OCT

The lamellar distribution of collagen in the anterior and peripheral corneal stroma adjacent to the Bowman layer has higher cohesive tensile strength compared with the posterior stroma, presenting the sub-Bowman region as the strongest area of the cornea.[37,38,39] As a result, femtosecond laser–assisted LASIK flaps that are thin and planar, and particularly small-incision lenticule extraction procedures, minimize biomechanical changes in the cornea.[40,41,42,43] Residual stromal bed measurements are useful when planning LASIK enhancements to avoid deeper ablations into the posterior stroma. For these reasons, advanced imaging of the predictability of refractive procedures should be incorporated into clinical practice.

Spectral-domain OCT high-resolution cross-line scan of the add-on lens can easily identify the posterior edge of the LASIK flap. Traditionally, one-dimensional measurements of the distance between the anterior surface of the cornea and the flap-stroma interface using high-resolution cross-sectional scans are used to asses flap thickness.[44,45,46,47,48,49,50,51,52,53,54,55] Pachymetric LASIK flap maps can be generated by SD OCT. In our study, the flap boundaries were manually detected and inspected, and nine points were manually measured in eight meridians to generate the flap-thickness profile maps.[31] The automated algorithm built into the RTVue software was used to interpolate the high resolution scans. The color scale ranged from 20 to 80 µm for the epithelial thickness maps and from 70 to 140 µm for the flap thickness profile maps (▶ Fig. 10.4).

In correlation with the changes in epithelial thickness observed at 1 week, 1 month, 3 months, and 9 months after myopic LASIK, comparable variations in femtosecond laser flap thickness profiles were seen in both the IL and FS laser groups. Progressive thickening of the femtosecond LASIK flaps was observed up to 3 months after femtosecond LASIK (▶ Fig. 10.6). No statistically significant difference was found for the IL and FS lasers flaps at 1 week ($P = 0.08$) and 1 month postoperatively ($P = 0.07$). Femtosecond-LASIK flaps were thicker in the IL group compared with the FS group at 3 and 9 months postoperatively ($P = 0.003$ and $P = 0.005$, respectively).

10.4 Advances in Anterior-Segment Biometry and Intraocular Lens Calculation

The two main sources of error in intraocular lens (IOL) power calculation after refractive surgery are measurements of the postoperative corneal power by standard keratometry and topography and IOL formula limitations based on inaccurate estimation of the effective lens position (ELP),[56,57,58,59,60,61,62,63,64,65] which is the distance between the vertex of the cornea to the plane of the IOL. Keratometers and topographers do not precisely measure the central cornea power, and corneal tomographers extrapolate curvature data based on elevation measurements relative to a reference shape. As a result, measurements of the cornea power (K) after refractive surgery tend to overestimate the K readings after laser corrections for myopia and to underestimate for hyperopia. Third-generation formulas (e.g., SRK T, Holladay 1, Hoffer Q) predict the ELP based on the axial length and keratometry. Using these formulas, a flat K power will produce a false shallow postoperative ELP, resulting in underestimation of the calculated IOL power and a hyperopic error.

The measurement of both the anterior and posterior corneal surfaces and the anterior and posterior lens by SD OCT systems allows three-dimensional quantification of the cornea, anterior chamber depth, lens, and effective IOL

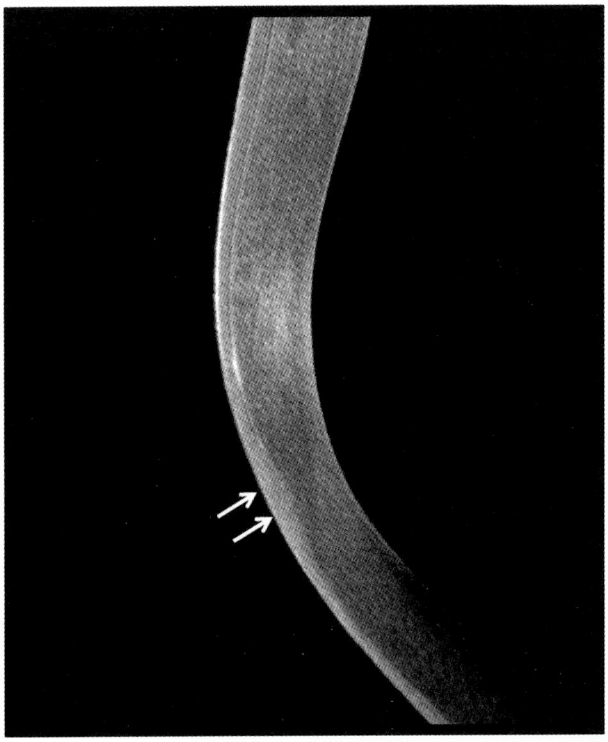

Fig. 10.3 Spectral-domain optical coherence tomography cross-sectional high resolution scans across the central 6-mm of the corneal apex in the vertical meridian in keratoconus. Regional epithelial thickness profile variability, with localized areas of thickened and thinned epithelium can be observed. Nasal (N), temporal (T), superior (S).

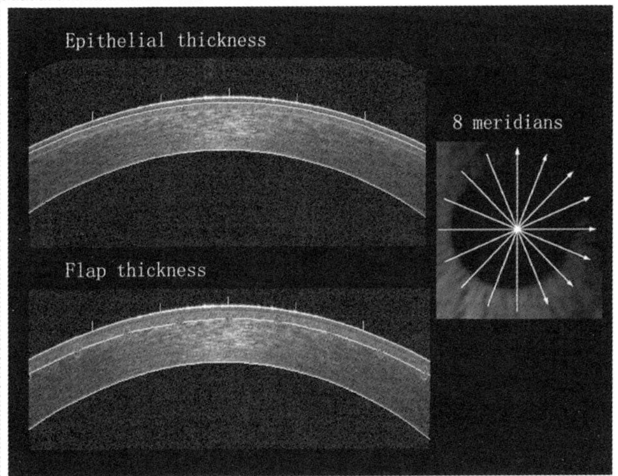

Fig. 10.4 Cross-sectional spectral-domain optical coherence tomography (SD OCT) high-resolution scans reveal epithelial and flap thickness profiles along eight radial meridians to generate epithelial thickness and femtosecond laser-assisted in-situ keratomileusis flap (LASIK) SD OCT maps (black arrows).

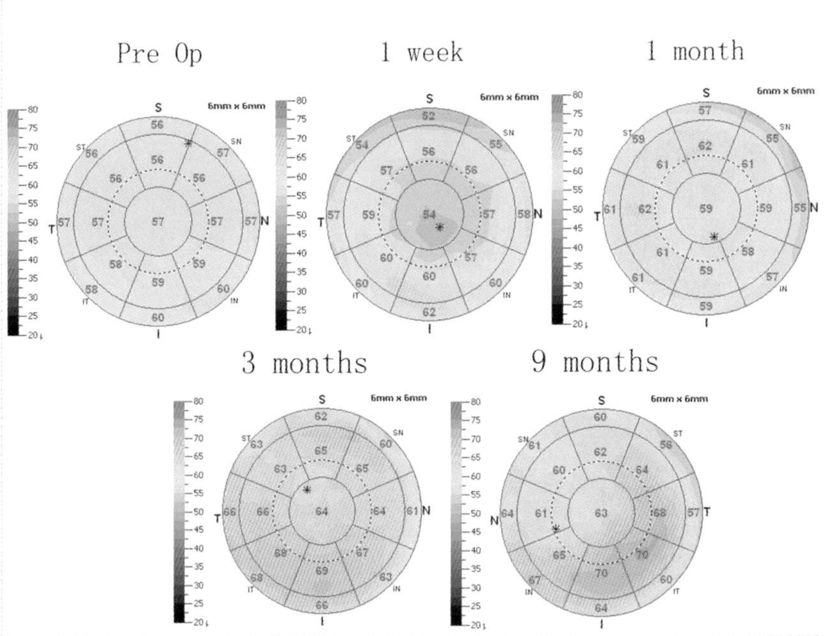

Fig. 10.5 Epithelial thickness profile mapping seen preoperatively, 1 week, 1 month, 3 and 9 months after femtosecond laser–assisted in-situ keratomileusis (LASIK) for myopia. SN, superonasal; ST, superotemporal. Nasal (N), temporal (T), superior (S), inferior (I).

position.[15,16] Additionally, SD OCT provides for the true corneal power calculation. SD OCT measurements of the central corneal power after myopic LASIK and radial keratotomy are lower than conventional keratometry; therefore, an OCT-based formula based on an optical vergence model of the eye (paraxial approximation of Gaussian optics) should be used.[66,67,68] In a pilot study, Tang et al showed that SD OCT–based IOL power calculation had better predictive accuracy than the clinical history method and was equivalent to the Haigis-L formula in postmyopic LASIK eyes.[66] 3-D OCT optical biometry and 3-D anterior segment reconstruction are promising tools for ELP, IOL tilt, and decentration evaluation.[16]

10.5 Advanced Spectral-Domain OCT Imaging: Case Report

A 42-year-old right-eye-dominant man was referred for evaluation of epithelial ingrowth in the right eye. The patient underwent myopic LASIK in both eyes in 2000 and LASIK flap lift enhancement in the right eye in March 2013 for mild myopic regression. At initial consultation, the patient reported blurred vision at distance and near in the right eye for about 1 week after the LASIK enhancement. Best-corrected visual acuity (BCVA) was 20/30 in the right eye and 20/15 in the left eye, with manifest refraction of −0.50 + 2.00@58 in the right eye and plano in the left eye. ▶ Fig. 10.7 shows the anterior-segment

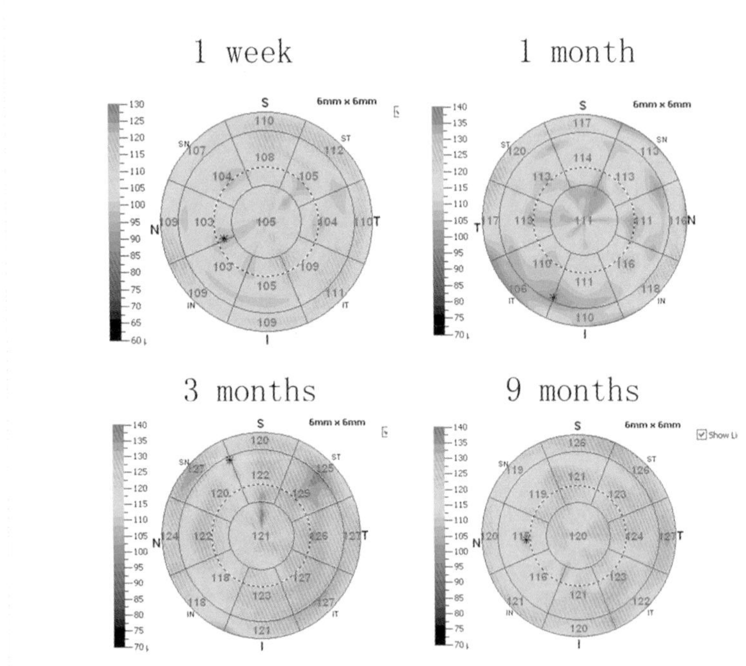

Fig. 10.6 Flap thickness profile mapping at 1 week, 1, 3, and 9 months post femtosecond laser-assisted in-situ keratomileusis (LASIK) for myopia. SN, superonasal; ST, superotemporal. Nasal (N), temporal (T), superior (S), inferior (I).

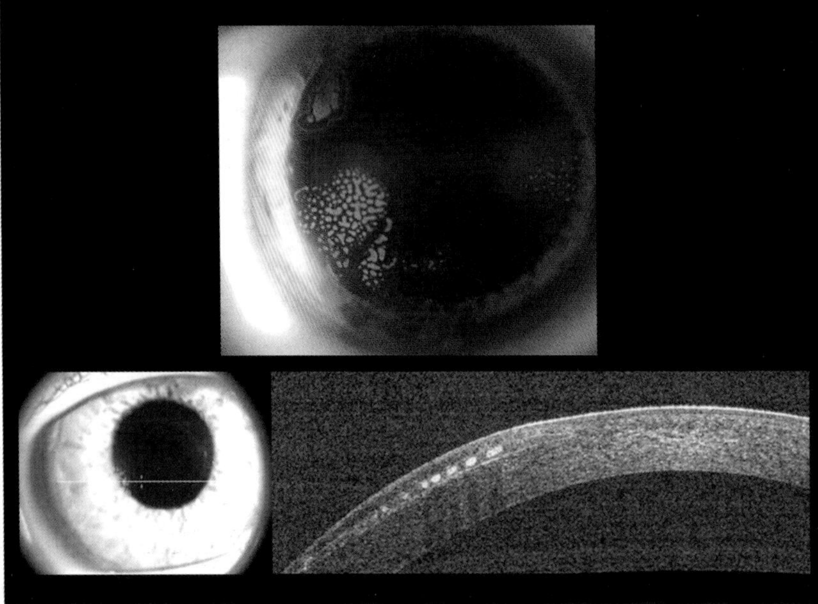

Fig. 10.7 Slit-lamp photograph and cross-sectional spectral-domain optical coherence tomography image of postoperative epithelial ingrowth.

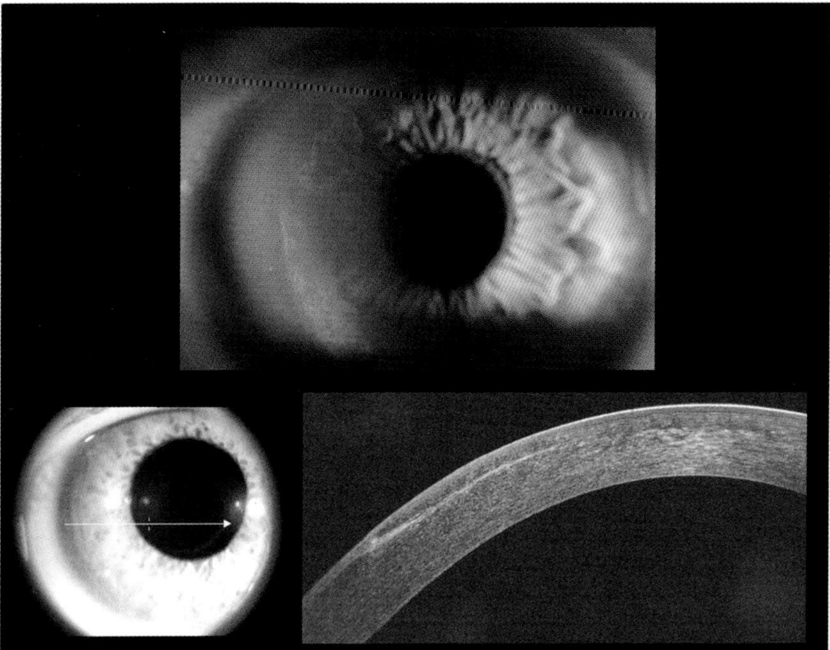

Fig. 10.8 Anterior-segment photograph and spectral-domain optical coherence tomography image 1 week after laser-assisted in-situ keratomileusis (LASIK) flap lift with extensive epithelial scraping of stromal bed and posterior surface of flap and beyond edge of flap edge. The white arrow shows the orientation of the high resolution cross-sectional scan.

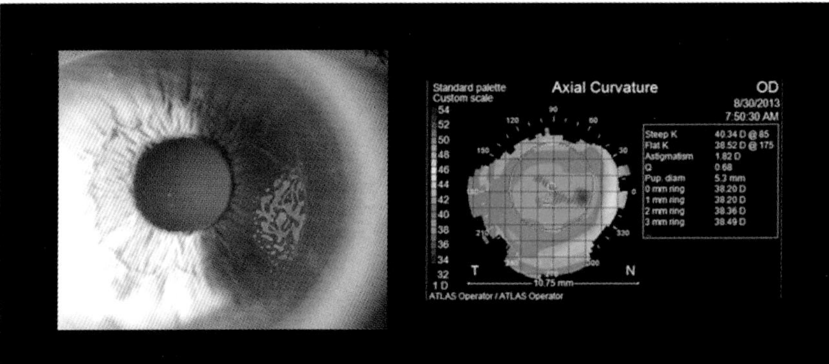

Fig. 10.9 Recurrence of epithelial ingrowth after flap lift and epithelial scraping (slit-lamp photograph and corneal topography axial map). OD, right eye. Nasal (N), temporal (T), corneal power (K).

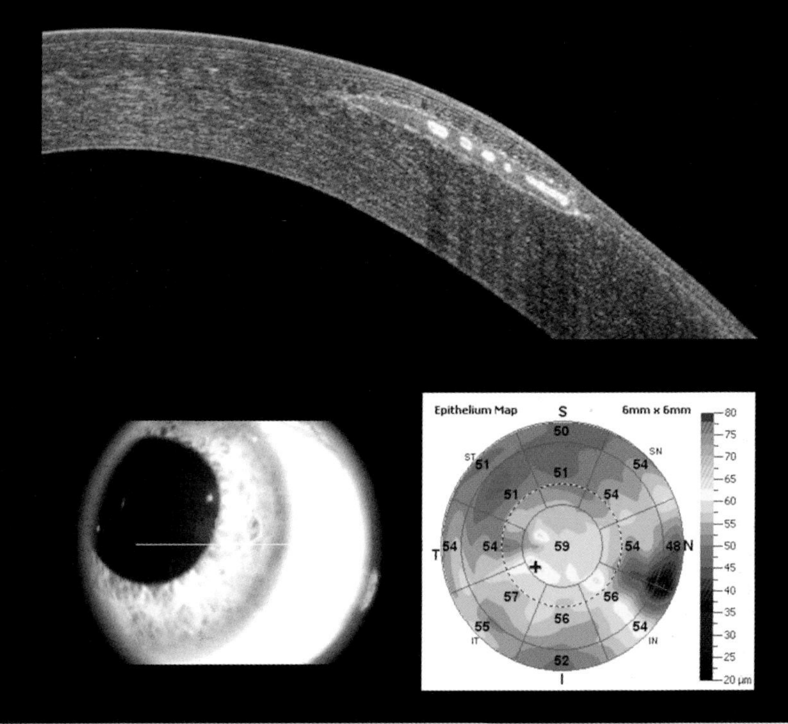

Fig. 10.10 Cross-sectional spectral-domain optical coherence tomography and epithelial thickness mapping demonstrating epithelial remodeling with thinning of the corneal epithelium overlying the area of epithelial ingrowth. IN, inferonasal; IT, infiltration thickness; SN, superonasal; ST, superotemporal.

photograph and cross-sectional high-resolution SD OCT image. Flap lift with extensive epithelial scraping of the stromal bed and posterior surface of the flap and beyond the flap edge was performed in the right eye. At 1 week after the flap lift in the right eye, BCVA was 20/20 with manifest refraction of − 2.00 + 1.00@45 (▶ Fig. 10.8 illustrates the slit-lamp photos and SD OCT). The patient returned for follow-up at 1 month after flap lift and epithelial scraping in the right eye; uncorrected visual acuity was 20/20, and the manifest refraction was plano, despite recurrence of the epithelial ingrowth from 3 to 4 o'clock (▶ Fig. 10.9). Cross-sectional high-resolution SD OCT scans and epithelial thickness mapping revealed epithelial remodeling with thinning of the epithelium overlying the area of epithelial ingrowth (▶ Fig. 10.10). Treatment options were discussed with the patient. At that point, the patient was asymptomatic, and his visual acuity had improved. We recommended observation. This case illustrates well the epithelial compensation overlying areas of stromal irregularities producing a smooth corneal surface.

In conclusion, SD OCT provides full assessment of all cornea layers and can be helpful in the diagnosis and management of complex refractive cases. High-resolution scans, total thickness, and epithelial and flap mapping add in to the interpretation of corneal topography and should be considered in the future planning of customized excimer laser ablation profiles. SD OCT 3-D reconstruction of the anterior segment and measurements of the corneal power are excellent tools for complex IOL calculation cases.

References

[1] Ortiz S, Siedlecki D, Pérez-Merino P, et al. Corneal topography from spectral optical coherence tomography (sOCT). Biomed Opt Express 2011: 3232–3247

[2] Karnowski K, Kaluzny BJ, Szkulmowski M, Gora M, Wojtkowski M. Corneal topography with high-speed swept source OCT in clinical examination. Biomed Opt Express 2011; 2: 2709–2720

[3] Radhakrishnan S, Goldsmith J, Huang D, et al. Comparison of optical coherence tomography and ultrasound biomicroscopy for detection of narrow anterior chamber angles. Arch Ophthalmol 2005; 123: 1053–1059

[4] Müller M, Dahmen G, Pörksen E, et al. Anterior chamber angle measurement with optical coherence tomography: intraobserver and interobserver variability. J Cataract Refract Surg 2006; 32: 1803–1808

[5] Dada T, Sihota R, Gadia R, Aggarwal A, Mandal S, Gupta V. Comparison of anterior segment optical coherence tomography and ultrasound biomicroscopy for assessment of the anterior segment. J Cataract Refract Surg 2007; 33: 837–840

[6] Radhakrishnan S, Rollins AM, Roth JE, et al. Real-time optical coherence tomography of the anterior segment at 1310 nm. Arch Ophthalmol 2001; 119: 1179–1185

[7] Gambra E, Ortiz S, Perez-Merino P, Gora M, Wojtkowski M, Marcos S. Static and dynamic crystalline lens accommodation evaluated using quantitative 3-D OCT. Biomed Opt Express 2013; 4: 1595–1609

[8] Huang D, Swanson EA, Lin CP, et al. Optical coherence tomography. Science 1991; 254: 1178–1181

[9] Keane PA, Bhatti RA, Brubaker JW, Liakopoulos S, Sadda SR, Walsh AC. Comparison of clinically relevant findings from high-speed fourier-domain and conventional time-domain optical coherence tomography. Am J Ophthalmol 2009; 148: 242–248, e1

[10] Sarunic MV, Asrani S, Izatt JA. Imaging the ocular anterior segment with real-time, full-range Fourier-domain optical coherence tomography. Arch Ophthalmol 2008; 126: 537–542

[11] Prakash G, Agarwal A, Jacob S, Kumar DA, Agarwal A, Banerjee R. Comparison of fourier-domain and time-domain optical coherence tomography for assessment of corneal thickness and intersession repeatability. Am J Ophthalmol 2009; 148: 282–290, e2

[12] Wojtkowski M, Srinivasan V, Ko T, Fujimoto J, Kowalczyk A, Duker J. Ultrahigh-resolution, high-speed, Fourier domain optical coherence tomography and methods for dispersion compensation. Opt Express 2004; 12: 2404–2422

[13] Ortiz S, Siedlecki D, Grulkowski I, et al. Optical distortion correction in optical coherence tomography for quantitative ocular anterior segment by three-dimensional imaging. Opt Express 2010; 18: 2782–2796

[14] Zhao M, Kuo AN, Izatt JA. 3D refraction correction and extraction of clinical parameters from spectral domain optical coherence tomography of the cornea. Opt Express 2010; 18: 8923–8936

[15] Ortiz S, Siedlecki D, Remon L, Marcos S. Three-dimensional ray tracing on Delaunay-based reconstructed surfaces. Appl Opt 2009; 48: 3886–3893

[16] Ortiz S, Pérez-Merino P, Durán S, et al. Full OCT anterior segment biometry: an application in cataract surgery. Biomed Opt Express 2013; 4: 387–396

[17] Ruggeri M, Uhlhorn SR, De Freitas C, Ho A, Manns F, Parel JM. Imaging and full-length biometry of the eye during accommodation using spectral domain OCT with an optical switch. Biomed Opt Express 2012; 3: 1506–1520

[18] Haque S, Jones L, Simpson T. Thickness mapping of the cornea and epithelium using optical coherence tomography. Optom Vis Sci 2008; 85: E963–E976

[19] Rabinowitz YS. Videokeratographic indices to aid in screening for keratoconus. J Refract Surg 1995; 11: 371–379

[20] Rabinowitz YS, Rasheed K. KISA% index: a quantitative videokeratography algorithm embodying minimal topographic criteria for diagnosing keratoconus. J Cataract Refract Surg 1999; 25: 1327–1335

[21] Schwiegerling J, Greivenkamp JE. Keratoconus detection based on videokeratoscopic height data. Optom Vis Sci 1996; 73: 721–728

[22] Kamiya K, Ishii R, Shimizu K, Igarashi A. Evaluation of corneal elevation, pachymetry and keratometry in keratoconic eyes with respect to the stage of Amsler-Krumeich classification. Br J Ophthalmol 2014; 98: 459–463

[23] Smadja D, Touboul D, Cohen A, et al. Detection of subclinical keratoconus using an automated decision tree classification. Am J Ophthalmol 2013; 156: 237–246, e1

[24] Ambrósio R Jr Caiado AL, Guerra FP, et al. Novel pachymetric parameters based on corneal tomography for diagnosing keratoconus. J Refract Surg 2011; 27: 753–758

[25] Belin MW, Ambrósio R. Scheimpflug imaging for keratoconus and ectatic disease. Indian J Ophthalmol 2013; 61: 401–406

[26] Saad A, Gatinel D. Topographic and tomographic properties of forme fruste keratoconus corneas. Invest Ophthalmol Vis Sci 2010; 51: 5546–5555

[27] Li Y, Meisler DM, Tang M, et al. Keratoconus diagnosis with optical coherence tomography pachymetry mapping. Ophthalmology 2008; 115: 2159–2166

[28] Qin B, Chen S, Brass R, et al. Keratoconus diagnosis with optical coherence tomography-based pachymetric scoring system. J Cataract Refract Surg 2013; 39: 1864–1871

[29] Rocha KM, Perez-Straziota CE, Stulting RD, Randleman JB. SD-OCT analysis of regional epithelial thickness profiles in keratoconus, postoperative corneal ectasia, and normal eyes. J Refract Surg 2013; 29: 173–179

[30] Rocha KM, Perez-Straziota CE, Stulting RD, Randleman JB. Epithelial and stromal remodeling after corneal collagen cross-linking evaluated by spectral-domain OCT. J Refract Surg 2014; 30: 122–127

[31] Rocha KM, Krueger RR. Spectral-domain optical coherence tomography epithelial and flap thickness mapping in femtosecond laser-assisted in situ keratomileusis. Am J Ophthalmol 2014; 158: 293–301

[32] Kanellopoulos AJ, Asimellis G. Longitudinal postoperative lasik epithelial thickness profile changes in correlation with degree of myopia correction. J Refract Surg 2014; 30: 166–171

[33] Sandali O, El Sanharawi M, Temstet C, et al. Fourier-domain optical coherence tomography imaging in keratoconus: a corneal structural classification. Ophthalmology 2013; 120: 2403–2412

[34] Reinstein DZ, Archer TJ, Gobbe M. Change in epithelial thickness profile 24 hours and longitudinally for 1 year after myopic LASIK: three-dimensional display with Artemis very high-frequency digital ultrasound. J Refract Surg 2012; 28: 195–201

[35] Reinstein DZ, Silverman RH, Raevsky T, et al. Arc-scanning very high-frequency digital ultrasound for 3D pachymetric mapping of the corneal epithelium and stroma in laser in situ keratomileusis. J Refract Surg 2000; 16: 414–430

[36] Li Y, Tan O, Brass R, Weiss JL, Huang D. Corneal epithelial thickness mapping by Fourier-domain optical coherence tomography in normal and keratoconic eyes. Ophthalmology 2012; 119: 2425–2433

[37] Dawson DG, Grossniklaus HE, McCarey BE, Edelhauser HF. Biomechanical and wound healing characteristics of corneas after excimer laser keratorefractive surgery: is there a difference between advanced surface ablation and sub-Bowman's keratomileusis? J Refract Surg 2008; 24: S90–S96

[38] Dupps WJ Jr Roberts C. Effect of acute biomechanical changes on corneal curvature after photokeratectomy. J Refract Surg 2001; 17: 658–669

[39] Randleman JB, Dawson DG, Grossniklaus HE, McCarey BE, Edelhauser HF. Depth-dependent cohesive tensile strength in human donor corneas: implications for refractive surgery. J Refract Surg 2008; 24: S85–S89

[40] Yao P, Zhao J, Li M, Shen Y, Dong Z, Zhou X. Microdistortions in Bowman's layer following femtosecond laser small incision lenticule extraction observed by Fourier-domain OCT. J Refract Surg 2013; 6: 1–7

[41] Zhao J, Yao P, Li M, et al. The morphology of corneal cap and its relation to refractive outcomes in femtosecond laser small incision lenticule extraction (SMILE) with anterior segment optical coherence tomography observation. PLoS ONE 2013; 8: e70208

[42] Reinstein DZ, Archer TJ, Randleman JB. Mathematical model to compare the relative tensile strength of the cornea after PRK, LASIK, and small incision lenticule extraction. J Refract Surg 2013; 29: 454–460

[43] Agca A, Ozgurhan EB, Demirok A, et al. Comparison of corneal hysteresis and corneal resistance factor after small incision lenticule extraction and femtosecond laser-assisted LASIK: a prospective fellow eye study. Cont Lens Anterior Eye 2014; 37: 77–80

[44] Stahl JE, Durrie DS, Schwendeman FJ, Boghossian AJ. Anterior segment OCT analysis of thin IntraLase femtosecond flaps. J Refract Surg 2007; 23: 555–558

[45] Kim JH, Lee D, Rhee KI. Flap thickness reproducibility in laser in situ keratomileusis with a femtosecond laser: optical coherence tomography measurement. J Cataract Refract Surg 2008; 34: 132–136

[46] von Jagow B, Kohnen T. Corneal architecture of femtosecond laser and microkeratome flaps imaged by anterior segment optical coherence tomography. J Cataract Refract Surg 2009; 35: 35–41

[47] Duffey RJ. Thin flap laser in situ keratomileusis: flap dimensions with the Moria LSK-One manual microkeratome using the 100-microm head. J Cataract Refract Surg 2005; 31: 1159–1162

[48] Kymionis GD, Portaliou DM, Tsiklis NS, Panagopoulou SI, Pallikaris IG. Thin LASIK flap creation using the SCHWIND Carriazo-Pendular microkeratome. J Refract Surg 2009; 25: 33–36

[49] Kim JH, Lee D, Rhee KI. Flap thickness reproducibility in laser in situ keratomileusis with a femtosecond laser: optical coherence tomography measurement. J Cataract Refract Surg 2008; 34: 132–136

[50] Miranda D, Smith SD, Krueger RR. Comparison of flap thickness reproducibility using microkeratomes with a second motor for advancement. Ophthalmology 2003; 110: 1931–1934

[51] Krueger RR, Dupps WJ Jr. Biomechanical effects of femtosecond and microkeratome-based flap creation: prospective contralateral examination of two patients. J Refract Surg 2007; 23: 800–807

[52] Li Y, Netto MV, Shekhar R, Krueger RR, Huang D. A longitudinal study of LASIK flap and stromal thickness with high-speed optical coherence tomography. Ophthalmology 2007; 114: 1124–1132

[53] Hood CT, Krueger RR, Wilson SE. The association between femtosecond laser flap parameters and ocular aberrations after uncomplicated custom myopic LASIK. Graefes Arch Clin Exp Ophthalmol 2013; 251: 2155–2162

[54] Rocha KM, Kagan R, Smith SD, Krueger RR. Thresholds for interface haze formation after thin-flap femtosecond laser in situ keratomileusis for myopia. Am J Ophthalmol 2009; 147: 966–972, e1

[55] Rocha KM, Randleman JB, Stulting RD. Analysis of microkeratome thin flap architecture using Fourier-domain optical coherence tomography. J Refract Surg 2011; 27: 759–763

[56] Aramberri J. Intraocular lens power calculation after corneal refractive surgery: double-K method. J Cataract Refract Surg 2003; 29: 2063–2068

[57] Arce CG, Soriano ES, Weisenthal RW, et al. Calculation of intraocular lens power using Orbscan II quantitative area topography after corneal refractive surgery. J Refract Surg 2009; 25: 1061–1074

[58] Yang R, Yeh A, George MR, Rahman M, Boerman H, Wang M. Comparison of intraocular lens power calculation methods after myopic laser refractive surgery without previous refractive surgery data. J Cataract Refract Surg 2013; 39: 1327–1335

[59] Awwad ST, Kilby A, Bowman RW, et al. The accuracy of the double-K adjustment for third-generation intraocular lens calculation formulas in previous keratorefractive surgery eyes. Eye Contact Lens 2013; 39: 220–227

[60] Saiki M, Negishi K, Kato N, et al. A new central-peripheral corneal curvature method for intraocular lens power calculation after excimer laser refractive surgery. Acta Ophthalmol (Copenh) 2013; 91: e133–e139

[61] Javadi MA, Feizi S, Malekifar P. Intraocular lens power calculation after corneal refractive surgery. J Ophthalmic Vis Res 2012; 7: 10–16

[62] Kwitko S, Marinho DR, Rymer S, Severo N, Arce CG. Orbscan II and double-K method for IOL calculation after refractive surgery. Graefes Arch Clin Exp Ophthalmol 2012; 250: 1029–1034

[63] Awwad ST, Kelley PS, Bowman RW, Cavanagh HD, McCulley JP. Corneal refractive power estimation and intraocular lens calculation after hyperopic LASIK. Ophthalmology 2009; 116: 393–400, e1

[64] Awwad ST, Manasseh C, Bowman RW, et al. Intraocular lens power calculation after myopic laser in situ keratomileusis: estimating the corneal refractive power. J Cataract Refract Surg 2008; 34: 1070–1076

[65] Gimbel HV, Sun R. Accuracy and predictability of intraocular lens power calculation after laser in situ keratomileusis. J Cataract Refract Surg 2001; 27: 571–576

[66] Tang M, Wang L, Koch DD, Li Y, Huang D. Intraocular lens power calculation after previous myopic laser vision correction based on corneal power measured by Fourier-domain optical coherence tomography. J Cataract Refract Surg 2012; 38: 589–594

[67] Tang M, Li Y, Huang D. An intraocular lens power calculation formula based on optical coherence tomography: a pilot study. J Refract Surg 2010; 26: 430–437

[68] Huang D, Tang M, Wang L, et al. Optical coherence tomography-based corneal power measurement and intraocular lens power calculation following laser vision correction (an American Ophthalmological Society thesis). Trans Am Ophthalmol Soc 2013;111:34–45

11 Descemet Membrane Detachment: Classification and Management

Soosan Jacob and Amar Agarwal

Posterior capsular rupture can result in various complications, including corneal damage.[1,2,3,4,5,6,7,8,9,10,11,12,13,14,15,16,17,18,19,20,21,22,23,24,25,26,27,28,29,30,31,32] Corneal damage can be due to the ensuing vitreous loss, manipulations by the surgeon, or the implantation of a suboptimal intraocular lens (IOL) in terms of its design, material, or location. It is important for the surgeon to understand the ramifications of corneal damage that can occur and how to manage it.

11.1 Descemet Membrane Detachment

Descemet membrane detachment is a complication patients occasionally face after surgery.[7,8] Various techniques have been proposed as treatment for detachment of the Descemet membrane, including observation,[9] viscoelastic injection,[10] air injection, the use of long-acting intracameral gas,[11,12] and insertion of transcorneal mattress sutures.[13] A detached Descemet membrane can be diagnosed on slit-lamp examination as a clear optical space between the stroma and the Descemet membrane.

Trypan blue dye may be injected into the anterior chamber to stain the Descemet membrane and aid in visualization. The anterior chamber is then irrigated with balanced salt solution (BSS) to wash away excess trypan blue and to study the dynamics of the detached Descemet membrane (▶ Fig. 11.1). An air bubble is then injected to appose the Descemet membrane to the corneal stroma. Gases, such as sulphur hexafluoride (SF6) or perfluoropropane (C3F8), can also be used in more severe or long-standing cases.

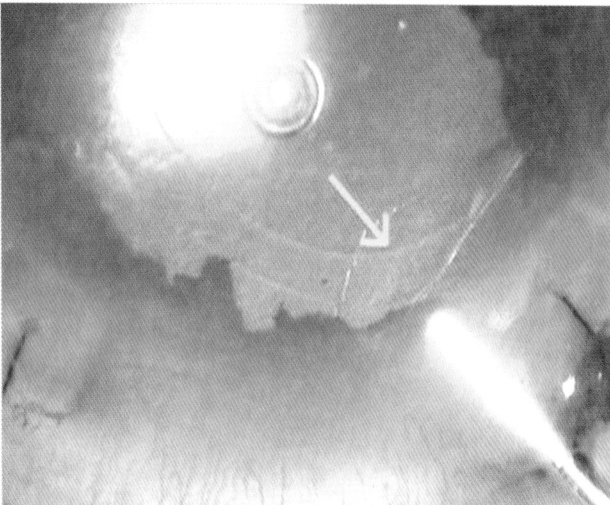

Fig. 11.1 A stripped Descemet membrane is shown. It is typically seen near incisions, and it lies loose, floating in the anterior chamber. It may have a crumpled or rolled-up edge with an undulating appearance on anterior segment optical coherence tomography (OCT), and it flutters on irrigating the anterior chamber with balanced salt solution (BSS). Yellow arrow indicates the detached descemet membrane.

11.2 New Classification of Descemet Membrane Detachment

Based on pathological features, in 1928, Samuels classified Descemet membrane detachment as *active* (pushed back) or *passive* (pulled back and torn away) owing to differences in elasticity between the parenchyma and the glass membrane.[6] Samuels also stated that this classification was more relevant pathologically and no great importance could be ascribed to these forms of detachment from the surgical standpoint. Descemet membrane detachment has also been previously classified as *planar* (a 1-mm or smaller gap between the Descemet membrane and the stroma) or *nonplanar* (a gap of 1 mm or larger) between the Descemet membrane and the stroma) based on morphology.[7]

Dr. Soosan Jacob proposed a new classification of Descemet membrane detachment based on the clinicomorphologic, etiologic, tomographic, and intraoperative features and proposed a new treatment algorithm for detachment of the Descemet membrane based on its classification. This classification is analogous to the classification of retinal detachment. The Descemet membrane is a vital layer of the cornea and is necessary for maintaining the clarity of the cornea, just as the neurosensory retina is required for visual perception. Because retinal detachment can be rhegmatogenous retinal detachment (RRD [secondary to hole, tear, or dialysis]), tractional retinal detachment (TRD), or bullous/exudative retinal detachment (BDD), we would classify Descemet membrane detachment as RDD, TRD (or TDD), BDD, or complex detachment (CDD) (▶ Table 11.1).

An RDD generally occurs as an intraoperative event when there is a break in the Descemet membrane with fluid accumulation between the Descemet membrane and overlying stroma. Analogous to an RRD, an RDD can be secondary to a hole (e.g., a double anterior chamber after perforation during deep anterior lamellar keratoplasty) or a tear (e.g., Descemet membrane detachment occurring during insertion of blunt instruments or IOL implantation during phacoemulsification). RDD can also occur secondary to dialysis of the Descemet membrane from its attachment at the Schwalbe line, a complication that is sometimes seen during trabeculotomy, punch insertion in trabeculectomy, or anterior-chamber maintainer insertion or if stripping of the Descemet membrane accidentally extends toward the periphery during endothelial keratoplasty of the Descemet membrane.

The Descemet membrane may also become detached secondary to an inflammatory or fibrotic process, resulting in TDD, which is analogous to a TRD. This could occur secondary to incarceration of the Descemet membrane in an inflammatory process (e.g., in peripheral anterior synechiae or within the

Table 11.1 Differentiating features of types of Descemet Membrane (DM) Detachments

Rhegmatogenous Descemet detachment		Tractional Descemet detachment	Bullous Descemet detachment	Complex Descemet detachment
Time of onset	Mostly intraoperative	Mostly postoperative	Secondary to disease process; sometimes intraoperative	Intraoperative or postoperative
History	History of surgery	History of inflammation, trauma, or surgery	History specific to underlying cause	Generally, history of surgery
Cause	Tear, hole, or dialysis	Incarceration of DM in inflammation, fibrosis, peripheral anterior synechiae, within the graft host junction, in wound suture with subsequent contraction Long-standing RDD becoming adherent to intraocular contents with secondary TDD.	Disease process, infection, or inflammation Intraoperative complication (e.g., blood or accidental injection of viscoelastic)	Poorly positioned DM endothelial keratoplasty graft combination of other DM detachments
Clinical findings	Undulating membrane lying loose in the anterior chamber. Folds present, Undulating movements seen on irrigating anterior chamber with balanced salt solution.	Stretched out tight like a trampoline between points of attachment. No folds. Immobile or sharp, fluttering movements seen on forcible irrigation with balanced salt solution	Convex membrane bulging into the anterior chamber with no break	Complex configurations or combination features of others
Anterior-segment OCT	Undulating linear hyperreflective signal in the anterior chamber Arc length of overlying stroma is similar to length of detached DM	Straight taut linear hyperreflective signal between two points of attachment Arc length of cornea is more than length of detached DM	Convex hyperreflective signal bulging into anterior chamber from overlying stroma. Space filled with exudate, pus, blood, viscoelastic, air, etc.	Complex configurations or combination features of others
Prognosis	Good if residual endothelial function adequate	Good if residual endothelial function adequate	Prognosis depending on cause	Depending on cause

RDD: Rhegmatogenous descemet's detachment, TDD: Tractional descemet's detachment

graft-host junction in large-diameter grafts) or secondary to incarceration in a wound or suture with subsequent contraction, resulting in a TDD. A long-standing RDD could also sometimes adhere to intraocular contents with secondary fibrosis, thus turning into a TDD. A BDD can occur secondary to a disease process, such as posterior corneal abscess, tumor, infection, or inflammation (analogous to bullous retinal detachment). In this type of Descemet membrane detachment, a separation and convex bulging of the Descemet membrane into the anterior chamber occur in the absence of a break in the Descemet membrane. The space between the stroma and the Descemet membrane is filled with pus, exudates, fluid, viscoelastic, or air, depending on the cause of BDD. This configuration of Descemet membrane can also be seen as part of the Anwar "big bubble" technique in deep anterior lamellar keratoplasty, which detaches the Descemet membrane from the stroma and sometimes occurs from accidental injection of viscoelastic into the pre-Descemetic space.[33] Clinically, an RDD is usually seen as an undulating membrane lying loose in the anterior chamber. It may also be scrolled or crumpled, depending on the extent of detachment. It has folds and is mobile, similar to an RRD. On the other hand, a TDD is stretched out tight, like a trampoline, between the points of attachment. It has no folds and is not mobile. A BDD is seen as a convex membrane bulging into the anterior chamber, similar to a bullous retinal detachment. A complex Descemet detachment shows complex folds or scrolls or shows a combination of features of others and can be seen sometimes in a poorly attached Descemet membrane endothelial keratoplasty (DMEK) graft.

11.3 Anterior-Segment OCT Features

In all cases of Descemet membrane detachment, there is generally overlying corneal epithelial and stromal edema, which may make visualization difficult. In this case, the anterior-segment OCT is useful for diagnosing this condition, as well as differentiating between various types of Descemet membrane detachment. An RDD is seen as an undulating linear hyperreflective signal in the anterior chamber, whereas a TDD is seen as a straight, taut linear signal between two points of attachment (▶ Fig. 11.2). In TDD, the arc length of the cornea, if measured, is found to be more than the length of the detached Descemet membrane, unlike in RDD, where the arc length of the overlying corneal stroma is similar to the length of the detached Descemet membrane. A BDD is seen as a convex, hyperreflective signal bulging into the anterior chamber from the overlying stroma, with the space between filled with exudate, pus, fluid, or air, depending on the cause of the Descemet membrane detachment. A CDD shows complex configurations on anterior-segment OCT.

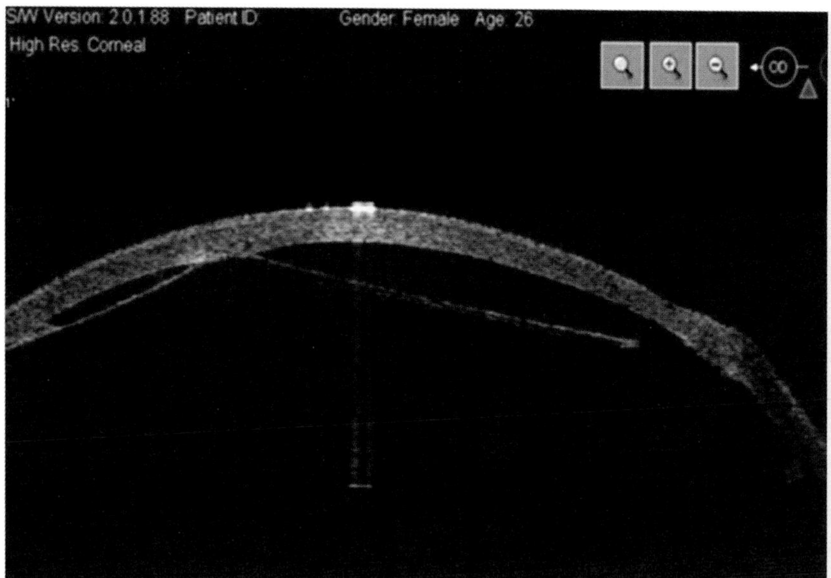

Fig. 11.2 A taut Descemet membrane detachment is seen stretched out between points of attachment on anterior-segment optical coherence tomography (OCT). It appears as a taut, linear, hyperreflection. Intraoperatively, it does not show much movement on irrigating the anterior chamber with balanced salt solution.

Intraoperatively, TDD can be verified by its more immobile nature and the absence of the typical undulating movement that is associated with an RDD on irrigating the anterior chamber with BSS. A taut Descemet membrane does not move with the undulations seen in an RDD, although with BSS it might show some sharp, small, fluttery movements on forcible irrigation.

11.4 Relaxing Descematotomy

Relaxing retinotomy is an established surgical technique in vitreoretinal surgery for periretinal traction and retinal foreshortening that does not allow the retina to settle down. Similar traction on the Descemet membrane secondary to inflammation or fibrosis or the Descemet membrane becoming incarcerated in a wound or suture leading to a TDD may not respond to the classic management strategies for Descemet membrane detachment. Injecting air or long-acting gas into the anterior chamber in an eye with TDD will not appose it to the corneal stroma because of the foreshortening. Jacobs developed a technique called *relaxing descemetotomy*, which is based on a principle similar to relaxing retinotomy, as a solution for this scenario.[34]

11.5 Treatment for Descemet Membrane Detachment Based on Classification

Treatment of the aforementioned conditions also differs from one to the next. Although both RDD and TDD require internal gas tamponade or pneumodescemetopexy and sub-Descemet fluid drainage—which is analogous to internal tamponade and subretinal fluid drainage in retinal detachments—TDD also requires relief or removal of the element of traction for the Descemet membrane to settle onto the stroma. This procedure can be done by relaxing descemetotomy incisions. In the presence of synechiae causing TDD, it may also require synechiolysis and membrane peeling to remove tractional fibrotic bands that pull on the Descemet membrane. Sub-Descemet fluid drainage is carried out by injecting gas from the side opposite to the tear (internal drainage) or, in some cases, by making a small stab incision in the cornea overlying the Descemet membrane detachment to drain the fluid externally.

Relaxing descemetotomy can be performed with the anterior chamber filled with viscoelastic or air. The tip of a 26-gauge needle is bent in the reverse direction, as in a capsulotomy needle, and is introduced into the anterior chamber to make the relaxing descemetotomy incisions (▶ Fig. 11.3). The extent of the incision is determined during surgery by assessing the degree of foreshortening that still remains. If foreshortening is not completely relieved, the incisions are further extended until the Descemet membrane is able to lie fully apposed against the stroma. These incisions are made in the peripheral cornea, avoiding the pupillary plane and the visual axis. Postoperative tamponade with nonexpansile concentration of C3F8 (14%) or SF6 (20%) is administered with face-up positioning of the patient for 1 hour (▶ Fig. 11.4). A reattachment might not occur in all cases, depending on the extent of inflammatory fibrotic damage to the endothelium, in which case the patient may require a posterior lamellar or full-thickness graft.

The term *descemetotomy* was first used by Lowenstein in 1993.[21,22,23,24] It was used with reference to a procedure in which the neodymium:yttrium-aluminum garnet (Nd:YAG) laser was used in the postoperative period to perform descemetotomy to create communication between the anterior chamber and the supernumerary chamber after intentionally retaining the Descemet membrane during keratoplasty for bullous keratopathy. The authors of those studies found that the membrane was resistant to Nd:YAG laser and required the use of high energy levels and multiple pulses. Steinemann et al[25] and Masket and Tennen[26] also used the Nd:Yag laser to create a central opening in an inadvertently retained opacified host Descemet membrane after penetrating keratoplasty. Chen et al[27] surgically removed a similarly retained host Descemet membrane after keratoplasty.

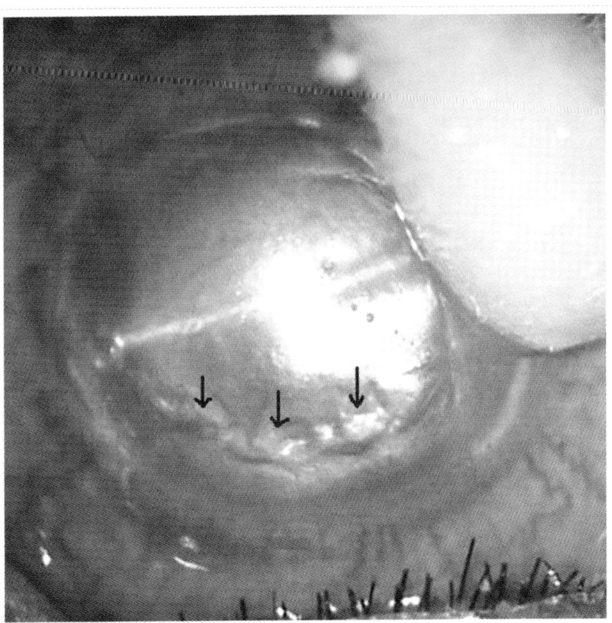

Fig. 11.3 Relaxing descemetotomy is done to relieve the tension and stress forces acting on the TDD. Once the relaxing descemetotomy cuts are made (arrows), the Descemet membrane becomes lax and can be apposed to the overlying corneal stroma by injecting an air bubble.

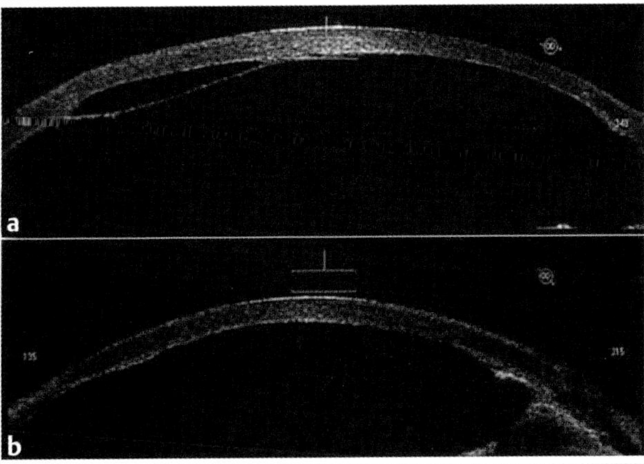

Fig. 11.4 (a) Preoperative optical coherence tomography (OCT) shows a tractional retinal detachment. (b) Postoperative OCT shows the Descemet membrane attached after relaxing descematotomy was performed.

These authors had previously used the term *iatrogenic descemetorhexis*[14] to describe a case in which accidental descemetorrhexis occurred in a patient during phacoemulsification. A similar case was also reported by Pan and Au Eong.[15] Descemetorrhexis has been described as part of endothelial keratoplasty procedures, in which the central Descemet membrane is intentionally removed from the host cornea.[28,29,30,31,32] The term *relaxing descemetotomy*, which the authors coined, differs from the aforementioned terms in that it describes a therapeutic procedure that relieves the traction forces and decreases foreshortening of the Descemet membrane in a procedure similar to that of relaxing retinotomy. The relaxing descemetotomy incisions break the stress forces acting on the Descemet membrane. The tautness of the Descemet membrane is relieved, and an air or gas bubble is able to appose the now lax Descemet membrane against the overlying corneal stroma. A long-acting gas, such as C3F8 or SF6, may be preferable over an air bubble to provide a longer period of tamponade, especially in RDD.[11,12]

11.6 Intraocular Lens Implantation in the Presence of Corneal Damage

We prefer to use the glued IOL technique with Descemet stripping automated endothelial keratoplasty (DSAEK) in cases with aphakic corneal decompensation. We have also used it in cases requiring full-thickness keratoplasty as well as DMEK. It is important to make the anterior segment stable when combining posterior lamellar keratoplasty techniques with glued IOL implantation. A pupilloplasty may be required for widely dilated, nonconstricting pupils to attain a good air fill in the anterior chamber at the end of surgery, as well as to avoid donor graft dislocation. Intracameral Miochol-E (acetylcholine chloride) should be instilled after implanting the glued IOL to constrict the pupil. This allows a good compartmentalization of the eye into a bicameral structure, allowing a greater support for the donor tissue. In our experience of DSAEK combined with glued IOL implantation, no incidence of donor dislocation into the posterior segment has occurred. The difference from sutured secondary posterior chamber IOLs lies in the rigid, nonelastic attachment of the IOL to the sclera with the glued IOL technique. The crystalline lens-bag-zonule complex—because of its 360-degree attachment to the ciliary area—is a trampoline-like structure (▶ Fig. 11.5). However, the Prolene sutures (2 or 4, depending on the technique) used for suture fixating an IOL to the sclera act as a hammock, which provides less torsional stability than the natural state. The glued IOL reduces the torsional and oscillatory freedom of the implant because the resultant IOL-haptic-sclera complex is more stable than the IOL-haptic-suture-sclera complex of the suture-fixated IOLs. This same biomechanical model is the reason for lesser pseudophacodonesis seen after glued IOL compared with suture-fixated IOL. The learning curve for the glued IOL procedure is fairly simple for most surgeons working with the anterior segment, and the detailed steps for the surgery have been provided earlier in the literature, as well as in this book (Chapter 17). Other authors also have noted the disastrous complications of the donor lenticule falling into the vitreous in aphakic eyes.[35] The placement of a glued IOL in situ before placement of the lenticule compartmentalizes the aphakic eye from a unicameral to bicameral environment, which will produce less instability in the anterior segment and will also act as a rigid barrier to prevent the donor lenticule from falling into the vitreous.

11.7 Descemet Membrane Endothelial Keratoplasty with Glued Intraocular Lenses

Descemet membrane endothelial keratoplasty has been described by Melles et al[36] for pseduophakic bullous keratopathy

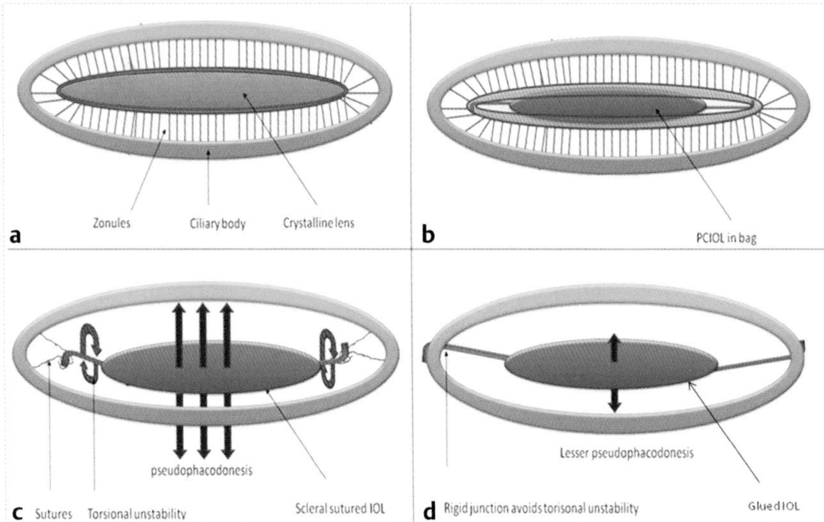

Fig. 11.5 Intraoperative lens (IOL) implantation and posterior capsular (PC) rupture. **(a)** Schematic diagram showing normal trampoline line arrangement of the ciliary body, zonules, and crystalline lens in a normal eye. **(b)** Schematic diagram showing the change in the case of a pseduophakic eye with an in-the-bag posterior-chamber PC IOL. **(c)** Schematic diagram showing a pseudophakic eye with a sutured scleral-fixated IOL with increased torsional instability and increased pseudophacodonesis due to sclera-suture-haptic-optic attachment. **(d)** Schematic diagram showing a pseudophakic eye with a glued IOL and reduced torsional instability and lesser pseudophacodonesis resulting from rigid sclera-haptic-optic attachment.

(▶ Fig. 11.6a). The basic technique consists of preparing the donor graft by partially trephining it and using a Sinskey hook (Appasamy Associates, Chennai, India) to lift up the edge of the cut Descemet membrane. After an adequate edge is lifted, a nontoothed forceps is used to gently grab the Descemet membrane at its very edge, and the graft is separated from the underlying stroma in a capsulorrhexis-like circumferential manner (▶ Fig. 11.6b). These steps are performed using the SCUBA technique described by Gimbel.[37,38] The DMEK graft is then stained with trypan blue and replaced in the sterile corneal storage medium while the recipient eye is prepared.

An anterior chamber maintainer is inserted, and two points are marked on the sclera exactly 180 degrees apart. Two 2.5 × 2.5-mm lamellar scleral flaps are created on either side, centered on the marks. Trypan blue is used to stain the patient's Descemet membrane before scoring and stripping it from approximately 8.5-mm diameter (as marked from above the corneal surface) using a reverse Sinskey hook. A 20-gauge needle is used to create a sclerotomy approximately 1 to 1.5 mm from the limbus under each scleral flap, and a 23-gauge vitrector introduced through the sclerotomy performs anterior vitrectomy. If a posterior chamber IOL is in the anterior chamber, it is repositioned in a closed-globe manner by exteriorizing its haptics through the sclerotomies (▶ Fig. 11.7a,b). If there is an anterior-chamber IOL, it is explanted and a new IOL is implanted by performing the conventional glued IOL technique. In aphakic eyes, a foldable IOL is injected into the anterior chamber, and its haptics are exteriorized through the sclerotomy. In all situations, once both haptics are exteriorized, the Scharioth tuck is used to tuck them into scleral tunnels made at the edge of the scleral flaps using a 26-gauge needle. Intracameral pilocarpine is then used to constrict the pupil; if necessary, a pupilloplasty is performed. The graft is then carefully loaded into a Visian implantable contact lens injector (STAAR Surgical, Monrovia, CA), with the cartridge tip held occluded with a finger. It is then injected gently into the anterior chamber by plunging the soft-tipped injector, taking care not to fold the graft (▶ Fig. 11.7c). Wound-assisted implantation is avoided, and the anterior-chamber maintainer flow is titrated carefully to prevent backflow and extrusion of the graft through the incision. The graft orientation is then checked, and it is unfolded gently (▶ Fig. 11.7d). Once unfolded, an adequately tight air bubble is injected under the graft to float it up against the stroma (▶ Fig. 11.7e). Finally, fibrin glue is used to seal the lamellar scleral flaps, conjunctiva, and the clear corneal incisions.

In patients with aphakia, loss of bicamerality of the eye because of absence of an iris-lens diaphragm is seen, leading to poor tamponade effect and posterior migration of the injected air. A disastrous complication can be dislocation of the lenticule into the vitreous cavity. These problems are solved when combining endothelial keratoplasty with a glued IOL.

This technique (endothelial keratoplasty with glued IOL) combines the advantages of stable fixation of the IOL, as well as the advantages of lamellar keratoplasty. In contrast, an anterior-chamber IOL has the disadvantage of decreased IOL-endothelial distance, which can cause long-term graft failure when combined with penetrating keratoplasty. It becomes especially disadvantageous when combined with DSAEK, in which the endothelium with donor stroma also occupies space within the anterior chamber, thereby bringing the anterior surface of the anterior-chamber IOL close to the DSEK lenticule. Hence, these patients require explantation of the anterior-chamber IOL with secondary IOL fixation and corneal transplantation.

Sutured scleral-fixated IOLs can be combined with endothelial keratoplasty, but the disadvantage of this combination is a longer open-sky period, making the patient more vulnerable to potential complications such as expulsive hemorrhage. In addition, more pseudophakodonesis is associated with sutured IOLs, as the fixation to the sclera is via sutures at two points. In the glued IOL technique, the haptic of the IOL itself is anchored to the sclera along a significant portion of its length. This stability of the glued IOL can, in our opinion, lead to a decreased rate of graft dislocation compared with a sutured scleral-fixated IOL, which has more intraocular mobility. The glued IOL also offers the ability to adjust the centration of the IOL anytime during surgery simply by adjusting the degree of tuck of the haptics into the scleral tunnel, unlike the longer and more tedious procedure that would be required to recenter a decentered sutured scleral-fixated IOL, thus eliminating all suture-related

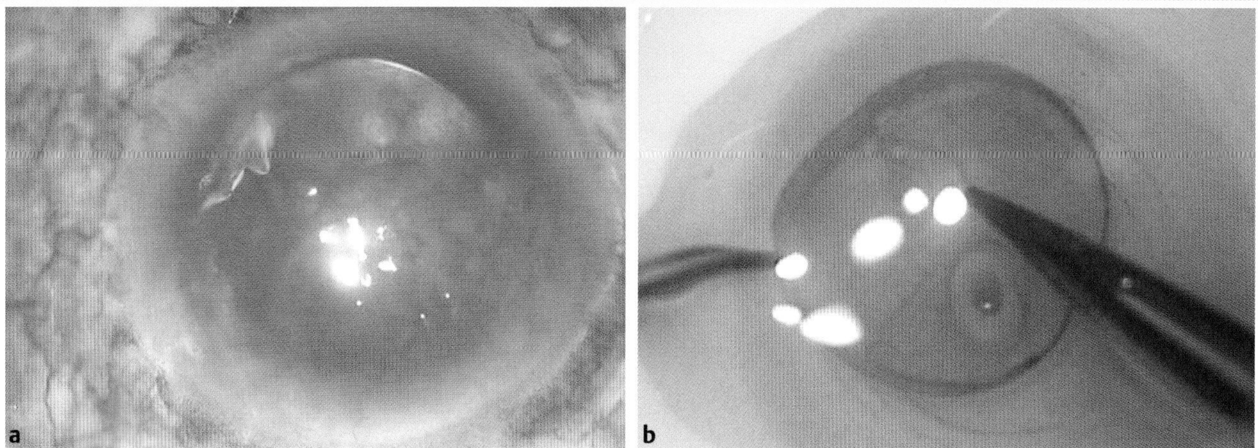

Fig. 11.6 (a) Preoperative pseudophakic bullous keratopathy. Note the posterior-chamber intraocular lens is implanted in the anterior chamber. (b) Preparation of a Descemet membrane endothelial keratoplasty graft.

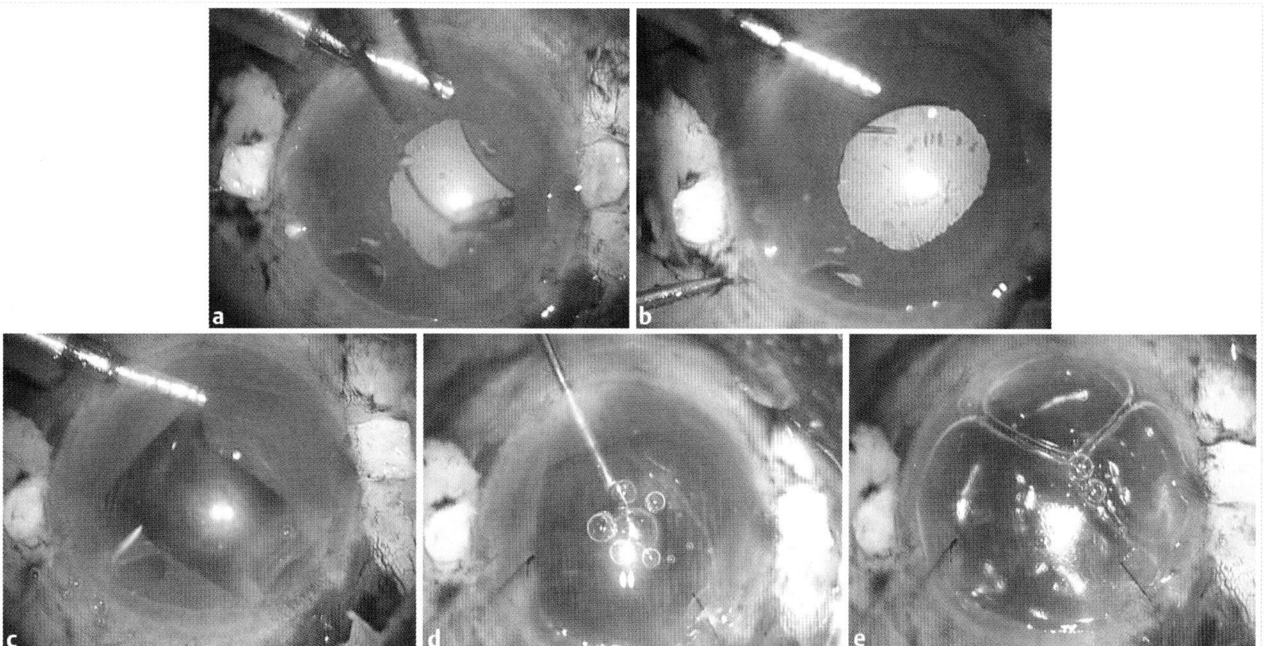

Fig. 11.7 Descemet membrane endothelial keratoplasty (DMEK) with glued intraoperative lens (IOL). (a) Posterior-chamber IOL implanted in anterior chamber, leading to corneal decompensation. The same posterior-chamber IOL is being relocated into the posterior chamber using a closed-globe, glued IOL technique. The haptic is grabbed from over the iris using an end-gripping forceps and, using a handshake technique and is transferred between the two hands until the tip of the haptic is held. (b) The haptic is exteriorized through the sclerotomy made under the scleral flap. The same procedure is followed for the second haptic, which is exteriorized through a sclerotomy under a second scleral flap created 180 degrees away from the first. Each haptic is then tucked into a scleral tunnel created at the edge of the scleral flap. (c) The DMEK graft is loaded into a Visian implantable contact lens injector and injected into the anterior chamber. (d) The DMEK graft is unrolled. (e) An air bubble is used to appose it against the overlying stroma.

complications, such as erosion, degradation, and exposure. The fibrin glue seals the flaps hermetically over the haptics and makes the procedure safe.

References

[1] Machemer R. [Cutting of the retina: a means of therapy for retinal reattachment (author's transl from German)] Klin Monatsbl Augenheilkd 1979; 175: 597–601

[2] Machemer R. Retinotomy Am J Ophthalmol 1981; 92: 768–774

[3] Machemer R, McCuen BW II de Juan E Jr. Relaxing retinotomies and retinectomies. Am J Ophthalmol 1986; 102: 7–12

[4] Alturki WA, Peyman GA, Paris CL, Blinder KJ, Desai UR, Nelson NC Jr. Posterior relaxing retinotomies: analysis of anatomic and visual results. Ophthalmic Surg 1992; 23: 685–688

[5] Bovey EH, De Ancos E, Gonvers M. Retinotomies of 180 degrees or more. Retina 1995; 15: 394–398

[6] Samuels B. Detachment of Descemet's membrane. Trans Am Ophthalmol Soc 1928;26:427–437 http://www.ncbi.nlm.nih.gov/pmc/articles/pmx1316706/pdf/taos00073-0462.pdf Accessed November 15 2011

[7] Mackool RJ, Holtz SJ. Descemet membrane detachment. Arch Ophthalmol 1977; 95: 459–463

[8] Kim T, Sorenson A. Bilateral Descemet membrane detachments. Arch Ophthalmol 2000; 118: 1302–1303

[9] Minkovitz JB, Schrenk LC, Pepose JS. Spontaneous resolution of an extensive detachment of Descemet's membrane following phacoemulsification. Arch Ophthalmol 1994; 112: 551–552

[10] Hoover DL, Giangiacomo J, Benson RL. Descemet's membrane detachment by sodium hyaluronate. Arch Ophthalmol 1985; 103: 805–808

[11] Zusman NB, Waring GO III Najarian LV, Wilson LA. Sulfur hexafluoride gas in the repair of intractable Descemet's membrane detachment. Am J Ophthalmol 1987; 104: 660–662

[12] Kim T, Hasan SA. A new technique for repairing descemet membrane detachments using intracameral gas injection. Arch Ophthalmol 2002; 120: 181–183

[13] Amaral CE, Palay DA. Technique for repair of Descemet membrane detachment. Am J Ophthalmol 1999; 127: 88–90

[14] Agarwal A, Jacob S, Agarwal A, Agarwal S, Kumar M A. Iatrogenic descemetorhexis as a complication of phacoemulsification. J Cataract Refract Surg 2006; 32: 895–897

[15] Pan JC, Au Eong KG. Spontaneous resolution of corneal oedema after inadvertent 'descemetorhexis' during cataract surgery. Clin Experiment Ophthalmol 2006; 34: 896–897

[16] Dirisamer M, Dapena I, Ham L, et al. Patterns of corneal endothelialization and corneal clearance after descemet membrane endothelial keratoplasty for fuchs endothelial dystrophy. Am J Ophthalmol 2011; 152: 543–555, e1

[17] Jacobi C, Zhivov A, Korbmacher J, et al. Evidence of endothelial cell migration after descemet membrane endothelial keratoplasty. Am J Ophthalmol 2011; 152: 537–542, e2

[18] Balachandran C, Ham L, Verschoor CA, Ong TS, van der Wees J, Melles GRJ. Spontaneous corneal clearance despite graft detachment in descemet membrane endothelial keratoplasty. Am J Ophthalmol 2009; 148: 227–234, e1

[19] Stewart RMK, Hiscott PS, Kaye SB. Endothelial migration and new descemet membrane after endothelial keratoplasty. Am J Ophthalmol 2010; 149: 683–684, author reply 683–684

[20] Cursiefen C, Kruse FE. [DMEK: Descemet membrane endothelial keratoplasty] [article in German] Ophthalmologe 2010; 107: 370–376

[21] Lazar M, Loewenstein A, Geyer O. Intentional retention of Descemet's membrane during keratoplasty. Acta Ophthalmol (Copenh) 1991; 69: 111–112

[22] Loewenstein A, Geyer O, Lazar M. Intentional retention of Descemet's membrane in keratoplasty for the surgical treatment of bullous keratopathy. Acta Ophthalmol (Copenh) 1993; 71: 280–282

[23] Loewenstein A, Lazar M. Deep lamellar keratoplasty in the treatment of bullous keratopathy. Br J Ophthalmol 1993; 77: 538

[24] Loewenstein A, Geyer O, Lazar M. Descemetotomy. J Cataract Refract Surg 1996; 22: 652

[25] Steinemann TL, Henry K, Brown MF. Nd:YAG laser treatment of retained Descemet's membrane after penetrating keratoplasty. Ophthalmic Surg 1995; 26: 80–81

[26] Masket S, Tennen DG. Neodymium:YAG laser optical opening for retained Descemet's membrane after penetrating keratoplasty. J Cataract Refract Surg 1996; 22: 139–141

[27] Chen YP, Lai PC, Chen PY, Lin KK, Hsiao CH. Retained Descemet's membrane after penetrating keratoplasty. J Cataract Refract Surg 2003; 29: 1842–1844

[28] Dapena I, Ham L, Moutsouris K, Melles GR. Incidence of recipient Descemet membrane remnants at the donor-to-stromal interface after descemetorhexis in endothelial keratoplasty. Br J Ophthalmol 2010; 94: 1689–1690

[29] Mehta JS, Hantera MM, Tan DT. Modified air-assisted descemetorhexis for Descemet-stripping automated endothelial keratoplasty. J Cataract Refract Surg 2008; 34: 889–891

[30] Wylęgała E, Tarnawska D, Dobrowolski D, Janiszewska D. [Outcomes of endothelial keratoplasty with descemetorhexis (DSEK)] [article in Polish] Klin Oczna 2007; 109: 287–291

[31] Bradley JC, McCartney DL, Busin M. Donor corneal disk insertion techniques in descemetorhexis with endokeratoplasty. Ann Ophthalmol (Skokie) 2007; 39: 277–283

[32] Nieuwendaal CP, Lapid-Gortzak R, van der Meulen IJ, Melles GJ. Posterior lamellar keratoplasty using descemetorhexis and organ-cultured donor corneal tissue (Melles technique). Cornea 2006; 25: 933–936

[33] Javadi MA, Feizi S. Deep anterior lamellar keratoplasty using the big-bubble technique for keratectasia after laser in situ keratomileusis. J Cataract Refract Surg 2010; 36: 1156–1160

[34] Agarwal A, Jacob S. Relaxing descemetotomy relieves stress forces in taut Descemet's membrane detachment. The technique allows the Descemet's membrane to become lax and apposed to the overlying corneal stroma. COMPLICATIONS CONSULT. Ocular Surgery News U.S. Edition, October 10, 2010

[35] Singh A, Gupta A, Stewart JM. Posterior dislocation of descemet stripping automated endothelial keratoplasty graft can lead to retinal detachment. Cornea 2010; 29: 1284–1286

[36] Melles GR, Ong TS, Ververs B, van der Wees J. Descemet membrane endothelial keratoplasty (DMEK). Cornea 2006; 25: 987–990

[37] SCUBA technique for DMEK donor preparation. www.youtube.com/watch?v=vpToO8PFsvI

[38] Giebel AW, Price FW. Descemet membrane endothelial keratoplasty (DMEK): The bare minimum. In DSEK: What you need to know about endothelial keratoplasty. By Francis W Price & Marianne O Price. SLACK Incorporated. Thorofore. Edition 2009. Chapter 10. Pg 121-124

12 Optical Coherence Tomography in Endothelial Keratoplasty

Yuri McKee, Evan Schoenberg, and Francis Price, Jr

First described by Huang et al[1] in 1991, the application of optical coherence tomography (OCT) in the measurement and imaging of ophthalmic systems has revolutionized the approach to many aspects of eye disease. As a noncontact imaging modality, OCT confers a distinct advantage over ultrasound and confocal biomicroscopy. The rapid, noninvasive, and high-resolution qualities of modern OCT make it an excellent adjunct to the diagnostic modalities available to the modern corneal surgeon. In this chapter, we use a case-based approach to demonstrate the use of OCT in the management of endothelial keratoplasty (EK).

The initial iteration of anterior-segment (AS) OCT was labeled time-domain (TD) OCT. Carl Zeiss Meditec (Dublin, OH) introduced the Visante TD-OCT as a tool for precise AS imaging in 2005. The Visante uses a 1310-nm wavelength that can penetrate the cornea and some limbal structures to give a limbus-to-limbus view of the AS with spatial resolution as fine as 15 µm. The Visante can demonstrate two-dimensional corneal shape, corneal opacities, corneal pachymetry, anterior-chamber depth, iris-corneal angle anatomy, iris anatomy, and structures adjacent to the anterior lens capsule, such as phakic intraocular lens (IOLs). Newer Fourier-domain (FD) OCT devices (e.g. Avanti, OptoVue, Freemont, CA; Cirrus, Carl Zeiss Meditec) use an 830-µm wavelength that is popular for retinal imaging. Although resolution improves up to 5 µm, the scan length is more limited. Special attachment lenses are required to image the AS with most models of FD OCT. Although current technology does not allow FD OCT to span the entire corneal diameter, the improved resolution of corneal and angle structures is quite useful.

In recent years, EK has rapidly gained in popularity worldwide for the treatment of cornea endothelial dysfunction. First described by Melles et al,[2] EK confers significant advantages over penetrating keratoplasty (PK), such as stronger postoperative integrity of the globe, less induced astigmatism, faster visual recovery, and significantly reduced episodes of immune graft rejection.[3] With the advances in EK technique have come challenges in securing the posterior corneal graft to the host cornea. Preoperative, intraoperative, and postoperative imaging of the AS with OCT has proven critical in many cases. Currently, the two most popular iterations of EK are Decsemet stripping automated endothelial keratoplasty (DSAEK) and Descemet membrane (DM) endothelial keratoplasty (DMEK). In our practice, DMEK is the preferred EK technique because of the vastly lower rejection rates, smaller incision size, rapid visual recovery, and better visual potential. DMEK is technically more difficult than DSAEK and thus is not suitable for eyes with a discontinuous iris-lens diaphragm, aphakia, aniridia, or extensive posterior corneal irregularity that may preclude DMEK graft adhesion. Unless a surgeon is highly experienced in DMEK technique, DSAEK may also be preferable in eyes with a history of filtering glaucoma surgery, PK, vitrectomy, and significant corneal edema that limits the view of the anterior chamber.

12.1 Preoperative OCT Imaging

In the presence of significant corneal edema, AS OCT may provide critical information regarding the anatomy of the AS and the suitability for EK surgery in a particular eye. Significant peripheral anterior synechia, a shallow anterior chamber, large iris defects, and posterior corneal irregularities may all increase the complexity of EK surgery. In eyes where slit-lamp examination is limited by media opacities, an AS OCT can demonstrate these potential problems preoperatively and assist in proper surgical planning. When treating endothelial failure of a previous PK graft, AS OCT provides valuable information about the potential for posterior apposition of the graft to the host, which can guide surgical planning and help predict postoperative difficulties with adherence. Some authors have suggested a role for AS OCT to determine the DSAEK graft diameter.[4] In cases of failed PK we prefer DMEK in most cases but will choose DSAEK if there is a significant graft-host mismatch as evidenced on AS-OCT.

12.2 Intraoperative OCT Imaging

The use of OCT during ophthalmic surgery has been previously reported by using a handheld OCT device or an OCT device attached to a C-arm in the operative suite. Use of OCT in this manner required a pause in surgery and repositioning of the surgical microscope to allow for OCT imaging.[5,6] Another approach to intraoperative OCT was described by Geerling et al, who coupled a TD OCT unit with a dielectrical mirror to a surgical microscope, producing two-dimensional images with a number of limitations, including difficulty orienting the image and poor light penetration, but it served as a proof of concept.[7] More recently, OCT was incorporated into a commercially available surgical microscope in the Haag-Streit iOCT system (Haag-Streit AG, Bern, Switzerland). This device allows for real-time images of the anterior or posterior segment during surgical maneuvers as the OCT scanning beam is incorporated into the microscope and projected though the main objective lens. A small liquid crystal display (LCD) screen near the surgeon allows for easy viewing of the OCT image with minimal head movement during surgery. Intraoperative OCT confers advantages in many different aspects of ophthalmic surgery. Specific advantages during EK include visualization of interface fluid during DSAEK, determination of proper graft orientation in DMEK, and visualization of posterior corneal deformities that may preclude proper graft positioning or adherence in either iteration of EK.[8]

12.3 Postoperative OCT Imaging

The most popular use for OCT in EK is evaluation of the graft postoperatively. Corneal edema may preclude a detailed slit-lamp view of graft position or adhesion. OCT is commonly used to evaluate the cause of graft detachment,[9] confirm proper graft orientation,[10] and guide postoperative decision making in cases of graft malfunction. OCT can also accurately check graft and host thickness during the immediate postoperative period[11,12] or later during episodes of graft rejection or graft failure. Other potential complications, including epithelial ingrowth,[13] interface opacification,[14] and retained DM,[15] may also be elucidated with AS OCT.

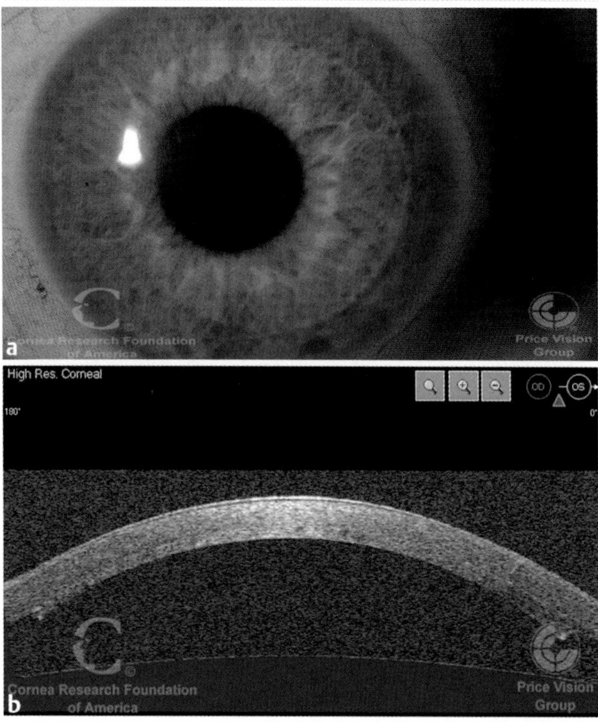

Fig. 12.1 (a) Color photograph of a normal Descemet-stripping endothelial keratoplasty (DSAEK) after complete healing. **(b)** Time-domain optical coherence tomography of a normal DSAEK.

A recent study by Melles et al[2,16] evaluated the predictive value of AS OCT in DMEK graft attachment, comparing graft attachment on AS OCT at 1 hour, 1 week, and 1 month postoperatively with attachment at 6 months. This study, in which no air reinjection was performed at any time point, concluded that DMEK graft attachment at 1 week had excellent predictive value for continued attachment through 6 months. Grafts that were attached at 1 hour but significantly detached at 1 week were likely to reattach spontaneously, whereas grafts detached at both time points were less likely to undergo spontaneous reattachment.[16] These findings provide insight into the evolution of graft adherence and may guide decision making in certain circumstances. It is worth noting that in our practice we reinject air for any significant detachment rather than awaiting spontaneous clearance. In our analysis of 673 eyes with at least 6 months' follow-up, this practice achieves visual improvement sooner and is not associated with decreased endothelial cell counts or increased incidence of any complications.[17]

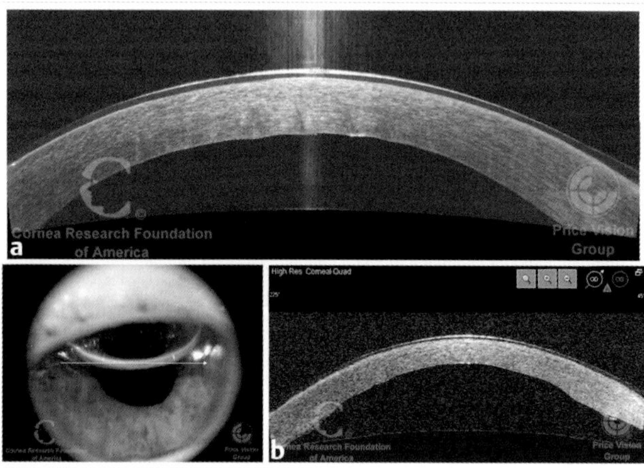

Fig. 12.2 (a) Postoperative day 1 Descemet membrane endothelial keratoplasty (DMEK) as seen on Fourier-domain optical coherence tomography (OCT). The air bubble is not visible on this image of the OCT, but the edge of a bubble can be seen in certain frames. Do not confuse the edge of an air bubble with an inverted graft or a graft detachment. **(b)** A normal DMEK on time-domain OCT at postoperative day 5. OD, right eye; OS, left eye.

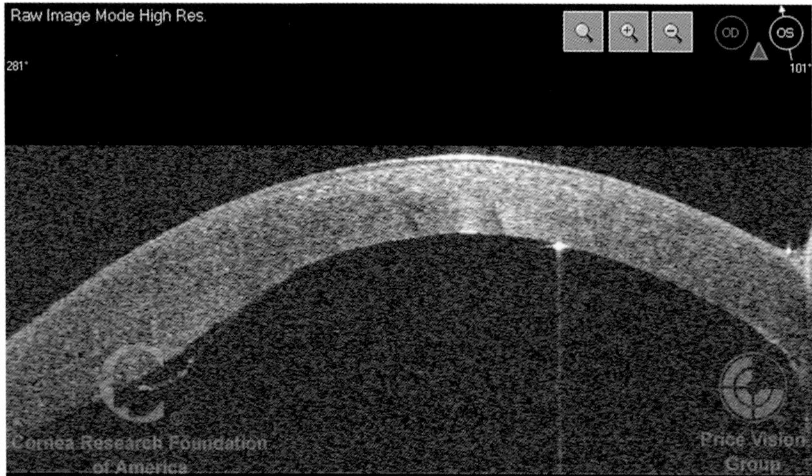

Fig. 12.3 A small peripheral Descemet membrane endothelial keratoplasty (DMEK) graft detachment demonstrated by time-domain OCT. This can be observed at normally scheduled visits. OD, right eye; OS, left eye.

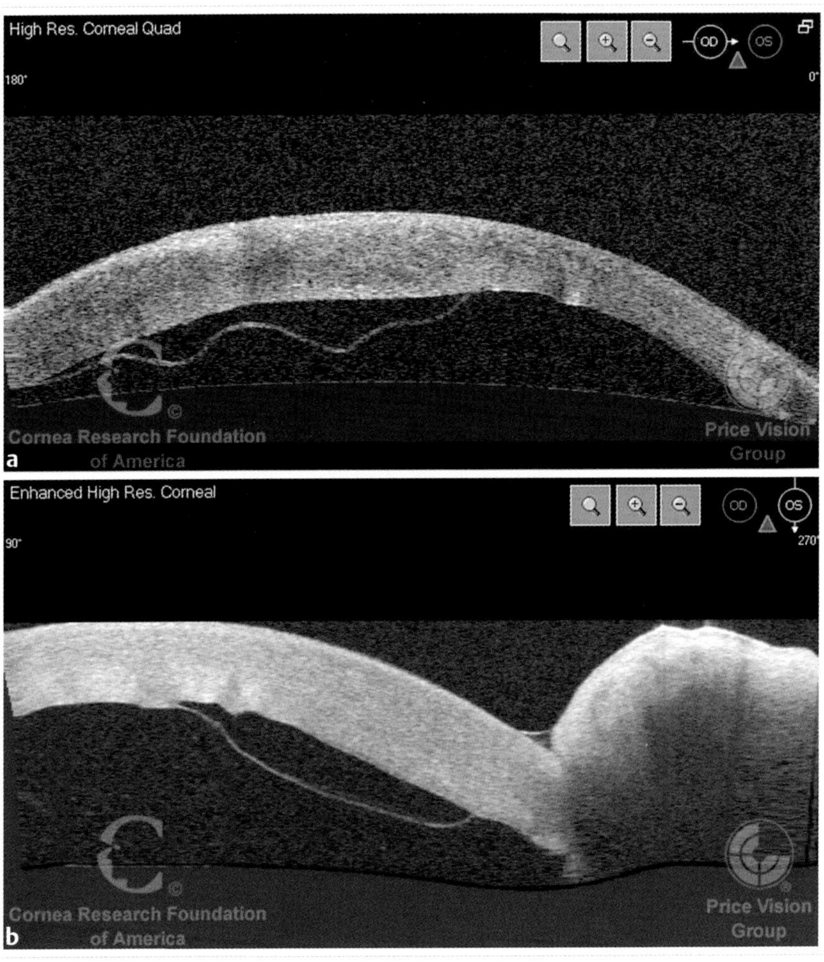

Fig. 12.4 **(a)** A large temporal Descemet membrane endothelial keratoplasty (DMEK) detachment that resolved with a repeat air injection. **(b)** A DMEK graft with a large inferior detachment that required sulphur hexafluoride (SF6) to resolve the detachment. The patient was carefully monitored after injection of SF6 owing to the presence of a trabeculectomy, which can be occluded by inert nonexpansile gases. OD, right eye; OS, left eye.

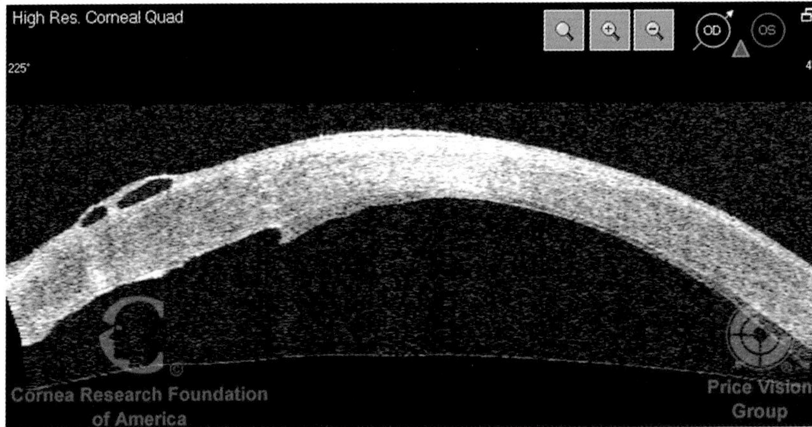

Fig. 12.5 Corneal edema and epithelial bullae due to superior displacement of the graft as demonstrated by time-domain optical coherence tomography. OD, right eye; OS, left eye.

12.4 Case Studies of OCT in Epithelial Keratoplasty

12.4.1 Case 1: Uncomplicated Normal DSEK

In this case, a normal postoperative DSEK is demonstrated (▸ Fig. 12.1). The central cornea is clear, and there is a thin, well-centered graft without folds or detachment. The graft edge is clearly seen by slit lamp and on OCT. Graft and host thickness can be measured individually on OCT. Ultrasonic pachymetry will yield only the total thickness of the graft-host complex. The Visante TD-OCT demonstrates the entire width of the graft and easily penetrates deep into the anterior chamber with the longer 1310-nm wavelength. Some detail is lost in the lower resolution with the longer wavelength. Graft and host thickness can be easily measured at any point using the "Flap Tool" function

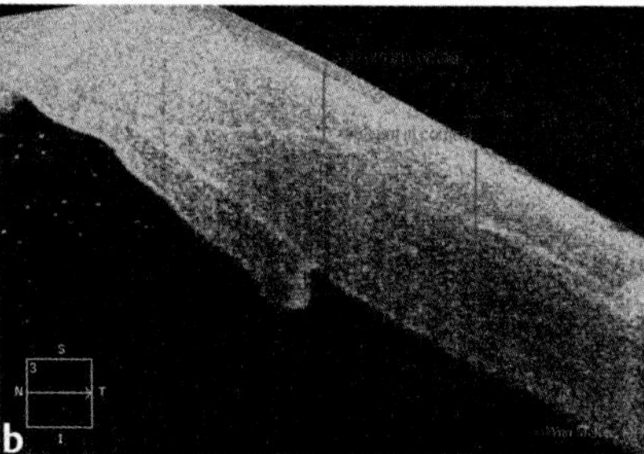

Fig. 12.6 (a) A peripheral Descemet-stripping endothelial keratoplasty (DSAEK) graft detachment near the main surgical wound resulting from a curl of posterior stroma and Descemet membrane (DM). **(b)** After surgical removal of the residual DM tissue and an additional air injection, the temporal graft detachment rapidly cleared along with the host stromal edema. This optical coherence tomography also demonstrates our preferred wound construction for a DSAEK with a short triplanar corneal tunnel and overlap of the inner lip of the wound with the DSAEK graft.

(not shown) that was originally designed to measure LASIK (laser-assisted in-situ keratomileusis) flap thickness.

12.4.2 Case 2: Uncomplicated DMEK

In this case, a postoperative day 1 DMEK (▶ Fig. 12.2) is still supported by an air bubble and fully attached as demonstrated by the Avanti FD OCT (Optovue, Freemont, CA). Note that the maximum scan diameter is 8 mm instead of 12 mm as in a Visante scan, accompanied by a corresponding decrease in scan depth. The FD OCT imparts higher resolution as a result of the shorter 830-nm wavelength of the scanning source. The DMEK graft adheres in such a seamless manner that it is nearly impossible to notice a difference between a graft and a virgin cornea.

This Visante TD-OCT demonstrates the normal appearance of a postoperative DMEK graft with good graft adhesion, centration, and function. This patient has no air left in the anterior chamber and a contact lens still in place, consistent with a postoperative day 5 OCT. The faint edge lift noted superiorly is inconsequential and may be observed in the course of normally scheduled postoperative visits. The surface hyperreflectivity in the AS OCT is due to the bandage contact lens placed at the conclusion of surgery because the patient underwent simultaneous superficial keratectomy.

12.4.3 Case 3: Small DMEK Detachment Requiring Observation Only

Two days after uncomplicated DMEK, this patient was found to have a localized inferior detachment of the graft (▶ Fig. 12.3). Small detachments such as this one are common and typically inferiorly where the air bubble spends less time, even with good reported compliance to supine positioning. The detachment was fully resolved by postoperative day 5. TD OCT provides visualization of even subtle detachments and may be used to objectively follow their extent. Note the gentle curve of the detached portion of the DMEK graft toward the stroma, confirming that the graft is in the proper orientation.

12.4.4 Case 4: DMEK Detachment Requiring Air

In this example, 3 days after DMEK, a large undulating DMEK graft detachment is demonstrated under an area of corneal edema (▶ Fig. 12.4a). This patient had an immediate benefit from an additional air injection and supine positioning. Careful inspection of the detached graft edge reveals a slight upward curl toward the corneal stroma. This finding confirms that the graft is in the correct orientation with endothelium facing the iris. In general, our criteria for air reinjection for DMEK are the following:

- An absence of adequate chamber air bubble to cover completely a detachment (typically < 30 to 40% air bubble)
- Graft detachment greater than two clock hours or an expanding detachment
- Significant edema over a graft detachment
- Graft detachments that threaten the visual axis

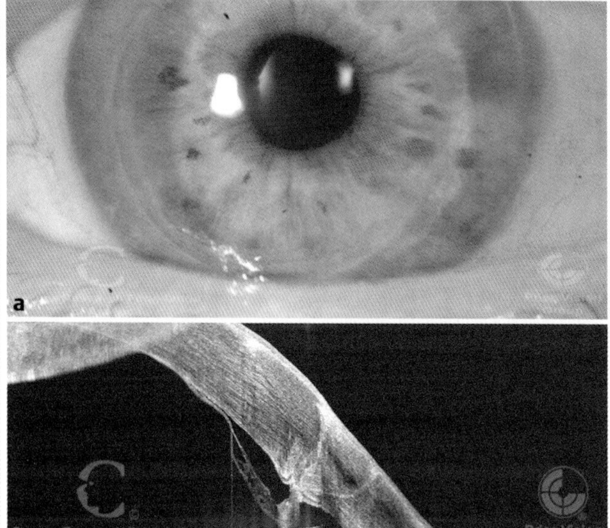

Fig. 12.7 (a) In this postoperative photograph, the central cornea is clear and the Descemet membrane (DM) endothelial keratoplasty (DMEK) graft is functioning well. A small inferotemporal area of haze in the old penetrating keratoplasty represents a stable chronic graft detachment that stabilized after the second air injection. **(b)** The Optovue Fourier-domain optical coherence tomography (OCT) clearly demonstrates a small piece of tissue at the graft-host interface that is causing the detachment. The OCT also demonstrates the chronic nature of the detachment as DM and endothelium have separated and become fibrotic. This stable detachment is unlikely to cause future problems and can simply be observed. Further air injection is unlikely to result in resolution of this detachment.

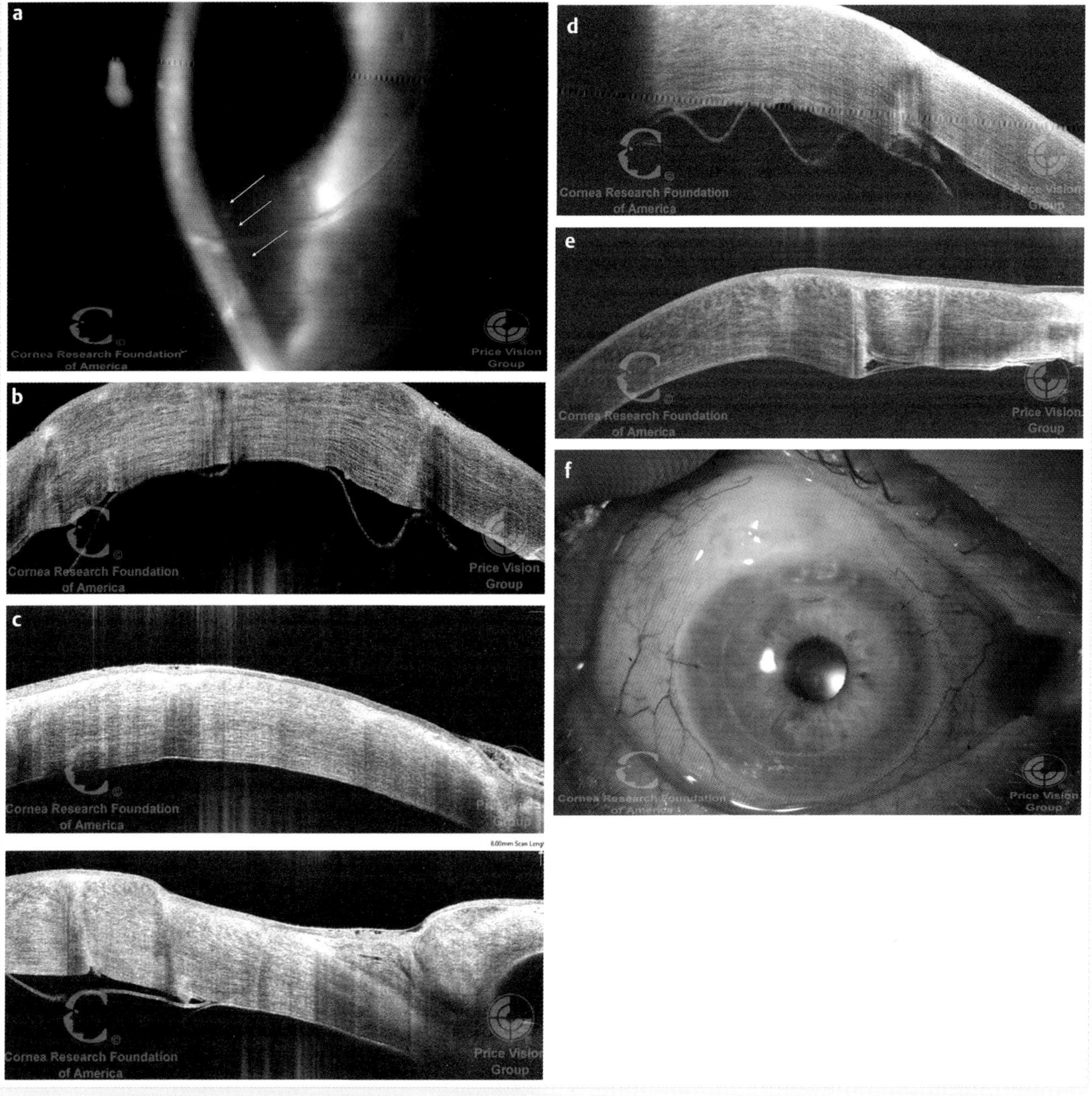

Fig. 12.8 (a) Slit-lamp photograph of an inferior graft detachment in an early postoperative Descemet membrane endothelial keratoplasty (DMEK) under a penetrative keratoplasty (PK). The air rapidly dissipated because of a well-functioning trabeculectomy. The white arrows indicate an inferior DMEK detachment. **(b)** Optovue Fourier-domain optical coherence tomography (FD-OCT) demonstrating a transverse plane view of a superior graft detachment in the early postoperative period as a result of rapid dissipation of the air bubble. **(c)** Optovue FD-OCT after injection of sulphur hexafluoride (SF6). This figure demonstrates transverse (top image) and vertical (bottom image) planes of the superior cornea. The glaucoma bleb filled with gas can be seen in the vertical plane. **(d,e)** An undulating temporal graft detachment before SF6 injection **(d)** supported by SF6 injection **(e)**. **(f)** The failed PK is now clear with a well-attached DMEK graft. The healing time was 2 weeks, and the risk of graft rejection is now less than 1%. A small bubble of SF6 is still present in the anterior chamber in this photograph.

Small, nonprogressive, peripheral detachments without overlying stromal edema that do not threaten the visual axis may be safely observed.

In another example, a DMEK was done in a patient (▶ Fig. 12.4b) who had a history of pars plans vitrectomy and a well-functioning trabeculectomy. The inability to shallow the anterior chamber during surgery in a patient without a vitreous body greatly increases the complexity and operating time of DMEK. In addition, a well-functioning trabeculectomy can quickly cause dissipation of even a full air fill, which can leave little air contact time for the graft and increase the chance of a need for repeat air injection. The use of 16% sulphur hexafluoride (SF6, a nonexpansile concentration) helps to increase the graft contact time of the inert gas, but caution must be used in the setting of a trabeculectomy. The inert gas absorbs much more slowly and can occlude the sclerostomy or fill the bleb with gas, resulting in a dangerous elevation of intraocular pressure. Inferior graft detachments are the most common, as patients often have trouble abiding by a strict supine positioning regimen. When upright, the bubble will continue to support the superior graft, but the inferior graft will be supported only when the patient is supine. Occasionally, supine positioning with a chin-up posture is required to ensure that the inferior aspect of the graft is fully supported by the air bubble. Face-down positioning should be avoided because it can lead to air migrating posterior to the iris.

12.4.5 Case 5: Postoperative Bullae after DSAEK

Bullae and stromal edema can make evaluation of graft position difficult, especially with a thin-cut DSAEK or DMEK. If the involved area is covered by the graft, graft dysfunction or failure may be indicated. On the other hand, if the involved area is outside the graft, observation and temporizing measures, such as hypertonic saline drops, should be advised because endothelial cells may migrate from the graft over time. AS OCT can demonstrate the graft position, even through a hazy cornea, while also visualizing the bullae themselves (▶ Fig. 12.5). In this case, inferior corneal edema after a DSAEK proved to be related to a superior displacement of the graft, but no graft detachment was noted. Observation and conservative measurements eventually resulted in resolution of the edema.

12.4.6 Case 6: Persistent DSAEK Detachment

This patient in case 6 underwent a combined phacoemulsification, IOL insertion, and DSAEK procedure for cataract and Fuchs endothelial dystrophy. The central corneal edema quickly cleared, but a persistent area of temporal corneal edema over the surgical wound persisted. Most DSAEK detachments spontaneously clear without additional air injection over a few days to a few weeks at most. Although the patient achieved excellent vision, she reported a slight visual distortion temporally as well as a foreign-body sensation associated with the edema. When the edema failed to clear, an AS OCT was done using a Cirrus FD-OCT (Carl Zeiss Meditec). Although the scan size is much less with FD OCT, the resolution is much greater, allowing for the visualization of details that might be missed on TD OCT. This detachment was shown to be the result of a curl of the host DM and likely a small amount of posterior stroma that was repelling the edge of the DSAEK graft (▶ Fig. 12.6a). Corneal edema over the graft detachment precluded visualization of the true nature of this problem. The OCT images proved that a repeat air injection would not resolve this detachment. The patient was taken back to the operating room, where the offending tissue scroll was removed with microforceps, and then an air bubble was placed to promote graft edge adhesion (▶ Fig. 12.6b). Postoperatively, the patient reported rapid resolution of discomfort and visual disturbance.

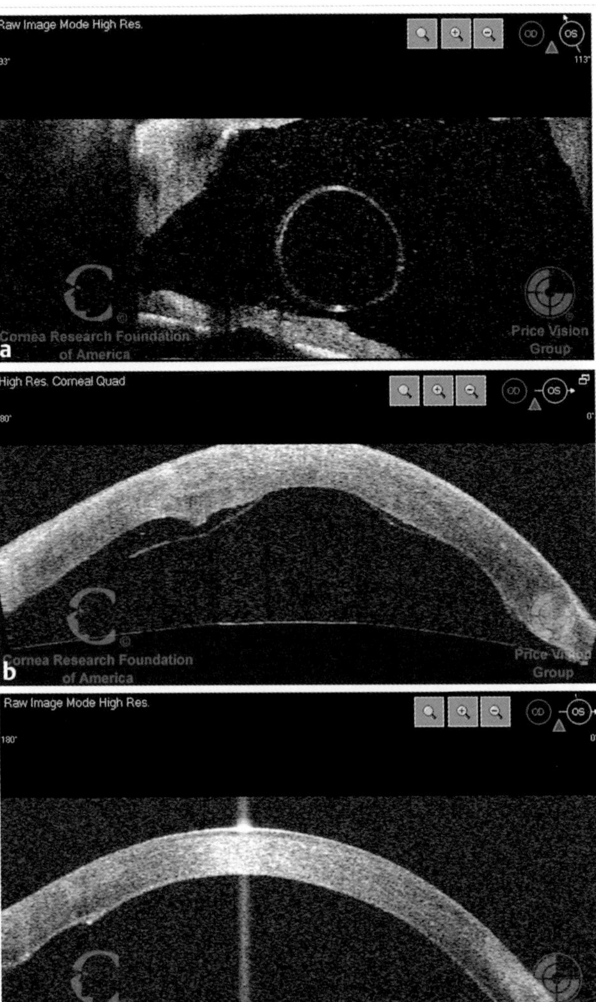

Fig. 12.9 (a) The graft was imaged with time-domain optical coherence tomography in its natural, endothelium-out, scrolled configuration against the iris, en face, with the peripheral cornea visible on the top-left side of the image. **(b)** The repeat Descemet membrane endothelial keratoplasty (DMEK) graft with a detachment over the graft-host junction of the previous penetrating keratoplasty (PK); a graft detachment requiring repeat air injection is noted. **(c)** Complete attachment of the DMEK under the PK after air reinjection. OD, right eye; left eye.

12.4.7 Cases 7 and 8: DMEK under Penetrating Keratoplasty

Placing a DMEK graft under a failed PK confers many advantages over replacing the entire graft, including a lower rejection rate, small incision, and quick recovery. Thus, rescuing a PK from endothelial failure becomes a much lower-risk surgery with a better long-term rejection profile. As a tradeoff, placing a DMEK under a PK requires significant experience with the surgical technique and closer postoperative follow-up resulting from the higher risk of graft edge detachment. The use of SF6 gas to increase the contact time of the anterior-chamber gas bubble may be useful in cases of DMEK under PK, especially when a significant posterior contour discrepancy exists in the graft-host interface. Preoperative evaluation of the graft-host interface can assist with surgical planning. A significant posterior discontinuity may be a reason for using a graft with a diameter equal to or less than the original PK graft; however, we have observed that using EK grafts smaller than 8 mm may lead to a higher rate of failure, presumably as a result of fewer overall endothelial cells in smaller grafts. Consequently, DMEK grafts may need to bridge the graft-host interface, leading to challenges in promoting graft edge adhesion. In questionable cases, the surgeon may opt for a DSAEK graft instead of a DMEK graft under a PK because the surgical technique is less demanding and obtaining stable graft adhesion may be less difficult. The following cases demonstrate some challenges in placing a DMEK under PK and how AS OCT can be useful in management of these cases.

Case 7

The first patient was referred for a slowly failing PK that was placed more than 20 years previously. The falling endothelial cell count and increasing graft thickness confirmed that graft failure was imminent. A DMEK graft was successfully placed. Although the graft did have good central adhesion, a small, persistent inferior-temporal graft detachment was present within the borders of the original PK graft (▸ Fig. 12.7). Because this detachment had shown some enlargement in the first 2 weeks after surgery, an additional air injection was placed and the patient resumed supine positioning for 3 days. A surgeon should decide whether a DMEK detachment requires additional air or gas injection within the first month after surgery because the detached portion of the graft can become fibrotic and inflexible beyond this time. Additional considerations include the area of intended host DM stripping because the retained DM is a risk factor for DMEK graft nonadhesion. DM should not be stripped across an old PK wound, which is one of the strongest points of adhesion between the graft and the host in a healed PK. Additionally, this can lead to additional posterior stromal irregularities for a DMEK graft to negotiate.

Case 8

In this second example of DMEK under PK, a man had a history of DSAEK placed under a failed PK. Several months after surgery, the DSAEK graft suffered an immune-related graft failure. The failed DSAEK extended beyond the margin of the old PK. Although DSAEK does not require full stripping of the DM, removal of a DSAEK often results in concurrent removal of all DM under the graft and in a margin beyond the original EK. Furthermore, in our experience, retained DM is a risk factor for DMEK detachment. To complicate this case further, the patient had a previous pars plans vitrectomy and a well-functioning trabeculectomy with an average intraocular pressure (IOP) of 5 to 8 mm Hg. In eyes with an absent vitreous body, the anterior chamber is difficult to shallow during surgery, increasing the intraoperative difficulty of DMEK. Eyes with very low IOP present a challenge in postoperative adhesion of EK grafts. Additionally, in eyes with a well-functioning trabeculectomy, the intraoperative air bubble can quickly dissipate via the sclerostomy into the bleb (▸ Fig. 12.8). The choice of air or inert, nonexpansile gas in this setting can be a dilemma. Inert gas may last more than twice as long as air in the normal eye, promoting graft adhesion, but it may occlude the sclerostomy of the trabeculectomy, causing a dangerous elevation in IOP.

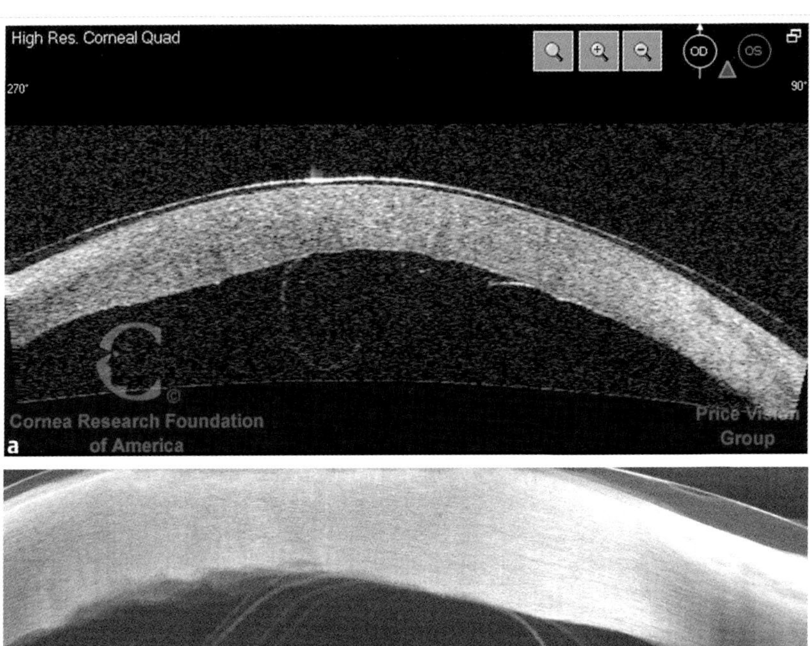

Fig. 12.10 **(a)** Visante time-domain optical coherence tomography (OCT) demonstrated that the graft was curling away from the stroma. **(b)** An Optovue Fourier-domain OCT of the inverted graft. The improved resolution (but narrower acquisition width) of this modality is evident. The ghosting images surrounding the Descemet membrane endothelial keratoplasty graft are the result of movement artifact. OD, right eye; OS, left eye.

12.4.8 Case 9: Complete DMEK Detachment

This patient had a history of PK had endothelial graft failure and cataract. Combined phacoemulsification, IOL placement, and DMEK were performed. On postoperative day 1, the cornea was diffusely edematous and IOP 4 mm Hg. With slit-lamp examination, it was impossible to determine whether or not the DMEK graft was attached. AS OCT allowed for rapid localization of the fully detached DMEK graft resting against the iris in the anterior chamber (▶ Fig. 12.9a). It was clear from the AS OCT that an additional air injection was not going to help with graft attachment.

The next day, the patient returned to surgery for repeat DMEK. An attempt could have been made to reposition the existing graft, but concern for a decreased cell count after manipulation trauma was the rationale for removal of the previous graft and placement of a new DMEK graft. On postoperative day 1, after repeat DMEK, the graft showed scattered small areas of detachment and significant nasal detachment, which did not clear on day 2 despite continued supine positioning. The AS OCT shows a mismatch between the host cornea and the existing PK graft, which interferes with DMEK adherence, resulting in a small temporal and larger nasal DMEK detachment (▶ Fig. 12.9b). Based on the degree of detachment, a repeat air fill to 80% air was performed in the minor procedure room. Three days after the air reinjection, the patient had spent the first 2 days in a supine position with slight left face turn for at least 10 hours per day; an AS OCT demonstrated excellent graft adherence to the PK (▶ Fig. 12.9c). The posterior curvature mismatch continued to discourage complete adherence outside the graft. Once this degree of attachment is obtained, observation alone is typically sufficient.

12.4.9 Case 10: Inverted DMEK Graft

A patient with a history of Fuchs endothelial dystrophy underwent DMEK. On postoperative day 1, he was found to have a posteriorly curling inferior graft detachment. A DMEK graft always scrolls with the endothelium to the outside. A graft curling away from the host cornea indicates that the graft is inverted (▶ Fig. 12.10). This problem is handled in the operating room by repositioning or replacing the graft.

12.4.10 Case 11: DSAEK Graft Detachment under Prior Corneoscleral Graft

This patient initially had bacterial keratitis involving the cornea, limbus, and limbal sclera that did not respond to aggressive antibacterial therapy. A 15-mm corneoscleral anterior lamellar graft was performed. To decrease the risk of intraocular spread of the infection, the patient's own DM and endothelium were not violated during this procedure. Postoperatively, the infection cleared, and the patient had a dense cataract and retrocorneal membrane. Phacoemulsification, IOL placement, and removal of the membrane (which corresponded to fibrosis surrounding the host Descemet) were performed without complication. Subsequently, however, the host endothelium failed. The patient underwent DSAEK under the corneoscleral graft.

On postoperative day 2, slit-lamp evidence of a large supranasal graft detachment of unclear cause was seen. Conventional management would suggest repeat air injection to float the graft back into position; however, AS OCT revealed that the graft margin was actually stuck on an iris root remnant from the corneoscleral graft (▶ Fig. 12.11a). Further air injections would not be likely to resolve the detachment. The next day, the patient returned to the surgical suite, and the graft was

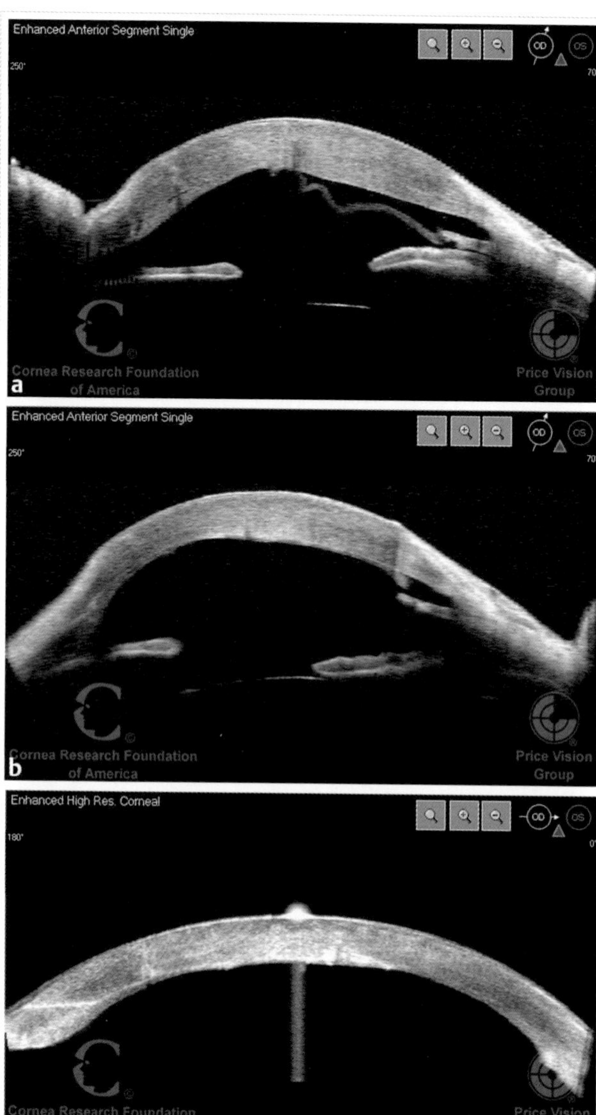

Fig. 12.11 (a) The Descemet-stripping endothelial keratoplasty (DSAEK) graft edge held out of the proper position by the iris root of the prior corneoscleral graft. (b) Postoperative day 1 from DSAEK reposition. The DSAEK graft is now in good position and fully attached. (c) One year after DSAEK, the cornea is clear and the graft well attached. OD, right eye; OS, left eye.

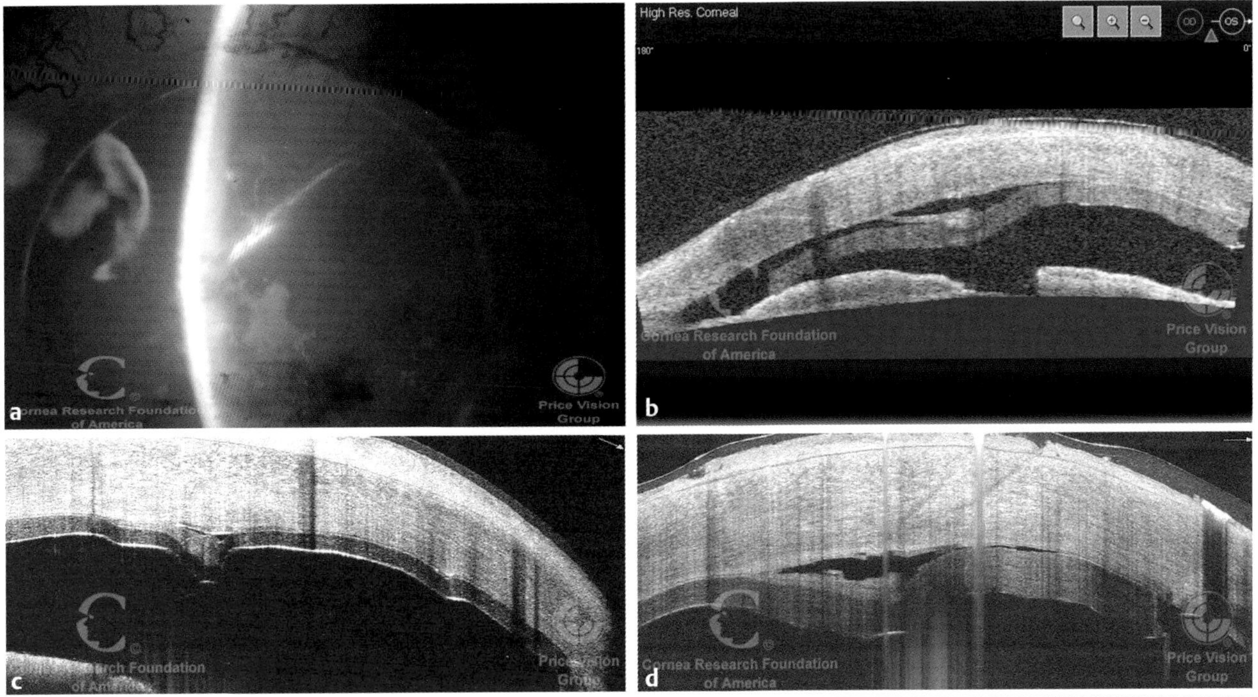

Fig. 12.12 (a) Slit-beam photograph of Descemet-stripping endothelial keratoplasty (DSAEK) under old forceps delivery injury (b) On postoperative day 1, the graft showed poor apposition to the host cornea, especially in the area of posterior corneal fibrosis. (c) Under a 95% air fill, the DSAEK graft conformed well to the host corneal deformity. (d) One week later, after air was no long pressing the graft into place, the graft could be seen conforming to the fibrotic Descemet remnant of the host. OD, right eye; OS, left eye.

repositioned. At postoperative week 1, the repositioned DSAEK graft was well positioned and fully attached (▶ Fig. 12.11b). The corneoscleral graft stroma remained edematous. At postoperative 1 year, the graft stroma was clear and of normal thickness (▶ Fig. 12.11c).

12.4.11 Case 12: DSAEK Graft Detachment with Posterior Corneal Fibrosis

A 58-year-old woman had a history of delivery forceps trauma that resulted in chronic corneal clouding. She was wearing bandage contact lenses for painful bullous keratopathy and band keratopathy, which developed 3 years previously. She underwent combined DSAEK and sodium-EDTA chelation. Descemet stripping was not attempted because of the poor view. After extensive manipulation, the graft was unfolded and positioned. A complete air fill for 8 minutes was followed by a reduction to a 50% bubble. On postoperative day 1, the cornea was significantly clearer than preoperatively, but a large inferior and nasal detachment of the graft was visible on slit-lamp examination. An oblique opacity could also be appreciated, but owing to the remaining corneal haze, it was unclear whether this was a result of host pathology or of a fold in the graft (▶ Fig. 12.12a).

The AS OCT demonstrated a relatively thick, opaque outcropping of tissue consistent with fibrosis of the patient's DM at the site of initial injury (▶ Fig. 12.12b). A laser inferior peripheral iridectomy was made, and the anterior chamber was filled 95% with air. Under air, closer apposition of the graft was achieved, as seen under the slit lamp and on AS OCT (▶ Fig. 12.12c,d).

12.4.12 Case 13: Intraoperative OCT with the Haag-Streit iOCT

Intraoperative OCT is a promising new technology that has now been integrated into the surgical microscope. In this example, a DMEK graft orientation is quickly and positively determined by OCT that is aimed through the main lens of the microscope. This results in real-time information being available to the surgeon without interrupting the surgical process (▶ Fig. 12.13).

12.5 Conclusion

Anterior-segment has radically changed the approach to evaluation and management of patients undergoing EK. Although preoperative evaluation can help guide surgical planning in difficult cases, postoperative availability to perform an AS OCT is critical in managing the inevitable graft detachments that occur in the typical postsurgical course of some patients. Intraoperative OCT is now becoming available and will further facilitate the surgical process, especially for DMEK. An understanding of the basic concepts, applications, and limitations of different OCT modalities is now a required skill for the modern corneal surgeon. As this technology rapidly advances, we should expect

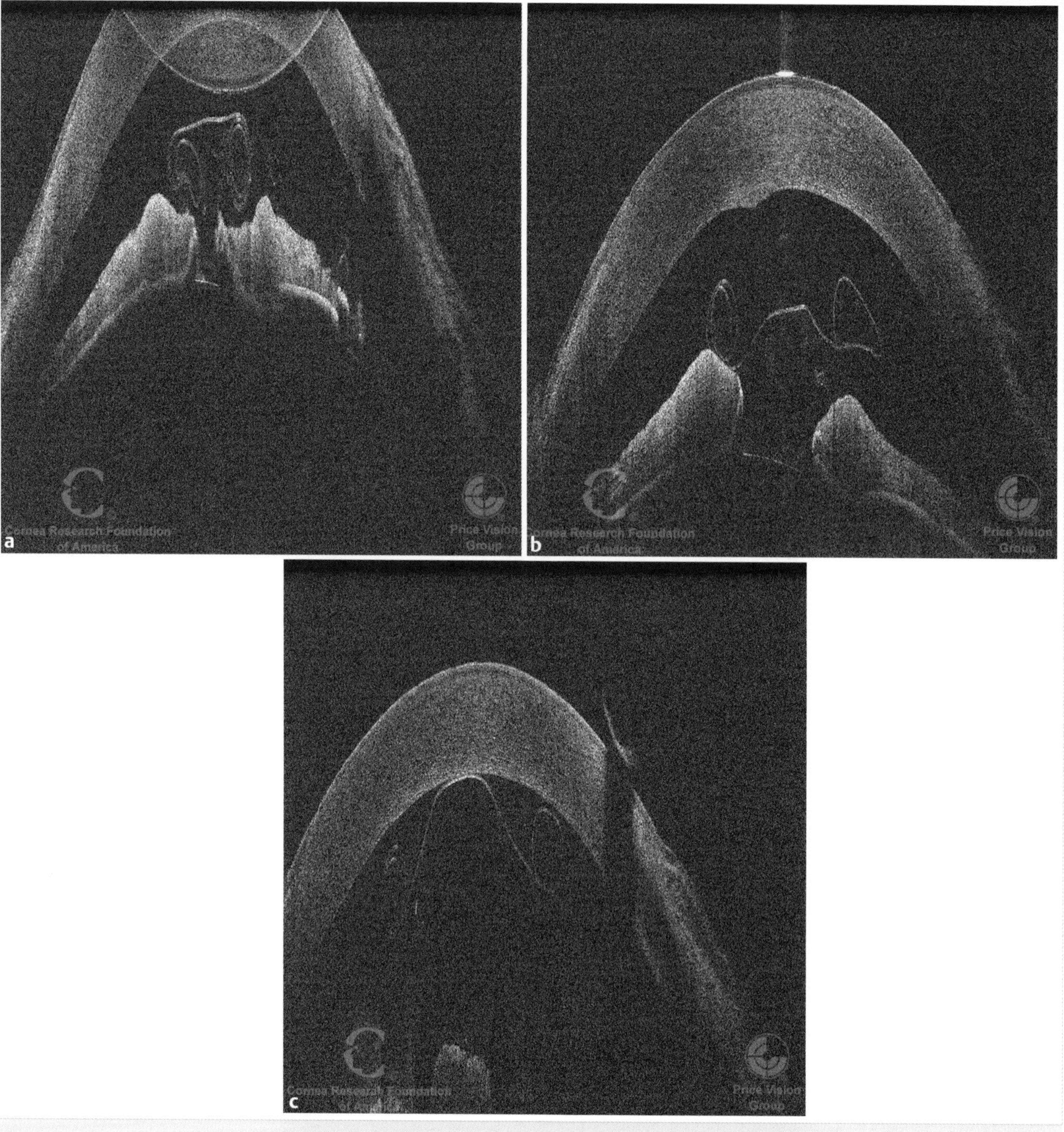

Fig. 12.13 (a) Intraoperative optical coherence tomography demonstrates an inverted Descemet membrane endothelial keratoplasty scroll after graft insertion. **(b)** The graft is flipped with a gentle burst of fluid and is now in the proper orientation. **(c)** The graft is suspended against the host stroma by an air bubble preventing accidental graft inversion and promoting graft opening.

further increases in scan width, depth, and resolution. Applying the information gleaned from this amazing technology will help guide the corneal surgeon to the correct diagnosis and treatment plan when offering EK to our patients.

References

[1] Huang D, Swanson EA, Lin CP, et al. Optical coherence tomography. Science 1991; 254: 1178–1181

[2] Melles GR, Eggink FA, Lander F, et al. A surgical technique for posterior lamellar keratoplasty. Cornea 1998; 17: 618–626

[3] Anshu A, Price MO, Price FW Jr. Risk of corneal transplant rejection significantly reduced with Descemet's membrane endothelial keratoplasty. Ophthalmology 2012; 119: 536–540

[4] Straiko MD, Terry MA, Shamie N. Descemet stripping automated endothelial keratoplasty under failed penetrating keratoplasty: a surgical strategy to minimize complications. Am J Ophthalmol 2011; 151: 233–237, e2

[5] Knecht PB, Kaufmann C, Menke MN, Watson SL, Bosch MM. Use of intraoperative fourier-domain anterior segment optical coherence tomography during descemet stripping endothelial keratoplasty. Am J Ophthalmol 2010; 150: 360–365, e2

[6] Ide T, Wang J, Tao A, et al. Intraoperative use of three-dimensional spectral-domain optical coherence tomography. Ophthalmic Surg Lasers Imaging 2010; 41: 250–254

[7] Geerling G, Müller M, Winter C, et al. Intraoperative 2-dimensional optical coherence tomography as a new tool for anterior segment surgery. Arch Ophthalmol 2005; 123: 253–257

[8] Steven P, Le Blanc C, Velten K, et al. Optimizing descemet membrane endothelial keratoplasty using intraoperative optical coherence tomography. JAMA Ophthalmol 2013; 131: 1135–1142

[9] Moutsouris K, Dapena I, Ham L, Balachandran C, Oellerich S, Melles GRJ. Optical coherence tomography, Scheimpflug imaging, and slit-lamp biomicroscopy in the early detection of graft detachment after Descemet membrane endothelial keratoplasty. Cornea 2011; 30: 1369–1375

[10] Saad A, Sabatier P, Gatinel D. Graft orientation, optical coherence tomography, and endothelial keratoplasty. Ophthalmology 2013; 120: 871–871, e3

[11] Di Pascuale MA, Prasher P, Schlecte C, et al. Corneal deturgescence after Descemet stripping automated endothelial keratoplasty evaluated by Visante anterior segment optical coherence tomography. Am J Ophthalmol 2009; 148: 32–37, e1

[12] Wong MHY, Chew A, Htoon HM, et al. Reproducibility of Corneal Graft Thickness measurements with COLGATE in patients who have undergone DSAEK (Descemet stripping automated endothelial keratoplasty). BMC Med Imaging 2012; 12: 25

[13] Suh LH, Shousha MA, Ventura RU, et al. Epithelial ingrowth after Descemet stripping automated endothelial keratoplasty: description of cases and assessment with anterior segment optical coherence tomography. Cornea 2011; 30: 528–534

[14] de Sanctis U, Brusasco L, Grignolo F. Wave like opacities at the interface after descemet stripping automated endothelial keratoplasty. Cornea 2012; 31: 1335–1338

[15] Suh LH, Yoo SH, Deobhakta A, et al. Complications of Descemet's stripping with automated endothelial keratoplasty: survey of 118 eyes at One Institute. Ophthalmology 2008; 115: 1517–1524

[16] Yeh R-Y, Quilendrino R, Musa FU, Liarakos VS, Dapena I, Melles GRJ. Predictive value of optical coherence tomography in graft attachment after Descemet's membrane endothelial keratoplasty. Ophthalmology 2013; 120: 240–245

[17] Feng MT, Price MO, Miller JM, Price FW Jr. Air reinjection and endothelial cell density in Descemet membrane endothelial keratoplasty: five-year follow-up. J Cataract Refract Surg 2014; 40: 1116–1121

13 Spectral-Domain Optical Coherence Tomography Evaluation of Pre-Descemet Endothelial Keratoplasty Graft

Ashvin Agarwal, Dhivya Ashok Kumar, and Amar Agarwal

Pre-Descemet endothelial keratoplasty (PDEK), a recent modification of endothelial keratoplasty, involves transplantation of the pre-Descemet layer (Dua layer) along with the Descemet membrane (DM) with endothelium. In this selective tissue transplantation, the pre-Descemet layer provides additional thickness to the thin DM. Dua and colleagues identified the pre-Descemet layer as a tough, fibrous layer about 10.15 ± 3.6 µm thick.[1] The principal advantages of the technique are easy intraoperative tissue handling and less injury to the donor harvested graft. The initial results showed good postoperative outcomes and fewer surgical complications.[2] The technique inherited the basic advantages of early visual rehabilitation and lowered graft rejection, similar to Descemet membrane endothelial keratoplasty (DMEK).[3,4] The postoperative graft position, although seen clinically by slit lamp, high-resolution spectral-domain optical coherence tomography (SD OCT) provides additional information for the configuration of endothelial grafts. In this chapter, we show the postoperative graft configuration using SD OCT.

13.1 Pre-Descemet Endothelial Keratoplasty

A corneoscleral disc with an approximately 2-mm scleral rim is dissected from the whole globe or obtained from an eye bank. A 30-gauge needle attached to a syringe is inserted from the limbus into the midperipheral stroma (▶ Fig. 13.1, upper left). Air is slowly injected into the donor stroma until a type 1 big bubble is formed (▶ Fig. 13.1, upper left and central). Trephination is done along the margin of the big bubble. The bubble wall is penetrated at the extreme periphery, and trypan blue is injected to stain the graft, which is then cut with a pair of corneoscleral scissors and covered with the tissue culture medium (▶ Fig. 13.1, upper right).

With the patient under peribulbar anesthesia, a trephine mark is made on the recipient cornea respective to the diameter of the DM to be scored on the endothelial side. A 2.8-mm tunnel incision is made at the 10 o'clock position near the limbus. The anterior chamber (AC) is formed and maintained by saline injection or infusion. The margin of recipient DM to be removed is scored with a reverse Sinskey hook and then peeled (▶ Fig. 13.1, middle left and central). Donor lenticule (endothelium-DM-pre-Descemet layer) roll is inserted in the custom-made injector (▶ Fig. 13.1, middle right) and injected in a controlled fashion into the AC (▶ Fig. 13.1, lower left). The donor graft is oriented endothelial side down and positioned onto the recipient posterior stroma by careful, indirect manipulation of the tissue with air and fluid (▶ Fig. 13.1, lower central). Once the lenticule is unrolled, an air bubble is injected underneath the lenticule to lift it toward the recipient posterior stroma (▶ Fig. 13.1, lower right). The AC is completely filled with air for the next 30 minutes, followed by an air-liquid exchange to pressurize the eye. The eye speculum is finally removed, and the AC is examined for air position. The patient is advised to lie in a strictly supine position for next 3 hours.

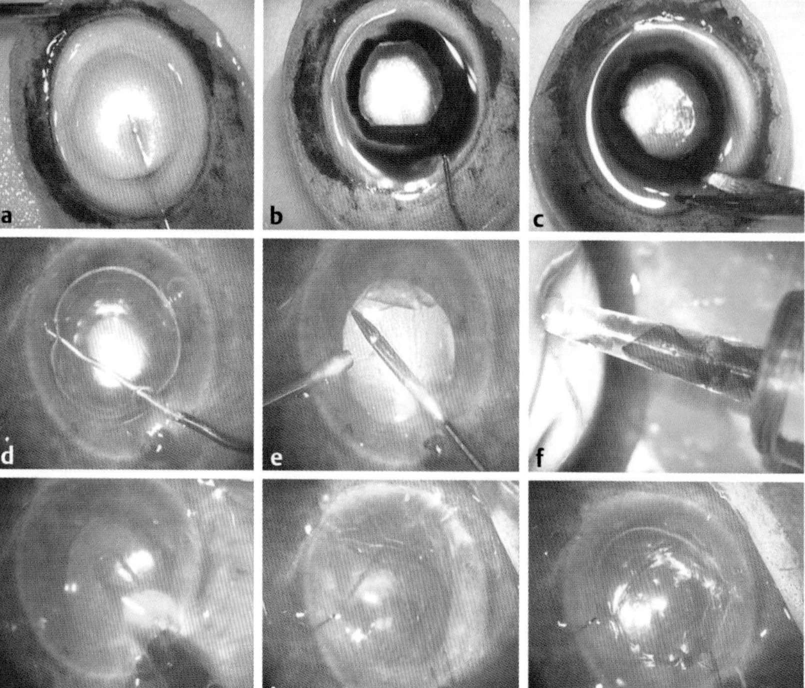

Fig. 13.1 (a) Pre-Descemet endothelial keratoplasty. **(b)** Type 1 bubble is formed in the donor cornea by injecting air via a 30-gauge needle. **(c)** Trypan blue is injected into the bubble. Trephination was done and the graft cut using a pair of corneal scissors. **(d,e)** Middle left and central: The margin of recipient Descemet membrane to be removed is scored using a reverse Sinskey hook and then peeled. **(f)** Donor lenticule roll is inserted in the custom-made injector and **(g)** injected in a controlled fashion into the anterior chamber. **(h)** The donor lenticule is positioned onto the recipient posterior stroma and unrolled with air and fluid. **(i)** Finally, an air bubble is injected underneath the lenticule to lift it toward the recipient posterior stroma and followed by air-fluid exchange.

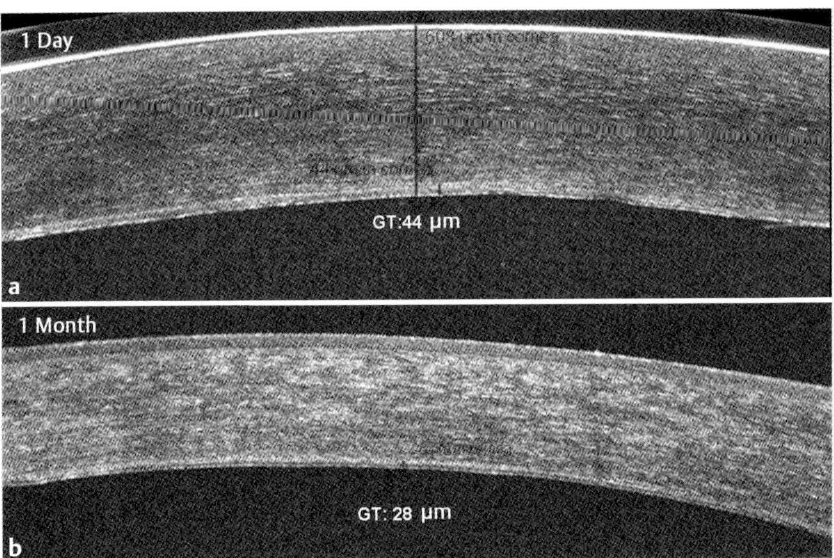

Fig. 13.2 Graft thickness shows significant reduction from the immediate postoperative period **(a)** to 1 month **(b)**.

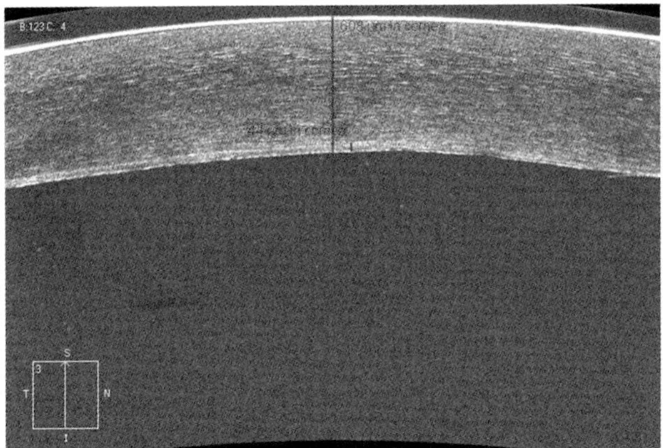

Fig. 13.3 Day 1 postoperative image of well-adhered graft seen in spectral-domain optical coherence tomography.

13.2 Spectral-Domain OCT

Postoperative SD OCT scans were performed by experienced examiner, and the scans were evaluated by expert ophthalmologists. An anterior-segment five-line raster pattern in an axis of 0 to 180 degrees and 90 to 270 degrees was used. The raster scan had five lines (length, 3 mm) and a distance of 250 µm between the lines. The scan was centered at the corneal vertex for a central 3-mm scan. Additional inferior, temporal, nasal, and superior positional scans were also taken. Graft thickness was measured in microns using the tool caliper in the SD OCT. Graft detachment was graded as group I when grafts were completely attached or with a minimal edge detachment; as group II for graft detachments less than one-third of the graft surface area, not affecting the visual axis; as group III when graft detachments comprised more than a third of the graft surface area; and as group IV when grafts were completely detached. Epithelial thickness and recurrence of bulla were noted. Graft-host junction was visualized for interface opacification. *Graft split* is defined as the separation of pre-Descemet layer and DM. Postoperative central corneal thickness (CCT) was also measured in all follow-ups. Twelve eyes of 12 patients whose mean age was 65 ± 3.8 years were evaluated (nine women, three men). The donor age ranged from 1 to 56 years. Graft size ranged from 7.5 to 8 mm. All eyes had preoperative pseudophakic bullous keratopathy as the indication for endothelial transplantation.

13.3 PDEK Graft in OCT

The mean graft thickness in PDEK was 37.3 ± 3.5 µm (range, 32–44 µm). The graft undergoes minimal dehydration in the postoperative period. The mean graft thickness on days 7, 30, and 90 was 35.5 ± 3.4 µm (32–40 µm), 33 ± 1.8 µm (32–36 µm), and 30.3 ± 2.6 µm (28–36 µm), respectively. The difference over the time period was significant (Friedman test, $P = 0.000$) (▶ Fig. 13.2), but there was no significant difference ($P = 1.000$) between the central (3 mm) and peripheral (4–6 mm) graft thickness.

The graft adhered well (▶ Fig. 13.3) in 9 of 12 eyes on day 1. Two eyes had group II detachment (▶ Fig. 13.4), and one eye had group III graft detachment (▶ Fig. 13.5). One eye with grade III detachment underwent air injection. The graft was well apposed on day 1 after air injection; however, there was redetachment on day 12, and rebubbling was done subsequently. In group I eyes with well-adhered graft, a small, shallow peripheral detachment was seen in the inferior (two eyes) and nasal quadrants (one eye). The mean detachment depth was 24.6 ± 8.3 µm. Descemet folds were noted in two eyes on day 1 (▶ Fig. 13.6), but they resolved on day 7 with medical management and supine position. Smooth concave configuration of the posterior cornea was obtained in all eyes by 1 month. None of the eyes had complete graft detachment or lenticule drop.

Eleven of 12 eyes had smooth graft-host interface. One eye had minimal interface haze by postoperative 1 month. After a course of intense steroid treatment, the graft-host interface haze decreased in one eye (▶ Fig. 13.7). Separation of graft into two linear hyperreflective lines was seen by OCT in two eyes. The posterior layer was 16 µm, and the anterior layer was 12 µm. Both eyes had mild corneal edema on day 1 that resolved with strict supine position and medical management.

All eyes had central epithelial defect on postoperative day 1. Epithelial healing was complete in all eyes by 48 hours. The mean epithelial thickness was 44.4 ± 9.8 µm by week 1 and reduced to 37.5 ± 6.2 µm in the last follow-up. There was a significant reduction in thickness ($P = 0.003$) over the time period. No difference in the central and peripheral epithelium was seen in 11 eyes. On postoperative day 1, mean CCT was 612 ± 46.4 µm. By day 7, significant resolution of corneal edema was noted ($P = 0.001$). Grade 3 cellular reaction was seen in one eye, and one eye had grade 4 fibrinous reaction. Shallow detachment was seen in the eye with fibrin (▶ Fig. 13.8). Intense steroid treatment attained good graft adherence by 2 weeks.

13.3.1 Correlations and Associations

No significant correlation was found between graft thickness and the best corrected vision at day 1 ($P = 0.409$) and day 90 ($P = 0.661$) or between the mean CCT reduction and the graft thickness reduction from day 1 to day 90 ($P = 0.645$, $r = 0.149$). No correlation was seen between the corneal edema and graft thickness on day 1 ($P = 0.374$, $r = 0.282$), nor was an association seen between the corneal thickness on day 1 and the graft detachment (chi-square test, $P = 0.285$). No association was found between the graft thickness on day 1 and the graft detachment (chi-square test, $P = 0.167$). There was strong association with graft adherence and best corrected visual acuity (chi-square, $P = 0.007$). Eyes with early detachment showed poorer visual outcome.

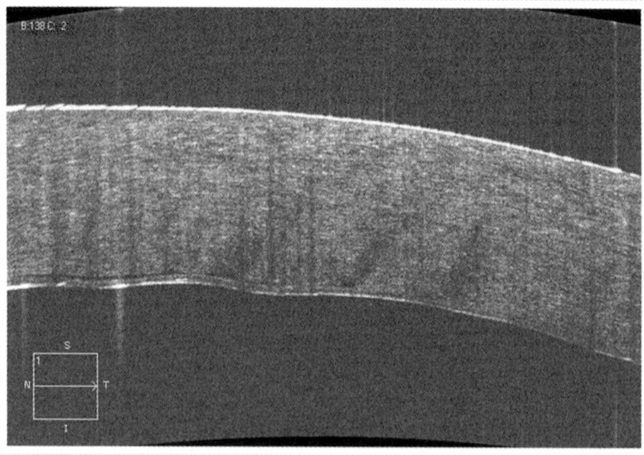

Fig. 13.4 Day 1 postoperative image showing shallow graft detachments in spectral-domain optical coherence tomography.

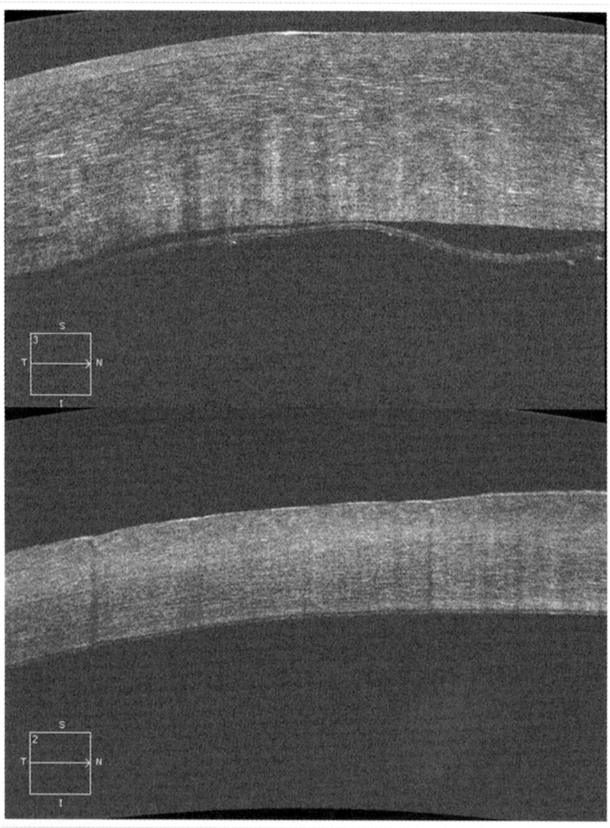

Fig. 13.5 Group III graft detachment after pre-Descemet endothelial keratoplasty **(a)** and reattachment after air injection **(b)**.

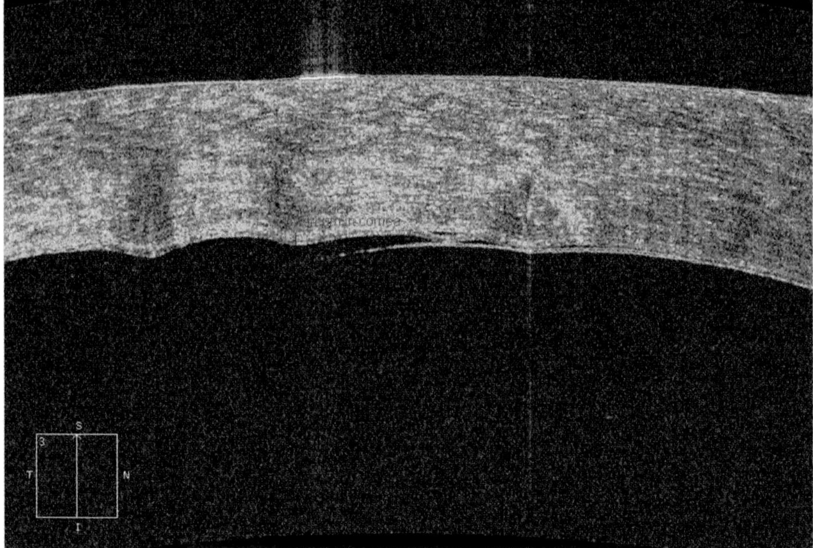

Fig. 13.6 Day 1 postoperative image showing Descemet membrane folds in spectral-domain optical coherence tomography with small shallow detachment.

13.3.2 OCT in Endothelial Keratoplasty

Anterior-segment OCT has been used in DMEK for predicting postoperative graft adherence.[5] It has also been used for intraoperative graft positioning.[6] In our study, we showed the behavior of PDEK graft in vivo in the postoperative follow-up.

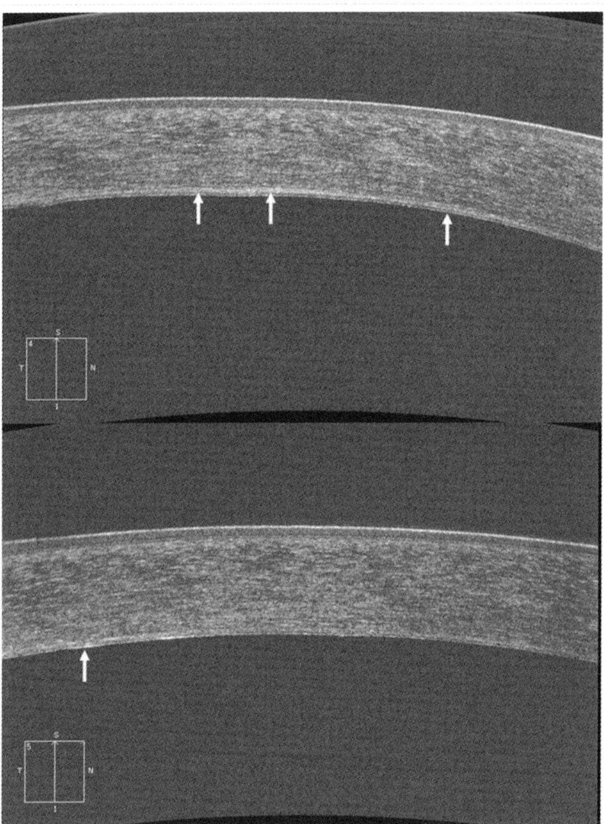

Fig. 13.7 Spectral-domain optical coherence tomography showing graft interface opacification (a, arrow) and resolution after treatment with intense steroids (b, arrow).

Yeh et al studied the predictability of OCT scan for graft attachment in DMEK.[5] They noted that the initial 1 hour showed the best predictive value in DMEK graft adherence. Because of graft edema and stromal edema in the immediate postoperative period, it might be difficult to localize detachments clinically by slit-lamp examination. Therefore, the anterior-segment OCT has been used to visualize those endothelial grafts (Descemet-stripping automated keratoplasty [DSAEK] or DMEK) under such situations. Although time-domain anterior-segment OCT[6,7,8] has been used for evaluating graft status after endothelial keratoplasties like DSAEK and DMEK, no studies have been reported on the evaluation of grafts by SD OCT. Clinically undetectable detachments can also be localized by SD OCT because of the higher resolution (5 µm).

13.3.3 PDEK Graft Versus Other Endothelial Grafts

The mean central graft thickness in ultrathin Busin graft was 78.28 ± 28.89 µm at 3 months postoperatively.[9] Shousha et al reported the thickness of a normal DM in elderly patients to be about 16 ± 2 µm (range, 13–20 µm) using ultrahigh-resolution OCT.[10] The mean graft thickness in our study was 37.3 ± 3.5 µm and was stabilized by 3 months (▶ Fig. 13.9). From our study, we noted that the PDEK grafts are thicker than DMEK grafts and thinner than ultrathin DSAEK grafts. The PDEK grafts were uniform, with no difference in the thickness from central to periphery as seen by OCT. Graft adherence has been a single important factor for better functional outcome after successful endothelial keratoplasty.[11,12] Graft detachment has been described as the common complication after endothelial keratoplasty techniques such as DMEK and DSAEK.[11,12,13,14] Although thinner grafts are more susceptible to incomplete graft adhesion after primary positioning, early visual recovery may be possible only with thin graft.[15] PDEK graft has the advantage of thinner grafts similar to DMEK, which can aid in easy intraoperative manipulation and at the same time postoperative adherence.

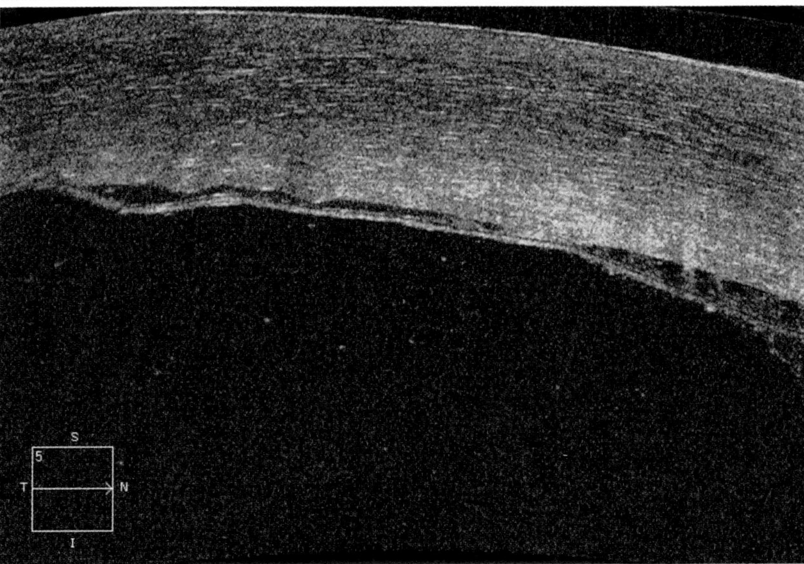

Fig. 13.8 Anterior-segment optical coherence tomography showing fibrin reaction with shallow detachment of pre-Descemet endothelial keratoplasty graft.

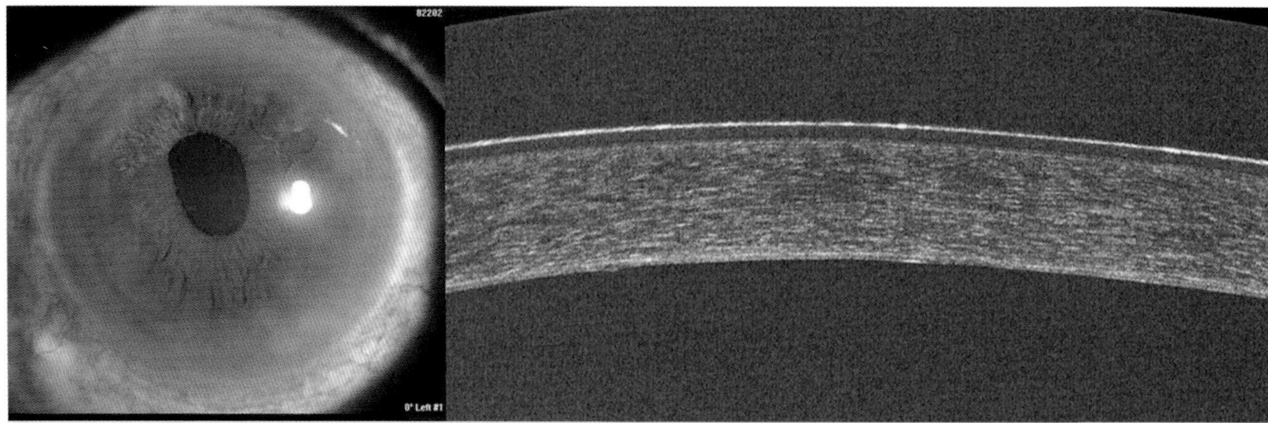

Fig. 13.9 Clinical photograph (a) and spectral-domain optical coherence tomography (b) 6 months after pre-Descemet endothelial keratoplasty with no interface haze.

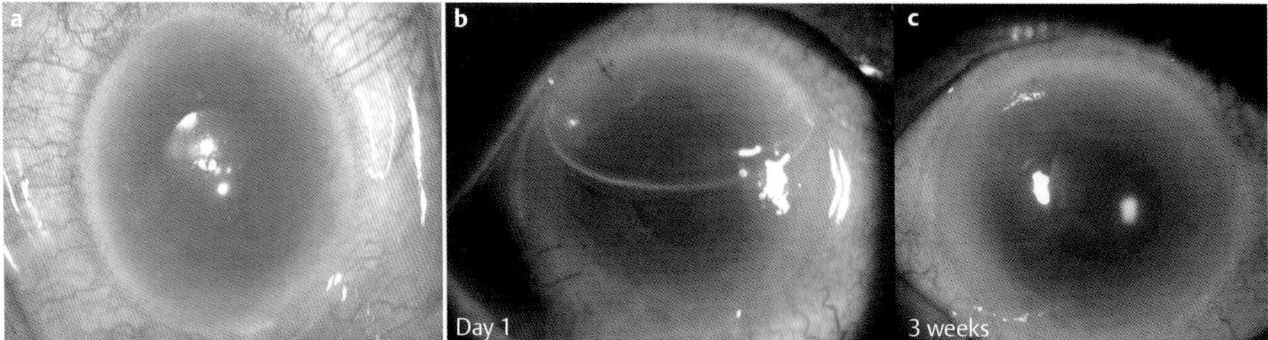

Fig. 13.10 Good postoperative corneal clarity was seen after pre-Descemet endothelial keratoplasty. (a) Preoperative, (b) immediate, (c) 3 weeks.

The two main factors that interfere with graft attachments are the intracorneal pressure and the interposition[15]; these factors are necessary for the PDEK grafts as well. Precut donor tissue over hydration, stromal edema (both donor and recipient), and irregular interface prevent graft adherence. In our study, the graft adhered well in 75% of the eyes. No eye had total graft detachment or lenticule drop in the AC.

The possibility of separation of corneal layers by pneumatic dissection has been proven and has been technically easier.[16,17] Hence, the preparation of PDEK lenticule is not difficult in the present clinical setup. The biggest challenge faced in DMEK is tissue loss in preparation and postoperative attachment. Price and Price reported that the recent advances in instrumentation and technique have reduced the learning curve of DMEK.[18] However, DMEK provides faster visual recovery without interface opacification.[19] The absence of interface reaction is one of the advantages of DMEK grafts compared with DSAEK grafts. Similarly, in PDEK graft analysis in OCT, less or no interface opacification was seen during the postoperative period (▶ Fig. 13.10). Dua et al reported the absence of keratocytes in the central region of the pre-Descemet layer, and this layer may be the factor that can potentially contribute to reduced haze, as air cleavage creates a smooth plane and lessened keratocyte activity.[1] The split in the graft that occurred in two eyes resolved spontaneously with strict supine position; however, those two eyes with graft split did not have graft detachment or corneal edema in the postoperative period. Nevertheless, the additional pre-Descemet layer attached to the DM is expected to provide a splinting effect to the DM in the graft and at the same time preserve the early visual rehabilitation of DMEK.

References

[1] Dua HS, Faraj LA, Said DG, Gray T, Lowe J. Human corneal anatomy redefined: a novel pre-Descemet's layer (Dua's layer). Ophthalmology 2013; 120: 1778–1785

[2] Agarwal A, Dua HS, Narang P, et al. Pre-Descemet's endothelial keratoplasty (PDEK). Br J Ophthalmol 2014 Sep; 98: 1181–5

[3] Melles GR, Ong TS, Ververs B, van der Wees J. Descemet membrane endothelial keratoplasty (DMEK). Cornea 2006; 25: 987–990

[4] Tourtas T, Laaser K, Bachmann BO, Cursiefen C, Kruse FE. Descemet membrane endothelial keratoplasty versus descemet stripping automated endothelial keratoplasty. Am J Ophthalmol 2012; 153: 1082–1090, e2

[5] Yeh RY, Quilendrino R, Musa FU, Liarakos VS, Dapena I, Melles GR. Predictive value of optical coherence tomography in graft attachment after Descemet's membrane endothelial keratoplasty. Ophthalmology 2013; 120: 240–245

[6] Steven P, Le Blanc C, Velten K, et al. Optimizing descemet membrane endothelial keratoplasty using intraoperative optical coherence tomography. JAMA Ophthalmol 2013; 131: 1135–1142

[7] Tan GS. 1, He M, Tan DT, Mehta JS. Correlation of anterior segment optical coherence tomography measurements with graft trephine diameter following Descemet stripping automated endothelial keratoplasty. BMC Med Imaging 2012; 12: 19

[8] Moutsouris K, Dapena I, Ham L, Balachandran C, Oellerich S, Melles GR. Optical coherence tomography, Scheimpflug imaging, and slit-lamp biomicroscopy in the early detection of graft detachment after Descemet membrane endothelial keratoplasty. Cornea 2011; 30: 1369–1375

[9] Busin M, Madi S, Santorum P, Scorcia V, Beltz J. Ultrathin Descemet's stripping automated endothelial keratoplasty with the microkeratome double-pass technique: two-year outcomes. Ophthalmology 2013; 120: 1186–1194

[10] Shousha MA. 1, Perez VL, Wang J, Ide T, Jiao S, Chen Q, Chang V, Buchser N, Dubovy SR, Feuer W, Yoo SH. Use of ultra-high resolution optical coherence tomography to detect in vivo characteristics of Descemet's membrane in Fuchs' dystrophy. Ophthalmology 2010; 117: 1220–1227

[11] Dirisamer M, van Dijk K, Dapena I, et al. Prevention and management of graft detachment in descemet membrane endothelial keratoplasty. Arch Ophthalmol 2012; 130: 280–291

[12] Guerra FP, Anshu A, Price MO, Giebel AW, Price FW. Descemet's membrane endothelial keratoplasty: prospective study of 1-year visual outcomes, graft survival, and endothelial cell loss. Ophthalmology 2011; 118: 2368–2373

[13] Shih CY, Ritterband DC, Rubino S, et al. Visually significant and nonsignificant complications arising from Descemet stripping automated endothelial keratoplasty. Am J Ophthalmol 2009; 148: 837–843

[14] Suh LH, Yoo SH, Deobhakta A, et al. Complications of Descemet's stripping with automated endothelial keratoplasty: survey of 118 eyes at one institute. Ophthalmology 2008; 115: 1517–1524

[15] Dapena I, Ham L, Melles GR. Endothelial keratoplasty: DSEK/DSAEK or DMEK —the thinner the better? Curr Opin Ophthalmol 2009; 20: 299–307

[16] Anwar M, Teichmann KD. Big-bubble technique to bare Descemet's membrane in anterior lamellar keratoplasty. J Cataract Refract Surg 2002; 28: 398–403

[17] Busin M. , Scorcia V, Patel AK, Salvalaio G, Ponzin D. Pneumatic dissection and storage of donor endothelial tissue for Descemet's membrane endothelialkeratoplasty: a novel technique. Ophthalmology 2010; 117: 1517–1520

[18] Price MO, Price FW Jr. Descemet's membrane endothelial keratoplasty surgery: update on the evidence and hurdles to acceptance. Curr Opin Ophthalmol 2013; 24: 329–335

[19] Ham L, Balachandran C, Verschoor CA, van der Wees J, Melles GR. Visual rehabilitation rate after isolated descemet membrane transplantation: descemet membrane endothelial keratoplasty. Arch Ophthalmol 2009; 127: 252–255

Part 3

Cataract Surgery

14 Optical Coherence Tomography Analysis in Cataract Surgery

Richard Packard

Optical coherence tomography (OCT) has extensive applications in the posterior segment (PS), and development of this technology for the anterior segment (AS) also has particular uses in cataract surgery.[1,2,3,4,5,6,7,8,9,10,11,12,13,14,15,16,17,18,19,20,21,22,23] It is interesting to note, however, that in a review article from 2011 on AS OCT, cataract surgery was not mentioned at all. Initially, OCT had been used to visualize the whole AS; then it was found that corneal wounds could be studied. More recently, with the use of the femtosecond laser for cataract surgery, OCT has found a vital role in imaging the AS to set the boundaries of laser activity in performing incisions, capsulotomy, and nuclear segmenting. Before we look at these in greater detail, remember the role of OCT retinal imaging to detect macular problems before cataract surgery. This is particularly important where multifocal intraocular lens (IOL) implantation is being considered. After cataract surgery, such macular changes as cystoid macular edema can be evaluated and the clinical course followed. AS OCT has also been used to study iris architecture, posterior capsular opacity, and anatomical changes in relation to specific postoperative issues.

14.1 Measuring the Anterior Segment

Anterior-segment OCT can be used to measure a number of different parts of the AS (▶ Fig. 14.1), which can be useful in cataract surgery as follows:

- Although the depth of the anterior chamber is generally measured as part of the biometry process, whether optically or with ultrasound, there is a place for OCT also. In a recent study, however, significant differences were found between the actual measurements recorded by different means. Partial coherence inferometry and Scheimpflug measurements were comparable, as were both manual and automated AS OCT but not each pair with the other.

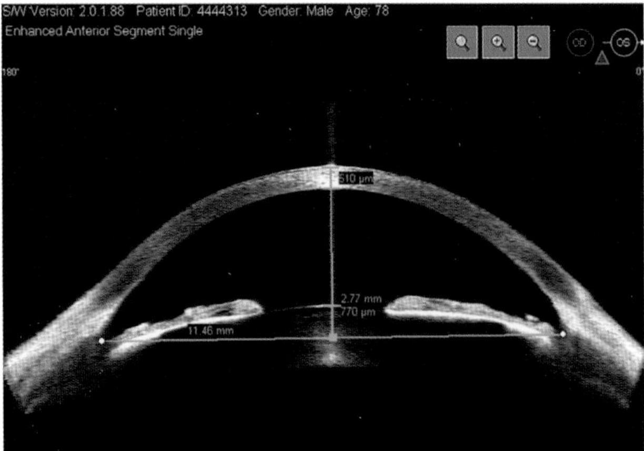

Fig. 14.1 Optical coherence tomography of whole anterior segment with size parameters. OD, right eye; OS, left eye.

- In addition to the depth of the anterior chamber, the curvature of the cornea, and thus its refractive power can be measured using AS OCT by matching curves to the anterior and posterior surfaces of the cornea. It has been found particularly useful for IOL calculations in patients who have had previous myopic laser refractive surgery. In a study comparing the use of AS OCT corneal measurements to obtain true corneal power with the Haigis-L formula (specifically for postmyopic laser patients), contact lens over refraction, and clinical history methods for the IOL calculation, the AS OCT results were much more accurate. The mean absolute error was 0.5 for AS OCT, 0.78 for Haigis-L, 1.46 for contact lens over refraction, and 1.78 for the clinical history method.
- Although toric IOLs are becoming more commonly used, keratotomies are still frequently used and ASOCT can be used for pachymetry of corneal thickness. This should help to prevent unexpected and certainly unwanted perforations. However, a difference was found when toric IOLs were compared with ultrasound measurements, and they cannot be used interchangeably because the AS OCT measured significantly less mean CCT of 536.9 ± 27.0 µm for OCT and 556.6 ± 30.5 µm for ultrasound.
- Lens thickness can also be measured with AS OCT, which is useful for hypermature cataracts before surgery to make the surgeon aware that the capsule may be under tension and the necessary precautions to avoid an anterior capsular tear can be implemented. With the advent of femtosecond laser–assisted cataract surgery (FLACS), the size of the lens is also vital. Most of the currently available lasers use AS OCT to visualize the lens in cross-section to set the extent of laser segmentation of the nucleus.

14.2 Observing Anatomical Changes in the Anterior Segment Caused by Cataract Surgery

A number of investigators have looked at the size, shape, and behavior of anterior chamber structures before and after cataract surgery using ASOCT:

- The appearance of the anterior chamber angle before and after phacoemulsification has been studied and showed, across a range patients aged between 15 and 91 years, that the angle-opening distance and the iris-trabecular space increased in all of them (▶ Fig. 14.2). Further, the amount of change was greater in older patients. The authors postulated that the greater lens volume with age might account for this finding.
- In another study to try to predict postoperative intraocular pressure (IOP), the iris cross-sectional area and convexity as seen with ASOCT proved useful predictors. A high cross-sectional area or convex hull of the iris segments was associated with lower postoperative IOP.

- It has been postulated that the timing and formation of the capsular bend around the sharp edge of an IOL may be important in preventing posterior capsular opacity. AS OCT has been used to study capsular bag closure in the early postoperative period; a one-piece hydrophobic IOL had earlier capsule bend formation at the optic edge than a three-piece silicone IOL.
- Late-onset capsular block syndrome occurs when milky-white liquid accumulates behind the IOL and reduces the patient's vision. The appearances before and after uneventful neodymium:yttrium-aluminum-garnet (Nd:YAG) laser capsulotomies were observed using AS OCT (▶ Fig. 14.3). Although the patient's best-corrected visual acuity (BCVA) improved in all cases, the IOL position and refraction did not change.

- The thickness of the posterior capsule with different IOL designs and materials has also been studied. A round-edged polymethylmethacrylate (PMMA) IOL was found to have the thickest posterior capsule, followed by a hydrophilic lens; the thinnest was the hydrophobic IOL. This correlated with BCVA.

More recently, with the use of the FLACS, OCT has found a vital role in AS imaging to set the boundaries of laser activity in performing incisions, capsulotomy, and nuclear segmenting. Considerable discussion has appeared in the peer-reviewed literature about the way different clear corneal incision (CCI) architectures behave during and after cataract surgery, and AS OCT has given us the tool to investigate this topic. Many aspects of the incision have now been studied from cross-sectional shape, dimensions, consistency, distortability, damage to corneal structures, ability to seal, effects of stromal hydration, long-term healing, comparison between laser and knife incisions, and many others. This part of the chapter presents an overview of the main findings.

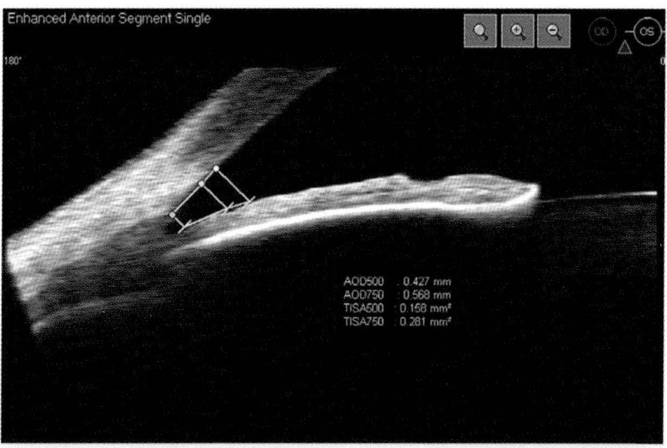

Fig. 14.2 **(a)** Preoperative and **(b)** postoperative view of the angle showing the increase in size.

14.3 Anterior-Segment OCT and the Cataract Incision

The first OCT study of corneal wounds in cataract surgery was done in 2006 using a modified retinal OCT; however, it demonstrated some of the possibilities in terms of imaging the cross-sectional architecture. The wounds were evaluated at 1, 3, and 30 days after surgery, and the most striking finding was that even though poor endothelial apposition was common, it did not lead to wound leakage even in these 3.2-mm incisions.

The following year, a study was reported using the first dedicated AS OCT, the Zeiss Visante. The object of this study was to study the profile of the wound created with different knives. Although the incisions were supposed to be uniplanar, all showed an arcuate configuration (▶ Fig. 14.4), described as being like a "tongue and groove" in the cornea that helped the incision to close. Further, with this arcuate profile, there was an extended arc of contact over a straight one.

This study had been performed 1 day after cataract surgery. Given that it is postulated that the early hours after surgery may be the time of greatest vulnerability for the wound, a study of early wound behavior seemed important. Patients were examined 1 hour after cataract surgery. The Visante was again used, and the essential features of the post-cataract surgical wound were defined. Five CCI architectural features were noted with the following frequencies: epithelial gaping (12%), endothelial gaping (41%), endothelial misalignment (65%), local detachment of Descemet membrane (DM) (62%), and loss of

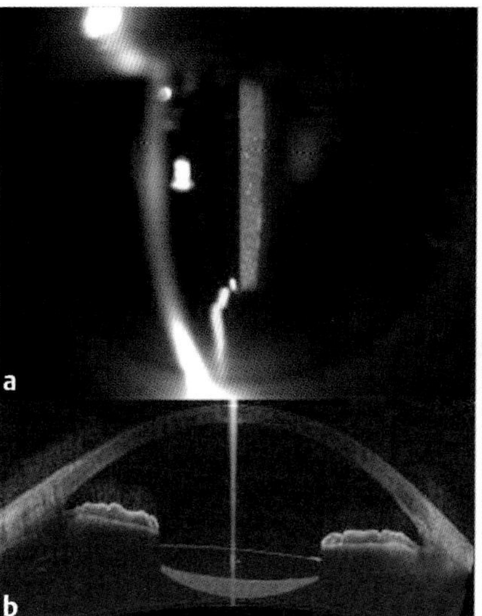

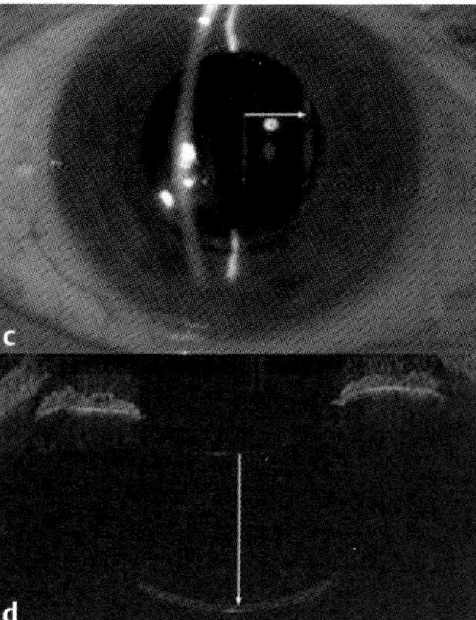

Fig. 14.3 **(a,b)** Pre- and **(c,d)** post-capsulotomy images of an eye with capsular block.

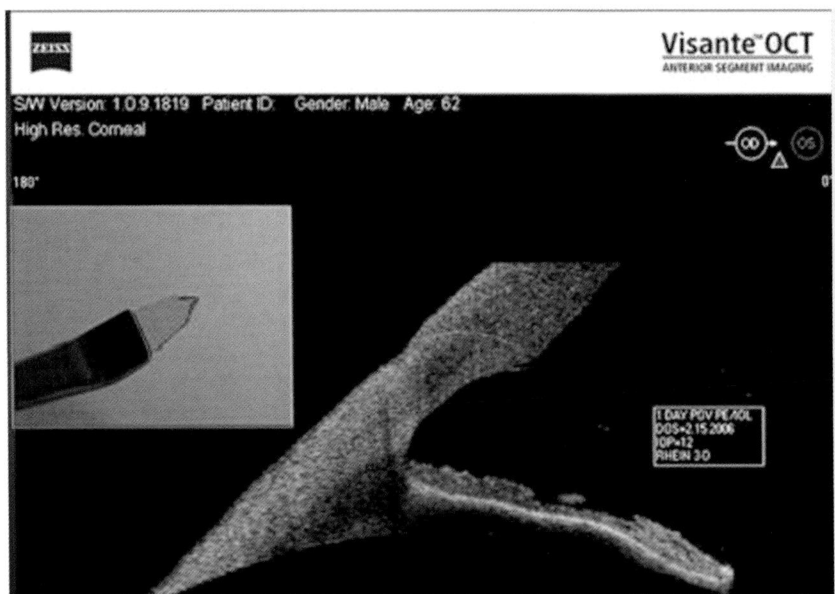

Fig. 14.4 Anterior-segment optical coherence tomography image of hydrated diamond knife incision at 1 day showing curved profile. OD, right eye; OS, left eye.

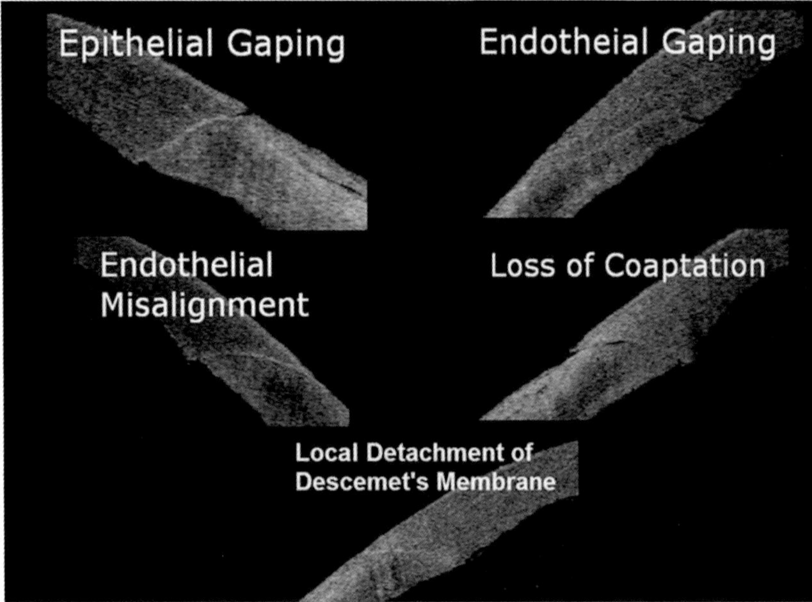

Fig. 14.5 Changes to cataract wound seen 1 hour postoperatively.

coaptation (9%) (▶ Fig. 14.5). This study was across four different wound sizes, from 3.2 to 2.2 mm. Interestingly, when IOP was measured at 1 hour, ranging from 3 to 46 mm Hg, the architectural features were related to IOP, not to wound width.

Multiple studies have now shown the repeatability of the dimensions of corneal wounds, such as chord length, incision angle, and corneal thickness at the incision (▶ Fig. 14.6). These findings, combined with observation of the architectural features mentioned already, have become the standards used for any AS OCT study of cataract incisions.

Several studies have now compared wounds in standard small-incision phacoemulsification using coaxial microincision cataract surgery with wounds using biaxial microincision cataract surgery. There seems to be some disagreement as to whether the biaxial or coaxial incisions cause more disturbances to the corneal architecture both in the short term or longer term, but none of these differences reach statistical significance.

As a further protection for the CCI in the early postoperative period, hydrogel materials have been developed to seal the wound. These are called *adherent ocular bandages* (AOBs), and AS OCT has been used to assess their behavior. In one study, patients who underwent coaxial microincision cataract surgery were allocated to an AOB group or to a control group. The CCIs were examined postoperatively within 2 hours, at 24 hours, and at 7 days using OCT imaging and a slit-lamp fluorescein 2% Seidel test. A significant difference was found in the mean immediate postoperative IOP compared with the control group (13.4 mm Hg ± 5.28 [SD]; range, 5–23 mm Hg) and the bandage group (19.4 ± 5.94 mm Hg; range, 11–29 mm Hg) ($P < 0.001$, t test). This finding may mean that the AOB was preventing microleaks (▶ Fig. 14.7). It was further found that the AOBs protected the incisions, selectively adhering to de-epithelialized areas and rapidly clearing from re-epithelialized areas.

So far, we have looked at incision architecture in single slices, which is useful for seeing the profile of a corneal wound; however, some machines now have a raster program that enables a block of tissue to be analyzed as a series of narrow slices right across the wound (▶ Fig. 14.8), providing the possibility to see whether the architecture that is normally observed at the midpoint of the wound is different at the edges. Indeed, this has proven to be so with three plane wounds becoming two planes at the edges. Also, if there is to be loss of coaptation, it is more likely to be found at the edges. This sort of study should be useful in designing better knives for corneal incisions. We carried out a study using AS OCT to analyze a consecutive cohort of 30 2.2-mm CCIs made with a new knife with novel blade configuration. It was possible to show that 29 of 30 were three plane incisions and the variability of wound length was only ± 0.12 mm.

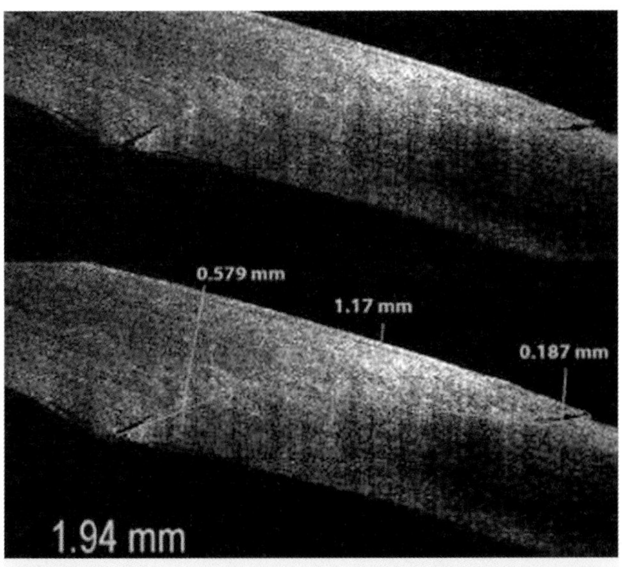

Fig. 14.6 Sizing the arc of contact within a clear corneal incision.

In addition, AS OCT has been used to assess corneal wound healing in the longer term. Images of wounds were obtained in consecutive eyes that had phacoemulsification 1 day to 180 months previously. The presence of DM detachment, posterior wound gape, and posterior wound retraction was assessed. The depth of wound retraction along the incision and the radial length of the incision were measured. The percentage of wound retraction relative to radial incision length was calculated. DM detachment and posterior wound gape appeared in the early postoperative period and persisted for up to 3 months, whereas posterior wound retraction developed later and was present in more than 90% of eyes after 3 years, indicating long-term wound remodeling (▶ Fig. 14.9).

The effect on a CCI by IOL injection has also been investigated using AS OCT in a study to analyze the effects of speed in lens insertion. Eyes that had phacoemulsification and Acrysof IQ IOL implantation using a screw-plunger type injector were randomly divided into two equally sized groups as follows: group F, fast IOL insertion (one revolution per second [rps]) plunger speed and group S, slow IOL insertion (¼ rps). When an injector system was used, slow IOL insertion affected clear corneal

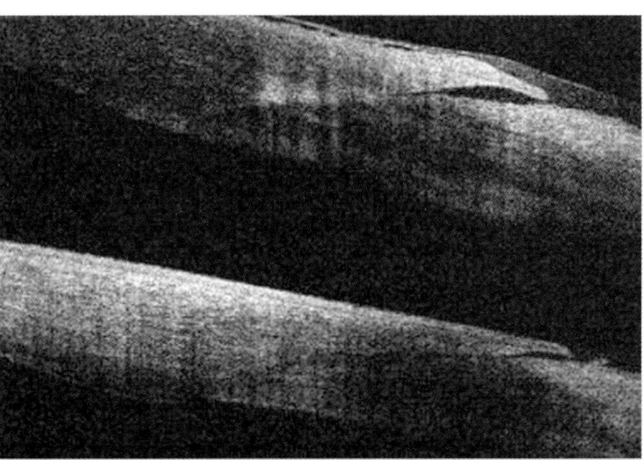

Fig. 14.7 Upper image shows adherent ocular bandage (AOB) covering epithelial defect with micro-leak contained. Lower image is wound without AOB and small epithelial defect.

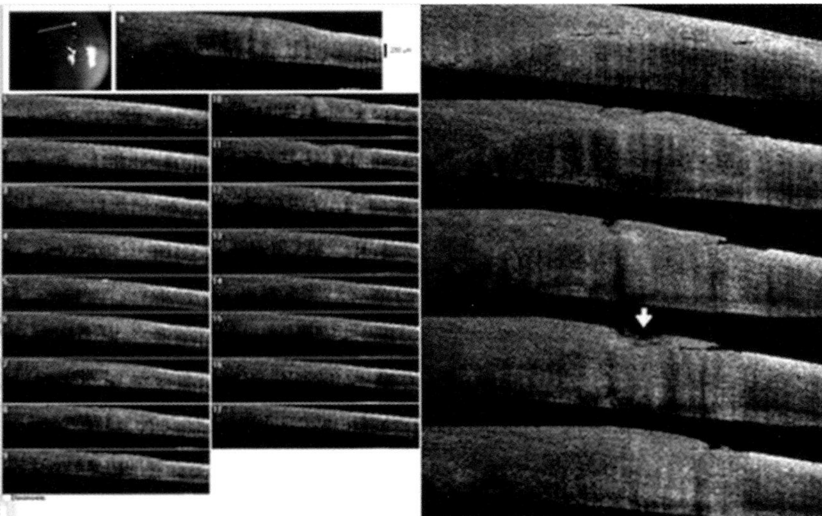

Fig. 14.8 Images from the raster program of the RTVue optical coherence tomography showing sequential slices across the wound. The white arrows show the loss of coaptation.

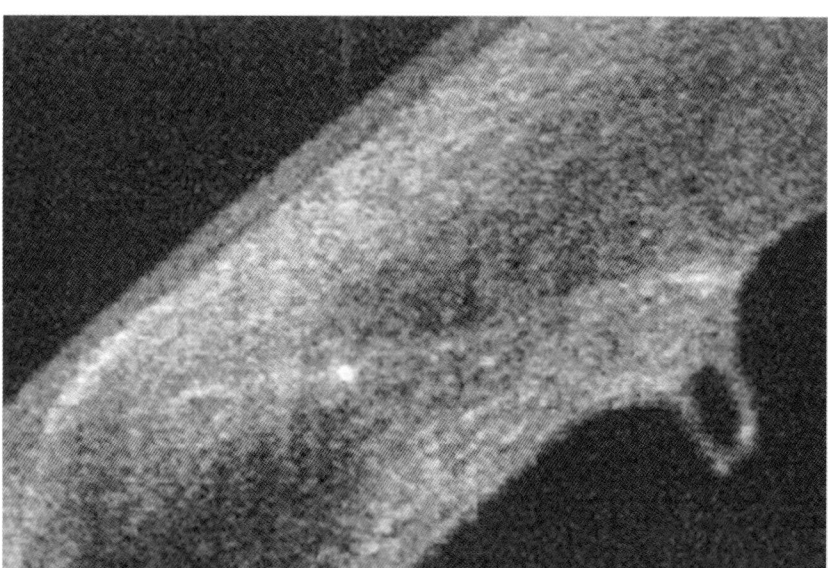

Fig. 14.9 Fully healed clear corneal incision at 3 months; Descemet detachment is still present.

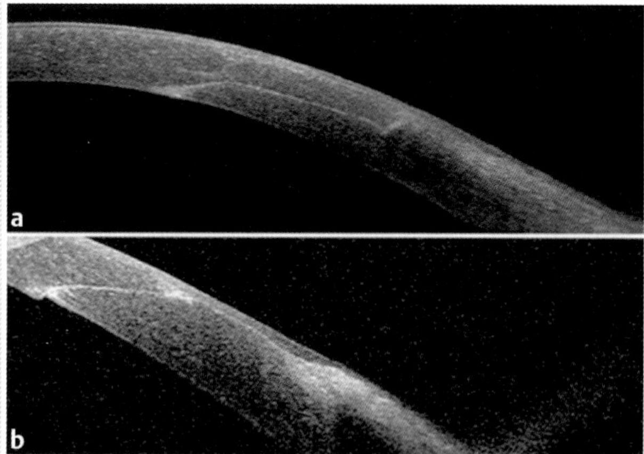

Fig. 14.10 **(a)** An incision created by a femtosecond laser. **(b)** A knife incision.

wound structure more than fast IOL insertion did, and twice as many eyes required stromal hydration (21 of 40 compared with 11 of 40). This was statistically significant ($P = 0.003$).[9]

Use of AS OCT with a raster program can assess wound size, and thus wound stretch, with great accuracy. In an unpublished study presented at the American Society of Cataract and Refractive Surgery in 2010, we examined at wound size 2 hours after phacoemulsification using the RTVue OCT. Seventeen slices at 15-µm intervals demonstrated in a 2.5-mm cube that the 2.2-mm incision was at that size and that any stretch from the surgery and lens implantation had gone. Interestingly, all the lenses were inserted with a wound-assisted technique using a one-handed injector and countertraction, which is appreciably faster than can be achieved with a screw injector.

The femtosecond laser, as we have seen, is now used to assist in cataract surgery, and AS OCT is an important part of imaging the AS in the process; but AS OCT has also been used to assess and compare the wounds created by this laser technology with incisions made with a steel blade (▶ Fig. 14.10).

It has been reported that femtosecond laser–generated CCIs had significantly lower endothelial gaping, endothelial misalignment, DM detachment, and posterior wound retraction than keratome-created CCIs and were within 10% of the intended length, depth, and angle measurements.[8] As far as outcomes were concerned, however, no difference was seen. Another study using cadaver eyes to test the sealability of CCIs made with either the laser or manually showed no difference in sealability despite the fact that the laser incisions were closer to target geometry and showed less variability than the manual ones.

14.4 OCT and the Femtosecond Laser in Cataract Surgery

For a femtosecond laser to assist in the steps of cataract surgery, good visualization of the AS structures is essential. Most of the manufacturers of femtosecond lasers use OCT to do this. To obtain sufficient penetration and resolution, this needs to be done with Fourier-domain OCT, which allows the corneal incision to be optimized, limbal relaxing incisions to be placed and of an appropriate depth, the capsulorhexis to be sized and centered, and the nucleus to be safely segmented by avoiding the posterior capsule. As we have shown, AS OCT has been used to evaluate postoperatively the corneal incisions made with a femtosecond laser and compare them with those made with a steel knife.

14.5 OCT in the Posterior Segment and Cataract Surgery

As is well known, cataract surgery can have an effect on the PS, and PS OCT is a useful tool to investigate these effects. Even before surgery, there is a role for OCT in imaging the posterior pole. Unrecognized epiretinal membranes can be seen as well as other pathologies, such as cystoid macular edema in diabetics or age-related macular degeneration. These findings are especially important if multifocal IOL implantation is contemplated because such posterior pole changes will degrade the

Table 14.1 Mean change in foveal thickness in patients with psuedoexfoliation syndrome, primary open-angle glaucoma, and pseudoexfoliation glaucoma after cataract surgery.

	Mean Change in Foveal Thickness (μm) ± SD				*P* Value*		
Postop Exam	Control	PXF	POAG	PXG	PXF Vs Control	POAG Vs Control	PXG Vs Control
1 wk	8.18 ± 9.86	6.63 ± 9.15	6.66 ± 8.04	6.23 ± 10.94	.56	.61	.50
2 wk	16.51 ± 15.32	16.86 ± 12.28	26.86± 19.16	25.64 ± 18.40	.9	.04	.05
4 wk	15.78 ± 16.24	15.45 ± 12.72	33.36 ± 21.97	39.70 ± 66.22	.9	.09	.01
8 wk	10.90 ± 12.65	11.22 ± 11.69	24.20 ± 15.04	23.35 ± 44.30	.9	.05	.06

POAG = primary open-angle glaucoma; PXF = pseudoexfoliation syndrome; PXG = pseudoexfoliation glaucoma
* Analysis of variance, least-signification-differences test for multiple comparisons

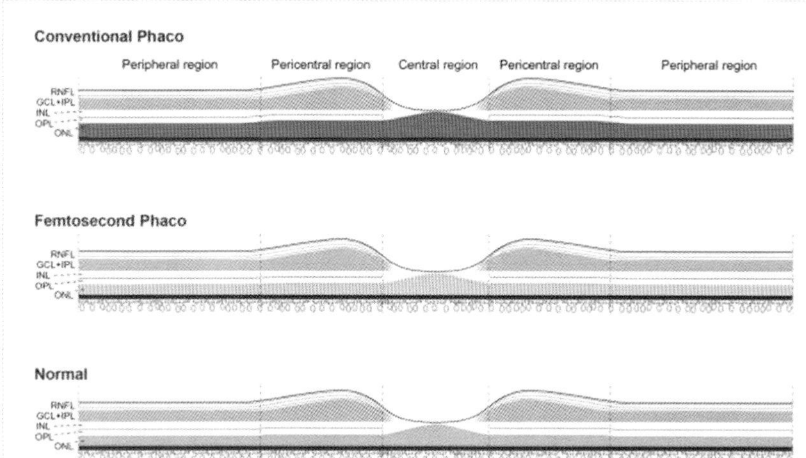

Fig. 14.11 Diagrams of macular area comparing thickness after conventional phacoemulsification and femtosecond laser–assisted cataract surgery. RNFL, retinal nerve fiber layer. GCL, Ganglion cell layer; INL, Inner nuclear layer; IPL, Inner plexiform layer; ONL, Outer nuclear layer; OPL, Outer plexiform layer.

image significantly and are thus a contraindication to the use of these lenses.

Several studies have investigated the postoperative changes in the PS using PS OCT.[17] Some of these findings have been surprising. It seems that choroidal thickness increases after cataract surgery, and the changes in choroidal thickness negatively correlated with the axial length (AL) in the late postoperative period. It was suggested that the fine changes in choroidal thickness after cataract surgery may affect the onset of AMD, and these effects may differ, depending on the AL. Nasal and inferior choroids were more affected.

Foveal thickness after cataract surgery is easily quantified using PS OCT. Although in a series of 41 eyes 11 had thickening, this result was not related to flare cell measurements but was present without evidence of breakdown of the blood aqueous barrier. Although it is not common, cystoid macular edema (CME) does occur after cataract surgery, and PS OCT has been used to look at this both to gauge frequency but also to assess the usefulness of prophylaxis with nonsteroidal anti-inflammatory (NSAIDs) drops preoperatively and postoperatively. In normal patients, in one study, the use of NSAIDs showed no significant difference in macular thickness. In patients with diabetes, however, using NSAIDs can reduce the incidence of CME and is recommended for 6 weeks after surgery. A further study looked at patients with primary open-angle glaucoma (POAG), pseudoexfoliation glaucoma (PXG), and pseudoexfoliation syndrome (PXF) with PS OCT to determine whether there were any differences in foveal thickness following cataract surgery. Although there was a significant increase in foveal thickness in all three groups compared with that found preoperatively, POAG and PXG patients had significantly greater increases than PXF patients (▶ Table 14.1). Furthermore, the incidence of CME was significantly greater in POAG and PXG as well. Where there is established CME, as in a diabetic patient, the use of intravitreal injections like triamcinalone or becacizumab at the time of cataract surgery can be assessed for efficacy with PS OCT.

With the advent of FLACS, there has been great interest in its effects on ocular tissues. One study investigated the macular thickness using PS OCT and found it was significantly less in patients having FLACS compared with standard phacoemulsification (▶ Fig. 14.11). It has been suggested that use of this technique might reduce the incidence of clinically significant CME.

14.6 Conclusion

Although cataract surgery is an extremely safe and successful surgery, the use of OCT in both the AS and the PS can give us insight into many aspects of the procedure and its effects on ocular tissues. The investigation of corneal incisions and their ability to seal and heal has changed our attitude about how we make our incisions and whether we use a knife or a laser. Ocular anatomy of the AS can be studied to see changes related to cataract surgery. PS OCT has shown us how our surgery can affect the PS and whether we can prevent complications like CME.

References

[1] Cavallini GM, Campi L, Torlai G, Forlini M, Fornasari E. Clear corneal incisions in bimanual microincision cataract surgery: long-term wound-healing architecture. J Cataract Refract Surg 2012; 38: 1743–1748D

[2] Doors M, Berendschot TTJM, de Brabander J, Webers CAB, Nuijts RMMA. Value of optical coherence tomography for anterior segment surgery. J Cataract Refract Surg 2010; 36: 1213–1229

[3] Fine IH, Hoffman RS, Packer M. Profile of clear corneal cataract incisions demonstrated by ocular coherence tomography. J Cataract Refract Surg 2007; 33: 94–97

[4] Elkady B, Piñero D, Alió JL. Corneal incision quality: microincision cataract surgery versus microcoaxial phacoemulsification. J Cataract Refract Surg 2009; 35: 466–474

[5] Wang L, Dixit L, Weikert MP, Jenkins RB, Koch DD. Healing changes in clear corneal cataract incisions evaluated using Fourier-domain optical coherence tomography. J Cataract Refract Surg 2012; 38: 660–665

[6] Torres LF, Saez-Espinola F, Colina JM, et al. In vivo architectural analysis of 3.2 mm clear corneal incisions for phacoemulsification using optical coherence tomography. J Cataract Refract Surg 2006; 32: 1820–1826

[7] Dupont-Monod S, Labbé A, Fayol N, Chassignol A, Bourges JL, Baudouin C. In vivo architectural analysis of clear corneal incisions using anterior segment optical coherence tomography. J Cataract Refract Surg 2009; 35: 444–450

[8] Grewal DS, Basti S. Comparison of morphologic features of clear corneal incisions created with a femtosecond laser or a keratome. J Cataract Refract Surg 2014; 40: 521–530

[9] Ouchi M. Effect of intraocular lens insertion speed on surgical wound structure. J Cataract Refract Surg 2012; 38: 1771–1776

[10] Teuma EV, Bott S, Edelhauser HF. Sealability of ultrashort-pulse laser and manually generated full-thickness clear corneal incisions. J Cataract Refract Surg 2014; 40: 460–468

[11] Calladine D, Ward M, Packard R. Adherent ocular bandage for clear corneal incisions used in cataract surgery. J Cataract Refract Surg 2010; 36: 1839–1848

[12] Schallhorn JM, Tang M, Li Y, Song JC, Huang D. Optical coherence tomography of clear corneal incisions for cataract surgery. J Cataract Refract Surg 2008; 34: 1561–1565

[13] Can I, Bayhan HA, Çelik H, Bostancı Ceran B. Anterior segment optical coherence tomography evaluation and comparison of main clear corneal incisions in microcoaxial and biaxial cataract surgery. J Cataract Refract Surg 2011; 37: 490–500

[14] Agarwal A, Kumar DA, Jacob S, Agarwal A. In vivo analysis of wound architecture in 700 microm microphakonit cataract surgery. J Cataract Refract Surg 2008; 34: 1554–1560

[15] Calladine D, Tanner V. Optical coherence tomography of the effects of stromal hydration on clear corneal incision architecture. J Cataract Refract Surg 2009; 35: 1367–1371

[16] Calladine D, Packard R. Clear corneal incision architecture in the immediate postoperative period evaluated using optical coherence tomography. J Cataract Refract Surg 2007; 33: 1429–1435

[17] Ohsugi H, Ikuno Y, Ohara Z, et al. Changes in choroidal thickness after cataract surgery. J Cataract Refract Surg 2014; 40: 184–191

[18] Nagy ZZ, Ecsedy M, Kovács I, et al. Macular morphology assessed by optical coherence tomography image segmentation after femtosecond laser-assisted and standard cataract surgery. J Cataract Refract Surg 2012; 38: 941–946

[19] Almeida DRP, Khan Z, Xing L, et al. Prophylactic nepafenac and ketorolac versus placebo in preventing postoperative macular edema after uneventful phacoemulsification. J Cataract Refract Surg 2012; 38: 1537–1543

[20] Almeida DRP, Johnson D, Hollands H, et al. Effect of prophylactic nonsteroidal antiinflammatory drugs on cystoid macular edema assessed using optical coherence tomography quantification of total macular volume after cataract surgery. J Cataract Refract Surg 2008; 34: 64–69

[21] Yüksel N, Doğu B, Karabaş VL, Cağlar Y NurşenYüksel. Foveal thickness after phacoemulsification in patients with pseudoexfoliation syndrome, pseudoexfoliation glaucoma, or primary open-angle glaucoma. J Cataract Refract Surg 2008; 34: 1953–1957

[22] Sourdille P, Santiago P-Y. Optical coherence tomography of macular thickness after cataract surgery. J Cataract Refract Surg 1999; 25: 256–261

[23] Cheema RA, Al-Mubarak MM, Amin YM, Cheema MA. Role of combined cataract surgery and intravitreal bevacizumab injection in preventing progression of diabetic retinopathy: prospective randomized study. J Cataract Refract Surg 2009; 35: 18–25

15 Optical Coherence Tomography Analysis of Wound Architecture in Sub-1-mm Cataract Surgery (700-µm Cataract Surgery)

Dhivya Ashok Kumar and Amar Agarwal

Clear corneal incisions are commonly used in cataract surgeries because of their self-sealing behavior and not requiring sutures. This self-sealing wound acts as a barrier for the ingress of microbes, thereby reducing the chance of postoperative infection. Clinically, cataract wounds are observed by the gold standard slit-lamp biomicroscopy. The nature of corneal wounds, however, has been well studied only by high-resolution imaging such as optical coherence tomography (OCT).[1] Wound architecture of a clear corneal wound includes the incision length or size, angle, epithelial alignment, stromal thickness, coaptation, and endothelial apposition. Microphakonit, a sub-1-mm cataract surgery, involves a clear corneal incision of less than 1 mm.[2,3] The smallest cataract incisions, reported in 2005, using 700-µm cataract surgical instruments has been termed *microphakonit*[2,3,4,5] to differentiate it from 0.9-mm phakonit.[6,7] In this chapter, we highlight the salient features and observations of cataract wound in microphakonit.

15.1 Microphakonit: 700-µm Cataract Surgery

With the patient under local anesthesia, a clear corneal sideport incision is made using a 0.8-mm keratome, and an ophthalmic viscosurgical device is injected. The main clear corneal phacoemulsification (phaco) incision is also made using a 0.8-mm microphakonit keratome at the intended position. A 5- to 6-mm capsulorhexis is performed with the 26-gauge needle bent to form a cystitome. A 25-gauge rhexis forceps (MicroSurgical Technology [MST], Redmond, WA) may also be used by those more accustomed to performing the rhexis using the capsulorhexis forceps. In the nondominant hand, a globe stabilization rod can be used to control the eye movements.

Cortical cleaving hydrodissection is performed, and the fluid wave under the nucleus and the rotation of the nucleus are checked. The advantage of microphakonit is that one can do hydrodissection from both incisions so that even the subincisional region can be easily hydrodissected. It is noteworthy, however, that because there is little escape of fluid, one should be careful during hydrodissection. If too much fluid is passed into the eye, a complication such as a posterior capsular rent may occur; therefore, it is necessary to decompress the anterior chamber during this maneuver by applying slight posterior pressure on the scleral lip while doing hydromaneuvers. The 22-gauge (0.7-mm) irrigating chopper (MST) is connected to the infusion line of the phaco machine and introduced using the foot pedal on position 1. The phaco probe is connected to the aspiration line, and the 0.7-mm phaco tip (without an infusion sleeve) is introduced through the clear corneal incision. Using the phaco tip and moderate ultrasound power, the center of the nucleus is directly embedded, starting from the superior edge of the rhexis, with the phaco probe directed obliquely downward toward the vitreous (▶ Fig. 15.1a). The settings at this stage are as follows: phaco power, 50%; aspiration flow rate, 20 cc/minute; and vacuum, 100 to 200 mm Hg. Using the karate-chop technique, the nucleus is chopped and removed. Cortical washup is then accomplished using the bimanual irrigation/aspiration (0.7-mm set) technique (▶ Fig. 15.1b).

One of the limitations in bimanual minimally invasive cataract surgery is destabilization of the anterior chamber during the surgery. This limitation has been overcome by the introduction of gas-forced infusion and the use of an antichamber collapser,[8,9] which injects air into the infusion bottle, pushing more fluid into the eye through the irrigating chopper and also preventing a surge. Thus, the use of 20/21-gauge irrigating chopper solves the problem of destabilization of the anterior chamber during surgery. Now, using a 22-gauge (0.7-mm) irrigating chopper, it is extremely essential that gas forced infusion, also called *external gas forced infusion*, be used in the surgery. When the surgeon uses the air pump contained in the same phaco machine, it is called *internal gas forced infusion*. Transmission of infective microbes is prevented by the use of a Millipore filter connected to the machine. The Stellaris machine made by Bausch & Lomb (Rochester, NY) has an inbuilt air pump to produce pressurized infusion.

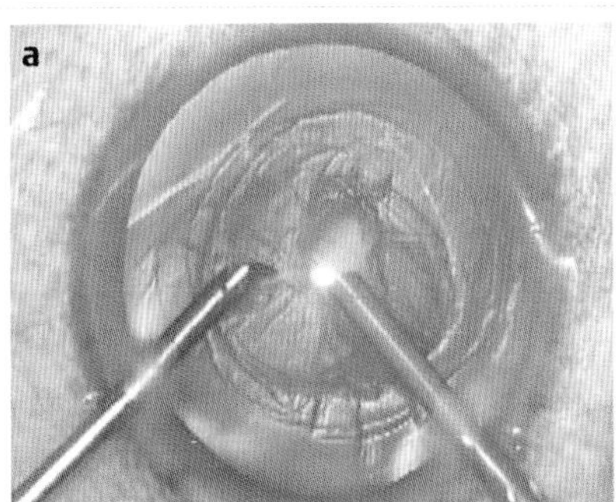

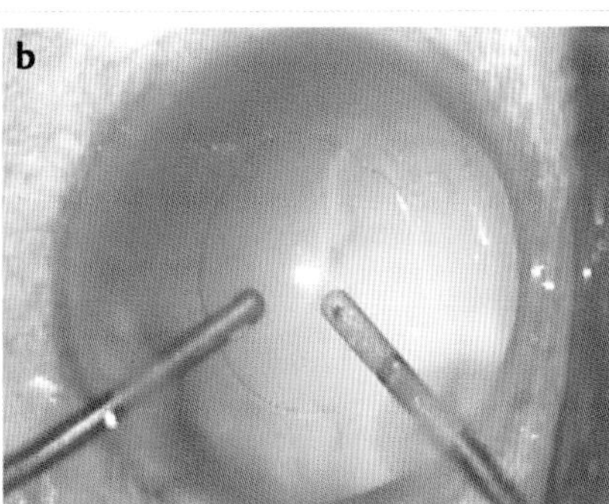

Fig. 15.1 (a) Microphakonit performed using 700-µm phaco needle and 700-µm irrigating chopper (MicroSurgical Technology, Redmond, WA). **(b)** Bimanual irrigation aspiration (I/A) done using a 700-µm bimanual I/A set (MicroSurgical Technology).

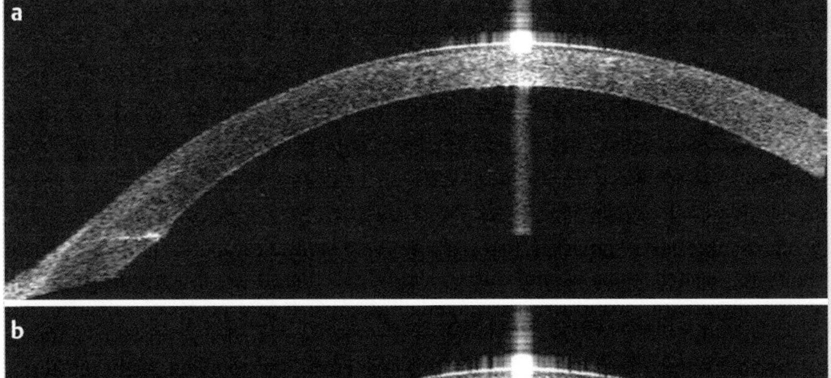

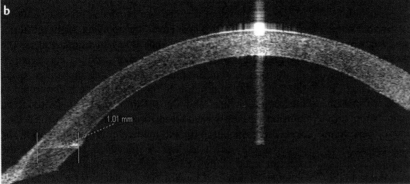

Fig. 15.2 Corneal high-resolution (10 mm × 3 mm) single-scan mode of anterior-segment optical coherence tomography of clear corneal incision (a) and the incision size measured by caliper tool (b)

15.1.1 Anterior Segment OCT Evaluation of Microphakonit Wound

Direct visualization of the wound can be achieved using anterior-segment (AS) OCT. Examination of postoperative wound morphology can be done using the prototype AS OCT (Carl Zeiss Meditec, Inc, Dublin, CA) Visante of 1310-nm wavelength. The method is noncontact and noninvasive. Corneal high-resolution (10 × 3 mm) single scan mode is preferred for wound examination. The axial resolution of AS OCT used is 18 µm, and transverse resolution is 60 µm. This noncontact method of imaging provides micrometer-scale cross-sectional images of the tissue. The patient is seated comfortably in the chair with the head positioned. The forehead and the chin of the patient are positioned in the headrest and the dual chin rest with automated right and left sensors, and the patient is advised to view the target through the examination eye. Then the examiner starts the scanning process by focusing with the video screen. Once the corneal vertex is observed on the screen, the clear corneal wound is traced. Usually, the wound will be seen as small opaque line across the cross-sectional cornea (▶ Fig. 15.2).

15.1.2 Features of Microphakonit Incision

Incision size

The size is measured from the epithelial to the endothelial side of the incision. Caliper tool is used for measuring the size across the cornea (▶ Fig. 15.2). The mean incision length of the microphakonit as measured with OCT is 1.13 ± 0.1 mm.[6] The mean angle of incision is 60.29 ± 11.4 degrees. A thick, dense apposition line is seen in 88.2% of the microphakonit wounds at 3 days postoperatively and in 100% at 7 days.

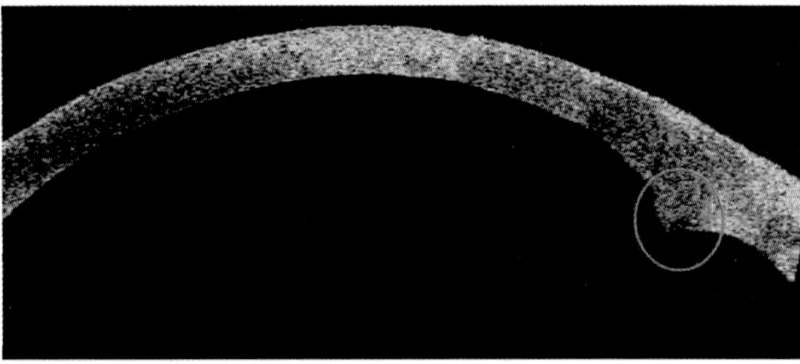

Fig. 15.3 Optical coherence tomography image showing the endothelial misalignment (circle).

Endothelial Alignment

The endothelium of both ends of the wound should be aligned. If there is gaping (▶ Fig. 15.3) of the wound on the endothelial side, then it is *misalignment*. There is positive correlation between wound gaping and endothelial misalignment.[6] Minimal misalignment with overriding can result from excess stromal hydration on one side, but it usually resolves within 48 hours. The microphakonit wound in the postoperative period showed good endothelial alignment on an average by day 3.

Coaptation

Coaptation literally means joining or reunion of two surfaces. In any corneal incision, coaptation is vital because it expresses the stability of the surface. Coaptation loss denotes that the two cut surfaces of the cornea have not united completely. The mean coaptation loss seen in microphakonit is 0.03 ± 0.06 mm in the immediate postoperative period.[6] A study reported that 70% of wounds have not had coaptation loss (▶ Fig. 15.4) in the immediate postoperative period.[6] We noted a significant positive correlation between the change in stromal hydration and

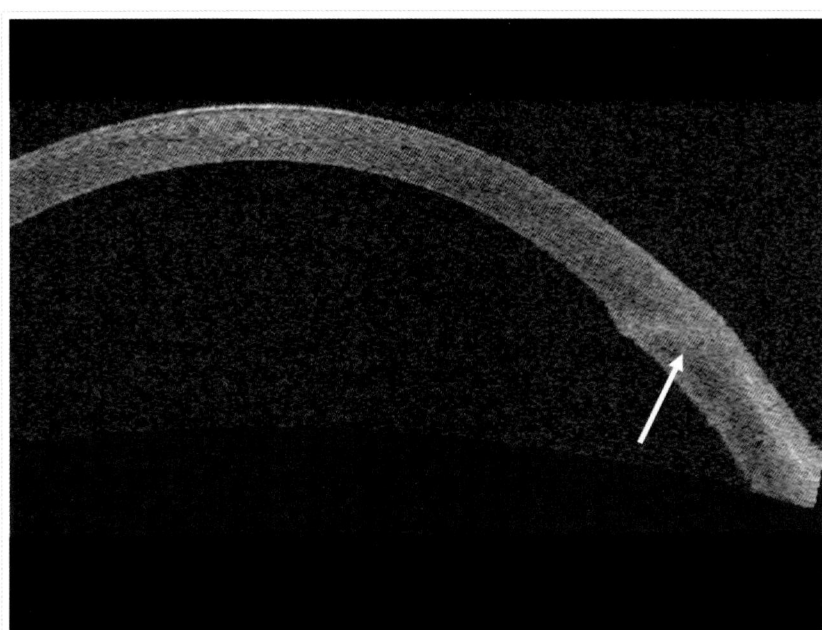

Fig. 15.4 Microphakonit wound with good apposition without coaptation loss (arrow).

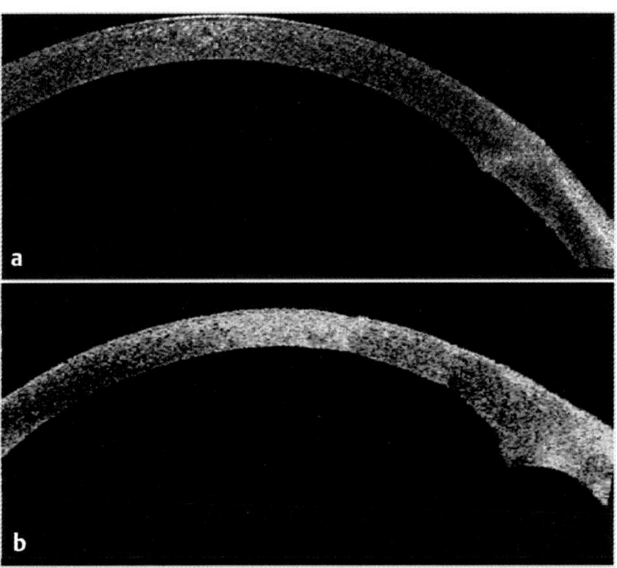

Fig. 15.5 Cross-sectional optical coherence tomography images of a wound at 1 day. **(a)** Microphakonit without extension. **(b)** Microphakonit with 2.8-mm extension.

coaptation loss in the postoperative period. No difference has been seen in the wound coaptation between the superior or temporal incisions. The effect of intraocular pressure (IOP) has been observed to be the same on both wounds (main or side port) in the same eye.

Epithelial Alignment

Normal epithelium is aligned in relation to the surface of the cornea. Whenever there is full thickness incision in the cornea, there is a break in the epithelium. This epithelium usually heals within 24 hours. One of our studies showed no epithelial misalignment on immediate, day 1, 3, and 7 postoperative periods. No fish-mouthing was seen in any of the microphakonit incisions.[6]

Descemet Membrane

Descemet membrane with the endothelium is usually identified as thick posteriormost layer in the OCT. In icrophakonit, the DM changes are very minimal. Descemet detachment in the main or side port wound has been noted to be less in eyes with sub-1-mm incision.

Stromal Hydration

Microincision cataract surgery wounds are always hydrated for good apposition. This gives good wound apposition and aids in apposition of the cut ends. Stromal hydration resolves within 24 to 48 hours.

15.2 Comparison of Microphakonit Incisions with and without Extension

Endothelial gaping has been noted in 57.1% of eyes with wound extension as compared to 0% in microphakonit without extension on day 7 (▶ Fig. 15.5). Twenty-eight percent of wounds with extension had persistent coaptation loss at 1 week; whereas 100% of the microphakonit wound without extension healed without coaptation loss at 1 week postoperative period[6] (▶ Fig. 15.6).

15.3 Advantages in Small Self-Sealing Incision

The microphakonit technique decreases the ingress of fluid and organisms from the ocular surface into the anterior chamber,

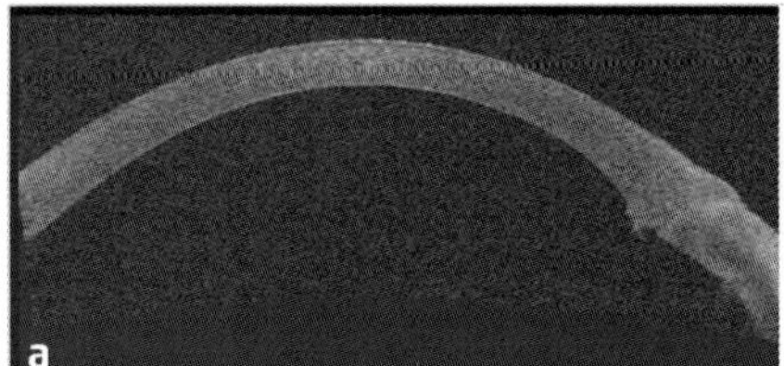

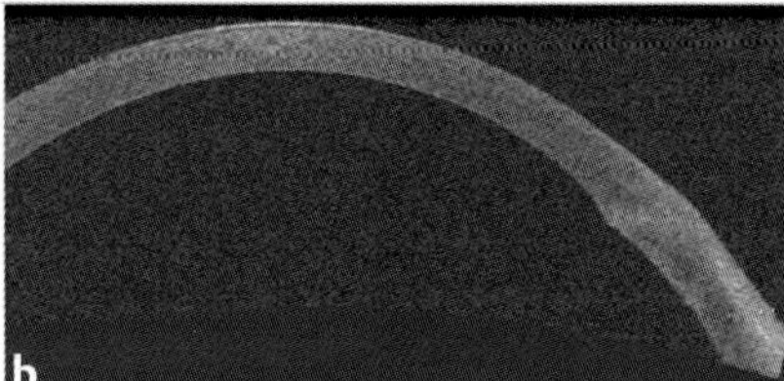

Fig. 15.6 Cross-section of the cornea in optical coherence tomography showing wound healing over time in microphakonit. **(a)** Endothelial misalignment is seen in the immediate postoperative period. **(b)** At 1 day, there is a well-formed apposition line and a decrease in endothelial misalignment.

thus decreasing the chances for endophthalmitis. We also observed no significant difference in the endothelial misalignment and coaptation loss in the wounds less than 10 mm Hg and more than 10 mm Hg, unlike the Calladine et al[9] study, which showed more endothelial misalignment in higher IOP. AS OCT images showed no external wound gaping as early as 1 day postoperatively and that the tunnels are well formed, reducing the risk of wound leak. Moreover, the wounds are so small and self-sealing that the chance of their opening as a result of lid or ocular movements is negligible.

15.4 Conclusion

Optical coherence tomography has been used widely for the evaluation of corneal wounds, either in the immediate or in the late postoperative period. Corneal wound construction and design play pivotal roles in the prevention of postoperative inflammation and infection. Small intricate details that are not visible to the naked eye are better seen using the high resolution of the OCT imaging. The noncontact and user-friendly nature of the method has attracted many innovative applications in this field. No doubt this method of wound evaluation will assist in understanding the dynamics of incisions and their relations to the postoperative outcomes.

References

[1] Calladine D, Packard R. Clear corneal incision architecture in the immediate postoperative period evaluated using optical coherence tomography. J Cataract Refract Surg 2007; 33: 1429–1435

[2] Agarwal A, Trivedi RH, Jacob S, Agarwal A, Agarwal S. Microphakonit: 700 micron cataract surgery. Clin Ophthalmol 2007; 1: 323–325

[3] Agarwal A, Jacob S, Sinha S, Agarwal A. Combating endophthalmitis with microphakonit and no-anesthesia technique. J Cataract Refract Surg 2007; 33: 2009–2011, author reply 2011

[4] Agarwal A, Jacob S, Agarwal A. Combined microphakonit and 25-gauge transconjunctival sutureless vitrectomy. J Cataract Refract Surg 2007; 33: 1839–1840, author reply 1840

[5] Agarwal A, Kumar DA, Jacob S, Agarwal A. n vivo analysis of wound architecture in 700 micron microphakonit surgery. J Cataract Refract Surg 2008; 34: 1554–1560

[6] Agarwal A, Agarwal A, Agarwal S, Narang P, Narang S. Phakonit: phacoemulsification through a 0.9 mm corneal incision. J Cataract Refract Surg 2001; 27: 1548–1552

[7] Pandey SK, Werner L, Agarwal A, et al. Phakonit. cataract removal through a sub-1.0 mm incision and implantation of the ThinOptX rollable intraocular lens. J Cataract Refract Surg 2002; 28: 1710–1713

[8] Agarwal A, Agarwal S, Agarwal A, Lal V, Patel N. Antichamber collapser. J Cataract Refract Surg 2002; 28: 1085–1086, author reply 1086

[9] Chaudhry P, Prakash G, Jacob S, Narasimhan S, Agarwal S, Agarwal A. Safety and efficacy of gas-forced infusion (air pump) in coaxial phacoemulsification. J Cataract Refract Surg 2010; 36: 2139–2145

16 Intraocular Lens Tilt

Kaladevi Satish, Dhivya Ashok Kumar, and Amar Agarwal

Intraocular lens (IOL) position in the postoperative period is commonly seen by slit-lamp examination. Ultrasound biomicroscopy (UBM) can be used to quantify the IOL position changes in the late postoperative period.[1] Clinical Purkinje image assessment has long been the method used in evaluating IOL position.[2] More recently, optical coherence tomography (OCT) has been used for this purpose.[3] OCT has its own advantages of being noncontact and less time consuming. High-speed anterior-segment (AS) OCT (Visante, Carl Zeiss Meditec, Dublin, CA) of 1310-nm wavelength has been used for IOL imaging.

16.1 Lens Position Module in OCT

Anterior-segment OCT (Visante, Carl Zeiss Meditec) has the option of including the type of scans that we require for evaluation in the specific mode as one module. As seen in ▶ Fig. 16.1, the lens position module includes the AS single mode raw mode and high-resolution raw mode, and normal AS scan mode can also be used. The limitation of normal AS scan mode is that whenever the vertex is not centered, the image capture does not happen. Hence, raw image mode is used.

16.2 Image Acquisition

The pupil should be dilated to at least 6 mm before examination. The headrest and the chin rest of the OCT are adjusted to guarantee a perpendicular position of the patient's head for each examination. Cross-sectional imaging of the IOL is carried out using the Visante AS OCT (Carl Zeiss Meditec). The eye is focused on the target in the viewing eyepiece of the patient. AS single-scan mode and high-resolution scans are taken in all four axes (0–180 degrees, 45–225 degrees, 315–135 degrees, and 270–90 degrees). In AS single scan, the examiner should capture the image when the reflection of the IOL is visible (▶ Fig. 16.1) and ensure that the corneal vertex is centered and the limbus is seen clearly. In high-resolution cornea mode, the reflection of the IOL with respect to the iris is seen. Iris pupillary margins are seen as high reflective edges, and the IOL convex surfaces are seen as a curved line of reflection (▶ Fig. 16.2).

16.3 Method to Calculate Intraocular Lens Tilt

The images then are analyzed using the caliper tools in the software of the AS OCT for iris vault (distance in millimeters between the iris margin and the anterior surface of the IOL at the pupillary plane [D1, D2]) (▶ Fig. 16.3). Using MatLab software version 7.1 (Mathworks, Natick, MA), AS single-scan images are analyzed. A straight line (L) passing through the limbus on either side of the image is marked as the reference line. A second line (1) passing through the horizontal axis of the IOL (▶ Fig. 16.4) is marked. The horizontal axis of the IOL is determined by the following method. The image from OCT is converted to binary for subsequent extraction of edge coordinates.

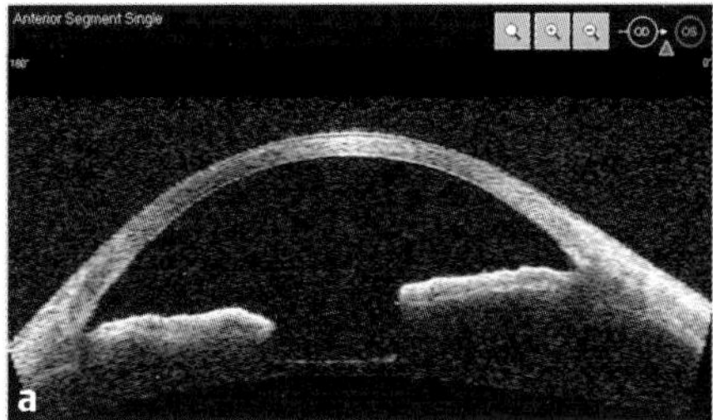

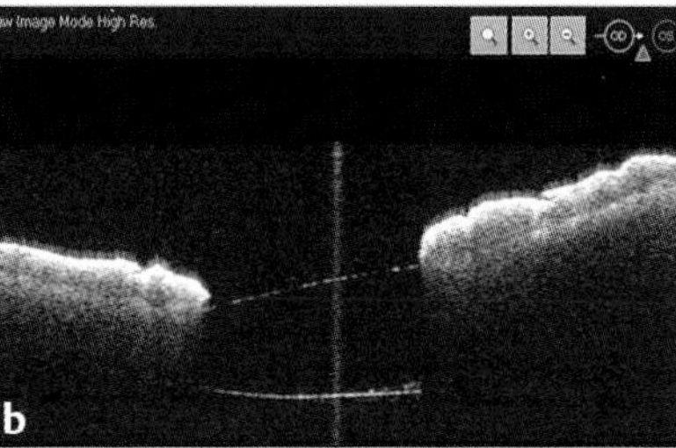

Fig. 16.1 **(a)** Anterior-segment single-scan raw mode and **(b)** high-resolution cornea raw mode for evaluation of intraocular lens position. OD, right eye; OS, left eye.

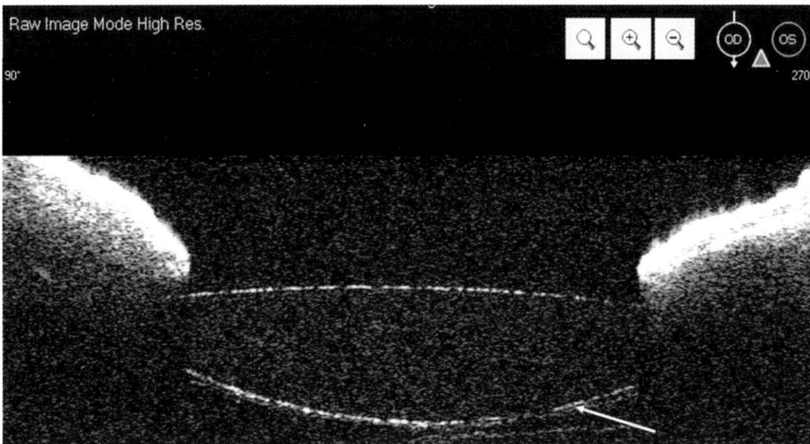

Fig. 16.2 High-resolution cornea raw mode showing the intraocular lens in the capsular bag (arrow). OD, right eye; OS, left eye.

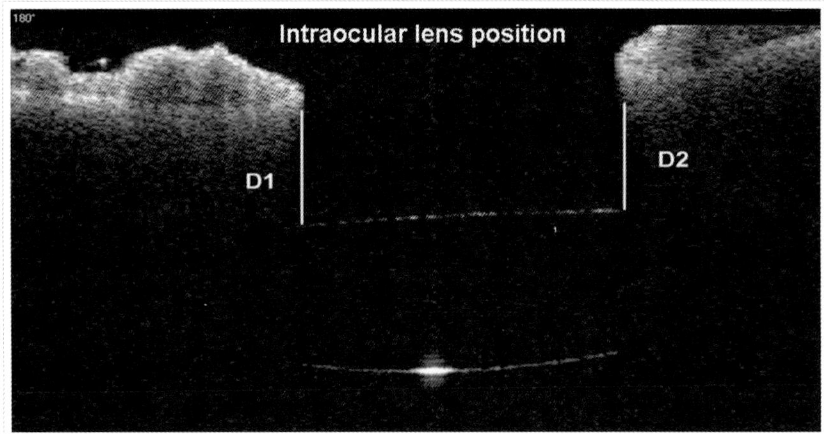

Fig. 16.3 Corneal high-resolution optical coherence tomography image showing intraocular lens (IOL) position. D1, D2 = distance in millimeters from iris margin to IOL optic edge at the pupillary plane.

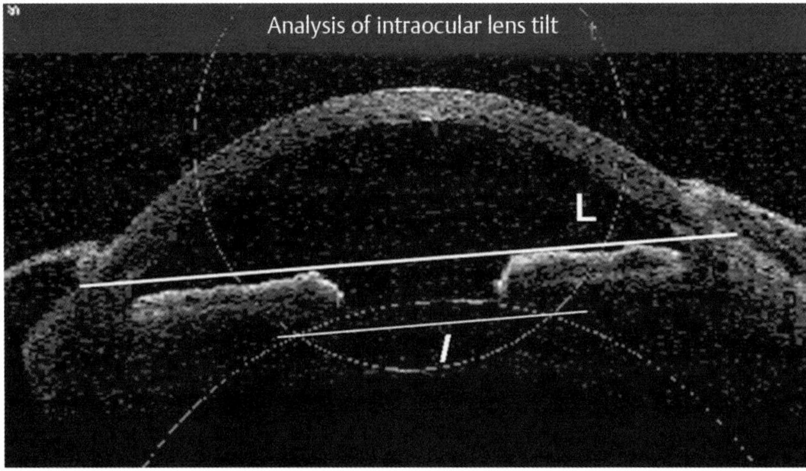

Fig. 16.4 Anterior-segment optical coherence tomography analysis of intraocular lens (IOL) tilt. L, slope of limbus; l, slope of IOL.

The selected points on the anterior and posterior arc edges of IOL are obtained. The mathematical representation to fit the anterior and posterior arc of IOL is derived from the equation of the circles passing through the given points (▶ Fig. 16.4). The intersection points of the two circles are joined to form the horizontal axis of the IOL. This is executed in all four quadrants (180–0 degrees, 225–45 degrees, 315–135 degrees, and 270–90 degrees). The slopes are calculated for both the straight lines (L,1). When the reference line along the limbus and the IOL optic are parallel, the optic is not considered to be tilted. The angle (θ) in degrees between the two lines (L and 1) is determined. The slope ratio is calculated by dividing the slope of IOL by the slope of the limbus.

16.3.1 Tilt in Normal Intraocular Lens

We reported the tilt of a normal IOL in the capsular bag to be 1.52 ± 0.9 degrees.[3] However, we noted that the tilt was not significant enough to affect the vision of the patients. The mean ocular residual astigmatism was 0.24 ± 0.47 diopters. No significant correlation was found between ocular residual astigmatism and postoperative best-corrected visual acuity. Of the four axes, the 180- to 0-degree axis showed the IOL contour completely in all 100% of the examined eyes (▶ Fig. 16.5). The mean distance D1 was 0.80 ± 0.6 mm, and the mean distance D2 was 0.83 ± 0.57 mm. On comparison with different types of IOLs, no significant difference in position was noted. There were three groups of IOLs: a single-piece acrylic IOL (Appasamy Associates, Chennai, India); a single-piece, foldable acrylic IOL (Akreos; Bausch & Lomb, Rochester, NY); and a single-piece PMMA (polymethylmethacrylate) IOL (Appasamy Associates). No significant difference was found among the IOL groups with respect to the slope ratio ($P = 0.431$, Kruskal-Wallis test), postoperative vision ($P = 0$ .935), and angle (θ; $P = 0.333$).

16.3.2 Intraocular Lens Decentration Estimation from Three-Dimensional Reconstruction of OCT

Wang et al identified the decentration of IOLs implanted within the capsular bag after uneventful phacoemulsification.[4] They used a separate algorithm for three-dimensional reconstruction of the IOL position. They noted that the mean IOL decentration in the x-axis and in the y-axis were 0.32 ± 0.26 mm and 0.40 ± 0.27 mm, respectively. The spatial distance of the IOL decentration was 0.56 ± 0.31 mm. No significant correlation between the ocular residual astigmatism and the tilted angle or the decentration distance was found.

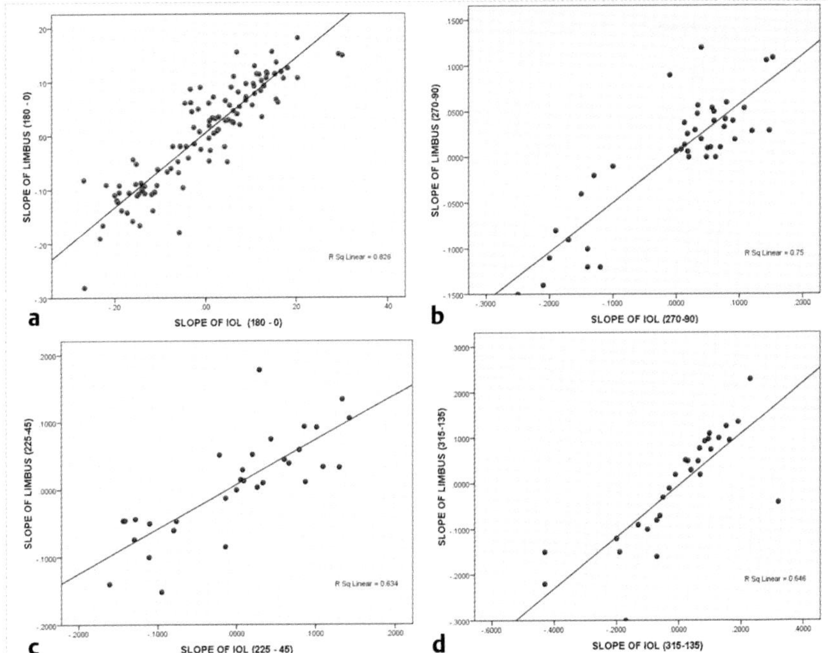

Fig. 16.5 Scatter plots showing the correlation of slope of intraocular lens (IOL) versus limbus at various axes **(a)** 180 to 0 degrees; **(b)** 270 to 90 degrees; **(c)** 225 to 45 degrees; **(d)** 315 to 135 degrees. The visibility of IOL contour was more in 180-0 axis scan. *x*-axis, slope of IOL; *y*-axis, slope of limbus.

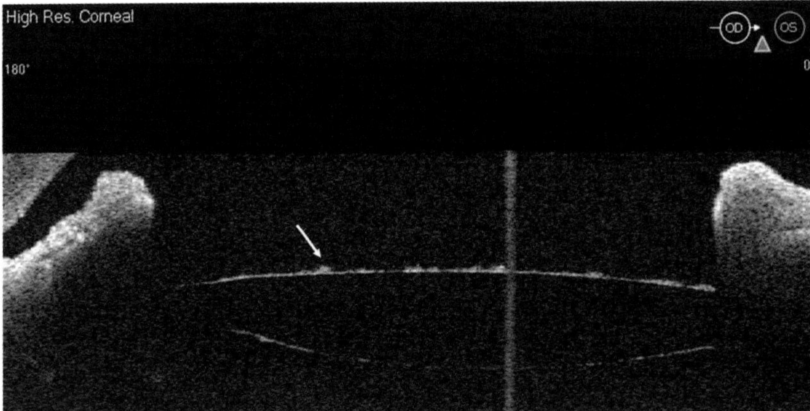

Fig. 16.6 Pigment dispersion is seen as hyper-reflective opacities on the surface of intraocular lens (white arrow). OD, right eye; OS, left eye.

16.3.3 Intraocular Lens Tilt in Trans-Scleral Fixation

Yamane et al used enhanced-depth imaging to obtain clearer images of the IOL.[5] The OCT instrument was pushed close enough to the eye to create an inverted image, and the inverted image was automatically reinverted to erect the image for the measurements. The angle of tilt of the IOL was determined by swept-source OCT (SS-1000 CASIA; Tomey Corporation, Nagoya, Japan). A standardized radial scan by the swept-source OCT was used after the pupil was dilated. The horizontal and vertical images of OCT were used to analyze the IOL tilt. A straight line passing through the iris-cornea angles on either side of the image was marked as a reference line. The angle between the reference line and the horizontal axis of IOL was taken to be the IOL tilt. The IOL tilt was measured in both the vertical and horizontal planes. The average of the IOL tilt in the vertical and horizontal planes was defined as the mean IOL tilt. The vertical and horizontal tilts were 2.2 ± 1.8 degrees and 2.5 ± 2 degrees respectively.

16.3.4 Changes Associated with Intraocular Lens Tilt

Capsule Changes

Anterior and posterior capsules usually adhere to the IOL in late postoperative eyes. Capsule opacification is seen as thick reflection from the posterior capsular bag behind the IOL.

Pigment Dispersion on IOL

Pigment dispersion is seen as clumping of cells or opacities on the surface of IOL (▸ Fig. 16.6). Dense pigment dispersion can prevent passage of light through it.

Iris Shaffing

The IOL may touch the pupillary margin iris epithelium, producing continuous friction (▸ Fig. 16.7).

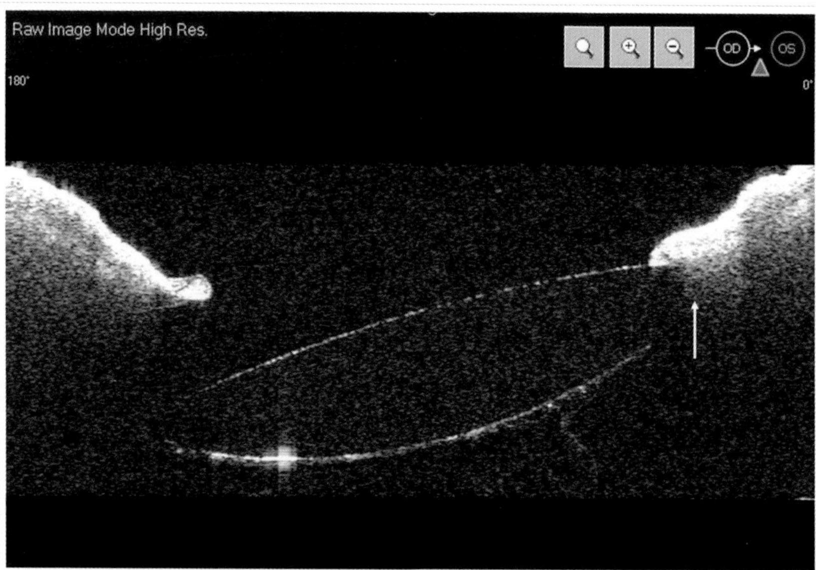

Fig. 16.7 Corneal high-resolution scan showing the iris-intraocular lens touch (white arrow).

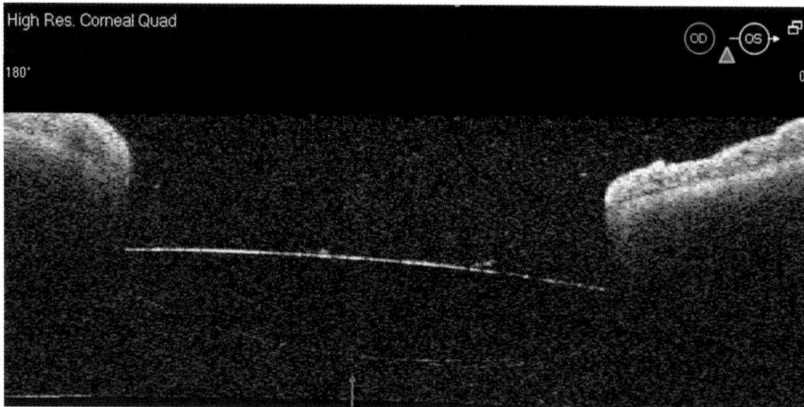

Fig. 16.8 Anterior surface of the intraocular lens is better seen than the posterior surface (red arrow). OD, right eye; OS, left eye.

Optic Capture

The IOL optic may be caught between the iris margin on one side and in the capsular bag. Optic capture may induce IOL tilt.

16.3.5 Limitations of Intraocular Lens Position Evaluation by OCT

Pupil dilatation is required for IOL position examination by OCT. IOL reflection may not be clearly visible in 100% of the IOL surfaces (▶ Fig. 16.8). Factors like variation in focus, depth, media clarity, and signal strength can affect the scan output. It may be difficult in patients who are uncooperative or having difficulty in focusing, but with the recent advances like hand-held OCT machines, the limitations associated with patient cooperation can be overcome. It is not possible to visualize the haptic position below the iris, which can be imaged with UBM.

16.3.6 How to Detect Presence of Intraocular Lens Tilt in Out Patient Department

1. Get a print of the anterior-segment single-scan OCT in four axes with measurements.
2. Check for the position of IOL in relation to the iris (D1,D2).
3. If there is difference in D1 and D2, there is tilt.
4. Check for the relation of IOL surface in relation to limbus. If the imaginary line (▶ Fig. 16.9) through the IOL center and limbus seems to intersect (not parallel), there is IOL tilt.

16.3.7 How to Detect Amount of Tilt

1. Quantify the amount of tilt by measuring the angles between the two axes.
2. Roughly, a simple protractor can also be used on the image to detect the approximate tilt from the axis

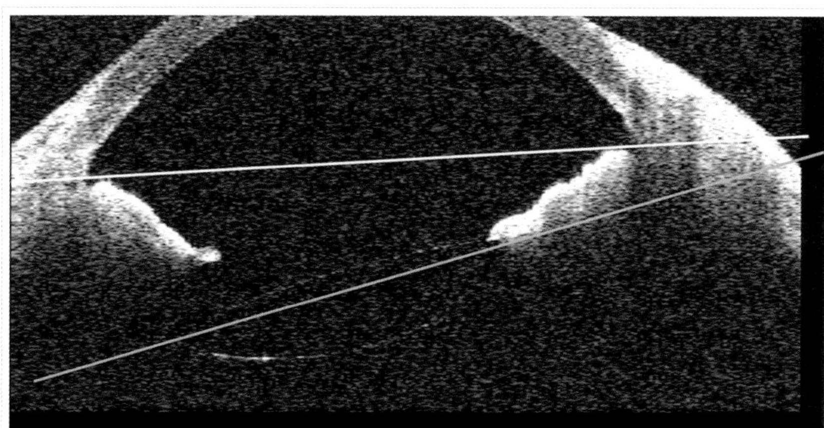

Fig. 16.9 Anterior-segment raw image of an eye with intraocular lens tilt.

16.3.8 Advantages of OCT Tilt Evaluation

The main advantage of OCT over UBM is its noninvasive (noncontact) nature, high resolution, and faster execution. There is no need for coupling fluid application or anesthesia for evaluation. Hence, this can be performed in the early postoperative period and in traumatized corneas. This process is patient friendly and easy for follow-up evaluation. Because the scans are stored, they can be recovered for prognosis as well. High-resolution of 18 μm gives the intricate IOL details that might not be detected by ultrasound-based instruments.

References

[1] Mura JJ, Pavlin CJ, Condon GP, et al. Ultrasound biomicroscopic analysis of iris-sutured foldable posterior chamber intraocular lenses. Am J Ophthalmol 2010; 149: 245–252, e2

[2] de Castro A, Rosales P, Marcos S. Tilt and decentration of intraocular lenses in vivo from Purkinje and Scheimpflug imaging: validation study. J Cataract Refract Surg 2007; 33: 418–429

[3] Kumar DA, Agarwal A, Prakash G, Jacob S, Saravanan Y, Agarwal A. Evaluation of intraocular lens tilt with anterior segment optical coherence tomography. Am J Ophthalmol 2011; 151: 406–412, e2

[4] Wang X, Dong J, Wang X, Wu Q. IOL tilt and decentration estimation from 3 dimensional reconstruction of OCT image. PLoS ONE 2013; 8: e59109

[5] Yamane S, Inoue M, Arakawa A, Kadonosono K.. Sutureless 27-gauge needle-guided intrascleral intraocular lens implantation with lamellar scleral dissection. Ophthalmology 2014; 121: 61–66

17 Glued Intraocular Lens Position: An Ocular Coherence Tomography Assessment

Athiya Agarwal, Dhivya Ashok Kumar, and Amar Agarwal

17.1 Background

Fibrin glue, which has been used for various indications in ophthalmology, has been known to provide good surgical adhesion.[1,2,3] Glued intraocular lens (IOL) technique is one such indication in which tissue glue has been used primarily for IOL implantation.[4] An anatomical position similar to a natural lens gives it an additional advantage compared with the anterior-chamber intraocular lenses. Maggi and Maggi pioneered the initial sutureless IOL fixation in eyes with deficient posterior capsule in 1997.[5] In 2006, Gabor Scharioth introduced transscleral needle fixation of IOLs in eyes with deficient capsules.[6] In 2007, Agarwal et al introduced the glued IOL technique, which comprised glued intrascleral haptic fixation of a posterior chamber IOL.[4] In this chapter, we analyze the position of glued IOL with high-speed anterior-segment optical coherence tomography (OCT).

17.2 Technique

Localized peritomy at the site of exit of the IOL haptics is done with the patient under peribulbar anesthesia. Two partial-thickness limbal-based scleral flaps about 2.5 × 2.5 mm are created exactly 180 degrees diagonally (use scleral marker) apart. An infusion cannula or anterior-chamber maintainer is inserted. One can use a 20- or 23-gauge trocar cannula for infusion. Positioning of the infusion cannula should be in the pars plana, about 3 mm from the limbus. Anterior-segment surgeons can use an anterior-chamber maintainer. Two straight sclerotomies with a 20-gauge needle are made about 1 to 1.5 mm from the limbus under the existing scleral flaps, followed by vitrectomy via pars plana or anterior route to remove all vitreous traction. A corneoscleral tunnel incision is then prepared for introducing the IOL in case of a nonfoldable IOL or a corneal incision with a keratome in the case of an injectable three-piece foldable IOL.

The IOL cartridge is passed into the anterior chamber. The glued IOL forceps (MicroSurgical Technology [MST], Redmond, WA) is then passed through the sclerotomy, and the tip of the haptic is grasped (▶ Fig. 17.1). The IOL is then gradually injected into the eye. Once the optic is unfolded, the glued IOL forceps is used to pull the haptic out and externalize it. The haptic is then held by an assistant or silicone ties. The surgeon now flexes the second haptic into the anterior chamber into the jaws of the glued IOL forceps introduced through the second sclerotomy using the handshake technique (▶ Fig. 17.2).[7] This haptic is also thus externalized. A limbus parallel scleral tunnel is made with a 26-gauge bent needle on either side at the point of haptic externalization. The haptic tips are then tucked into the intralamellar scleral tunnel.

Air is then injected into the anterior chamber, and the fluid from the infusion cannula is turned off, which helps to prevent hypotony and also keeps the area of the glue application dry. The reconstituted fibrin glue (Tisseel, Baxter, CA) prepared is injected under the scleral flaps. Local pressure is given over the flaps for about 10 to 20 seconds. The corneoscleral wound is closed using 10–0 monofilament nylon in a nonfoldable three-piece IOL, and in case of foldable IOL, the corneal incision is

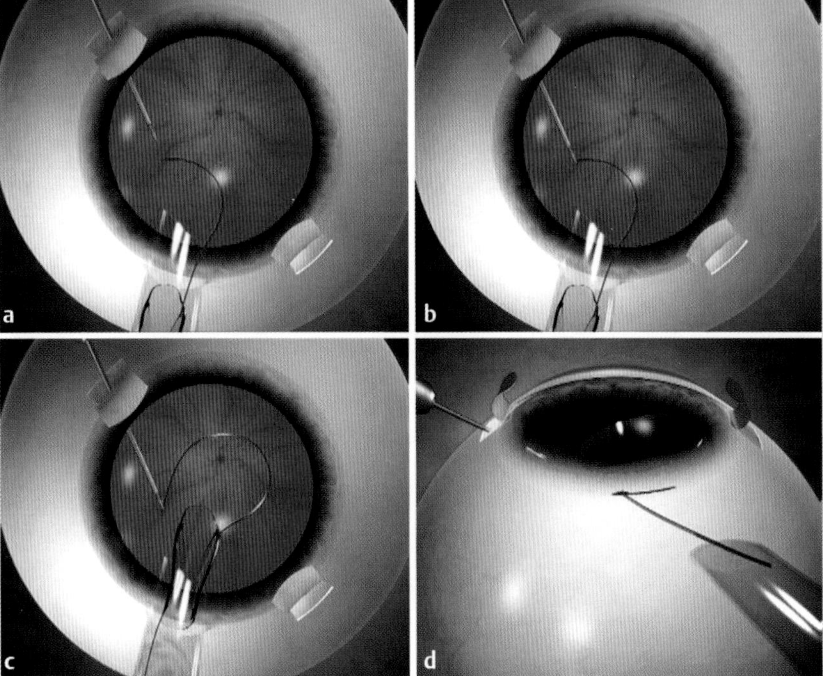

Fig. 17.1 (a) Haptic outside the cartridge. Glued-intraocular lens (IOL) forceps ready to grasp the haptic tip. **(b)** Haptic tip caught with the forceps. **(c)** Injection of the IOL continued until the optic unfolds inside the anterior chamber. **(d)** Haptic externalization started.

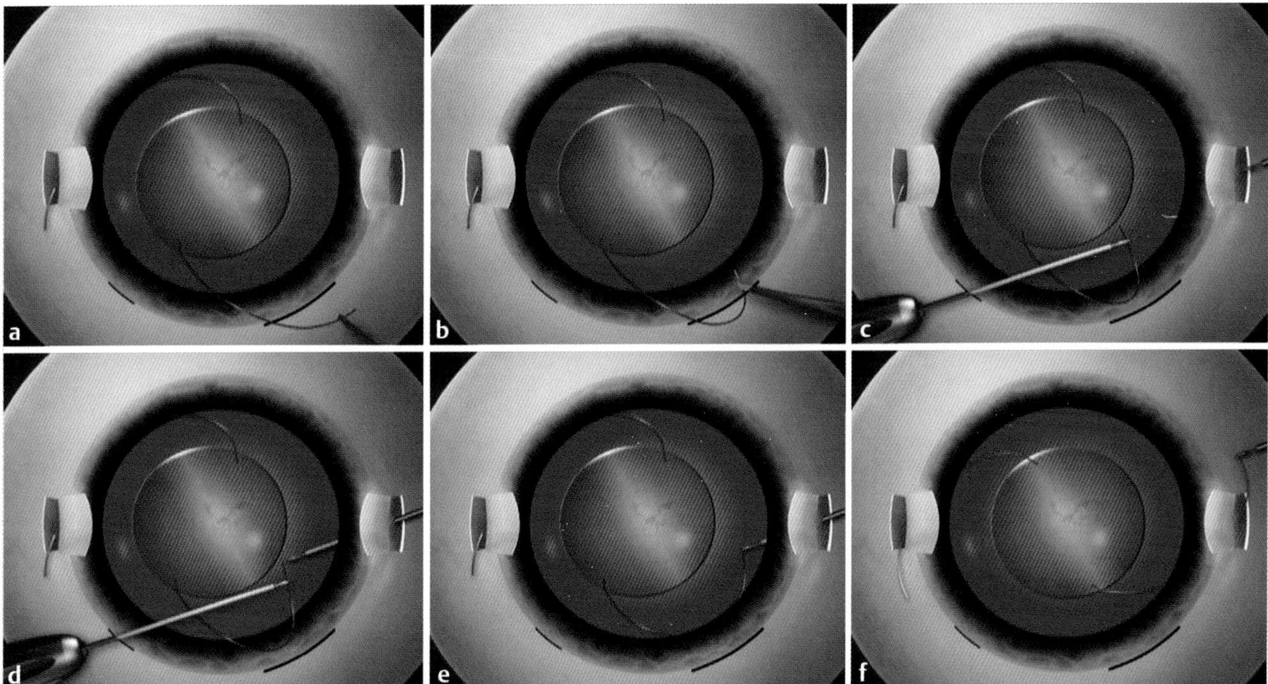

Fig. 17.2 **(a)** Trailing haptic caught with the first glued-intraocular lens (IOL) forceps. **(b)** Haptic flexed into the anterior chamber. **(c)** Haptic transferred from the first forceps to the second forceps using the handshake technique. The second forceps is passed through the side port. **(d)** First forceps is passed through the sclerotomy under the scleral flap. Haptic is transferred from the second forceps back to the first using the handshake technique. Haptic tip is grasped with the first forceps. **(e)** Haptic is pulled toward the sclerotomy. **(f)** Haptic externalized.

sealed with fibrin glue. The conjunctiva is closed with the fibrin glue in all eyes irrespective of the type of IOL.

17.3 Anterior-Segment OCT

Cross-sectional imaging of the IOL was done using Visante anterior-segment OCT (Carl Zeiss Meditec, Dublin, CA). Corneal high-resolution quad mode was used. Images were taken in four axes: 180 to 0 degrees, 90 to 270 degrees, 225 to 45 degrees, and 315 to 135 degrees. The optics of the IOL were imaged and referred with the position of iris. The images were then analyzed using the caliper tools in the software of anterior-segment OCT for iris vault. D1 and D2 were measured as the distances in millimeters between the iris margin and the anterior surface of IOL optic (▶ Fig. 17.3). The mean pupil size was kept at 6 to 7 mm in all the eyes by pharmacologic dilatation (0.5% tropicamide). For analysis purposes, OCT images in 180 to 0 degrees (horizontal) and 270 to 90 degrees (vertical) axes has been used. All patients underwent refraction (manifest and autorefractometer), retinoscopy, best-corrected spectacle vision (BCVA; Snellen distant vision acuity charts) and corneal topography (Orbscan, Bausch & Lomb, Rochester, NY). Slit-lamp examination (Topcon slit-lamp imaging system, 25 × magnification) was performed, and the IOL position was clinically examined by an experienced ophthalmologist. Ocular residual astigmatism (ORA) using the Alpins method was determined and graphical correlation performed.[8]

The inclusion criteria were the minimum 5-year follow-up and preoperative indications of surgical aphakia, posterior capsular rupture, and subluxated cataract; also, the patient's cooperation for OCT examination is required. Patients of pediatric age group or uncooperative were excluded.

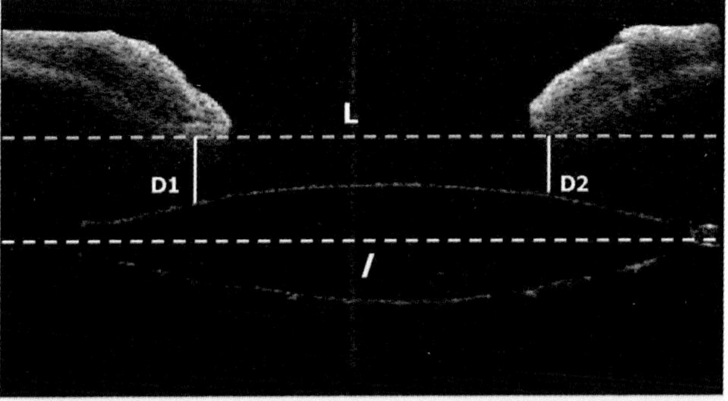

Fig. 17.3 Optical coherence tomography image showing the method of intraocular lens (IOL) optic position evaluation. L, slope of iris, l, slope of IOL; D1, D2, distance of IOL from iris.

17.4 Intraocular Lens Tilt Estimation in OCT

Using MatLab version 7.1 (The Mathworks, Inc., Natic, MA), the corneal high-resolution images were analyzed.[9] A straight line (L) passing through the iris pigment epithelium on either side of the image was marked as the reference line. A second line (*l*) passing through the horizontal axis of the IOL was marked.[10,11] The slopes were calculated for both straight lines (L, *l*). Slope ratio was obtained by dividing the slope of IOL by the slope of

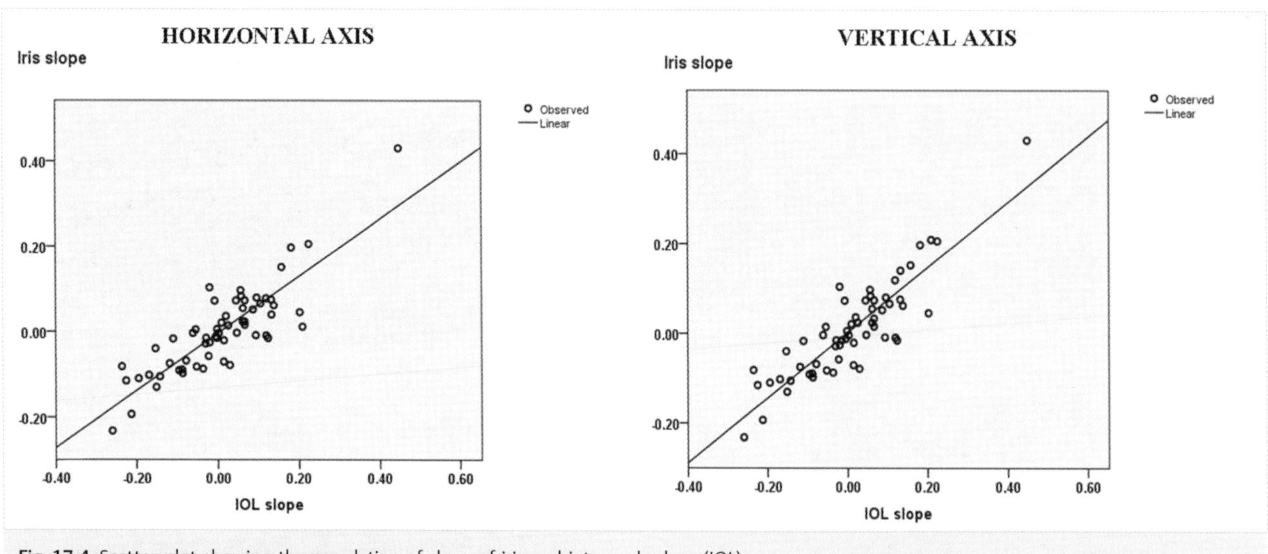

Fig. 17.4 Scatter plot showing the correlation of slope of iris and intraocular lens (IOL).

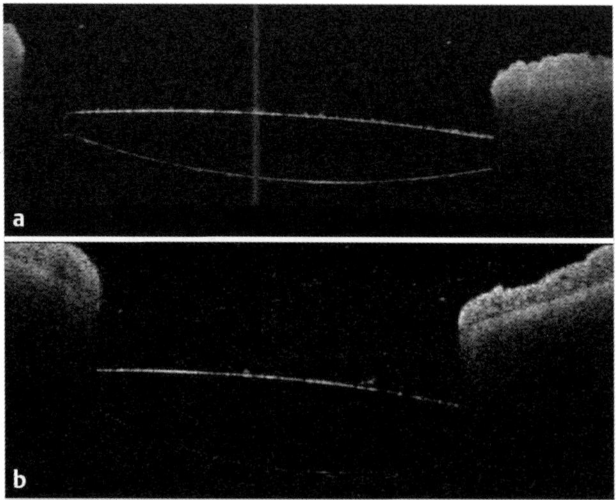

Fig. 17.5 Optical coherence tomography image with both optic surfaces clear **(a)** and only anterior surface clear **(b)**.

the iris. When the reference line along the iris (L) and the IOL optic (l) were parallel, the optic was not considered tilted. A difference of more than 100 µm between the two positions (D1 and D2) was considered optic tilt.[11]

17.4.1 Optic Position in Glued Intraocular Lens

The calculated mean slope of the IOL was 0.009 ± 0.1, and the slope of the iris was 0.002 ± 0.1 in 180 to 0 degrees (horizontal) axis. The calculated mean slope of the IOL was 0.008 ± 0.12, and the slope of the iris was 0.008 ± 0.10 in 90 to 270 (vertical) axes. There was significant correlation of slope of the iris with the IOL in both horizontal ($P = 0.000$, $r = 0.854$) and vertical axes ($P = 0.000$, $r = 0.880$) (▶ Fig. 17.4). The mean distance D1 and D2 was 0.94 ± 0.36 mm and 0.95 ± 0.36 mm, respectively. No difference was found between the D1 ($P = 0.131$) and D2 ($P = -0.181$) in the rigid IOL and foldable IOL groups (▶ Fig. 17.4). Both surfaces

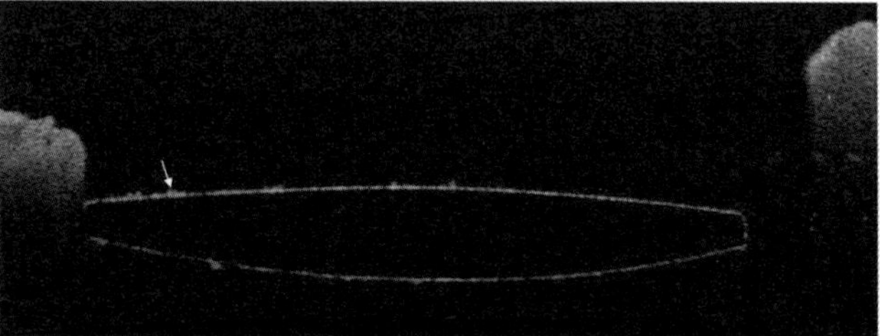

Fig. 17.6 Optical coherence tomography image showing an optic surface with pigment dispersion (arrow).

of the optic were seen in 50 eyes (83.3%) (▶ Fig. 17.5). Ten eyes (16.6%) had interrupted reflection from either of the surfaces (▶ Fig. 17.5). Ten (16.6%) of 60 eyes had pigment dispersed on the IOL surface, seen hyperreflective spots on the optic (▶ Fig. 17.6). Of 10 eyes with pigment dispersion, six were rigid and four were foldable IOLs. Iris adhesion to the optic was seen in four eyes (6.6%). Of 60 eyes, 21 (35%) had optic tilt detected on OCT, and 39 eyes (65%) had no optic tilt (▶ Fig. 17.7). No significant association was found between the IOL tilt and BCVA noted (chi-square test, $p = 0.468$).

17.4.2 Ocular Residual Astigmatism

The ORA was 0.53 ± 0.5 diopters. Significant correlation was noted between the ORA and total astigmatism ($r = 0.620$, $P = 0.000$), but no correlation was found between the IOL slope and the ORA ($r = 0.045$, $P = 0.730$) or of the ORA with the position of the IOL at D1 ($P = 0.494$) and D2 ($P = 0.791$). There was no association between ORA and optic tilt ($P = 0.326$), nor was a significant difference found in the ORA between the eyes with and without optic tilt ($P = 0.762$). The mean postoperative BCVA was 0.63 ± 0.2. There was a weak correlation ($P = 0.013$; $r = -0.363$) between the ORA and the BCVA (▶ Fig. 17.8) and no significant correlation of optic position at D1 ($P = 0.729$) and D2 ($P = 0.574$) with BCVA. No correlation was found between the slope ratio and BCVA ($P = 0.674$).

Fig. 17.7 Optical coherence tomography image showing a rigid intraocular lens implanted with no tilt.

17.4.3 Scleral Apposition with Glue

Fibrin glue provides airtight closure, and by the time the fibrin starts to degrade, surgical adhesions would have occurred in the scleral bed as shown in our follow-up anterior-segment OCT images in which postoperative perfect scleral flap adhesion (▶ Fig. 17.9) was observed as early as day 1 and was well sealed at 6 weeks.[4]

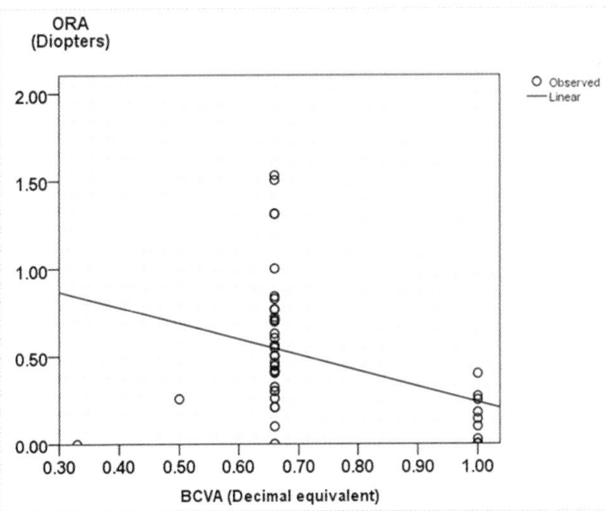

Fig. 17.8 Scatter plot showing the correlation of ocular residual astigmatism (ORA) with best-corrected visual acuity (BCVA).

17.4.4 Glued IOL in Various Indications

Glued IOL can be performed in eyes with postsurgical or traumatic aphakia. Eyes with subluxated cataract and intraoperative posterior capsular tear or zonular dialysis hindering IOL implantation are ideal candidates for glued IOL.[4,12] Congenital conditions like ectopia lentis and aniridia with lens subluxation are also indications for glued IOL implantation.[13,14] Glued IOL can be performed in eyes with postoperative IOL dislocation either anterior or posterior owing to weak zonules (▶ Fig. 17.10, ▶ Fig. 17.11).[15]

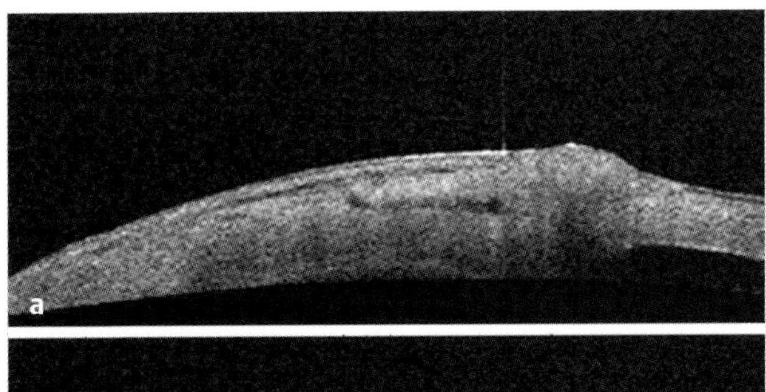

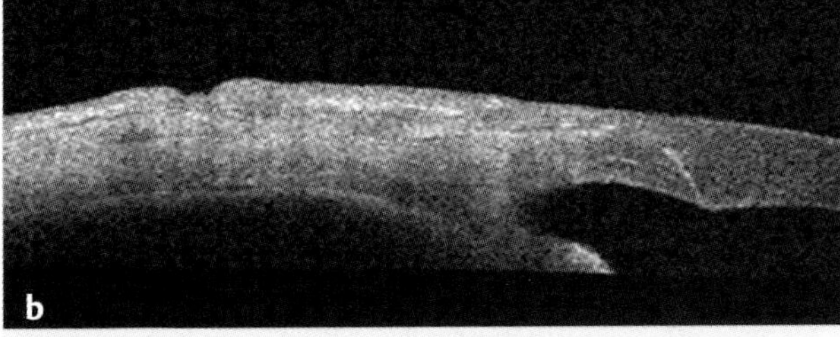

Fig. 17.9 Optical coherence tomography (OCT) section at the sclerotomy site showing the flaps. The scleral flap as seen by anterior segment OCT on day 1 **(a)** and well-sealed scleral flaps at 6 weeks **(b)**.

17.4.5 Comparison with Microscopic Tilt in Ultrasound Biomicroscopy

In the OCT study, we noted that 65% of the eyes had no microscopic tilt and 35% had microscopic tilt, which was not significant enough to cause vision loss. The incidence of optic tilt seen in this analysis was greater than that using UBM (17.4%), probably because of the greater axial resolution of OCT.[9] The limitation of OCT is that it needs to dilate the pupil each time for IOL visualization given that the iris pigment epithelium prevents

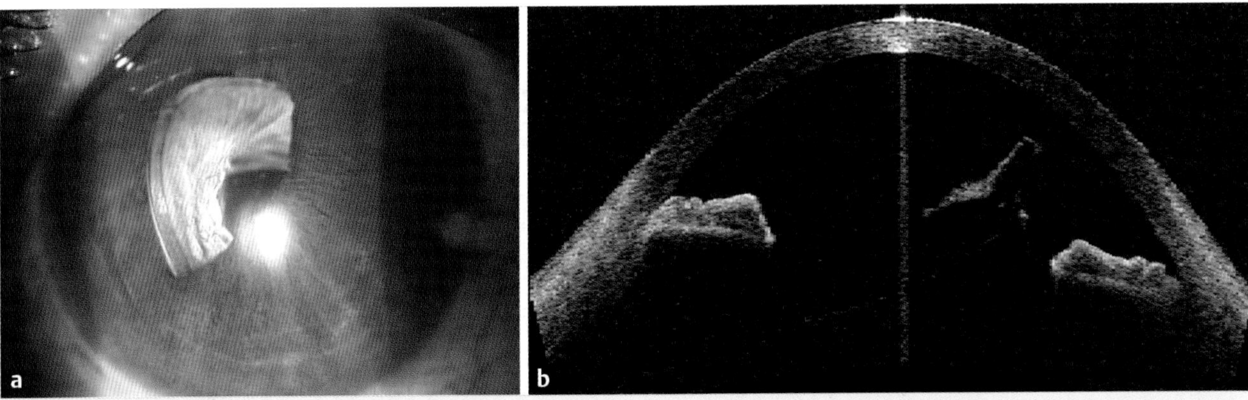

Fig. 17.10 **(a)** Partial anterior subluxation of the posterior chamber intraocular lens (IOL) and **(b)** the corresponding optical coherence tomography image.

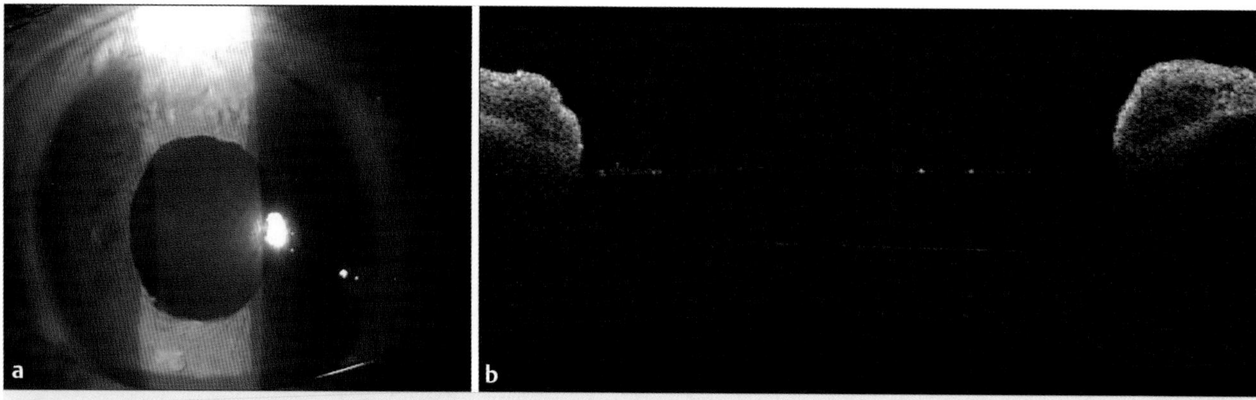

Fig. 17.11 (a) Same patient postoperatively after luxated intraocular lens (IOL) removal and transscleral glued IOL fixation performed and (b) the corresponding optical coherence tomography image showing the glued IOL.

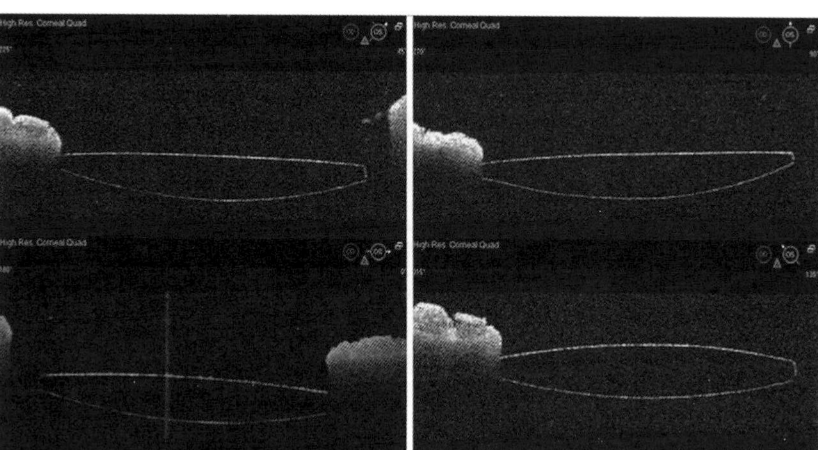

Fig. 17.12 Corneal high-resolution quad-mode anterior segment optical coherence tomography showing a 360-degree well-centered intraocular lens. OD, right eye; OS, left eye.

infrared wavelength transmission. However, OCT offers a noncontact method of evaluating the IOL position with higher resolution (▶ Fig. 17.12) compared with UBM, haptic visualization, and pars plicata or plana sclerotomy examination delineation.

17.4.6 Glued Intraocular Lens Versus Sutured Scleral Fixated Intraocular Lens

In the conventional sutured transscleral-fixated posterior capsular IOL technique, IOL tilt occurs because of the torque created by asymmetric suture placement on the IOL. Teichmann and Teichmann studied combinations of suture configurations and recommended looping the sutures symmetrically through the opposing eyelets.[16] Theoretically, tilt can also be eliminated using radial suture placement; this is anatomically undesirable, however, because one suture will exit through the ciliary body in transscleral suture fixation. Asymmetric attachment of the sutures to the haptics; failure to place the needles through the sclera 180 degrees apart; and suture loosening, breakage, or slippage on the haptics can also result in IOL tilt with suture-fixated posterior capsule IOLs. With glued IOLs, however, there is no anchoring of haptics with sutures; hence, no suture or haptic problems can occur. In the suture-fixated posterior-capsule IOL technique, the suture needle is blindly passed using the ab externo method; however, in the glued IOL method, the haptics come directly through the sclerotomies made in the measured position on direct visualization. The exact anatomical positioning of the sclerotomy is an important step in the glued IOL method.

17.5 Conclusion

Although the difference between the axial position of the glued IOL and the normal in-the-bag IOL was minimal, no significant association was found between the optic position and the BCVA noted. We noticed no difference between the foldable and nonfoldable types of IOLs with respect to the iris in axial position. Glued IOLs have shown good stability over the long term with no significant IOL tilt.

References

[1] Hovanesian JA, Karageozian VH. Watertight cataract incision closure using fibrin tissue adhesive. J Cataract Refract Surg 2007; 33: 1461–1463

[2] Lagoutte FM, Gauthier L, Comte PRM. A fibrin sealant for perforated and preperforated corneal ulcers. Br J Ophthalmol 1989; 73: 757–761

[3] Grewing R, Mester U. Fibrin sealant in the management of complicated hypotony after trabeculectomy. Ophthalmic Surg Lasers 1997; 28: 124–127

[4] Agarwal A, Kumar DA, Jacob S, Baid C, Agarwal A, Srinivasan S. Fibrin glue-assisted sutureless posterior chamber intraocular lens implantation in eyes with deficient posterior capsules. J Cataract Refract Surg 2008; 34: 1433–1438

[5] Maggi R, Maggi C. Sutureless scleral fixation of intraocular lenses. J Cataract Refract Surg 1997; 23: 1289–1294
[6] Gabor SG, Pavlidis MM. Sutureless intrascleral posterior chamber intraocular lens fixation. J Cataract Refract Surg 2007; 33: 1851–1854
[7] Agarwal A, Jacob S, Kumar DA, Agarwal A, Narasimhan S, Agarwal A. Handshake technique for glued intrascleral haptic fixation of a posterior chamber intraocular lens. J Cataract Refract Surg 2013; 39: 317–322
[8] Alpins NA, Goggin M. Practical astigmatism analysis for refractive outcomes in cataract and refractive surgery. Surv Ophthalmol 2004; 49: 109–122
[9] Kumar DA, Agarwal A, Packialakshmi S, Agarwal A. In vivo analysis of glued intraocular lens position with ultrasound biomicroscopy. J Cataract Refract Surg 2013; 39: 1017–1022
[10] Kumar DA, Agarwal A, Prakash G, Jacob S, Saravanan Y, Agarwal A. Evaluation of intraocular lens tilt with anterior segment optical coherence tomography. Am J Ophthalmol 2011; 151: 406–412, e2
[11] Loya N, Lichter H, Barash D, Goldenberg-Cohen N, Strassmann E, Weinberger D. Posterior chamber intraocular lens implantation after capsular tear: ultrasound biomicroscopy evaluation. J Cataract Refract Surg 2001; 27: 1423–1427
[12] Kumar DA, Agarwal A. Glued intraocular lens: a major review on surgical technique and results. Curr Opin Ophthalmol 2013; 24: 21–29
[13] Kumar DA, Agarwal A, Prakash D, Prakash G, Jacob S, Agarwal A. Glued intrascleral fixation of posterior chamber intraocular lens in children. Am J Ophthalmol 2012; 153: 594–601, e1–e2
[14] Kumar DA, Agarwal A, Jacob S, Lamba M, Packialakshmi S, Meduri A. Combined surgical management of capsular and iris deficiency with glued intraocular lens technique. J Refract Surg 2013; 29: 342–347
[15] Nair V, Kumar DA, Prakash G, Jacob S, Agarwal A, Agarwal A. Bilateral spontaneous in-the-bag anterior subluxation of PCIOL managed with glued IOL technique: a case report. Eye Contact Lens 2009; 35: 215–217
[16] Teichmann KD, Teichmann IAM. The torque and tilt gamble. J Cataract Refract Surg 1997; 23: 413–418

18 Use of Optical Coherence Tomography in Femtosecond Laser Lens and Cornea Surgery

Jason Philip Brinton and George O. Waring IV

Since its development in 2001, optical coherence tomography (OCT) has demonstrated increasingly wide use across a range of ophthalmic applications.[1,2] Although the technology was first described for imaging of the peripapillary retina and coronary artery, it has subsequently been used for evaluation of the cornea, iridocorneal angle, crystalline lens, vitreous, vitreoretinal interface, optic nerve, retina, choroid, and vasculature of the eye.[3] High-resolution, noninvasive imaging of these structures has imparted significant value to practitioners in a variety of clinical scenarios: (1) OCT has become the gold standard for establishing some diagnoses (e.g. macular pucker), (2) it can be used to follow the effects of treatment (e.g., for exudative age-related macular degeneration), and (3) it can guide decision making during surgery (e.g., with intraoperative assessment of macular hole closure).[4,5,6,7,8] In coupling OCT with femtosecond lasers, however, we find the first instance of OCT (4) forming the imaging basis for direct guidance of a surgical device.

In early 2001, the same year in which OCT was first described in the literature, the IntraLase Corporation (Irvine, CA) received 510k clearance from the U.S. Food and Drug Administration (FDA) to market a femtosecond laser for corneal flap creation. The primary virtue of femtosecond laser technology was that it had the capacity to precisely photodissect ophthalmic tissue without collateral photodisruption. The marriage of optical coherence and femtosecond laser technologies into an integrated diagnostic-therapeutic device was consummated 8 years later. In August 2009, the U.S. FDA granted 510k approval for an OCT-guided femtosecond laser for the fashioning of an anterior capsulotomy at the time of cataract surgery.

18.1 Femtosecond Lasers Using OCT Guidance

Three OCT-guided laser platforms are presently available for use in femtosecond laser lens surgery and laser-assisted in-situ keratomileusis (LASIK) surgery. The Lensx (Alcon Laboratories, Ft. Worth, TX), Catalys (Abbott Medical Optics, Santa Ana, CA), and Victus (Bausch & Lomb, Rochester, NY) technologies use a three-dimensional (3-D) spectral-domain OCT along with a video microscope to enable image-guided femtosecond laser application. These lasers can perform anterior capsulotomy, crystalline lens fragmentation, corneal incisions, and astigmatic keratotomy. Additionally, the Victus and Lensx platforms can be used for lamellar flap creation at the time of LASIK surgery.

18.1.1 Lensx

The Lensx was the first of these lasers introduced to the market. Its first commercial use was in December 2009 by Dr. Zoltan Nagy of Semmelweis University in Budapest, Hungary.[9] Lensx has received approval for anterior capsulotomy, phacofragmentation, partial- and full-thickness corneal incisions, and corneal flap creation in LASIK.

From an imaging standpoint, the Lensx laser system OCT uses spectral-domain OCT technology. It performs a high-resolution, cross-sectional tomographic scan of the internal microstructure of the eye by measuring backscattered light. It scans up to 8.5 mm deep to enable anterior-segment imaging from the anterior surface of the cornea to the posterior lens (▶ Fig. 18.1). The Lensx laser system uses a combination of circle scan and

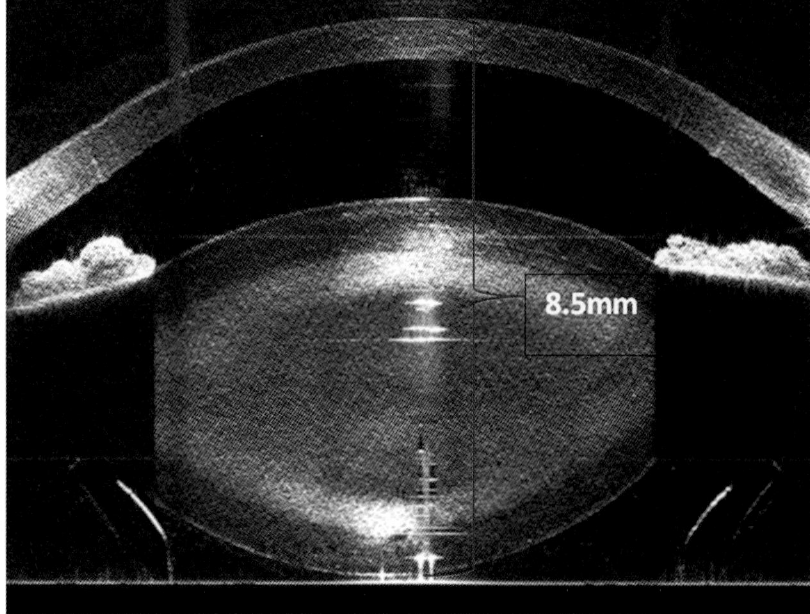

Fig. 18.1 Lensx laser optical coherence tomography scans up to 8.5 mm deep to enable imaging of the entire segment in one scan.

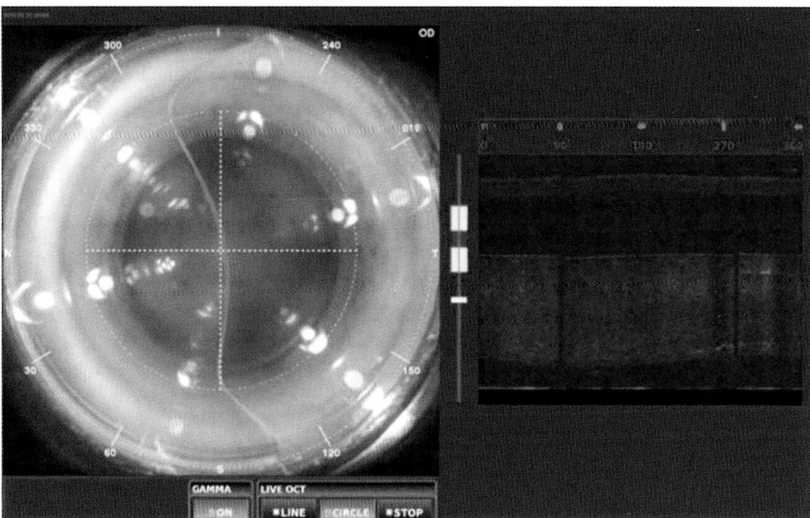

Fig. 18.2 Live circle scan can be seen on the left of the screen during the docking process. OCT, optical coherence tomography; OD, right eye.

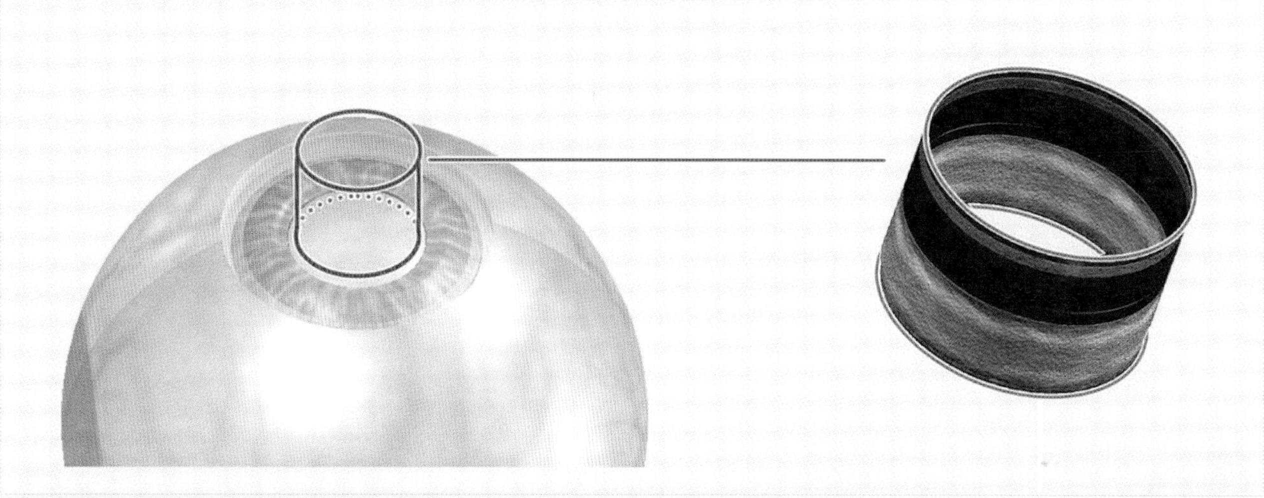

Fig. 18.3 The optical coherence tomography beam rotates about the laser system 360 degrees at a set diameter consistent with the capsulotomy.

line scan to identify anterior segment landmarks. On the video microscope OCT screen, the circle scan can be seen to the right of the video image during the docking process (▶ Fig. 18.2). The OCT beam rotates about the laser system 360 degrees at a set diameter consistent with the capsulotomy size (▶ Fig. 18.3). A column in the Z direction is collected at each point along the circumference of the circle scan; the summation of these points forms a cylinder. The cylinder is subsequently unwrapped, creating the displayed OCT image (▶ Fig. 18.4, ▶ Fig. 18.5). In the circle scan, several reference lines and control points are shown to indicate landmarks. The dotted crosshair identifies the highest and lowest points of the anterior capsule. The dotted vertical line identifies maximum lens tilt and dictates the position of the OCT line scan (▶ Fig. 18.6). The line scan is a cross-sectional image at the highest angular deviation or maximum lens tilt identified on the circle scan (▶ Fig. 18.7). Combination of the circle scan and line scan gives the 3-D corneal and lens alignment information. Image analysis algorithms assist users in identifying interfaces inside the anterior segment by prepositioning control points. The user must review and accept OCT images individually.

The Lensx OCT system is capable of imaging the posterior lens surface, even in patients with hypermature cataracts (▶ Fig. 18.8) and brunescent cataracts (▶ Fig. 18.9). In patients with subcapsular cataracts, the OCT gives high resolution and images that can assist the surgeon in planning lens removal in the operating room, even where cataract density prevents femtosecond laser phacofragmentation (▶ Fig. 18.10).

18.1.2 Catalys

Along with the other two platforms, the Catalys femtosecond laser system employs 3-D spectral-domain OCT to scan the anterior segment. Catalys computer guidance systems use these data to identify anterior-segment landmarks (▶ Fig. 18.11) and assist in treatment planning.

The system's 3-D OCT includes more than 10,000 A-scans of the anterior segment, which are completed in a spiral pattern,

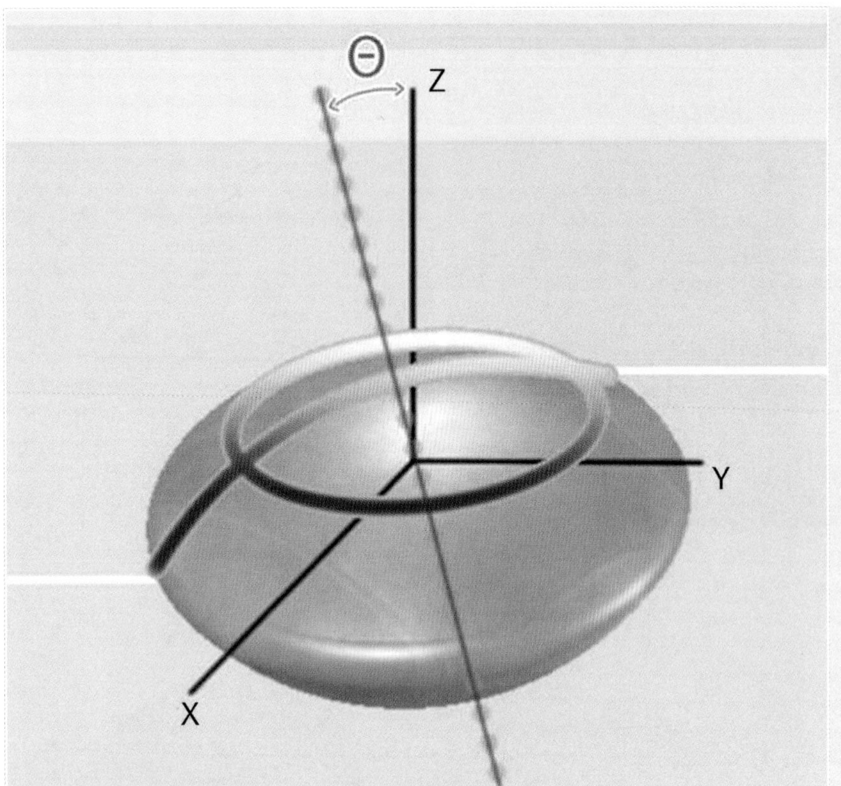
Θ
Z
Y
X

Fig. 18.4 A slice in the Z direction is collected at each point along the circumference of the circle scan and the summation of these points forms a cylinder.

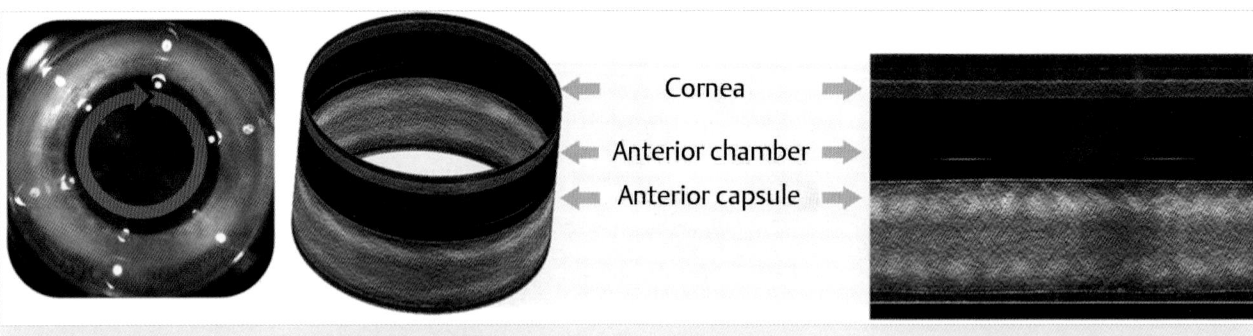
Cornea
Anterior chamber
Anterior capsule

Fig. 18.5 The cylinder is subsequently unrolled, creating the image.

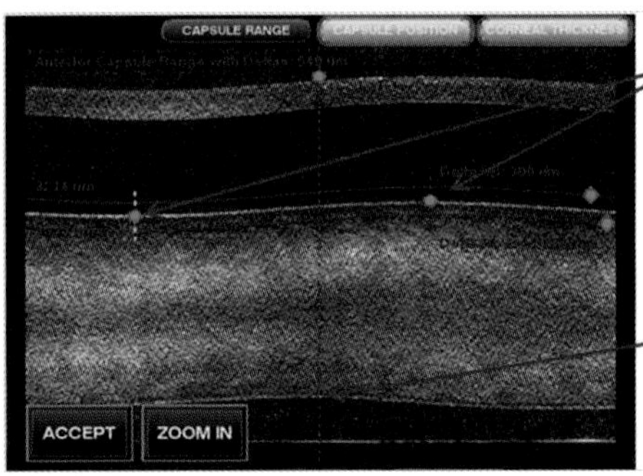
CAPSULE RANGE
ACCEPT
ZOOM IN
The pink cross hair identifies he highest point of the anterior capsule and the yellow cross hair identifies the lowest point of the anterior capsule.
The peak of the posterior capsule wave is the location of the maximum lens tilt and where the dotted vertical line is aligned.

Fig. 18.6 In the circle scan, the dotted crosshair identifies the highest and lowest points of the anterior capsule. The dotted vertical line is aligned with the highest point of the posterior capsule, which is identified as the maximum lens tilt and dictates the position of the line-scan optical coherence tomography.

as illustrated in ▶ Fig. 18.12. This extent of OCT imaging coverage is similar to that of the Victus laser but distinct from the Lensx laser, which uses OCT imaging only along a *z*-axis corresponding to the anterior capsulotomy diameter. The OCT operates at a wavelength of 820 to 930 nm with an axial resolution of 30 µm and a lateral resolution of 15 µm. Because of the unique laser wavelength and favorable signal-to-noise-ratio, the Catalys OCT can image through the posterior capsule. It has been reported as effective in the peer-reviewed literature and conference proceedings to achieve good visualization with intumescent[10] and brunescent[11] cataracts. It can effectively illustrate variations of normal anatomy, such as in the case of a thickened crystalline lens in a crowded anterior segment. It has also demonstrated good posterior capsule visualization for performing bag in-the-lens IOL implantation.

After OCT image acquisition, algorithms automatically map each surface (anterior cornea, posterior cornea, iris, limbus, anterior and posterior lens) and account for possible tilt. Catalys is the only platform to perform automatic mapping of these structures guided by OCT. The sagittal and axial cross-sections (▶ Fig. 18.13, ▶ Fig. 18.14, ▶ Fig. 18.15) demonstrate the presence of lens tilt with surface maps overlaid (▶ Fig. 18.16). Using ocular surface identification, the software can display central corneal thickness, aqueous depth, and anterior chamber depth, among other dimensions.

After the ocular surfaces are identified, safety zones and the incisions are calculated. In surface mapping guides, laser pulses are placed according to a specified pattern based on the full-volume scan without relying on manual surface selection. Catalys is unique among the laser platforms in that it is capable of compensating incisions for tilt, including capsulotomy, fragmentation, primary cataract incisions/side ports, and arcuate incisions. Each incision is confirmed independently on the cross-section and en face view (▶ Fig. 18.17). Once the incisions have been customized, the OCT images begin streaming at a frequency of 0.5 Hz, continuously refreshing with the overlays displayed (▶ Fig. 18.18). The surgeon has the capability to confirm the automated surface fits throughout the procedure, with the

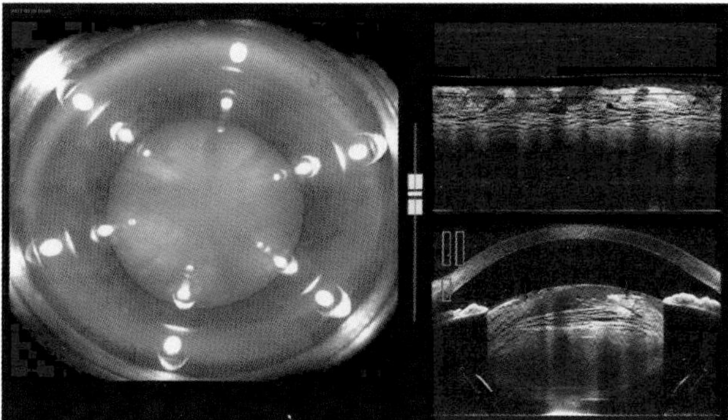

Fig. 18.8 Lensx optical coherence tomography image of hypermature cataract.

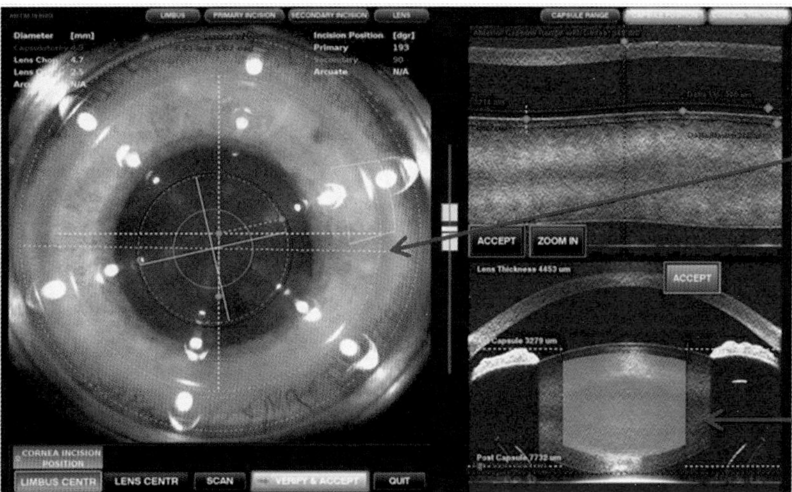

Fig. 18.7 The line scan is a cross-sectional image at the highest angular deviation or maximum lens tilt identified on the circle scan.

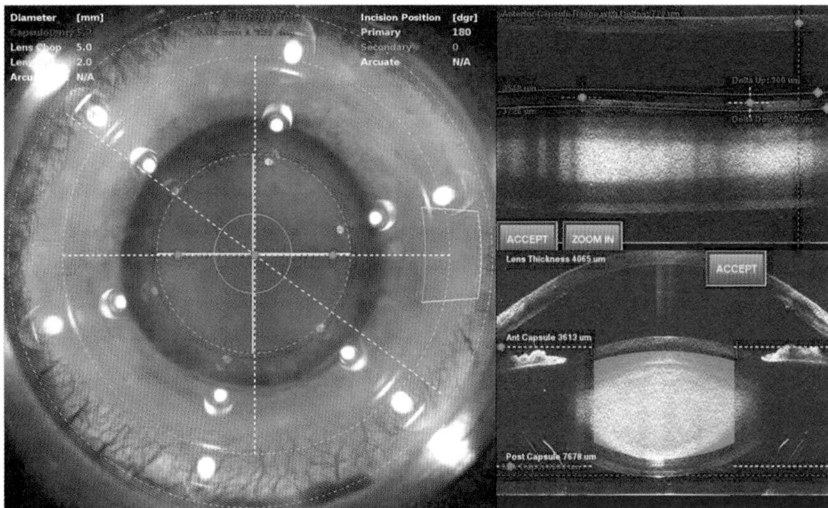

Fig. 18.9 Lensx optical coherence tomography image of brunescent cataract.

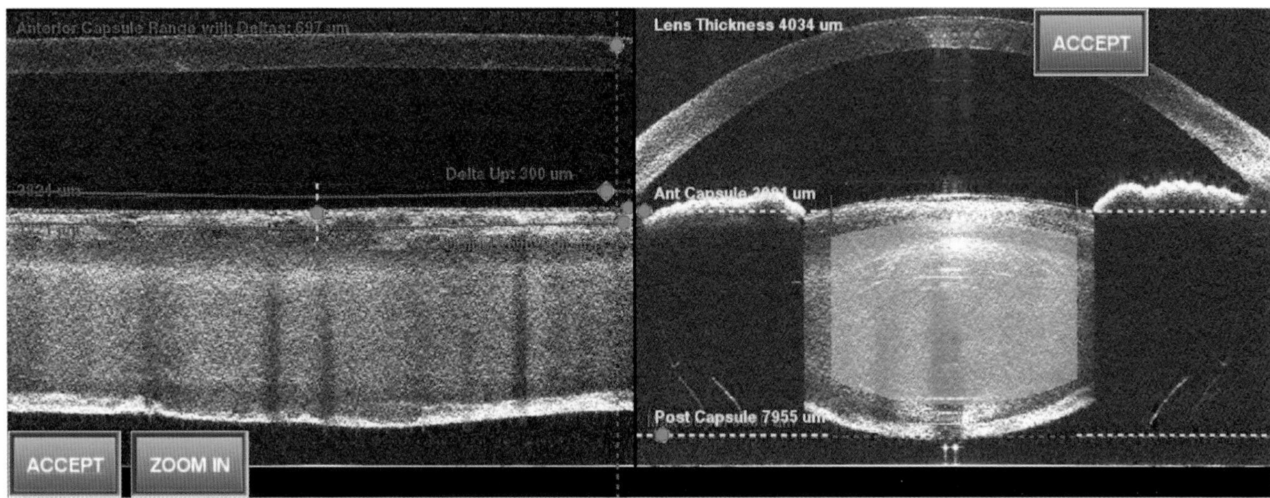

Fig. 18.10 Lensx optical coherence tomography image of subcapsular cataract.

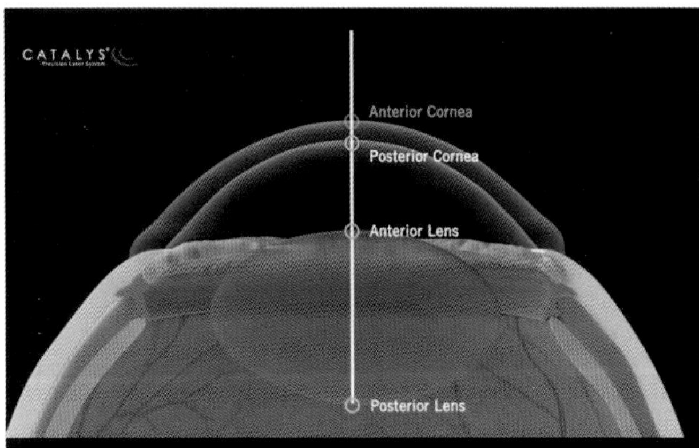

Fig. 18.11 Primary anterior segment landmarks identified by optical coherence tomography imaging.

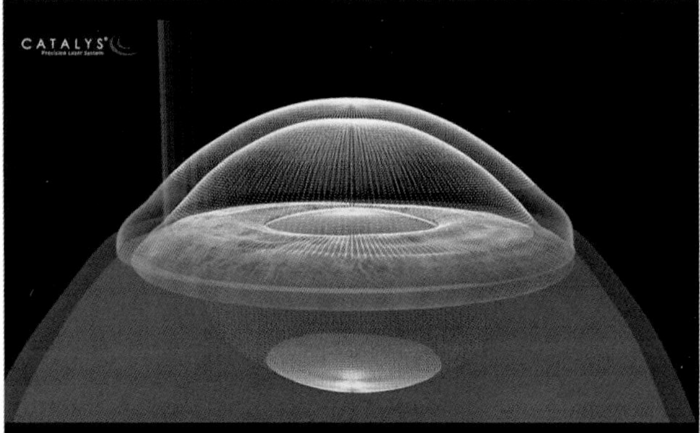

Fig. 18.12 Axial view illustrating how A-scans are completed in a spiral pattern to cover the full volume of the anterior segment.

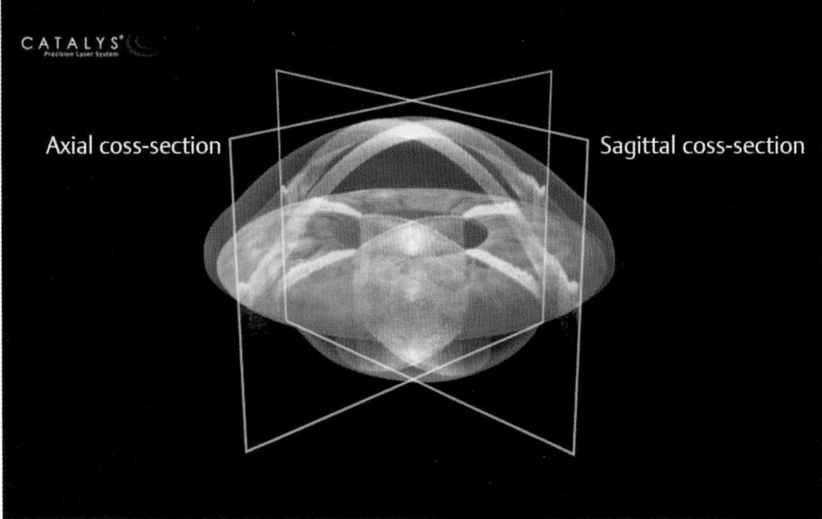

Fig. 18.13 Two cross-sectional scans are completed to provide axial and sagittal optical coherence tomography images.

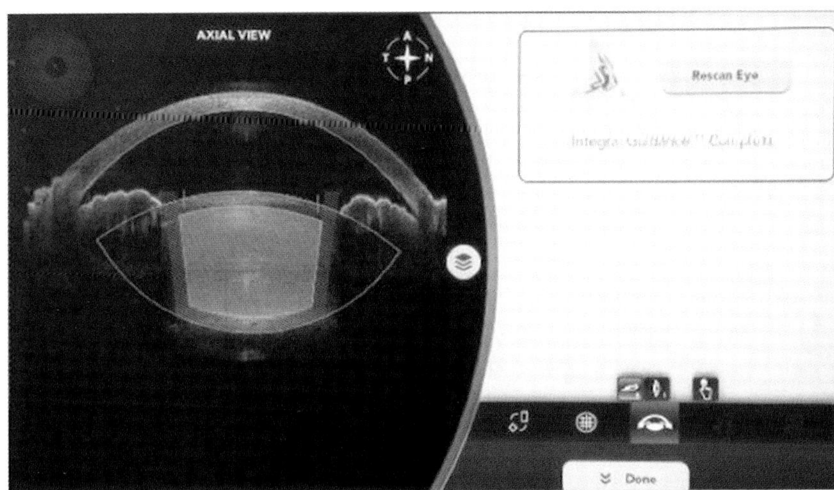

Fig. 18.14 Catalys optical coherence tomography image, axial view.

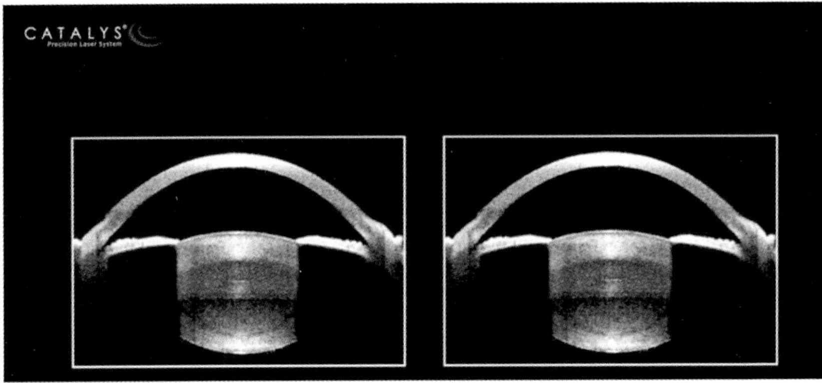

Fig. 18.15 Display of axial and sagittal optical coherence tomography images.

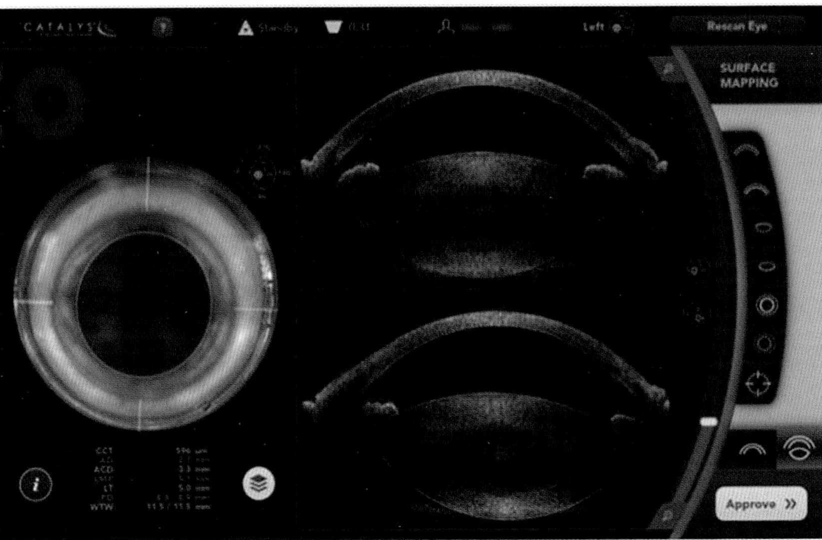

Fig. 18.16 Optical coherence tomography images showing lens tilt and dimensions. The pink crosshair identifies the highest point of the anterior capsule and the yellow crosshair identifies the lowest point of anterior capsule (upper arrows). The peak of the posterior capsule wave is the location of the maximum lens tilt and where the dotted vertical line is aligned (lower arrow).

OCT images streaming underneath for confirmation or detection of eye movement. Once confirmation of surfaces is complete, the surgeon confirms the incisions and fires the laser (▶ Fig. 18.19). The Catalys laser has received FDA approval for anterior capsulotomy, phacofragmentation, primary cataract incisions and side ports, and arcuate incisions.

18.1.3 Victus

The Victus femtosecond laser platform has been commercially available since 2011 and is European Confirmity (CE) marked for anterior capsulotomy, lens fragmentation, arcuate incisions, corneal incisions, LASIK flaps, intracorneal ring segments,

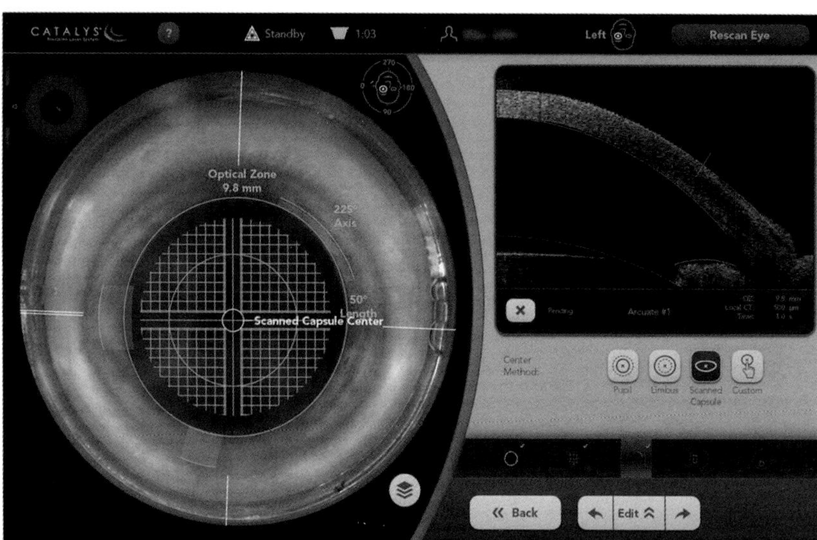

Fig. 18.17 Incision confirmation.

penetrating keratoplasty, lamellar keratoplasty, and pockets for crosslinking applications. In the United States, it received clearance for the creation of corneal flaps, anterior capsulotomy as part of cataract surgery, and corneal incisions. At the time of publication of this chapter, the platform referred to in the text is CE marked and not yet commercially available in the United States.

Victus incorporates a swept-source variant of spectral-domain OCT. It is based on the fast sweeping (multiple tens of thousands of Hertz) of the OCT wavelength around the average wavelength of 1.31 µm. Each wavelength sweep corresponds to an A-scan of any OCT image (i.e., cross-sectional scan, circle scan, or advanced trajectory), providing the user with an unprecedented responsive video rate OCT image at 25 Hz, covering cross-sectional scans of 12.5 mm width and 11.0 mm depth while achieving a resolution of less than 15 µm axially and 25 µm laterally. The OCT technology provides visualization with live imaging during the docking process and throughout the procedure. The complete range of interest between the cornea and the posterior lens surface can be displayed during a cataract procedure, including anterior capsulotomy, lens fragmentation, corneal side incisions, and arcuate incisions.

As an OCT-guided platform, Victus was designed to support the surgeon's decision-making process by guiding the surgeon's attention to the relevant OCT and camera images. The geometry of the displayed OCT scans (cross-sectional or circular scan), their range (cornea vs. full depth), and their magnification factor depend on the treatment and workflow stage. Although any treatment can be planned offline based on prior knowledge of parameters such as the cataract grade, lens thickness, and cornea thickness, some parameters will be adjusted based on image data collected at the time of docking. These parameters include the position, volume, and any possible tilt of the lens. Capsulotomy and lens fragmentation patterns are adjusted using software-supported recognition of the pupil and lens.

Accurate handling of a tilted lens and decentered pupil is a requirement to achieve a circular capsulotomy cut. In the following examples, we discuss two typical OCT-guided workflows with Victus to demonstrate the level of integration of video-rate OCT images into the surgeon's workflow.

Example 1: Flap Creation

At the time of docking, a video microscopic image and cross-sectional live OCT image are both displayed (▶ Fig. 18.20). These images assist the surgeon with docking and fixation of the eye. Proper docking is proceeding when the OCT cross-sectional scan shows direct contact between the cornea and patient interface at a defined pressure. The example chosen in ▶ Fig. 18.20 shows a pronounced air gap of approximately 200 µm.

In the next step, the thickness and position of the planned flap are overlaid onto the OCT image (▶ Fig. 18.21). At this stage, the surgeon can position the flap treatment in relation to the top view of the eye and adjust flap parameters, including flap thickness and diameter. During femtosecond laser application, the surgeon monitors progress via both video microscopic image and live cross-sectional OCT (▶ Fig. 18.22).

Example 2: OCT-Guided Femtosecond Laser Capsulotomy, Lens Fragmentation, and Arcuate Incisions

Before surgery, treatment parameters can be set in advance based on schematic cross-sections and top views of an eye (not shown). Docking proceeds as with flap creation (▶ Fig. 18.20). For cataract procedures, a dedicated "soft docking" mode is used. After docking, a treatment alignment display illustrates the planned location for capsulotomy and lens fragmentation (▶ Fig. 18.23) and highlights the relevant eye anatomy. The geometry of the proposed capsulotomy and lens fragmentation treatment is shown in relation to two OCT cross-sectional scans through the center of the pupil at 0 and 90 degrees, as well as a circular scan parallel to the pupil edge. Based on this information, the surgeon approves the planned treatment. An option for manual adjustment of the treatment is available via two "edit" buttons shown in ▶ Fig. 18.23.

After the treatment has been reviewed and approved, the surgeon is presented with the treatment screen (▶ Fig. 18.24). As femtosecond laser energy is applied to the eye, dissection of the capsular bag and lens can be followed on a magnified cross-sectional OCT image.

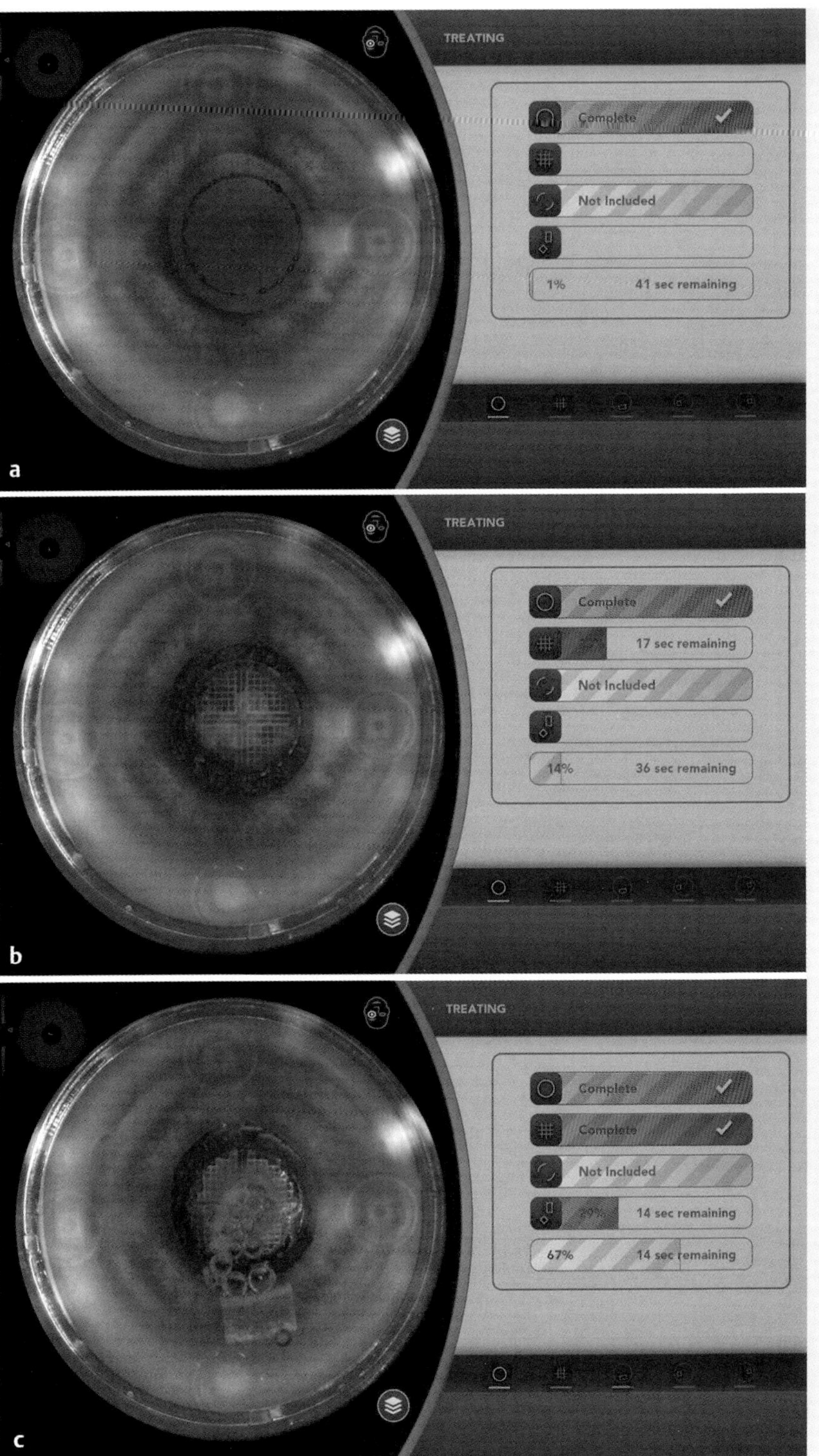

Fig. 18.18 (a) Laser treatment proceeds with capsulotomy, **(b)** lens fragmentation, and **(c)** corneal incisions.

Arcuate incision creation is also supported by OCT technology. ▶ Fig. 18.25 illustrates the position of arcuate incisions in relation to the pupil and limbus; depth is illustrated on OCT cross-sectional scans. The typical clinical workflow for the application of arcuate incisions involves a readout of the recommended parameters (angular width, depth ratio, diameter) from a nomogram based on the patient's keratometry or manifest astigmatism readings and pachymetry. The resulting values are programmed before the treatment with the femtosecond laser. After an OCT-guided workflow, the surgeon reviews the planned incision depth on magnified cross-sections of the cornea in the vicinity of the incision.

For corneas demonstrating varying thickness, treatment depth can be customized along the length of the planned arcuate to compensate for local pachymetry values. In this case, the surgeon is presented with a cross-sectional scan of the cornea (▶ Fig. 18.26), where the arcuate incision can be adjusted according to local pachymetry.

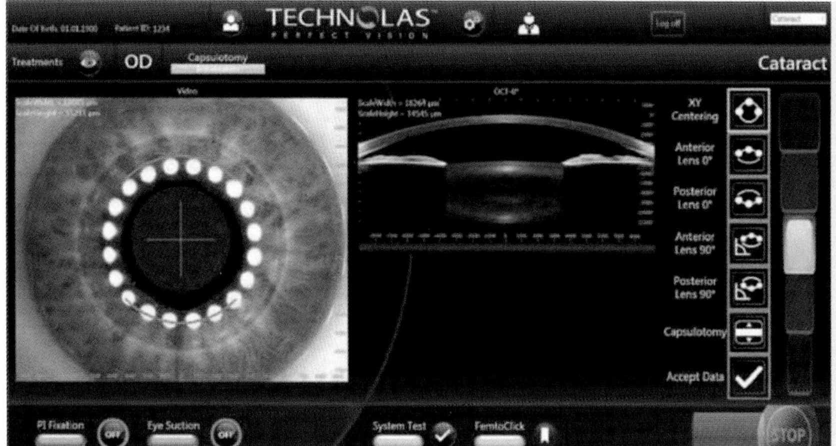

Fig. 18.19 Victus video microscopic image (left side) and optical coherence tomography image (right side). OD, right eye.

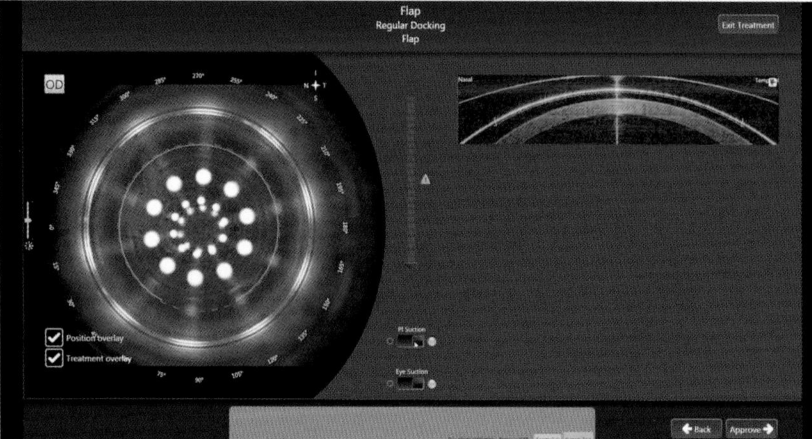

Fig. 18.20 Live images during docking of the patient: The patient's eye is positioned based on the surgeon's review of the live camera and optical coherence tomography cross-sectional image. Note the air gap visible while the eye is not in contact with the patient interface. OD, right eye.

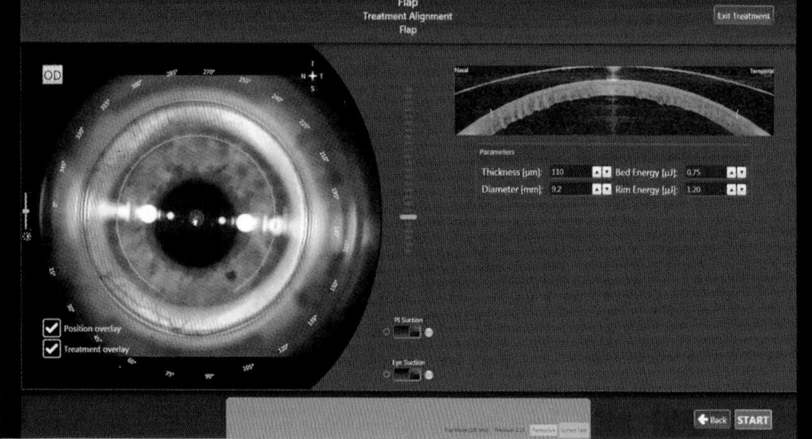

Fig. 18.21 Alignment of the flap treatment to the geometry of the patient's eye. Thickness, diameter, and lateral position of the flap are overlaid on the optical coherence tomography image. OD, right eye.

The Victus OCT imaging system provides surgeons with comprehensive information for completing the various surgical applications of the laser. During all phases of treatment, the surgeon benefits from live OCT images, which can cover the anterior segment from the cornea to the posterior lens surface.

18.2 Femtosecond Lasers Using Other Imaging Technologies

Other lasers perform comparable functions using different imaging modalities. The Lensar (Lensar, Orlando, FL) laser has

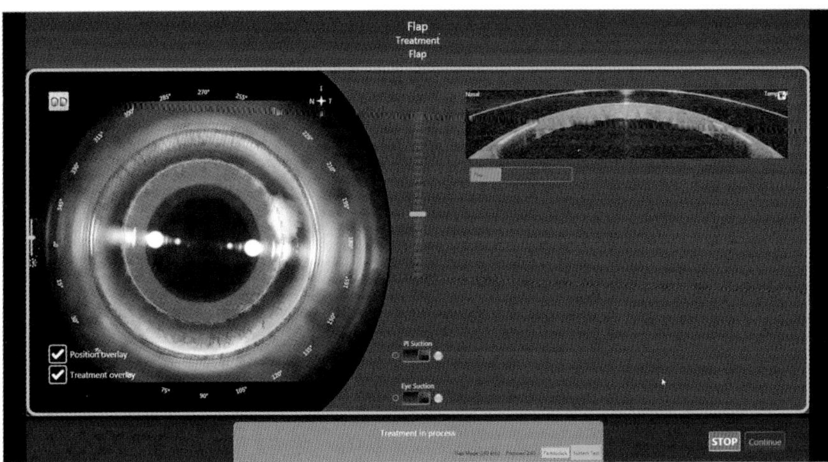

Fig. 18.22 Monitoring the progress of a lamellar flap cut during application of the femtosecond laser beam. The dissected corneal tissue along the cut (white lines within cross-section of cornea) throws a typical shadow toward the posterior corneal surface as a result of the different scattering of the optical coherence tomography beam. OD, right eye.

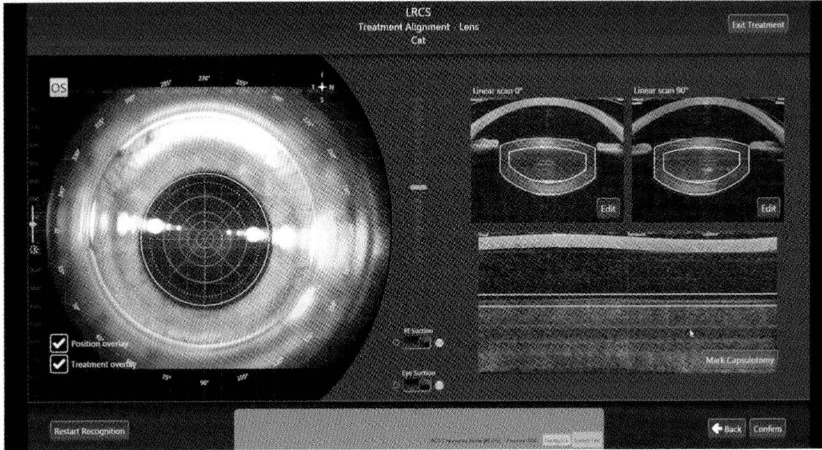

Fig. 18.23 Alignment screen for the capsulotomy and lens fragmentation treatments. The planned treatment is reviewed and approved by the surgeon based on this view. On the right side, optical coherence tomography cross-sections at 0 and 90 degrees as well as a circular scan along the edge of the capsulotomy are shown. Overlays indicate the boundaries of the capsulotomy and lens fragmentation treatments. On cross-sectional scans, the capsulotomy is indicated by a purple-colored rectangle. The lens fragmentation pattern fills the volume limited by the white lines, which maintain a defined distance to the detected anterior and posterior lens surfaces and to the pupil (indicated by yellow lines). Imaging effectively recognizes and compensates for lens tilt. OS, left eye. LRCS: Laser refractive cataract surgery.

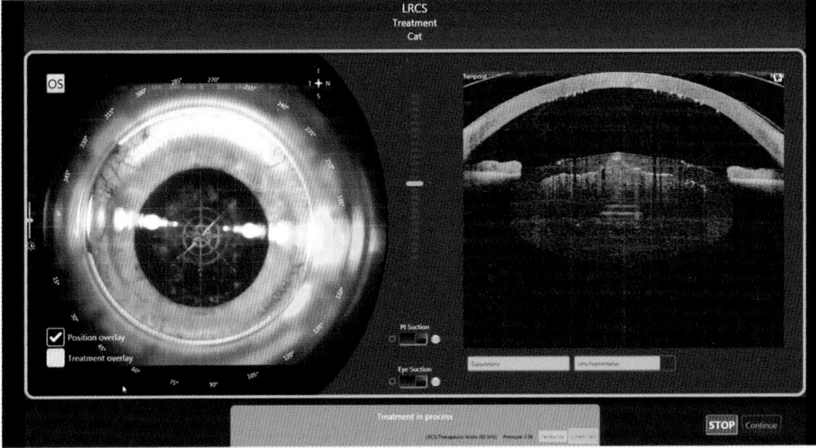

Fig. 18.24 Monitoring the progress of a capsulotomy and lens fragmentation treatment. Optical coherence tomography cross-section shows rising gas bubbles in the anterior chamber. This effect can be seen as the effects of phacofragmentation progress anteriorly and interact with aqueous. LRCS: Laser refractive cataract surgery.

been approved for anterior capsulotomy, phacofragmentation, corneal incisions, and astigmatic keratotomy. The Lensar platform is unique in that its imaging system uses 3-D ray-tracing confocal structural illumination rather than OCT. Upon docking with the patient interface, a super luminescent diode illuminates the eye with infrared light. A video camera records the resultant images using the Scheimpflug principle to guide surgical planning. Four additional femtosecond laser platforms are presently used to fashion lamellar flaps for LASIK surgery. The Intralase (Abbott Medical Optics),

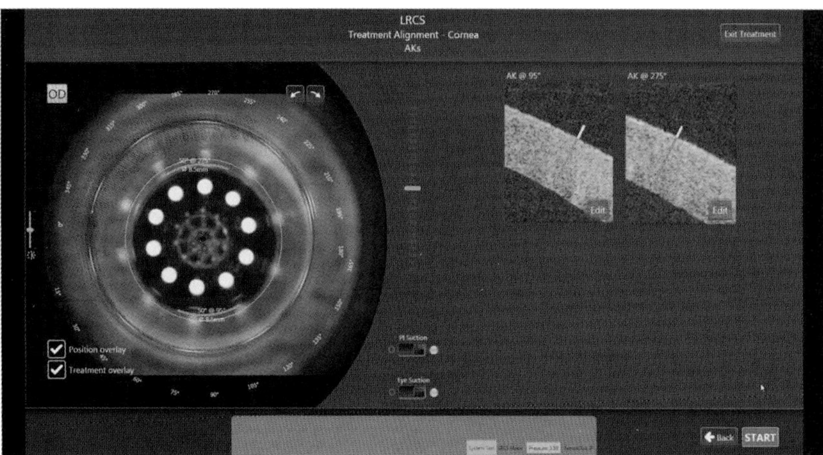

Fig. 18.25 Optical coherence tomography (OCT)-guided alignment of arcuate incisions. OCT cross-sectional scans reveal the depth and local contour of the cornea.

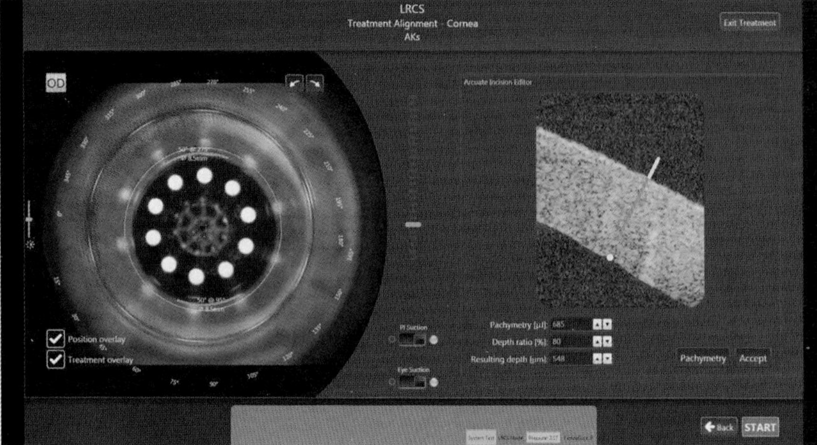

Fig. 18.26 Optical coherence tomography (OCT)-guided planning of arcuate incisions. A magnified OCT cross-sectional scan allows adjustment of incision depth to follow local pachymetry. OD, right eye. LRCS: Laser refractive cataract surgery; AK: Arcuate keratotomy.

Visumax (Carl Zeiss Meditec, Jena, Germany), Wavelight fs200 (Alcon), and Femto ldv (Ziemer Ophthalmic Systems, Port, Switzerland) lasers perform this function, among several additional applications; individual lasers in this group can create pockets for corneal inlays and channels for intrastromal corneal rings, fashion donor and host tissue for femtosecond laser-assisted keratoplasty, perform intrastromal corneal treatment for presbyopia, and perform astigmatic keratotomy.

18.3 Role of OCT in Select Femtosecond Laser Surgical Applications

18.3.1 Capsulotomy

Optical coherence tomography imaging is integral to the ability of the femtosecond laser to dissect an anterior lens capsule accurately and with a high degree of circularity. The surgeon first uses a video microscopic image to center the capsulotomy from an *x-y* axis standpoint. The OCT image is subsequently viewed to determine the depth of treatment along the *z*-axis. OCT imaging identifies and assists the user in compensating for lens tilt, ensuring that the capsulotomy is circular rather than effectively oval. OCT aids in distinguishing the anterior capsule, which contains a fibrogranular material made of type IV collagen and matrix proteins from the cells of the crystalline lens epithelium and outer cortex. A more narrowly tailored capsulotomy treatment avoids unnecessary laser pulses in the lens cortex, which potentially increase laser time and can further complicate the removal of anterior lens cortex with the irrigation and aspiration handpiece. Primary posterior laser-assisted capsulotomy has also been described to prevent posterior capsule opacification after cataract, particularly in the pediatric population.[12,13]

18.3.2 Lens Fragmentation Pattern

The anteroposterior width of the lens ranges from 3 mm at birth to 6 mm in the ninth decade of life. OCT imaging allows the surgeon to determine appropriately the anterior and posterior bounds of phacofragmentation with a high degree of accuracy. Placing laser pulses too close to the posterior capsule risks posterior capsule rupture, whereas leaving too large of a zone between the posterior extent of phacofragmentation and the posterior capsule can make phacofragmentation less effective, particularly in eyes with a dense posterior lens plate. Imaging allows surgeons to set a customized safety margin separating the posterior extent of phacofragmentation from the posterior capsule. Values in the range of 0.5 mm are commonly used.

18.3.3 Partial- and Full-Thickness Corneal Incisions

From an *x-y* axis standpoint, wound, paracentesis, and arcuate keratotomy placement are selected by the surgeon based on the laser videomicroscope image. OCT imaging assists in setting the depth (e.g. 100% for incisions, 80% for arcuate keratotomy), angle, and profile (e.g., planar vs. multiplanar) of these incisions. Accurate assessment of corneal thickness is essential to avoid poster extension of arcuate incisions and inadvertent corneal perforation. OCT imaging also allows the laser to fashion intrastromal arcuate incisions that do not extend anteriorly through the epithelium. Some surgeons favor this approach because it avoids epithelial disruption with its attendant discomfort, tear-film disruption, and risk of infection. Although arcuate incisions are typically fashioned at the time of femtosecond laser lens surgery, they have also been described for primary correction of mixed astigmatism, astigmatism correction during phakic intraocular lens surgery, and astigmatism correction after penetrating keratoplasty.

References

[1] Huang D, Swanson EA, Lin CP, et al. Optical coherence tomography. Science 1991; 254: 1178–1181

[2] Drexler W, Fujimoto JG, eds. Optical Coherence Tomography: Technology and Applications. Berlin: Springer; 2008

[3] Izatt JA, Hee MR, Swanson EA, et al. Micrometer-scale resolution imaging of the anterior eye in vivo with optical coherence tomography. Arch Ophthalmol 1994; 112: 1584–1589

[4] Wykoff CC, Berrocal AM, Schefler AC, Uhlhorn SR, Ruggeri M, Hess D. Intraoperative OCT of a full-thickness macular hole before and after internal limiting membrane peeling. Ophthalmic Surg Lasers Imaging 2010; 41: 7–11

[5] Ehlers JP, Ohr MP, Kaiser PK, Srivastava SK. Novel microarchitectural dynamics in rhegmatogenous retinal detachments identified with intraoperative optical coherence tomography. Retina 2013; 33: 1428–1434

[6] Pichi F, Alkabes M, Nucci P, Ciardella AP. Intraoperative SD-OCT in macular surgery. Ophthalmic Surg Lasers Imaging 2012; 43 Suppl: S54–S60

[7] Ray R, Barañano DE, Fortun JA, et al. Intraoperative microscope-mounted spectral domain optical coherence tomography for evaluation of retinal anatomy during macular surgery. Ophthalmology 2011; 118: 2212–2217

[8] Binder S, Falkner-Radler CI, Hauger C, Matz H, Glittenberg C. Feasibility of intrasurgical spectral-domain optical coherence tomography. Retina 2011; 31: 1332–1336

[9] Nagy Z, Takacs A, Filkorn T, Sarayba M. Initial clinical evaluation of an intraocular femtosecond laser in cataract surgery. J Refract Surg 2009; 25: 1053–1060

[10] Dick HB, Schultz T. Femtosecond laser-assisted cataract surgery in infants. J Cataract Refract Surg 2013; 39: 665–668

[11] Batlle, et al. Proceedings of the European Society of Cataract and Refractive Surgery (ESCRS) 2013. In: European Society of Cataract and Refractive Surgery. Amsterdam, Netherlands: ESCRS; 2013

[12] Dick HB, Canto AP, Culbertson WW, Schultz T. Femtosecond laser-assisted technique for performing bag-in-the-lens intraocular lens implantation. J Cataract Refract Surg 2013; 39: 1286–1290

[13] Dick HB, Schultz T. Primary posterior laser-assisted capsulotomy. J Refract Surg 2014; 30: 128–133

Part 4

Optical Coherence Tomography in Retinal Diseases

19 Optical Coherence Tomography Diagnosis of Retinal Diseases

Mandeep Lamba, Soosan Jacob, and Amar Agarwal

Optical coherence tomography (OCT) was developed through a collaborative effort between the New England Eye Center, Tufts University School of Medicine, the Department of Electrical Engineering and Computer Science at Massachusetts Institute of Technology (MIT), and Lincoln Laboratory, MIT. It is a new, noninvasive, noncontact, transpupillary imaging technology for in vivo evaluation of retinal structures and has a resolution of 10 to 17 µm. Similar to B-scan, it produces cross-sectional images of the retina, the difference being that it uses the optical backscattering of light unlike the sound waves, which are used in B-scan. It therefore uses the optical properties, rather than acoustic properties, of the tissues and therefore obtains a much higher axial resolution of approximately 10 µm. The anatomical layers of the retina can be differentiated, and retinal thickness can be measured. It can also be used for anterior-segment imaging to visualize the cornea, iris, lens, and angle.[1] Retinal imaging is performed using infrared light at approximately 800-nm wavelength, whereas for anterior-segment OCT, light of 1300-nm wavelength is used.

The image is displayed using a false color map that corresponds to detected backscattered light levels ranging between 4×10^{-10} to 10^{-6} of the incident light. Although retinal imaging is its most common application so far, OCT can be applied in a wide variety of fields other than ophthalmology.[2,3,4] The ability of OCT to perform a nonexcisional optical biopsy in real time while giving detailed qualitative and quantitative information is its main advantage. Compared with ultrasound, its main disadvantage is that light is highly scattered or absorbed by most biological tissues, all the more in case of opaque tissues. Hence, optical imaging is restricted to only the superficial tissues, which are optically accessible. The advantage of OCT is its axial resolution of about 10 µm, which is 10 to 20 times more than standard ultrasound B-mode imaging.[5] Research OCT imaging systems have even higher resolution of up to about 3 µm.[6] The axial resolution of OCT is determined by the physical properties of the light source, whereas transverse resolution is determined by the focused spot size of the optical beam and is generally around 20 to 25 µm. The absolute minimum spot size is limited by the optical aberrations of that particular eye, unlike in other imaging applications.[7] Image resolution also depends on the speed of acquisition, pixels in the image, and the basic resolution of the system.

19.1 Principle of OCT

Sir Isaac Newton first established the technique of low-coherence or white-light interferometry. OCT performs cross-sectional imaging based on low-coherence interferometry by using a continuous beam of low-coherence light. This light is back-reflected from different tissue boundaries, and the machine measures the echo-time delay and intensity of backscattered or back-reflected light from the microstructures inside the tissues. The light is backscattered differently from nonhomogeneous tissues, depending on their optical properties and refractive indices. Serial axial measurements are taken at different transverse positions. These signal intensities are processed by the computer and displayed as grayscale or as a false color-coded image. In grayscale, white corresponds to the strongest backscattered signal and black to the weakest one. Grayscale is not as informative as the false color-coded image because computer monitors have only 8-bit gray resolution, or 256 gray levels. Also, the eye has a limited ability to distinguish between subtle shades of gray.[7] Postprocessing of the image makes it possible to obtain measurements or to reconstruct topography maps. Software programs are available for different scan patterns and different image processing protocols. ▶ Table 19.1 describes the parts of the OCT machine.

19.2 Color Coding in OCT

A rainbow of colors is used for ophthalmic imaging (▶ Table 19.2). Images are displayed as grayscale/false color scale. Maximum intensity signal (50 dB) is displayed as white in grayscale and red in false color scale. Weakest intensity signal (95 dB) is displayed as black and blue.

Table 19.1 Parts of optical coherence tomography

Light source	Super luminescent diode
Partially reflecting mirror	Beam splitter splits the incident light beam into two parts and also receives the back-reflected reference optical beam
Photodetector	Measures the distance the light has traveled to and from the ocular structures. The light pulses will coincide if they are same and produce phenomenon of interference.
Interferometer	Constructed using fiber-optic coupler, which can precisely measure the echo structure of reflected light and perform high-resolution measurements of the distance and thickness of different structures
Computer	Signals are processed electronically and displayed on a computer.
Conventional slit-lamp biomicroscope and a fixed + 78 D condensing lens	Required for retinal examination
Infrared video camera	Required for viewing and scanning the probe beam on the fundus

19.3 Interpretation of OCT of the Normal Retina

The light beam of the OCT can be transmitted, absorbed, or scattered, depending on tissue properties. Tissues with high absorption or backscattering, such as hemoglobin and melanin, can cause shadowing of the underlying tissues.

As seen in ▶ Fig. 19.1, there is an increase in backscattering at the vitreoretinal interface. The fovea is seen as a thinner area where the inner layers disappear and the photoreceptor layer thickens. Only the outer nuclear layer (ONL) and photoreceptor layer are seen in the fovea. The nerve-fiber layer (NFL) is a highly scattering layer at the inner margin of the retina and is seen as red. It is thickest at the optic disc margins and absent at the fovea. All axonal layers, such as the NFL and the plexiform layers, are more backscattering (inner plexiform layer [IPL]), moderately backscattering (outer plexiform layer [OPL]), or highly backscattering (Henle fiber layer) and hence are seen as red. The nuclear layers (ganglion cell layer [GCL], inner nuclear layer [INL], and outer nuclear layer [ONL]) are poorly backscattering and are seen as blue-black. The GCL increases in thickness in the parafoveal region. The reflection between the inner and outer segments is seen immediately anterio pigment epithelium (RPE) as another highly scatte a result of the difference in the refractive index of the ment (IS) and the outer segment (OS), which contains sin. The IS and OS are thicker in the foveal region, which seen in the OCT. The external limiting membrane (ELM) sometimes be seen as a thin backscattering layer behind the ONL. The RPE and choriocapillaris are visualized as the posterior limit of the retina and are highly scattering, seen as red. The RPE, Bruch membrane, and the choriocapillaris cannot be identified separately. The light beam is relatively attenuated on passing through the retinal layers and the choriocapillaris so that structures posterior to this are not seen well because of shadowing.

Table 19.2 Color coding in optical coherence tomography (OCT)

Layers of retina	Backscattering	False color in OCT
Nerve-fiber and plexiform layers	High	Red
Nuclear layers	Weak	Blue to black
Ganglion cell layer	Weak	Blue to black
Outer plexiform layer	High	Red
Inner plexiform layer	Moderate	Green to yellow
Boundary between photoreceptor inner segments and outer segments	Thin high	Red
Retinal pigment epithelium	Strong	Red
Choriocapillaries	High	Red

19.4 Interpretation of OCT of the Optic Nerve Head

The optic disc shows a characteristic contour on OCT (▶ Fig. 19.2). The NFL is thickest near the disc rim, which is composed almost entirely of the NFL. The backscattering decreases as the fibers turn to enter the optic disc because they are no longer perpendicular to the light beam. The

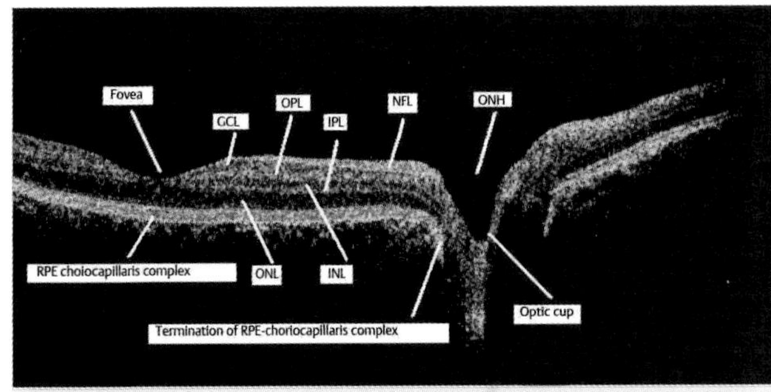

Fig. 19.1 Line scan showing normal retinal architecture. GCL, ganglion cell layer; INL, inner nuclear layer; IPL, inner plexiform layer; NFL, nerve-fiber layer; ONH, optic nerve head; OPH, outer plexiform layer; RPE, retinal pigment epithelium.

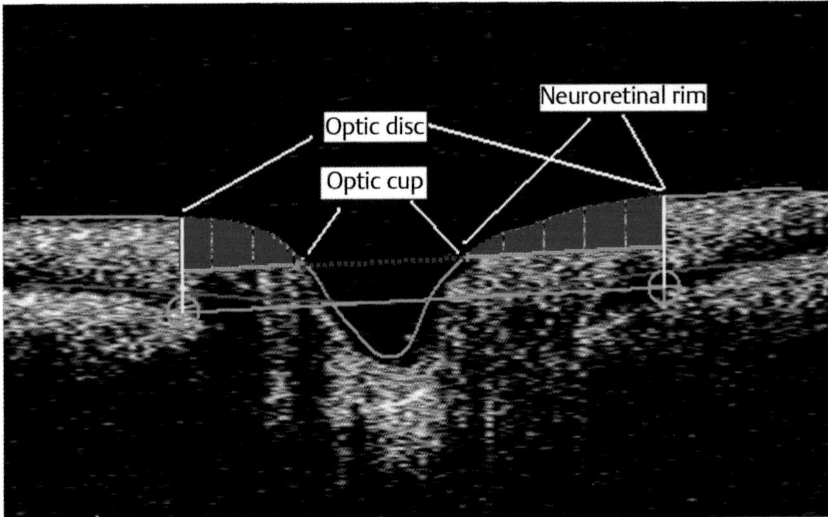

Fig. 19.2 Optic nerve head scan on optical coherence tomography (OCT) showing a normal nerve head.

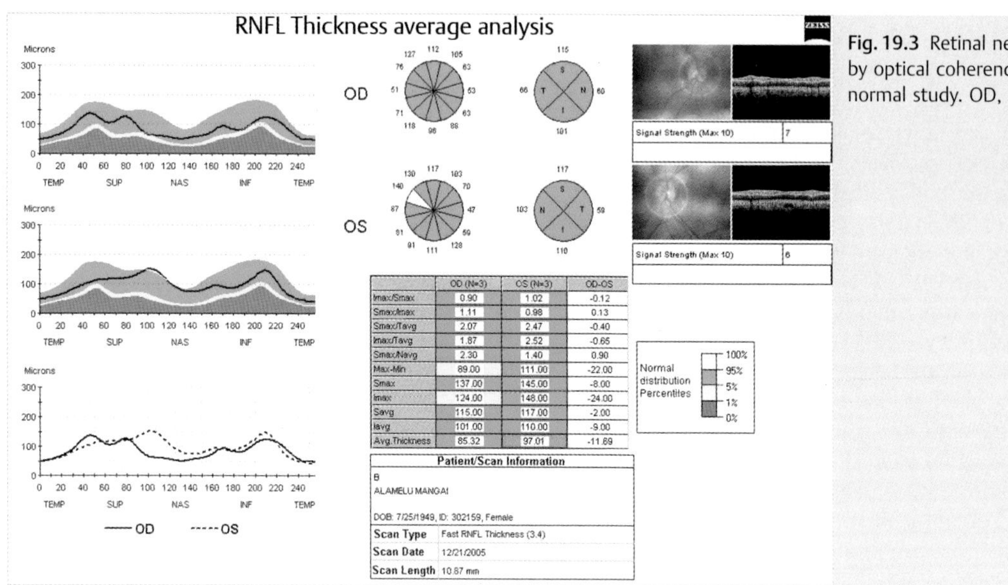

	OD (N=3)	OS (N=3)	OD-OS
Imax/Smax	0.90	1.02	-0.12
Smax/Imax	1.11	0.98	0.13
Smax/Tavg	2.07	2.47	-0.40
Imax/Tavg	1.87	2.52	-0.65
Smax/Navg	2.30	1.40	0.90
Max-Min	89.00	111.00	-22.00
Smax	137.00	145.00	-8.00
Imax	124.00	148.00	-24.00
Savg	115.00	117.00	-2.00
Iavg	101.00	110.00	-9.00
Avg.Thickness	85.32	97.01	-11.69

Patient/Scan Information
B
ALAMELU MANGAI
DOB: 7/25/1949, ID: 302159, Female

Scan Type	Fast RNFL Thickness (3.4)
Scan Date	12/21/2005
Scan Length	10.87 mm

Fig. 19.3 Retinal nerve-fiber layer (RNFL) analysis by optical coherence tomography showing a normal study. OD, right eye; OS, left eye.

photoreceptor layer, RPE, and choriocapillaris terminate at the lamina cribrosa.

19.5 Scanning Protocols

19.5.1 Circumpapillary OCT Scans

Boundary-detection software automatically detects the NFL, and its thickness is measured (▶ Fig. 19.3). The circumpapillary scan is "unwrapped," and the corresponding quadrants are marked. Normally, the thickest NFL layer is seen in the superotemporal and inferotemporal quadrants. The retinal vessels may be seen as they emerge from the disc as shadowing of the posterior layers.

19.5.2 Radial Scans through the Optic Nerve Head

A series of scans are taken radially, along different clock hours, all intersecting at the center of the optic nerve head. The orientation of each is shown on a corresponding fundus photograph. The contour of the disc can be studied in each meridian, which is especially useful in conditions such as glaucoma, optic atrophy, and papilledema. The computer software measures parameters such as diameter and area of the disc, cup, rim, cup:disc ratio, and so forth. The NFL thickness can be measured in each scan, and different areas can be compared. It is thickest along the vertical scan where the superior and inferior arcuate fibers enter the disc and thinnest along the horizontal scan, where correspondingly fewer fibers enter the disc.

19.5.3 Macular Raster Scans

These scans are useful for studying macular pathology. Six serial raster scans of the macula at fixed intervals are done, and each scan is shown on the corresponding fundus photograph.

19.5.4 Macular Radial Scans

This type of scan is also useful for studying macular pathology. Six serial radial scans through each clock hour are taken through the macula, all intersecting at the fovea, which allows the software to construct macular thickness maps.

19.6 Quantitative Analysis Algorithms

19.6.1 Retinal Thickness Measurement

Boundary-detection software detects the anterior border of the retina at the vitreoretinal interface and posterior boundary between the IS and OS of the photoreceptors and calculates the retinal thickness. Although this does not measure the exact anatomical boundaries of the retina, it has good consistency in repeated measurement and therefore is useful in follow-up of the patient.

19.6.2 Nerve-Fiber Layer Thickness Measurement and Analysis

The NFL thickness is measured directly from a circumpapillary scan at 3.4-mm diameter using an automated computer algorithm. The NFL and total retinal thickness are estimated at each clock hour and quadrant and overall mean thickness is measured. Various algorithms are used to analyze and display these measurements and comparisons, producing an age- and race-adjusted normative database. The advantage of OCT over other optic nerve head analyzers and confocal scanning laser ophthalmoscopes is that a reference plane is not required to determine NFL thickness. Instead, it provides an absolute cross-sectional measurement of retinal substructures from which the NFL thickness is calculated.

Table 19.3 Important uses of optical coherence tomography

Measurement of optic nerve head structure
Topographic retinal thickness mapping: Quantitatively assessing macular edema, central serous retinopathy, and diabetic maculopathy
Assessment of the size of macular hole and the presence of vitreomacular traction
Visualize the continuity of retinal pigment epithelium (RPE) and choriocapillary complex (e.g., RPE defect, RPE detachment, and age-related macular degeneration)
Retinal nerve-fiber analysis in evaluation of glaucoma

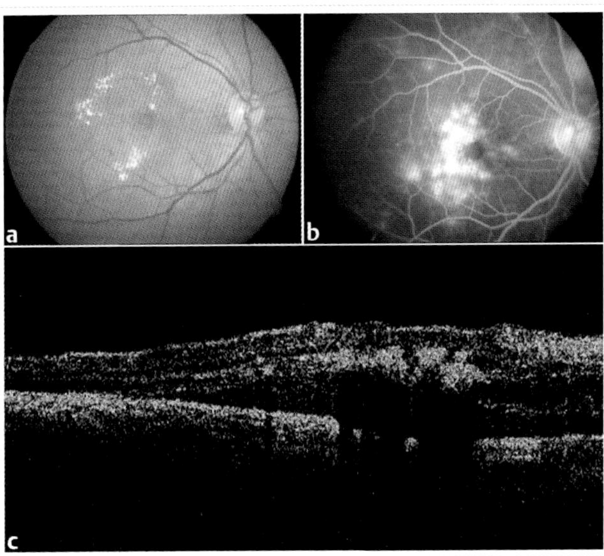

Fig. 19.5 Nonproliferative diabetic retinopathy. (a) Fundus photograph of nonproliferative diabetic retinopathy shows hard exudates arranged in a circinate pattern with thickening of macula correlating with clinically significant macular edema. Few scattered dot and blot hemorrhages are also seen. (b) Angiography shows diffuse leak from the perifoveal capillaries, giving a flower-petal pattern. Scattered areas of leaks are also seen in other areas. (c) Retinal thickening in the macular area with intraretinal fluid accumulation in cystic spaces is seen well on the right side. Hyperreflective areas seen with back-shadowing correspond to the hard exudates.

19.6.3 Optic Nerve Head Analysis

Radial optic nerve head scans through different meridia are analyzed by software to measure diameters as well as areas of the disc, cup, neuroretinal rim, and the cup:disc ratio along different meridia. The cup diameter is estimated by a line that is offset parallel and anteriorly by a standard amount to the line that defines the disc diameter.[8] The optic disc profile along different meridia can also be visualized.

19.7 Retinal Topography

Multiple scans can be combined to reconstruct a two-dimensional topographical map of the retina. The information is displayed as a false color-coded image, which can be directly compared with the observer's view of the retina.

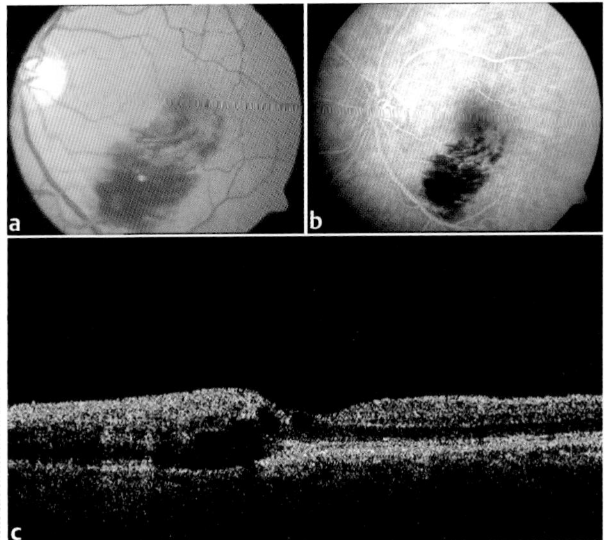

Fig. 19.4 Inferotemporal branch retinal vein occlusion (BRVO). (a) Fundus photograph of a nonischemic inferotemporal BRVO showing flame-shaped hemorrhages above the inferotemporal arcade extending to the macula. (b) Angiography shows blocked fluorescence corresponding to the area of hemorrhages. (c) Increased perifoveal thickness is seen on the left side along with retinal edema. Hyporeflective cystic spaces seen in the perifoveal and foveal regions are suggestive of macular edema. Loss of foveal contour is seen.

19.8 OCT in Different Situations

Optical coherence tomography is of great use in various ocular conditions (▶ Table 19.3).

19.8.1 Retinal Vein Occlusions

Optical coherence tomography is quite useful in evaluating retinal thickening and edema; the presence of macular edema; intraretinal, preretinal, and subhyaloid hemorrhages; and other pathologies associated with retinal vein occlusions. It is also of prime importance in deciding on management and monitoring response to treatment. ▶ Fig. 19.4 shows the color picture, fundus fluorescein angiogram, and OCT of an inferotemporal branch retinal vein occlusion.

19.8.2 Nonproliferative Diabetic Retinopathy

Hard exudates and hemorrhages (▶ Fig. 19.5), as well as retinal edema, are seen in nonproliferative diabetic retinopathy; these findings are of great importance in diagnosing diabetic macular edema, deciding on management, and evaluating the response to various modalities of management.

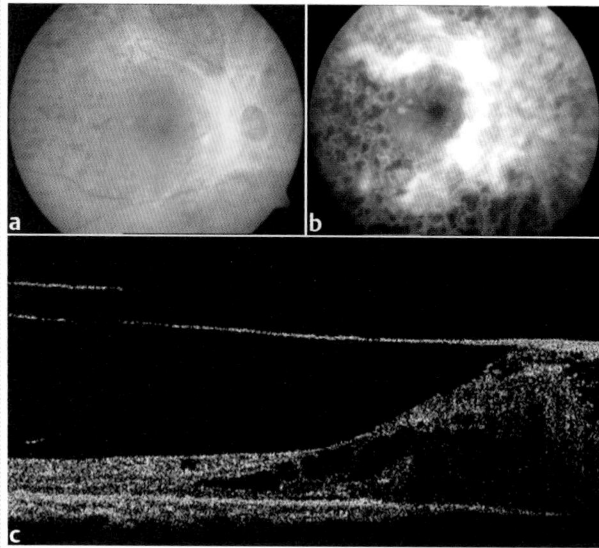

Fig. 19.6 Proliferative diabetic retinopathy. **(a)** Fundus photograph of proliferative diabetic retinopathy shows extensive fibrovascular proliferation extending anteriorly from the disc. Old laser marks are seen. **(b)** Angiography shows staining and leakage of the fibrovascular proliferation. Neovascularization of both the disc and elsewhere is seen. **(c)** Hyperreflective band in the preretinal area corresponding to the fibrovascular proliferation. Static Traction is seen on the retina with secondary retinal thickening and intraretinal fluid accumulation in cystic space, more on the right side.

Fig. 19.7 Cystoid macular edema (CME). **(a)** Color fundus photograph of cystoid macular edema shows cystic macular changes with retinal thickening in the macula. **(b)** Fluorescein angiography shows hyperfluorescent areas in the perifoveal region in a petalloid fashion, which is typical of CME. **(c)** Line scan of the macula shows loss of foveal contour. Increased retinal thickness in the macula with multiple large optically clear, low reflective cystic spaces with septae seen in the inner retina.

19.8.3 Proliferative Diabetic Retinopathy

Fibrovascular proliferations are seen as hyperreflective preretinal bands. The presence of vitreoretinal traction at the interface can be appreciated, as well as any secondary retinal changes (► Fig. 19.6).

19.8.4 Cystoid Macular Edema

Loss of foveal contour is seen with retinal edema, thickening, and fluid accumulation in the form of cystic spaces, predominantly in the outer plexiform and inner nuclear layers. Tissue bands, probably representing the stretched Müller cells, are seen between the cystic spaces (► Fig. 19.7).

19.8.5 Epiretinal Membrane

Epiretinal membranes (ERMs) are visible on OCT as a hyperreflective layer on the retinal surface and may be adherent throughout their extent or lying separated from the retina. Any edema or retinal structural distortion caused by the membrane can also be identified.[9] ERM with pseudohole can be differentiated from other similar entities. OCT is also helpful in planning for surgery[10] (► Fig. 19.8, ► Fig. 19.9).

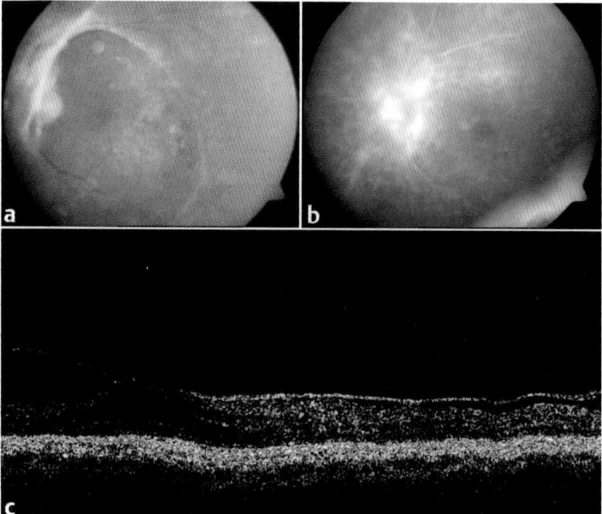

Fig. 19.8 **(a)** Color fundus photograph of epiretinal membrane (ERM) showing fibrous proliferation arising from the disc extending over both the arcades with contraction of the membrane seen over the macula. **(b)** Fluorescein angiography shows staining of the glial proliferation. **(c)** Horizontal line scan over the macula shows increased retinal thickness with an ERM covering the entire macular area with loss of foveal contour. Hyperreflecting ERM is seen over the neurosensory retina with hyporeflective spaces showing a well-defined area of separation between the inner retina and the ERM indicating that membrane peeling is possible.

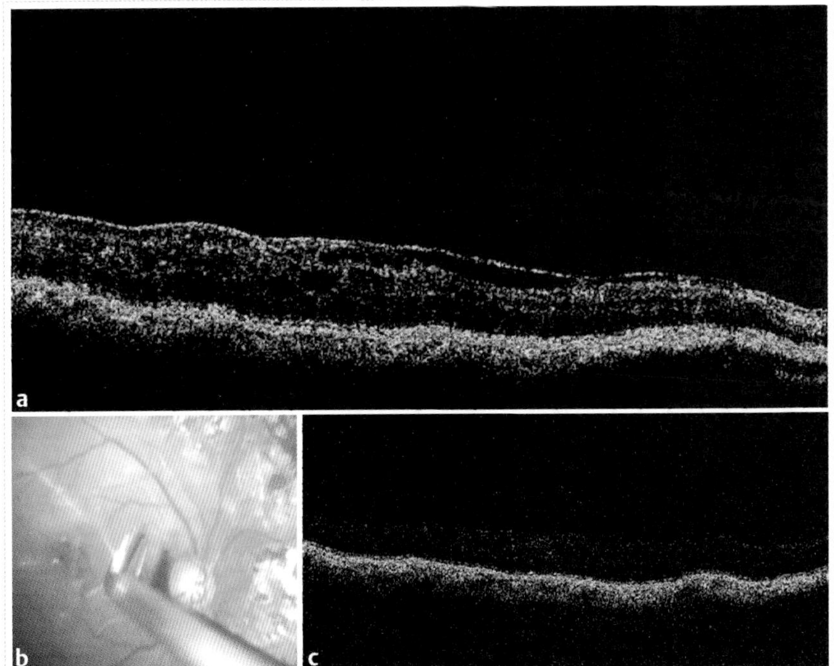

Fig. 19.9 **(a)** Preoperative horizontal line scan of the macula of another patient shows high reflecting epiretinal membrane (ERM). **(b)** Surgical removal of the ERM showing membrane peeling using forceps. **(c)** Horizontal line scan of the same patient 2 days postoperatively shows the absence of high reflective ERM after vitrectomy and membrane peeling. Some retinal thickening and edema are still seen.

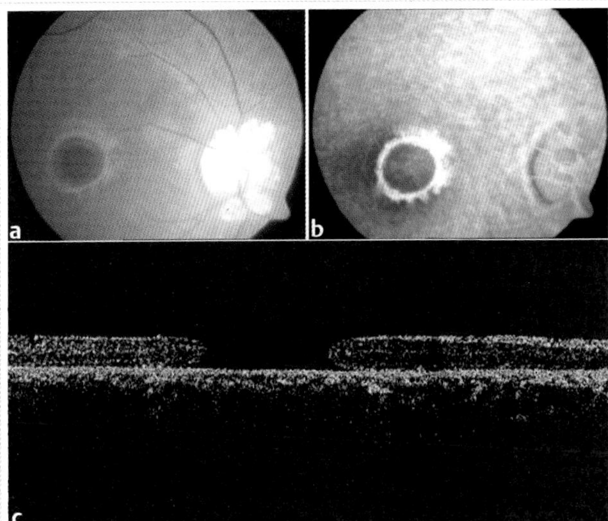

Fig. 19.10 Macular hole. **(a)** Color photograph shows a full thickness macular hole with a cuff of subretinal fluid (SRF) encircled by retinal pigment epithelium (RPE) defects. **(b)** Fluorescein angiography shows the ring of hyperfluorescence corresponding to the RPE defects seen in the color photograph. **(c)** Line scan through the macula shows full-thickness defect of all the retinal layers in the fovea with minimal SRF seen as a hyporeflective space at both edges of the hole. At the base of the hole, only RPE is seen, typical of a full-thickness hole.

19.8.6 Macular Hole

The various stages of macular hole can be identified by OCT. A pseudocyst formation[11,12] is the initial stage, followed by full-thickness dehiscence < 400 µm (stage 2), further enlargement to > 400 µm with subretinal and intraretinal edema at the edges (stage 3), and finally large full-thickness defects with posterior vitreous detachment in stage 4 holes (▶ Fig. 19.10).

19.8.7 Central Serous Retinopathy

On OCT, central serous retinopathy is seen as the retinal layers being elevated above an optically clear fluid-filled cystic space (▶ Fig. 19.11). A turbid central serous retinopathy is seen in ▶ Fig. 19.12. Any associated pigment epithelial detachment is seen as localized elevation of the hyperreflective RPE layer with shadowing of the choroidal signal behind it. Longitudinal follow-up of the patient can be done to aid in treatment (observation versus laser).

19.8.8 Age-Related Macular Degeneration

- *Drusen* are seen as alterations in the RPE-choriocapillaris complex that cause localized distortion of this hyperreflective layer.
- *Geographic atrophy* is seen as a well-defined area of chorioretinal degeneration, which unmasks the larger tape-shaped choroidal vessels (▶ Fig. 19.13).
- *Subretinal neovascular membrane* (SRNV): Findings vary depending on the type and stage of the SRNV. They usually include an enlargement or thickening, generally fusiform, of the RPE-choriocapillaris complex. Tenting of this layer is also seen as also sometimes splitting. Hemorrhages and fluid-filled spaces may be seen, along with disorganization of the overlying neurosensory retina (▶ Fig. 19.14).

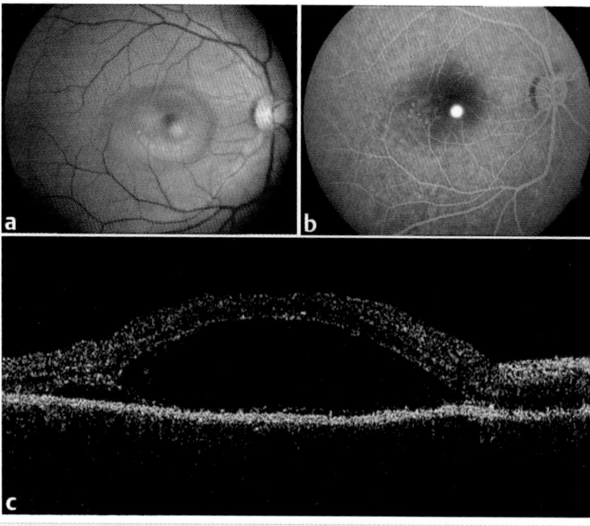

Fig. 19.11 Central serous retinopathy (CSR). **(a)** Color photograph of a fundus with CSR shows an oval area of serous elevation of the neurosensory retina in the macula. **(b)** Fluorescein angiography shows an ink-blot hyperfluorescent leak in the early phase. **(c)** Optical coherence tomography confirms the serous separation of the neurosensory retina in the macula, seen as an optically clear zone between the neurosensory retina and the RPE.

19.8.9 Choroidal Nevus

For choroidal nevus, OCT is especially important in the follow-up of high-risk patients by monitoring the thickness and size of the nevus as well as associated secondary changes (▶ Fig. 19.15).

19.8.10 Optic Atrophy

Retinal nerve-fiber layer (RNFL) analysis shows thinning of the NFL; the site and the amount of thinning are determined by the type and extent of optic atrophy (▶ Fig. 19.16).

19.8.11 Glaucoma

In early diagnosis of glaucoma, RNFL analysis is extremely useful before perimetric loss. Loss of the double-hump pattern is seen in RNFL analysis. Thinning of the RNFL is seen, first in the superotemporal and inferotemporal quadrants. Age- and race-matched statistical analysis is also done (▶ Fig. 19.17). Optic nerve head analysis uses boundary detection algorithms to quantify cup, disc, and neuroretinal rim parameters. (▶ Fig. 19.18)

19.8.12 Myelinated Nerve-Fiber Layer

Myelinated NFL can be seen as a hyperreflective area with shadowing of the underlying layers. An increase in the thickness of the RNFL in that quadrant is also seen (▶ Fig. 19.19).

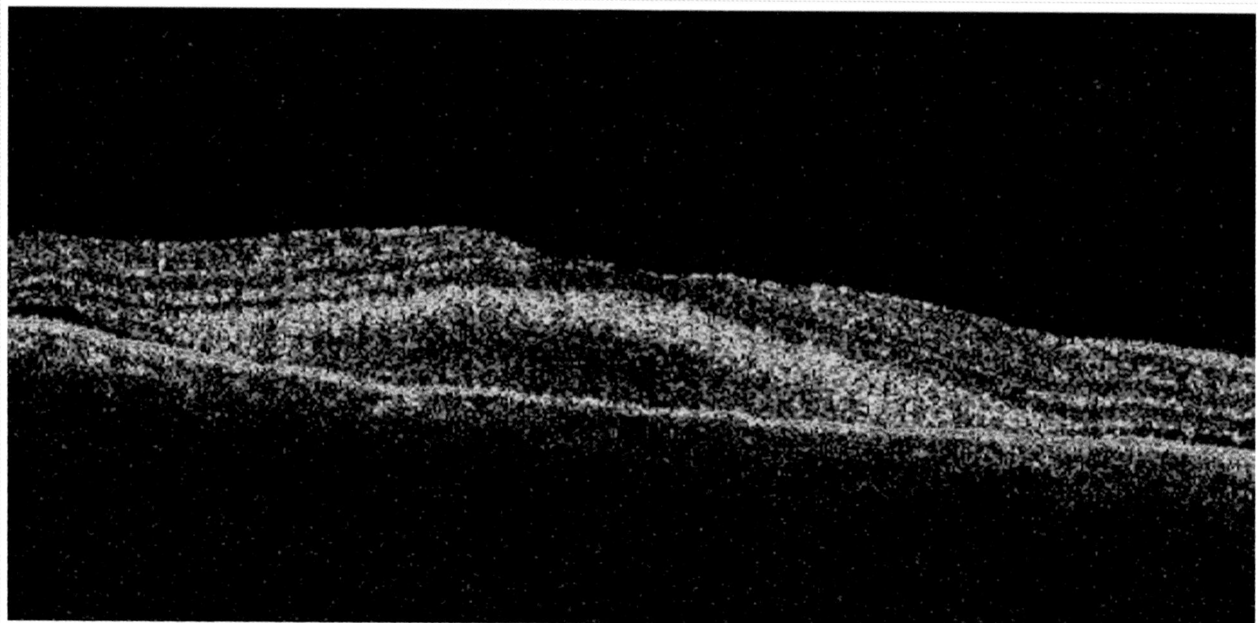

Fig. 19.12 Optical coherence tomography shows a turbid central serous retinopathy recognized as intermediate reflective signals seen in the subretinal space.

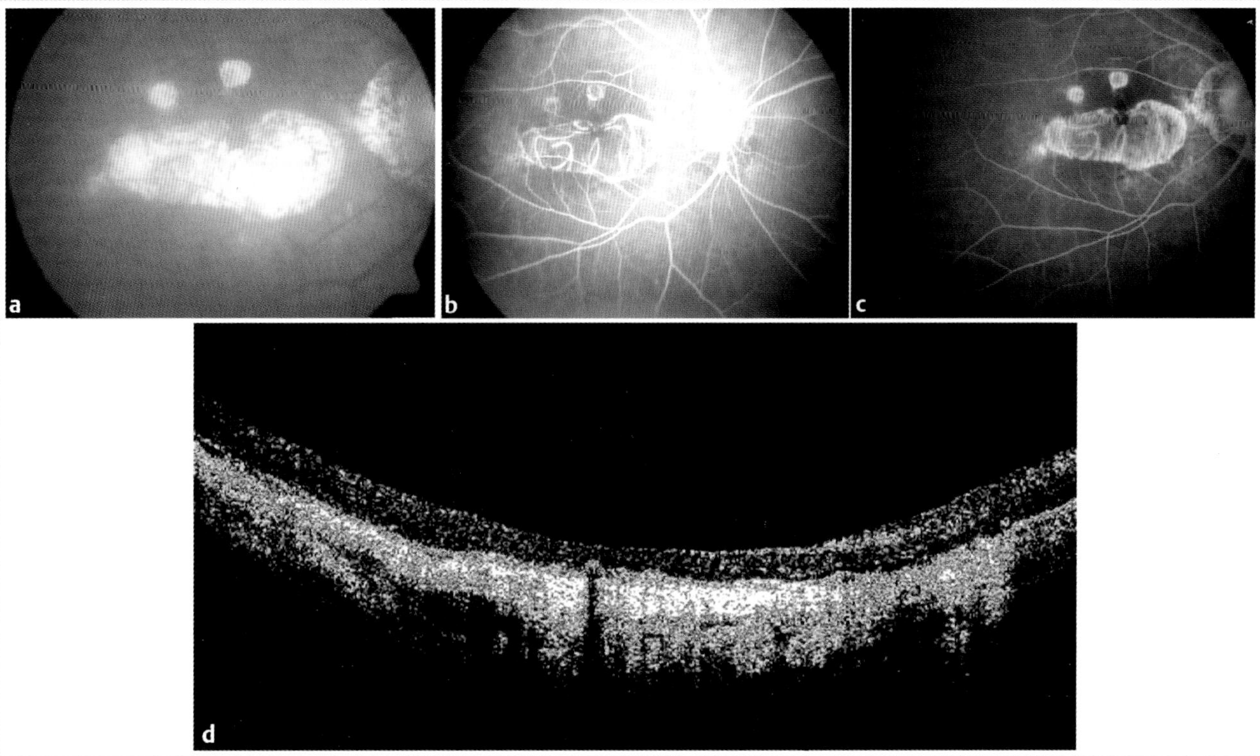

Fig. 19.13 **(a)** Color fundus photograph shows a well-defined area of geographic atrophy in the macular area. **(b,c)** Fluorescein angiogram shows a well-defined area of hyperfluorescence with late staining but no leakage. **(d)** Line scan through the area of geographic atrophy shows thinning of the overlying retina with increased signal seen from the underlying choroid resulting from attenuation of the retinal pigment epithelium choriocapillaris complex.

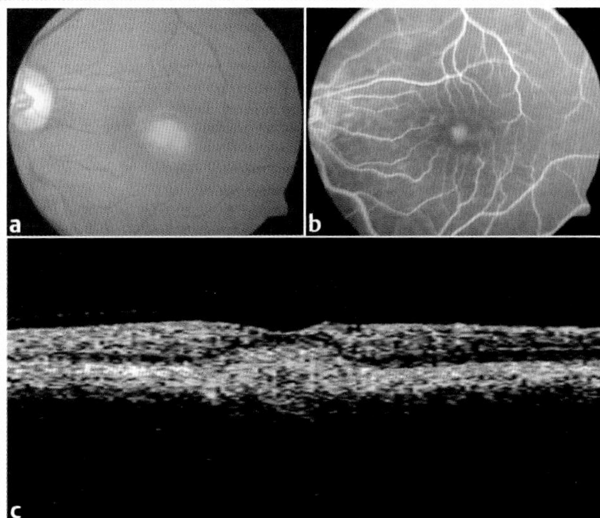

Fig. 19.14 Subretinal neovascular membrane (SRNV). **(a)** Color fundus photograph is suggestive of an SRNV membrane. **(b)** Fundus fluorescein angiography shows a fuzzy area of leak in the foveal avascular zone in the early phase, suggestive of an occult SRNV. **(c)** Optical coherence tomography shows fusiform enlargement of the retinal pigment epithelium-choriocapillaris complex with blunting of the foveal contour. A posterior hyaloid detachment is also seen on the left side as an intermediate reflective membrane.

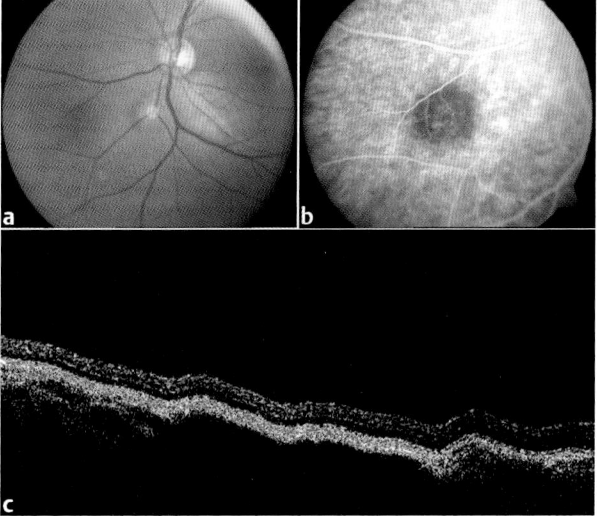

Fig. 19.15 Choroidal nevus. **(a)** Fundus photograph shows hyperpigmented, oval choroidal nevus in the inferonasal region with normal overlying retina. **(b)** Fluorescein angiography shows blocked choroidal fluorescence in the region of choroidal nevus with normal overlying retinal vessels. **(c)** Line scan through the choroidal nevus shows the thickened retinal pigment epithelium-choriocapillaris complex with increased hyperreflectivity seen in the same area.

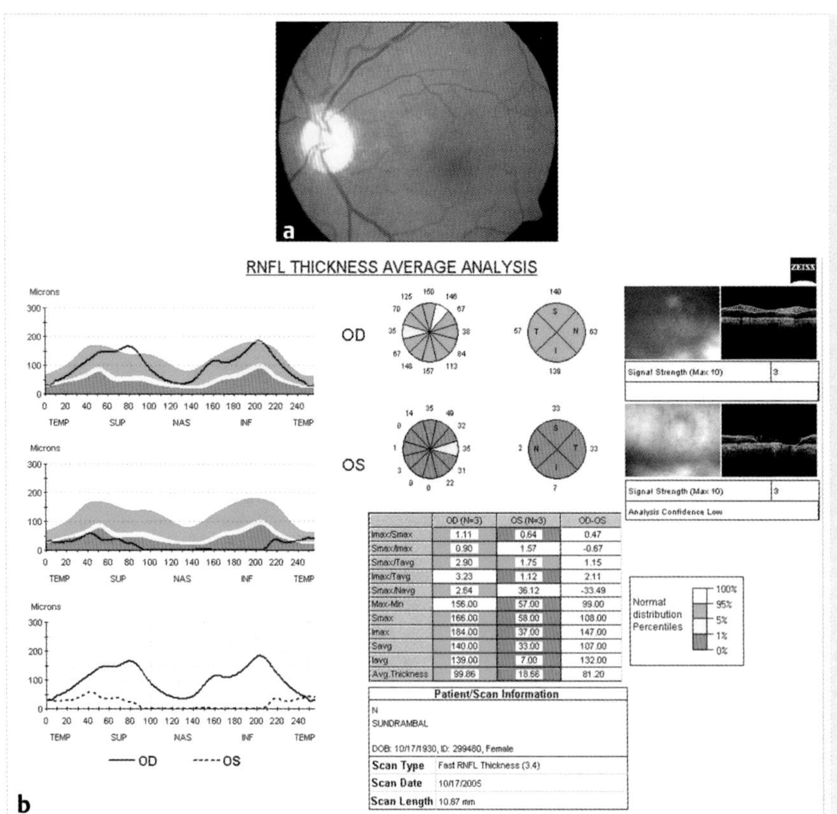

	OD (N=3)	OS (N=3)	OD-OS
Imax/Smax	1.11	0.64	0.47
Smax/Imax	0.90	1.57	-0.67
Smax/Tavg	2.90	1.75	1.15
Imax/Tavg	3.23	1.12	2.11
Smax/Navg	2.64	36.12	-33.49
Max-Min	156.00	57.00	99.00
Smax	166.00	58.00	108.00
Imax	184.00	37.00	147.00
Savg	140.00	33.00	107.00
Iavg	139.00	7.00	132.00
Avg.Thickness	99.86	18.66	81.20

Patient/Scan Information	
N SUNDRAMBAL DOB: 10/17/1930, ID: 299480, Female	
Scan Type	Fast RNFL Thickness (3.4)
Scan Date	10/17/2005
Scan Length	10.87 mm

Fig. 19.16 (a) Color fundus photograph of optic atrophy shows marked disc pallor. **(b)** Marked thinning of the retinal nerve-fiber layer (RNFL) is seen in all quadrants. Statistical analysis shows almost all parameters to be grossly abnormal.

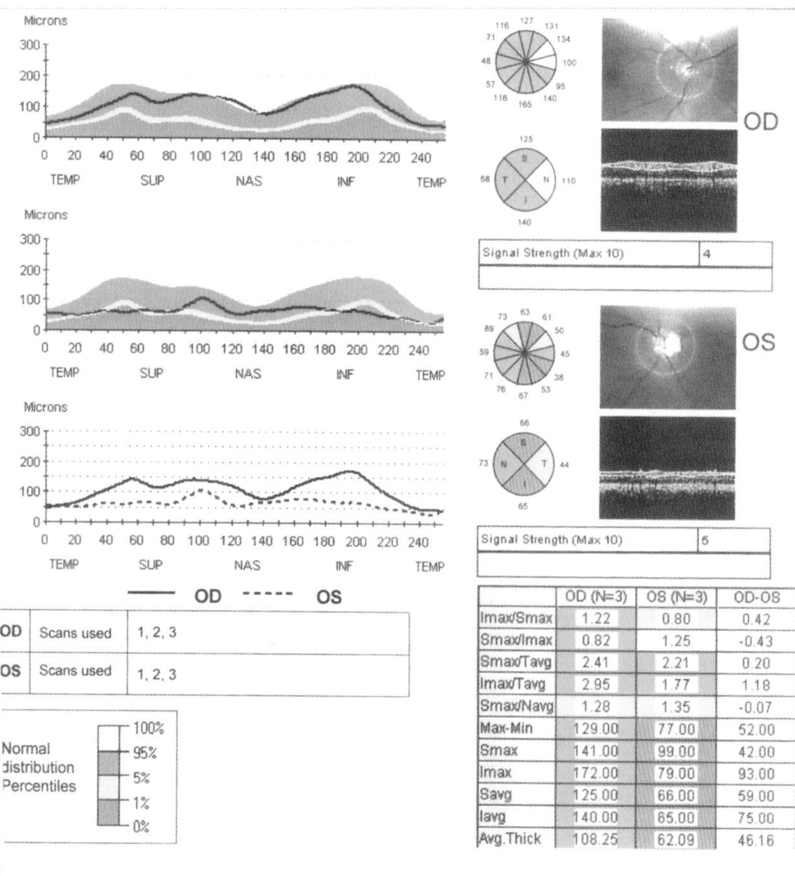

	OD (N=3)	OS (N=3)	OD-OS
Imax/Smax	1.22	0.80	0.42
Smax/Imax	0.82	1.25	-0.43
Smax/Tavg	2.41	2.21	0.20
Imax/Tavg	2.95	1.77	1.18
Smax/Navg	1.28	1.35	-0.07
Max-Min	129.00	77.00	52.00
Smax	141.00	99.00	42.00
Imax	172.00	79.00	93.00
Savg	125.00	66.00	59.00
Iavg	140.00	65.00	75.00
Avg.Thick	108.25	62.09	46.16

Fig. 19.17 Retinal nerve-fiber layer (RNL) analysis of the right eye (OD) is within normal limits, whereas the left eye shows marked loss of retinal nerve fibers, predominantly in the superior and inferior quadrants and also mild loss in the temporal quadrant. There is loss of the double-hump pattern in the plotting of the RNFL of the left eye (OS).

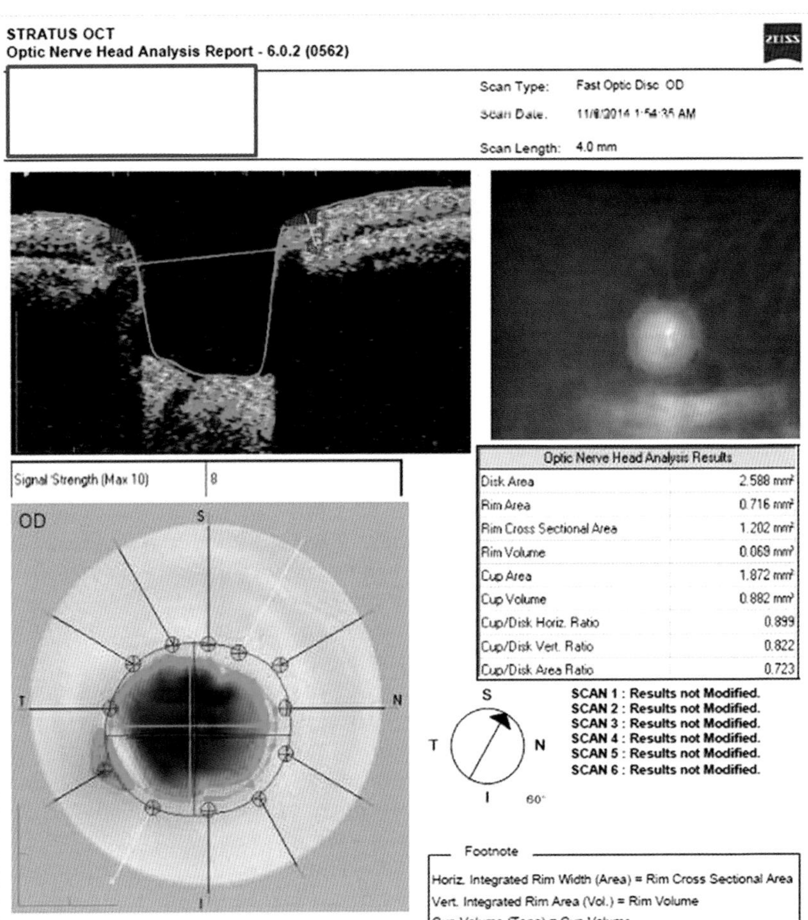

Fig. 19.18 Optic nerve head analysis shows large cup:disc ratio of around 0.8 with correspondingly decreased neuroretinal rim area. OD, Right eye.

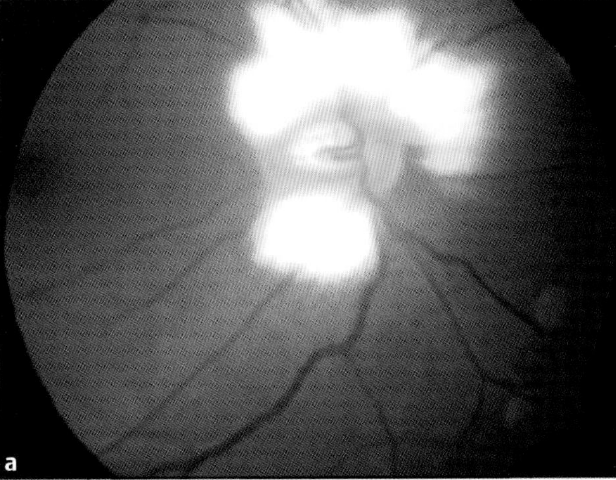

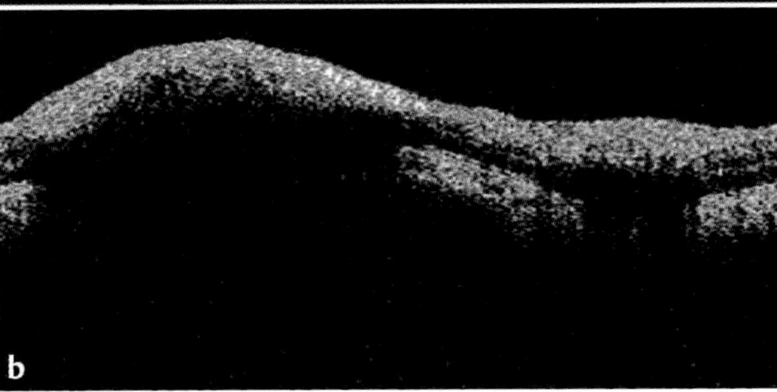

Fig. 19.19 **(a)** Large areas of myelinated nerve-fiber layer are seen around the disc. **(b)** Hyperreflective signal with shadowing of the posterior layers is seen in the area of myelination.

References

[1] Izatt JA, Hee MR, Swanson EA, et al. Micrometer-scale resolution imaging of the anterior eye in vivo with optical coherence tomography. Arch Ophthalmol 1994; 112: 1584–1589

[2] Fujimoto JG, Pitris C, Boppart SA, Brezinski ME. Optical coherence tomography: an emerging technology for biomedical imaging and optical biopsy. Neoplasia 2000; 2: 9–25

[3] Fujimoto JG. Optical coherence tomography for ultrahigh resolution in vivo imaging. Nat Biotechnol 2003; 21: 1361–1367

[4] Fujimoto JG, Brezinski ME, Tearney GJ, et al. Optical biopsy and imaging using optical coherence tomography. Nat Med 1995; 1: 970–972

[5] Hee MR, Izatt JA, Swanson EA, et al. Optical coherence tomography of the human retina. Arch Ophthalmol 1995; 113: 325–332

[6] Drexler W, Morgner U, Ghanta RK, Kärtner FX, Schuman JS, Fujimoto JG. Ultrahigh-resolution ophthalmic optical coherence tomography. Nat Med 2001; 7: 502–507

[7] Fujimoto JG, Hee MR, Huang D, et al. Principles of optical coherence tomography. In: Optical Coherence Tomography of Ocular Diseases, 2nd ed. Thorofare, NJ: Slack Inc; 2009

[8] Wollstein G, Folio LS, Nevins JE, Ishikawa H, Puliafito CA, Fujimoto JG, Schuman J. In: Schumann J, Puliafito CA, Fujimoto J, Duker S III. Optical Coherence Tomography of Ocular Diseases. 3rd ed. Thorofare, NJ: SLACK, Inc.; 2012

[9] Wilkins JR, Puliafito CA, Hee MR, et al. Characterization of epiretinal membranes using optical coherence tomography. Ophthalmology 1996; 103: 2142–2151

[10] Azzolini C, Patelli F, Codenotti M, Pierro L, Brancato R. Optical coherence tomography in idiopathic epiretinal macular membrane surgery. Eur J Ophthalmol 1999; 9: 206–211

[11] Gaudric A, Haouchine B, Massin P, Paques M, Blain P, Erginay A. Macular hole formation: new data provided by optical coherence tomography. Arch Ophthalmol 1999; 117: 744–751

[12] Haouchine B, Massin P, Gaudric A. Foveal pseudocyst as the first step in macular hole formation: a prospective study by optical coherence tomography. Ophthalmology 2001; 108: 15–22

20 Vitreomacular Traction and Optical Coherence Tomography Classification

Mehreen Adhi and Jay S. Duker

Diseases of the vitreomacular interface (VMI) are broadly classified as vitreomacular traction (VMT), full-thickness macular hole (FTMH), lamellar macular hole (LMH), and epiretinal membrane (ERM).[1,2,3,4,5] Over the past few years, an understanding of the anatomical changes at the VMI in both normal and pathological states has become possible with the widespread availability of optical coherence tomography (OCT). Recent advances in OCT technology, as well as innovations in surgical techniques and the recent availability of pharmacologic vitreolysis, have coalesced to enormously increase clinicians' interest and understanding of diseases of the VMI.

Using spectral-domain (SD) OCT, multiple studies have characterized the findings associated with both the normal features of vitreous aging and the abnormal changes in VMI disease.[1,2,3,4] However, much of the clinical practice and evaluation of emerging surgical and pharmacological therapies for these conditions have been hindered by a lack of a consistent and uniform nomenclature surrounding these conditions. Considering this unmet need, an international group of macular disease experts was convened in 2012 to develop a consensus system for classification of VMI conditions using SD OCT.[5] The result of this collaborative study is a new anatomical OCT-based classification of the VMI conditions: the International Vitreomacular Traction Study (IVTS) Group Classification System.[5] This anatomical, OCT-based classification of VMI findings and diseases permits a consistent terminology for these conditions such that a standardized reporting system is established,[5] and the diagnosis and management of VMI conditions using OCT are facilitated. It does not take into account the symptoms or clinical findings, however, and is strictly anatomically based using OCT.

20.1 OCT-Based Classification of Vitreomacular Adhesion

In the normal state, all eyes have a complete adhesion of the vitreous to the inner retinal surface at birth. As the eye ages, a complex series of events causes the vitreous cortex to detach from the inner retina. This phenomenon is called *posterior vitreous detachment* (PVD) and is a normal aging process.[1,2,5,6] However, it can be accelerated by blunt trauma, inflammation, and intraocular surgery. PVD usually begins in the perifoveal region and progresses over many years to involve multiple sites in the peripheral fundus before finally coalescing into a complete separation of the vitreous cortex from the macula and the optic nerve, with the appearance of the Weiss ring. For the most part, this is a nonpathological process. In some eyes, the vitreous cortex detaches inadequately or incompletely from the inner retinal surface. This phenomenon is termed an *anomalous* PVD.[5,6,7]According to the IVTS Group Classification System,[5] an anomalous PVD is defined as a partial vitreous detachment with an anomalous persistent attachment in the macular region resulting in tractional distortion of the retina. An anomalous PVD may then lead to pathological features of VMI disease.[5,6,7]

In the anatomical OCT-based IVTS Group Classification System, vitreomacular adhesion (VMA) is equivalent to a stage 1 PVD in the Uchino, Gaudric, and Johnson classification systems.[1,2,6,8] The anatomical OCT-based IVTS Group Classification System[5] defines VMA as a specific stage of vitreous separation (▶ Table 20.1, ▶ Fig. 20.1). It is defined as a perifoveal separation of the vitreous cortex with continuing VMA within a 3-mm radius of the foveal center, associated with a completely normal retinal morphology. The detached posterior hyaloid may appear on or above the retinal surface. If it is above the retinal surface, the angle between the detached vitreous cortex and the inner retinal surface is *acute*. VMA is usually asymptomatic and appears as a normal finding on OCT during the natural course of the progression of PVD. Over time, the vitreous usually separates completely from the inner retinal surface as part of the normal physiologic aging process.

Using the anatomical OCT-based classification system,[5] VMA is subclassified by the size of the VMA as measured using the caliper function tool on OCT into (1) *focal* VMA, where the size of the VMA is ≤ 1500 µm; or (2) *broad* VMA, where the size of adhesion measures more than 1500 µm (▶ Table 20.1, ▶ Fig. 20.1). The area of VMA is measured roughly parallel to the retinal pigment epithelium, and small regions of dehiscence (< 1 mm) between the vitreous and the inner retina that may be present within the zones of a broad VMA are disregarded. When VMA is not associated with any other ocular disease, it is termed *isolated* VMA. In cases where VMA is associated with other macular abnormalities, such as diabetic macular edema, age-related macular degeneration, or retinal vein occlusion, it is termed *concurrent* VMA (▶ Table 20.1, ▶ Fig. 20.1). It should be noted that this OCT-based definition of VMA[5] does not take into account the symptoms, as specific visual symptoms may be subjective and may be caused by a separate disease process.

Table 20.1 Anatomic optical coherence tomography based classification of vitreomacular adhesion (VMA), vitreomacular traction (VMT), and full-thickness macular hole (FTMH) according to the International Vitreomacular Traction Study Group classification system

Classification	Subclassification
VMA	Size: Focal (≤ 1500 µm) or broad (> 1500 µm) Isolated or concurrent
VMT	Size: Focal (≤ 1500 µm) or broad (> 1500 µm) Isolated or concurrent
FTMH	Size: small (≤ 250 µm), medium (> 250– ≤ 400 µm) or large (> 400 µm) Status of vitreous: With or without VMT Cause: Primary or secondary

Source: Duker JS, Kaiser PK, Binder S, et al. The International Vitreomacular Traction Study Group classification of vitreomacular adhesion, traction, and macular hole. Ophthalmology 2013;120 (12):2611–2619.

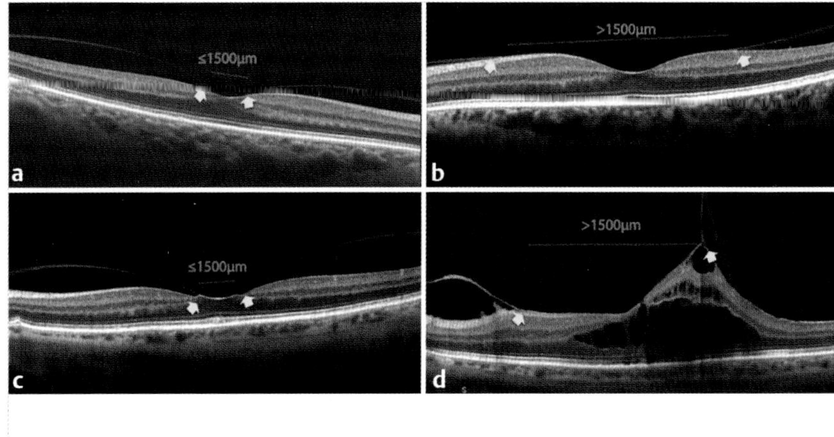

Fig. 20.1 Optical coherence tomography images showing the anatomical classification of vitreomacular adhesion (VMA) **(a,b)** and vitreomacular traction (VMT) **(c,d)**. **(a)** Focal VMA. Yellow arrows mark the sites of vitreomacular attachment. The area of attachment is less than 1500 µm (red line and green numbers), and there is no detectable change in contour and morphology of underlying foveal tissue. **(b)** Broad VMA. Yellow arrows mark the sites of vitreomacular attachment. The area of attachment is > 1500 µm (red line and green numbers), and there is no detectable change in contour and morphology of underlying foveal tissue. **(c)** Focal VMT. The yellow arrows mark the sites of vitreomacular attachment. The area of attachment is less than 1500 µm (red line and green numbers), and the foveal morphology is abnormal. **(d)** Broad MT. Yellow arrows mark the sites of vitreomacular attachment. The area of attachment is more than 1500 µm (red line and green numbers), and the foveal morphology is abnormal with associated cystoid macular edema possibly due to the traction on the retina caused by the anomalous vitreous detachment.

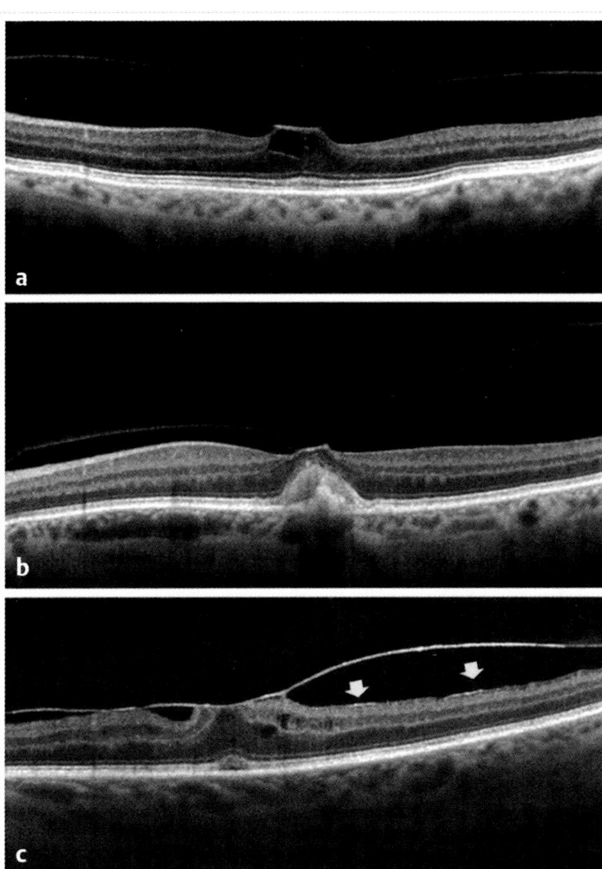

Fig. 20.2 Optical coherence tomography images showing vitreomacular traction (VMT). **(a)** Focal VMT with an intraretinal pseudocyst formation. **(b)** Focal VMT with concomitant occurrence of a secondary disease process, most likely pattern dystrophy. **(c)** Focal VMT with an associated epiretinal membrane (yellow arrows).

20.2 OCT-Based Classification of Vitreomacular Traction

During an anomalous progression of PVD,[5,6,7] excessive traction on the macula can result and cause changes in the foveal contour, compromising vision.[9] The anatomical OCT-based IVTS Group Classification System[5] defines VMT as a perifoveal vitreous separation with continuing vitreomacular attachment within a 3-mm radius of the foveal center, associated with an abnormal retinal morphology (▶ Table 20.1, ▶ Fig. 20.1, ▶ Fig. 20.2). An abnormal retinal morphology may involve distortion of the fovea, intraretinal structural changes such as pseudocyst formation (▶ Fig. 20.2), macular schisis, cystoid macular edema (CME), subretinal fluid, elevation of the fovea above the retinal pigment epithelium, or any combination of these. Unlike VMA, where the vitreous separation is virtually always related to a normal physiologic process, VMT is the result of an anomalous progression of PVD.

Using the anatomical OCT-based classification system,[5] VMT is subclassified by the size of vitreomacular attachment as measured using the caliper function tool on OCT into (1) focal VMT, where the size of vitreomacular attachment measures ≤ 1500 µm; or (2) broad VMT, where the size of vitreomacular attachment measures > 1500 µm (▶ Table 20.1, ▶ Fig. 20.1). As with VMA, when VMT is not associated with any other ocular disease, it is termed *isolated* VMT. In cases where VMT is associated with other macular abnormalities, it is termed as *concurrent* VMT (▶ Table 20.1, ▶ Fig. 20.2).

As PVD progresses, residual cortical vitreous may be left on the retinal surface, even in the setting of a complete, or stage 4, PVD with Weiss ring. This occurrence is termed *vitreoschisis*.[10,11] The residual vitreous remnant may serve as a nidus for proliferation, thus forming an epiretinal membrane (ERM). ERM typically contains glial cells and histiocytes that collect and attach to the vitreous remnant on the retinal surface.[12]Contracture of an ERM may cause further traction on the macula, resulting in distortion of the retinal morphology. Sometimes, VMT and ERM are seen on OCT simultaneously (▶ Fig. 20.2).

20.3 OCT-Based Classification of Full-Thickness Macular Hole

The Gass classification of macular holes is widely used clinically and was based on careful clinical examination; this classification predates both the invention of OCT and the use of vitrectomy to repair macular holes. It divides macular holes into four stages (▶ Table 20.2).[13,14] Over the past few years, OCT has increased the understanding of the anatomy and progression of macular holes. The anatomical OCT-based IVTS Group Classification System[5] defines a full-thickness macular hole (FTMH) as an anatomical defect in the fovea that involves an interruption of all the neurosensory retinal layers from the inner limiting membrane (ILM) to the retinal pigment epithelium. This definition requires such a detection on at least one OCT B-scan. Sometimes, small FTMHs are missed by examining only one OCT B-scan, and so, a series of closely spaced OCT B-scans is a more appropriate way to examine for an FTMH on OCT.

Using the anatomical OCT-based classification system,[5] an FTMH is subclassified based on the following parameters: (1) size of the hole, (2) status of the vitreous, and (3) cause of FTMH.

Table 20.2 Comparison of the commonly used clinical stages of macular hole and the anatomical optical coherence tomography (OCT)-based classification of vitreomacular adhesion, vitreomacular traction, and macular hole according to the International Vitreomacular Traction Study Group classification system)[5]

Macular hole stages in common clinical use	Anatomic OCT-based classification
Stage 0	VMA
Stage 1: Impending macular hole	VMT
Stage 2: Small hole	Small or medium FTMH with VMT
Stage 3: Large hole	Medium or large FTMH with VMT
Stage 4: FTMH with PVD	Small, medium or large FTMH without VMT

Abbreviations: FTMH, full-thickness macular hole; PVD, posterior vitreous detachment; VMA, vitreomacular adhesion; VMT, vitreomacular traction.

Source: Duker JS, Kaiser PK, Binder S, et al. The International Vitreomacular Traction Study Group classification of vitreomacular adhesion, traction, and macular hole. Ophthalmology 2013;120 (12):2611–2619.

20.3.1 Size

Using the caliper function tool on OCT, the aperture size of the FTMH is measured roughly parallel to the retinal pigment epithelium at the narrowest opening of the hole in the mid retina or at the photoreceptor tips (▶ Table 20.1, ▶ Fig. 20.3). Using this function, FTMH is classified as small, medium, or large based on its aperture size on OCT. OCT-based measurements of the aperture size of FTMH predict medical and surgical treatment outcomes.[15,16,17] A *small* FTMH is defined as a FTMH with an aperture size measuring ≤ 250 µm (▶ Table 20.1, ▶ Fig. 20.3). This cutoff is obtained from studies showing that small FTMHs are associated with a small rate of spontaneous closure and a rate of closure approaching 100% with vitrectomy.[16] Small FTMHs are also associated with the best response (approximately 60%) to pharmacologic vitreolysis.[16] A medium FTMH is defined as an FTMH with an aperture size measuring > 250 µm and ≤ 400 µm (▶ Table 20.1, ▶ Fig. 20.3). Postsurgical FTMH closure rates for medium FTMHs approach approximately 90% with complete removal of the residual hyaloid, with or without peeling of the inner limiting membrane.[15,17] Compared with small FTMHs, *medium* FTMHs have a lower response rate (approximately 50%) to pharmacologic vitreolysis.[18] A *large* FTMH is defined as an FTMH with an aperture size measuring > 400 µm(▶ Table 20.1, ▶ Fig. 20.3). Roughly half the FTMHs are large FTMHs at diagnosis. They have a 90 to 95% closure rate afater vitrectomy with inner limiting membrane peeling and a 75% closure rate after vitrectomy without inner limiting membrane peeling.[19] Pharmacologic vitreolysis has been tried in a few eyes with large FTMHs, but no anatomical success has been reported so far in this group.[16]

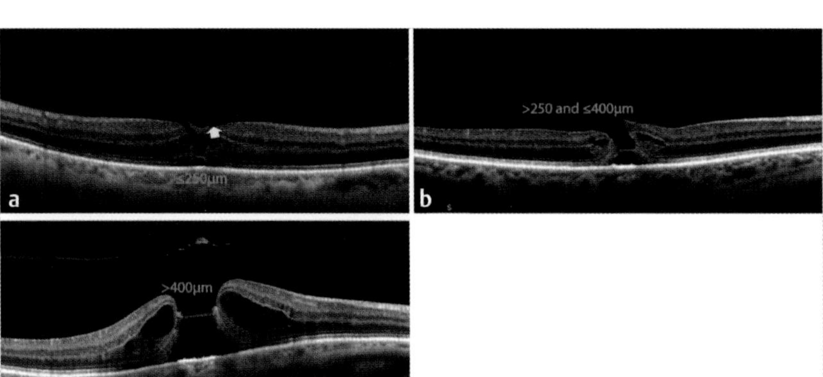

Fig. 20.3 Optical coherence tomography (OCT) images showing the anatomical classification of full-thickness macular hole (FTMH), defined anatomically as a full-thickness interruption all the retinal layers from the inner limiting membrane to the retinal pigment epithelium. **(a)** Small FTMH (≤ 250 µm) associated with vitreomacular traction (yellow arrow). The aperture size is measured using the OCT caliper function as a line drawn roughly parallel to the retinal pigment epithelium (red line and green numbers) at the narrowest hole width in the mid retina or at the photoreceptor tips. **(b)** Medium FTMH (> 250 µm ≤ 400 µm) as measured using the OCT caliper function (red line and green numbers). **(c)** Large FTMH (> 400 µm) as measured using the OCT caliper function (red line and green numbers).

20.3.2 Status

Full-thickness macular holes are categorized secondarily based on the presence or absence of VMT (▸ Table 20.1, ▸ Fig. 20.3)

20.3.3 Cause

Full-thickness macular holes are categorized as either *primary* or *secondary* based on their cause. Primary FTMH was previously referred to as idiopathic macular hole. It is defined as FTMH that is initiated by VMT. Secondary FTMH is defined as FTMH that is caused by other pathologies and did not have demonstrable preexisting or concurrent VMT. These pathologies include, but are not limited to, blunt trauma,[20,21,22,23] high myopia,[24,25] macular schisis,[26] macular telangiectasia type 2,[27] surgical trauma,[28,29] and macroaneurysm.[30,31] FTMH can occur in the presence of macular edema associated with conditions such as diabetic macular edema, age-related macular degeneration, vascular occlusions, and uveitis.[32,33] Such cases are classified as primary FTMH if they have a preexisting or concurrent VMT. In cases where an FTMH develops after vitrectomy for retinal detachment or lens removal,[34,35] the FTMH is classified as secondary FTMH because the vitreous has obviously been removed before the FTMH develops.

20.4 OCT-Based Classification of Impending Macular Hole

Previously, for circumstances where an FTMH is observed in one eye and the fellow eye reveals a VMA or VMT, the fellow eye was referred to as a *stage 0 macular hole*, probably because the fellow eye in such a circumstance is shown to have an increased risk of developing a FTMH.[36] The anatomical OCT-based IVTS Group Classification System[5] defines this condition as an *impending macular hole* in the fellow eye. It is possible that the FTMH that is threatened in the fellow eye may resolve spontaneously, or it may progress to another disease of the VMI, such as ERM or LMH.

20.4.1 OCT-Based Classification of Lamellar Macular Hole

Gass first described LMH as a macular lesion resulting from CME.[37] On slit-lamp biomicroscopy, an LMH appears as a well-circumscribed reddish, round lesion. LMH is a partial-thickness defect in the fovea and is difficult to detect using slit-lamp biomicroscopy alone. At present, the understanding of the evolution of LMH is limited.[38] It is thought to arise from an incomplete FTMH formation, traction from an ERM overlying the inner retina, or both. Forces from the ERM or the posterior vitreous acting in the anteroposterior and tangential directions on the macula may lead to formation of LMH.[39,40] Most patients with LMH have limited central vision loss, and reading vision may deteriorate over time possibly from the concurrent ERM.

Using the anatomical OCT-based classification system,[5,40] LMH is defined by the following features: (1) an irregular foveal contour; (2) a defect in the inner fovea with or without actual loss of tissue; (3) intraretinal splitting (schisis), typically between the outer plexiform and outer nuclear layers; and (4) the presence of an intact photoreceptor layer (▸ Fig. 20.4). LMH can be distinguished fairly easily from FTMH on OCT by the presence of an intact photoreceptor layer in LMH and an interruption of this layer in an FTMH.

20.5 OCT-Based Classification of Macular Pseudohole

Macular pseudohole is a clinical diagnosis made at the slit lamp, not an OCT diagnosis. It appears as a discrete, reddish, round lesion approximately 200 to 400 µm in diameter and, as the name implies, strongly resembles an FTMH. A characteristic feature on clinical examination is the presence of a concomitant ERM that distorts the foveal contour and an altered light reflex. OCT shows that ERM plays a central role in formation of a macular pseudohole, as its contraction pulls the underlying retinal

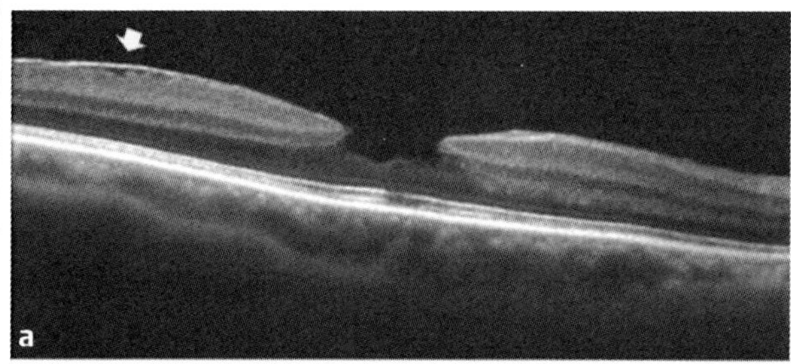

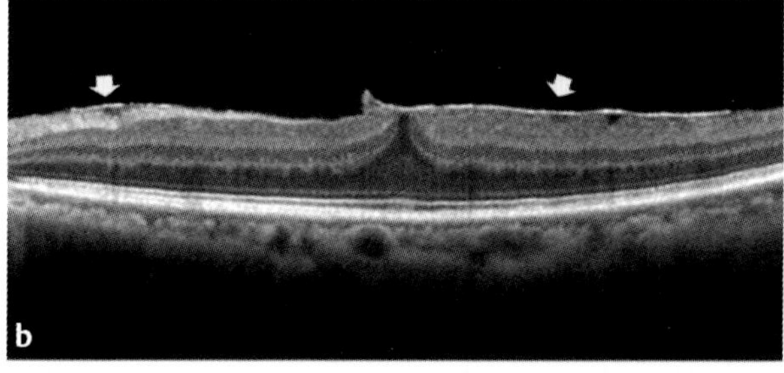

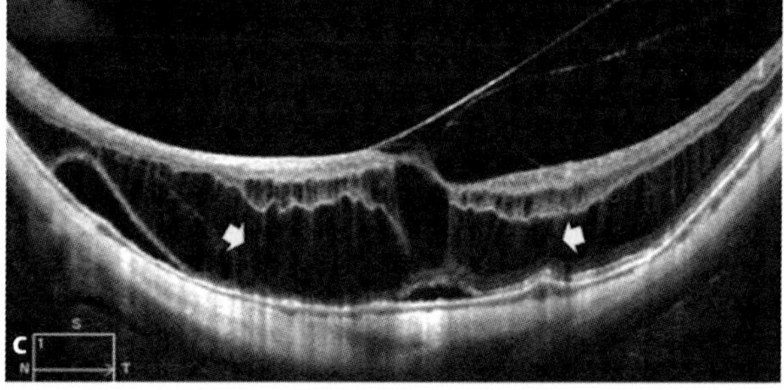

Fig. 20.4 Optical coherence tomography (OCT) image of a lamellar macular hole **(a)** with an associated epiretinal membrane (yellow arrow). Note that there is a maintenance of the photoreceptor layer, which is not seen in a full-thickness macular hole. **(b)** OCT image illustrating anatomical features of a macular pseudohole associated with an epiretinal membrane (yellow arrows). Note that there is no loss of foveal tissue. **(c)** OCT of macular schisis (intraretinal splitting) between the outer plexiform and outer nuclear layers asscociated with focal vitreomacular traction. Note the thick inner retinal layer and a thin outer retinal layer separated by a wide hyporeflective space. There is bridging tissue connecting the two split layers (yellow arrows).

Table 20.3 Summary of the anatomic optical coherence tomography (OCT)-based classification of vitreomacular interface conditions (according to the International Vitreomacular Traction Study Group Classification System)

Anatomic state	Anatomic OCT-based classification of vitreomacular interface conditions

VMA	Definition
	• Perifoveal vitreous detachment
	• Vitreomacular attachment within a 3-mm radius of the foveal center
	• Normal foveal morphology
	Classification
	• By size of vitreomacular attachment
	  ○ Focal (≤ 1500 µm)
	  ○ Broad (> 1500 µm, parallel to the RPE and may include areas of dehiscence)
	• By the presence of concurrent retinal conditions
	  ○ Isolated
	  ○ Concurrent

VMT	Definition
	• Perifoveal vitreous detachment
	• Vitreomacular attachment within a 3-mm radius of the foveal center
	• Associated changes in the foveal morphology, intraretinal structural changes, and/or elevation of the fovea above the RPE
	• No full-thickness interruption of all retinal layers
	Classification
	• By size of vitreomacular attachment
	  ○ Focal (≤ 1500 µm)
	  ○ Broad (> 1500 µm, parallel to the RPE; may include areas of dehiscence)
	• By the presence of concurrent retinal conditions
	  ○ Isolated
	  ○ Concurrent

FTMH	Definition
	• Full-thickness foveal lesion involving interruption of all retinal layers from ILM to RPE
	Classification
	• By aperture size (measured horizontally across the hole at the narrowest point of the hole or the photoreceptor tips, not the ILM)
	  ○ Small (≤ 250 µm)
	  ○ Medium (> 250 µm to ≤ 400 µm)
	  ○ Large (> 400 µm)
	• By status of vitreous
	  ○ Presence of VMT
	  ○ Absence of VMT
	• By cause
	  ○ Primary (initiated by VMT)
	  ○ Secondary (directly due to associated disease or trauma known to cause macular hole in the absence of prior VMT)

LMH	Definition • Irregular foveal contour • Defect in the inner fovea with or without actual loss of retinal tissue • Intraretinal splitting (schisis), typically between the outer plexiform and outer nuclear layers • Intact photoreceptor layer
Macular pseudohole	Definition • Invaginated or heaped up foveal margins • Concomitant ERM with a central opening • Steep macular contour to the central fovea with a near-normal central foveal thickness • No loss of retinal tissue

Abbreviations: ERM, epiretinal membrane; FTMH, full-thickness macular hole; ILM, inner limiting membrane; LMH, lamellar macular hole; RPE, retinal pigment epithelium; VMA, vitreomacular adhesion; VMT, vitreomacular traction.
Source: Duker JS, Kaiser PK, Binder S, et al. The International Vitreomacular Traction Study Group classification of vitreomacular adhesion, traction, and macular hole. Ophthalmology 2013;120(12):2611–2619.

tissue toward the foveal center,[41] which results in an invagination of the perifoveal retinal tissue into a shape that mimics an FTMH on clinical examination but in fact does not contain any actual loss of retinal tissue characteristic of FTMH. OCT is 100% sensitive in revealing the specific morphologic features that accurately rule out the presence of FTMH and establish the diagnosis of a macular pseudohole.[5,39,41]

Using the anatomical OCT-based classification system,[5] macular pseudohole is defined as having the following features: (1) invaginated or heaped-up foveal margins, (2) concomitant ERM with a central opening, (3) steep macular contour to the foveal center with close to normal foveal thickness, and (4) no loss of foveal tissue (which is typically seen with LMH and FTMH) (▶ Fig. 20.4).

20.6 OCT-Based Classification of Myopic Retinal Schisis

Macular schisis or intraretinal splitting is a well-known complication of high myopia. On slit-lamp biomicroscopy, schisis can rarely have a stellate foveal appearance[42]; however, typically it is hard to ascertain schisis on slit-lamp biomicroscopy. Benhamou et al described the OCT characteristics and evolution of macular schisis associated with high myopia and showed two patterns of macular schisis on OCT: *outer retinal schisis* and *inner retinal schisis*.[43] In outer retinal schisis, which is more common, the retina is split into a thicker inner layer and a thinner outer layer. Inner retinal schisis is defined as splitting of the retina such that it is divided into a thinner inner layer and a thicker outer layer.[43] Retinal schisis may result in the formation of an LMH or FTMH.[43]

On OCT, macular schisis typically appears as an intraretinal splitting that involves a thick inner retinal layer and a thin outer retinal layer that are usually separated by a wide hyporeflective space. It is associated in some cases with bridging tissue connecting the two split layers (▶ Fig. 20.4).

20.7 Conclusion

An easy to remember and simple anatomical definition of VMI conditions on OCT is important for a better clinical application, execution and analysis of clinical studies and predicting outcomes of surgical and pharmacologic therapies. Such an OCT-based anatomical classification of VMI conditions allows clinicians and trainees to speak the same language when discussing VMI conditions and is summarized in ▶ Table 20.3. As the OCT technology advances and as the understanding of VMI conditions broadens, these anatomical OCT-based definitions are subject to further improvement and change.

References

[1] Uchino E, Uemura A, Ohba N. Initial stages of posterior vitreous detachment in healthy eyes of older persons evaluated by optical coherence tomography. Arch Ophthalmol 2001; 119: 1475–1479

[2] Johnson MW. Perifoveal vitreous detachment and its macular complications. Trans Am Ophthalmol Soc 2005; 103: 537–567

[3] Sonmez K, Capone A Jr Trese MT, Williams GA. Vitreomacular traction syndrome: impact of anatomical configuration on anatomical and visual outcomes. Retina 2008; 28: 1207–1214

[4] Koizumi H, Spaide RF, Fisher YL, Freund KB, Klancnik JM Jr Yannuzzi LA. Three-dimensional evaluation of vitreomacular traction and epiretinal membrane using spectral-domain optical coherence tomography. Am J Ophthalmol 2008; 145: 509–517

[5] Duker JS, Kaiser PK, Binder S, et al. The International Vitreomacular Traction Study Group classification of vitreomacular adhesion, traction, and macular hole. Ophthalmology 2013; 120: 2611–2619

[6] Johnson MW. Posterior vitreous detachment: evolution and complications of its early stages. Am J Ophthalmol 2010; 149: 371–382, e1

[7] Sebag J. Anomalous posterior vitreous detachment: a unifying concept in vitreo-retinal disease. Graefes Arch Clin Exp Ophthalmol 2004; 242: 690–698

[8] Gaudric A, Haouchine B, Massin P, Paques M, Blain P, Erginay A. Macular hole formation: new data provided by optical coherence tomography. Arch Ophthalmol 1999; 117: 744–751

[9] Johnson MW. Posterior vitreous detachment: evolution and role in macular disease. Retina 2012; 32 Suppl 2: S174–S178

[10] Kishi S, Demaria C, Shimizu K. Vitreous cortex remnants at the fovea after spontaneous vitreous detachment. Int Ophthalmol 1986; 9: 253–260

[11] Seabag J. Vitreoschisis. Graefes Arch Clin Exp Ophthalmol 2008; 246: 329–332

[12] Snead DR, James S, Snead MP. Pathological changes in the vitreoretinal junction 1: epiretinal membrane formation. Eye (Lond) 2008; 22: 1310–1317

[13] Gass JD. Reappraisal of biomicroscopic classification of stages of development of a macular hole. Am J Ophthalmol 1995; 119: 752–759

[14] Gass JD. Idiopathic senile macular hole. Its early stages and pathogenesis. Arch Ophthalmol 1988; 106: 629–639

[15] Ip MS, Baker BJ, Duker JS, et al. Anatomical outcomes of surgery for idiopathic macular hole as determined by optical coherence tomography. Arch Ophthalmol 2002; 120: 29–35

[16] Stalmans P, Benz MS, Gandorfer A, et al. MIVI-TRUST Study Group. Enzymatic vitreolysis with ocriplasmin for vitreomacular traction and macular holes. N Engl J Med 2012; 367: 606–615

[17] Ullrich S, Haritoglou C, Gass C, Schaumberger M, Ulbig MW, Kampik A. Macular hole size as a prognostic factor in macular hole surgery. Br J Ophthalmol 2002; 86: 390–393

[18] Trese MT, Williams GA, Hartzer MK. A new approach to stage 3 macular holes. Ophthalmology 2000; 107: 1607–1611

[19] Chang S. Controversies regarding internal limiting membrane peeling in idiopathic epiretinal membrane and macular hole. Retina 2012; 32 Suppl 2: S200–S203, discussion S203–S204

[20] Arevalo JF, Sanchez JG, Costa RA, et al. Optical coherence tomography characteristics of full-thickness traumatic macular holes. Eye (Lond) 2008; 22: 1436–1441

[21] Oehrens AM, Stalmans P. Optical coherence tomographic documentation of the formation of a traumatic macular hole. Am J Ophthalmol 2006; 142: 866–869

[22] Rossi T, Boccassini B, Esposito L, et al. The pathogenesis of retinal damage in blunt eye trauma: finite element modeling. Invest Ophthalmol Vis Sci 2011; 52: 3994–4002

[23] Yu W, Zheng L, Zhang Z, Dai R, Dong F. Spectral-domain optical coherence tomography characteristics of macular contusion trauma. Ophthalmic Res 2012; 47: 220–224

[24] Ripandelli G, Rossi T, Scarinci F, Scassa C, Parisi V, Stirpe M. Macular vitreoretinal interface abnormalities in highly myopic eyes with posterior staphyloma: 5-year follow-up. Retina 2012; 32: 1531–1538

[25] Singh AJ, Muqit MM, Woon WH. Is axial length a risk factor for idiopathic macular hole formation? Int Ophthalmol 2012; 32: 393–396

[26] Shukla D, Naresh KB, Rajendran A, Kim R. Macular hole secondary to X-linked retinoschisis [Letter]. Eye (Lond) 2006; 20: 1459–1461

[27] Shukla D. Evolution and management of macular hole secondary to type 2 idiopathic macular telangiectasia [Letter]. Eye (Lond) 2011; 25: 532–533

[28] Fabian ID, Moisseiev E, Moisseiev J, Moroz I, Barak A, Alhalel A. Macular hole after vitrectomy for primary rhegmatogenous retinal detachment. Retina 2012; 32: 511–519

[29] Garcia-Arumi J, Boixadera A, Martinez-Castillo V, Zapata MA, Fonollosa A, Corcostegui B. Macular holes after rhegmatogenous retinal detachment repair: surgical management and functional outcome. Retina 2011; 31: 1777–1782

[30] Sagara N, Kawaji T, Koshiyama Y, Inomata Y, Fukushima M, Tanihara H. Macular hole formation after macular haemorrhage associated with rupture of retinal arterial macroaneurysm. Br J Ophthalmol 2009; 93: 1337–1340

[31] Sato R, Yasukawa T, Hirano Y, Ogura Y. Early-onset macular holes following ruptured retinal arterial macroaneurysms. Graefes Arch Clin Exp Ophthalmol 2008; 246: 1779–1782

[32] Taylor SR, Lightman SL, Sugar EA, et al. The impact of macular edema on visual function in intermediate, posterior, and panuveitis. Ocul Immunol Inflamm 2012; 20: 171–181

[33] Tsukada K, Tsujikawa A, Murakami T, Ogino K, Yoshimura N. Lamellar macular hole formation in chronic cystoid macular edema associated with retinal vein occlusion. Jpn J Ophthalmol 2011; 55: 506–513

[34] Papathanassiou M, Alonistiotis D, Petrou P, Theodossiadis P, Vergados I. Macular hole formation following phacoemulsification cataract surgery. Clin Exp Optom 2011; 94: 112–114

[35] Besirli CG, Johnson MW. Traction-induced foveal damage predisposes eyes with pre-existing posterior vitreous detachment to idiopathic macular hole formation. Eye (Lond) 2012; 26: 792–795

[36] Chan A, Duker JS, Schuman JS, Fujimoto JG. Stage 0 macular holes: observations by optical coherence tomography. Ophthalmology 2004; 111: 2027–2032

[37] Gass JD. Lamellar macular hole: a complication of cystoid macular edema after cataract extraction: a clinicopathologic case report. Trans Am Ophthalmol Soc 1975; 73: 231–250

[38] Takahashi H, Kishi S. Tomographic features of a lamellar macular hole formation and a lamellar hole that progressed to a full-thickness macular hole. Am J Ophthalmol 2000; 130: 677–679

[39] Haouchine B, Massin P, Tadayoni R, Erginay A, Gaudric A. Diagnosis of macular pseudoholes and lamellar macular holes by optical coherence tomography. Am J Ophthalmol 2004; 138: 732–739

[40] Witkin AJ, Ko TH, Fujimoto JG, et al. Redefining lamellar holes and the vitreomacular interface: an ultrahigh-resolution optical coherence tomography study. Ophthalmology 2006; 113: 388–397

[41] Allen AW Jr Gass JD. Contraction of a perifoveal epiretinal membrane simulating a macular hole. Am J Ophthalmol 1976; 82: 684–691

[42] Menchini U, Brancato R, Virgili G, Pierro L. Unilateral macular retinoschisis with stellate foveal appearance in two females with myopia. Ophthalmic Surg Lasers 2000; 31: 229–232

[43] Benhamou N, Massin P, Haouchine B, Erginay A, Gaudric A. Macular retinoschisis in highly myopic eyes. Am J Ophthalmol 2002; 133: 794–800

21 Optical Coherence Tomography Diagnosis of Macular Diseases

J. Fernando Arevalo, Andres F. Lasave, and Fernando A. Arevalo

Optical coherence tomography (OCT) provides new morphologic, qualitative, and quantitative data of all retinal layers that are valuable for diagnosis, development of the best treatment strategy, and monitoring treatment in most macular diseases.

The objective of this chapter is to review the use of OCT as a diagnostic tool in the most common macular diseases, such as vitreoretinal interface disorders of the posterior pole including macular hole, lamellar macular hole and pseudohole, epiretinal membrane (ERM), vitreomacular traction syndrome, and age-related macular degeneration (AMD).

21.1 Vitreoretinal Interface Disorders

21.1.1 Macular Hole

Idiopathic macular hole is a retinal disease characterized by a full-thickness defect of the foveal area with associated visual acuity reduction, metamorphopsia, and a central scotoma. OCT has improved the understanding and management of idiopathic macular hole. Its incidence is around 3 in 1000, and it is more common in women between the sixth and seventh decades of life.[1] The pathophysiology of the development of idiopathic macular hole has been extensively studied.[2,3,4] In the 1970s, recent posterior vitreous detachment was usually noted in eyes with macular holes, whereas eyes with preexisting vitreous detachment rarely developed a macular hole. This observation led to the conclusion that vitreous traction plays an important role in macular hole formation.[5] In 1983, Avila et al suggested that the main cause of macular hole formation is anteroposterior traction exerted by vitreous fibers on the center of the fovea.[5] In 1988, Gass[2] introduced the concept of tangential traction of the vitreous cortex at the foveolar edges as the cause of macular hole. Immediately, foveal dehiscence was followed by centripetal retraction of retinal elements.[2] The posterior hyaloid face of the vitreous remained attached to the foveola and surrounding macular region at the initial stages of hole formation.[6] In 1995, the same author suggested that most full-thickness macular holes arise from an umbo dehiscence without loss of foveal tissue.[7]

Although slit-lamp observations and photographic documentation were provided, adequate imaging of the posterior hyaloid detachment and retinal layers was impossible before the OCT era. With the help of OCT, other investigators have proposed that the hole formation involves vitreoretinal separation with vitreofoveal adhesion exerting oblique traction on the fovea, followed by foveal cysts or foveal detachment, foveal dehiscence, and finally full-thickness hole formation.[2,3]

With some modification, OCT staging can parallel the staging of macular holes with biomicroscopic examination. OCT has demonstrated changes in the vitreomacular interface that are not visible using biomicroscopy (▶ Fig. 21.1). This imaging method has provided further detailed structure changes and improved our understanding of the mechanism of macular hole formation. It is now widely accepted that the early event leading to macular hole is the persistent adherence of the cortical vitreous to the fovea with adjacent vitreoretinal separation. The resultant traction on the fovea causes foveal detachment or an intraretinal space termed *pseudocyst*. Further traction leads to dehiscence of foveal tissue, resulting in full-thickness macular hole formation.[8,9]

Classification of idiopathic macular holes as proposed by Gass[2,4] has always been the standard in staging macular holes. However, sometimes determination of the developmental stage of macular holes has been difficult to assess clinically. Since the introduction of the OCT, staging of macular holes has changed, especially with respect to the early stages.

The Gass classification[2,4] indicates that stage 1 holes (foveal detachment) can be distinguished by reduced or absent foveal pit and the presence of an optically clear space beneath the fovea suggesting a foveolar detachment. Vitreomacular traction is present as a result of posterior incomplete vitreous detachment lifting the foveal area and the formation of an impending macular hole. Clinically, this appears as a yellowish spot on the fovea. Depending on how soon the patient is examined after the onset of symptoms and the degree of elevation of the retina, either a yellow spot 100 to 200 µm in diameter (stage 1A) or a yellow ring approximately 200 to 350 µm in diameter (stage 1B) is present in the foveolar area. As the foveolar retinal detachment (stage 1A) progresses to foveal retinal detachment (stage 1B), the progressive stretching and thinning of the foveolar center may cause redistribution of the xanthophyll pigment into a ring configuration.

Stage 2 holes are those in the early formation stage. In most patients, the yellow ring enlarges, and a full-thickness retinal dehiscence will develop within several weeks or months. This stage shows a partial break on the surface of the retina, but the operculum is still attached to the retina or separated from the underlying retina with a small full-thickness loss of retinal tissue of less than 400 µm in diameter.

Stage 3 holes have a full-thickness retinal dehiscence with a complete break in the outer retinal tissue and variable amounts

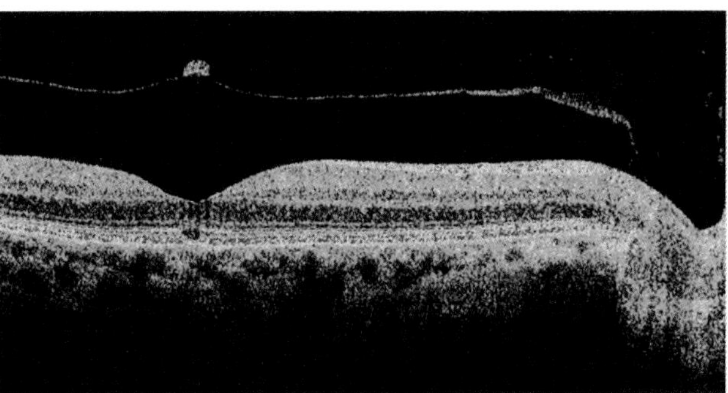

Fig. 21.1 Optical coherence tomography has demonstrated changes in the vitreomacular interface not visible with biomicroscopy.

of surrounding macular edema that increase retinal thickness and decrease reflectivity in the outer retinal layers. In this stage, separation of the operculum from the underlying retina is complete; hole diameter is greater than 400 µm.

Stage 4 holes are characterized by the complete loss of tissue greater than 400 µm in diameter and a complete posterior vitreous detachment with release of the anteroposterior tractional forces.

Stage 1 and 2 macular holes are difficult to differentiate ophthalmoscopically, and high-resolution OCT images can help to classify them. Stage 2 often progresses to stage 3 with some visual loss; therefore, appropriate staging with OCT can help to determine when surgery is indicated.[10]

Vitreoretinal traction is important in the pathogenesis of macular holes, and it can be identified by OCT.[11] Duker et al[12] found vitreoretinal interface abnormalities by OCT in 21% of fellow eyes. Furthermore, OCT may be a useful method of assessing the risk for hole formation in the fellow eye of patients with a unilateral macular hole. Considering that the probability of developing a macular hole in the contralateral eye is 13% in 48 months,[13] it is then mandatory to perform bilateral tomographic imaging in patients affected by this pathology for early detection in the other eye. However, the concept of surgery in the normal contralateral eye of patients with macular holes is not acceptable.

For stage 2-4 macular holes, OCT is effective, and quantitative information may be directly extracted from the OCT tomograms, including the status of the vitreoretinal interface, the diameter of the hole, and the extent of surrounding subretinal fluid accumulation.[11] OCT is useful in differentiating simulating lesions and in allowing better counseling of patients regarding their disorder.

In addition, accurate assessment of macular hole size is important for both research studies and to guide clinical management. The size of a macular hole has been shown to affect anatomical and visual success. Macular hole size and postoperative resolution can be evaluated by OCT.[14,15,16,17,18]

Altaweel and Ip[14] published the latest staging of idiopathic macular holes based on OCT findings. In stage 1A, OCT demonstrates perifoveal posterior vitreous detachment with continued foveolar adherence. Tractional forces are anteroposterior and tangential. Retinal tissue remains at the base of the pseudocyst. Pseudocyst formation (hyporeflective image on OCT) occurs without affecting all retinal layers and with an intact outer retina. In stage 1B, the foveal pseudocyst affects all retinal layers, including the photoreceptor layer with an intact roof. There is incomplete posterior vitreous detachment with persistent adhesion onto the fovea in stages 1A and 1B (▶ Fig. 21.2). In stage 2A, the roof of the pseudocyst has been torn open and continues to have traction exerted by the vitreous attachment. There is persistent traction of the posterior hyaloid that is firmly attached to the inner retina. A break in the roof of the pseudocyst gives rise to a full-thickness macular hole. In stage 2B, the roof of the pseudocyst has completely separated from the retina. At this point, there is release of the anteroposterior tractional forces. The distance between the edges of the hole is less than 400 µm. In stage 3, the prefoveal operculum can still be appreciated, but the distance between the hole edges is greater than 400 µm. The posterior hyaloid is completely detached from the inner retina, as opposed to the description of Gass,[2] wherein the former remains attached to the perifoveal area. In stage 4, vitreous detachment is complete which cannot be seen tomographically and can be confirmed only by slit-lamp biomicroscopy or ultrasonography (▶ Fig. 21.3, ▶ Fig. 21.4, ▶ Fig. 21.5, ▶ Fig. 21.6).

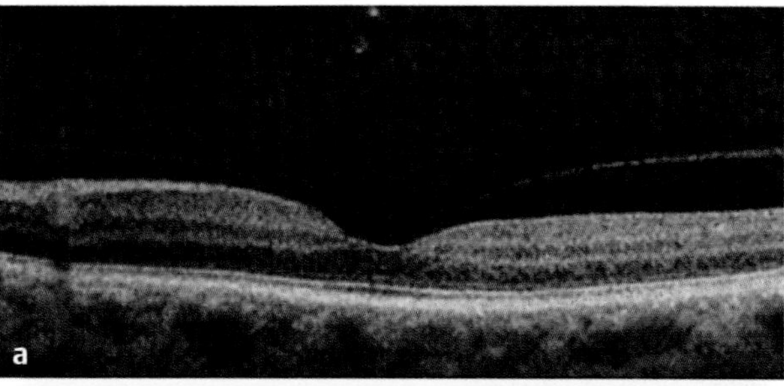

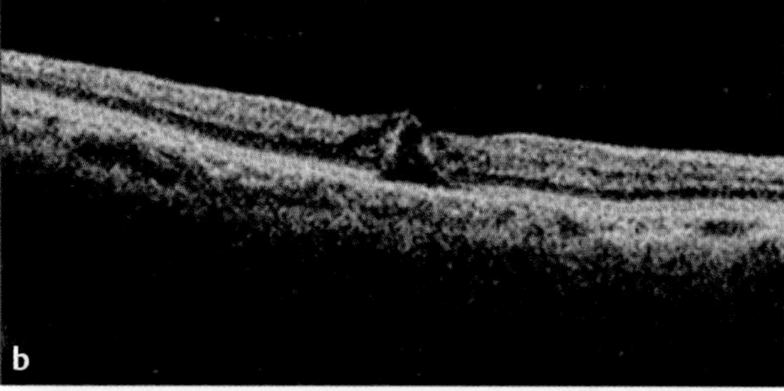

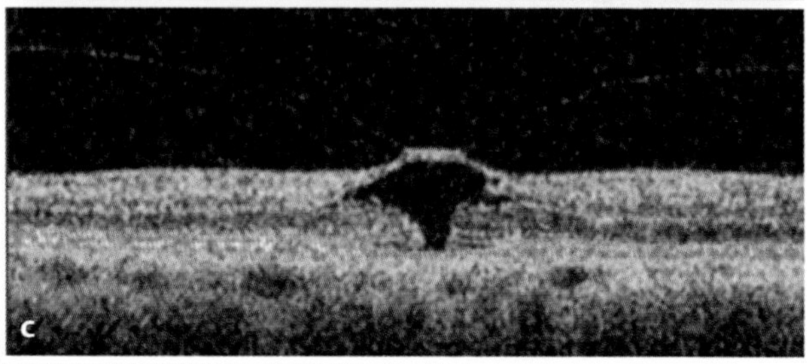

Fig. 21.2 Full-thickness macular hole classification. **(a)** Stage 0: Preimpending hole. **(b)** Stage 1A: Optical coherence tomography demonstrates perifoveal posterior vitreous detachment with continued foveolar adherence. Tractional forces are anteroposterior and tangential. Retinal tissue remains at the base of the pseudocyst. **(c)** Stage 1B: In this stage, the pseudocyst enlarges and extends to the retinal pigment epithelium. Foveolar detachment (impending hole) is present.

The main differences between the biomicroscopic and the OCT staging of idiopathic macular holes are the presence of a tight focal foveolar adherence of the posterior hyaloid versus a perifoveal vitreomacular detachment, the formation of a foveal pseudocyst versus a detachment in Gass' stage 1 hole, and the subdivision of stage 2 into two distinct anatomical types.

In cases with a base diameter less than 400 µm as measured by OCT, an anatomical closure was achieved in 92%, and in those with a base diameter greater than 400 µm, this value decreased to 56%. Several variables—like preoperative visual acuity, symptoms' duration, hole diameter by OCT (as a single variable), and stereoscopic funduscopy—may predict the final visual outcome.[15,16] One study demonstrated that OCT measurement is predictive not only of the possibility for anatomical closure but also of postoperative visual acuity outcome. By

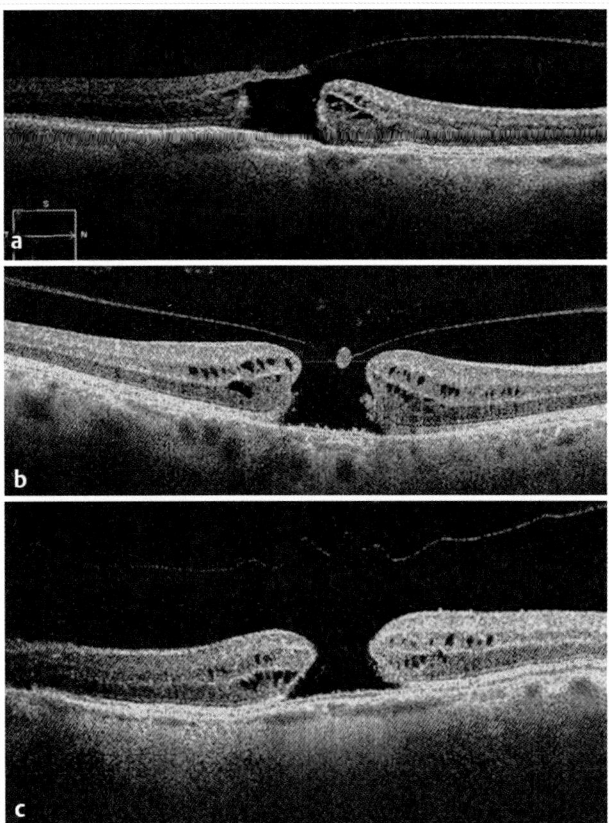

Fig. 21.3 Full-thickness macular hole classification. (a) Stage 2A: The roof of the pseudocyst has been torn open and continues to have traction exerted by the vitreous attachment. (b) Stage 3: Image shows a full-thickness retinal dehiscence with a complete break in the outer retinal tissue. There is complete separation of the operculum from the underlying retina, with a hole diameter of more than 400 µm. Full-thickness macular hole (>400 µm); (c) Stage 4: A complete loss of tissue of >400 µm is seen with a complete detachment of the posterior vitreous and release of the anteroposterior tractional forces. Full-thickness macular hole plus complete vitreous detachment.

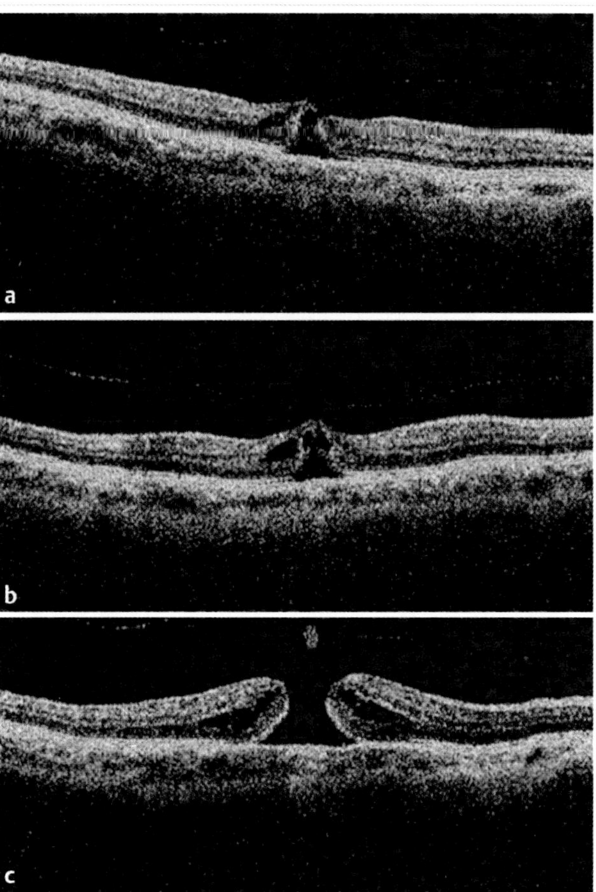

Fig. 21.4 Sequential foveal tomographic images by time-domain optical coherence tomography. (a) At the initial visit, small intrafoveal splits are seen between the inner and outer retina of a typical stage 1A macular hole with the posterior hyaloid reflecting a perifoveal posterior vitreous detachment with continued foveolar adherence that progresses to stage 1B at 1-month follow-up (b). After intravitreal injection of tissue plasminogen activator, a full-thickness macular hole was present (c).

using the maximum hole diameter, minimum hole diameter, and height as reference values, the authors use a formula to infer macular hole prognosis.[16]

Likewise, OCT is useful in evaluating anatomical closure after macular hole surgery (▶ Fig. 21.7). The flattening of the retina and the disappearance of the retinal cysts may be appreciated postoperatively. Closure of the horizontal component of a hole wherein there is complete detachment usually takes place in the first postoperative days. Absence of closure within the first postoperative month entails poor prognosis.[7] In the normal course of an idiopathic macular hole, in about 2% of cases, the macular hole may close by itself spontaneously when there is release of vitreomacular traction. In such cases, the photoreceptors may be affected as a result of the previously existing traction and, as a consequence, may give rise to an absolute central scotoma.

In conclusion, OCT imaging is a highly important tool in the diagnosis, in evaluation of the etiopathogenesis, for postoperative follow-up, and as a predictive factor in the prognosis of idiopathic macular holes.

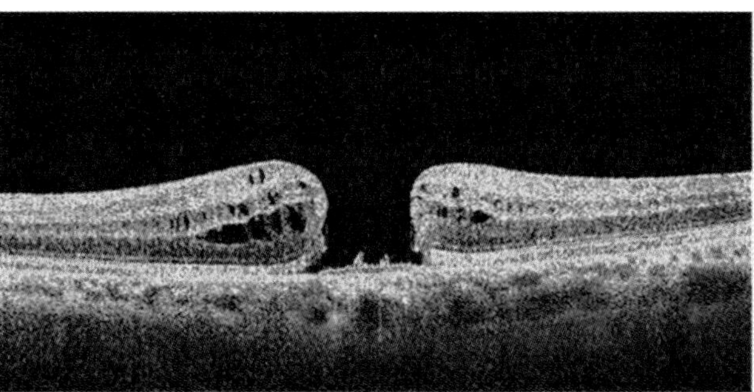

Fig. 21.5 Optical coherence tomography image showed a full-thickness macular hole with complete vitreous detachment.

21.1.2 Non–Full-Thickness Macular Holes

The description and pathogenesis of non–full-thickness macular holes have been better understood with the advent of OCT.

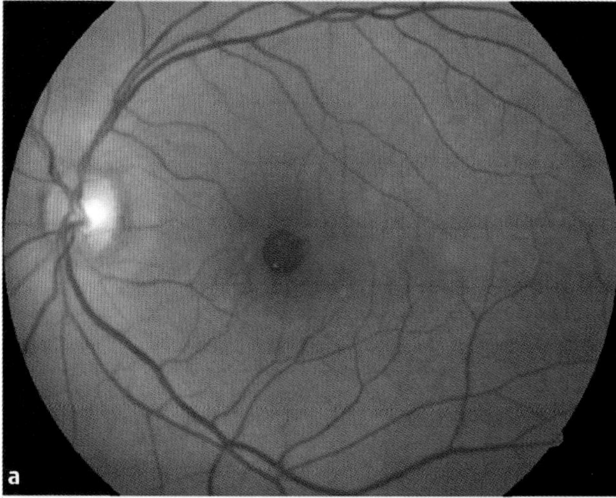
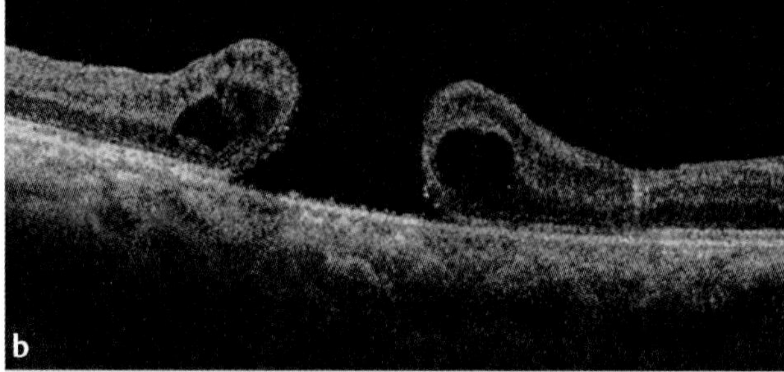

Fig. 21.6 A case of a stage 4 macular hole. (a) Color picture of a full-thickness macular lesion. (b) Optical coherence tomography image demonstrates a surrounding macular edema that increase retinal thickness and decrease reflectivity in the outer retinal layers. Full-thickness macular hole and complete vitreous detachment are observed.

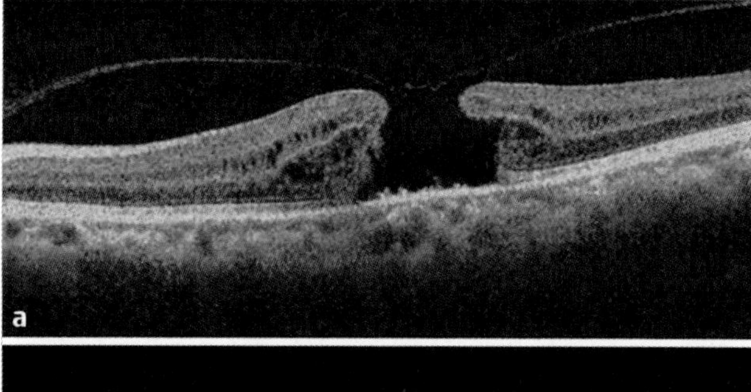
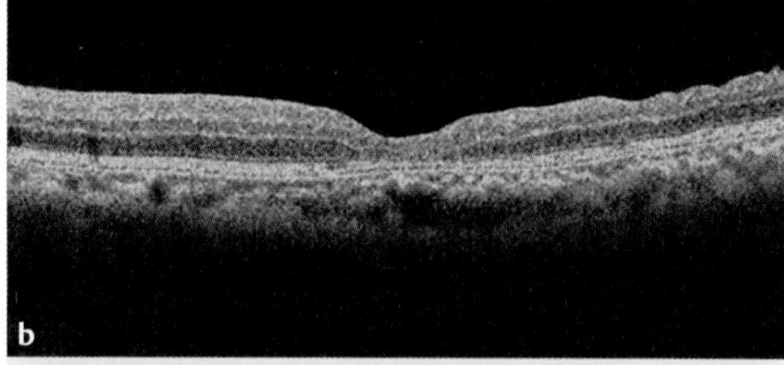

Fig. 21.7 Spectral-domain optical coherence tomographic images of a 68-year-old patient with a full-thickness macular hole before surgery (a). Six months after surgery (b), good foveal contour was achieved, and the visual acuity improved from 20/200 to 20/80.

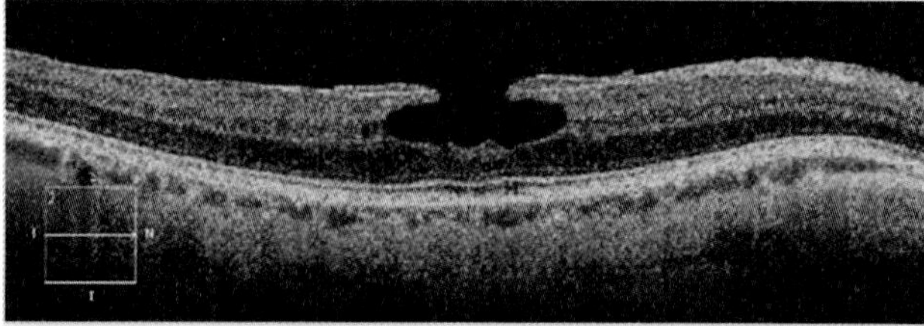

Fig. 21.8 Spectral-domain optical coherence tomographic image shows a stable lamellar hole. A thick epiretinal membrane is evident. Central foveal thickness remained stable throughout 12 months of follow-up. Outer nuclear layer is intact and visible centrally.

Lamellar macular hole (LMH) and macular pseudohole (MPH) can be different clinical manifestations of the same disease.

Lamellar macular hole was first described by Gass[17] in 1975 as an abortive process of full-thickness macular hole formation resulting from deroofing of cystoid macular edema. Instead, MPH was described as being caused by centripetal contraction of previously present ERM, which surrounds but does not cover the foveal area.[18] However, coexistence and possible evolution from a MPH to lamellar macular hole after progressive ERM contraction are possible.[19]

Since the development of OCT, interest in diagnosis of LMHs has been renewed because high-resolution images can detect a lamellar macular defect that is not always visible clinically.[20,21] Data based on OCT proved that only 28% to 37% of LMHs are correctly diagnosed by biomicroscopy.[21,22] OCT enables clear differentiation between macular pseudoholes (MPHs) and LMHs.[21]

In OCT, LMHs have been described as non–full-thickness defects of the macula having an irregular foveal contour with a dehiscence in the inner fovea, separation of the inner from the outer retinal layers, and absence of a full-thickness foveal defect with intact outer retinal layers at the base of the hole[22] (▶ Fig. 21.8, ▶ Fig. 21.9).

In OCT, MPH has been described as having a steep fovea contour and a normal or slightly increased central and paracentral retinal thickness[22] (▶ Fig. 21.10, ▶ Fig. 21.11). Thus, before the OCT era, many cases might have been misdiagnosed. In full-thickness macular holes, the percentage of coexisting ERMs confirmed with SDOCT is about 13%.[23] Different authors have reported on ERMs coexisting with LMH in 62 to 73% of cases using OCT.[24]

Witkin et al[21] reported that with ultrahigh-resolution optical coherence tomography, ERMs are visible in 89% of LMH cases. Other observations demonstrate the presence of a hyperreflective linear structure in all the cases of LMH.[25] LMH is generally regarded as a clinically stable disorder. Theodossiadis et al[26] studied 41 patients with LMH and reported a mean decline of 6.4% in visual acuity after 37.1 months of observation. Indications for surgical treatment of LMH remain controversial. Only a limited number of reports on vitrectomy results in LMH patients have been published, and most studies reported favorable outcomes.[19,27,28,29] Recent reports on vitrectomy with removal of the ERM-ILM with or without gas injection demonstrated benefit both functionally and morphologically.[30,31]

Bottoni et al[32] support previous indications[26] in planning treatment strategies; thus, vitrectomy could be indicated in LMHs showing a progressive thinning of foveal thickness and/or

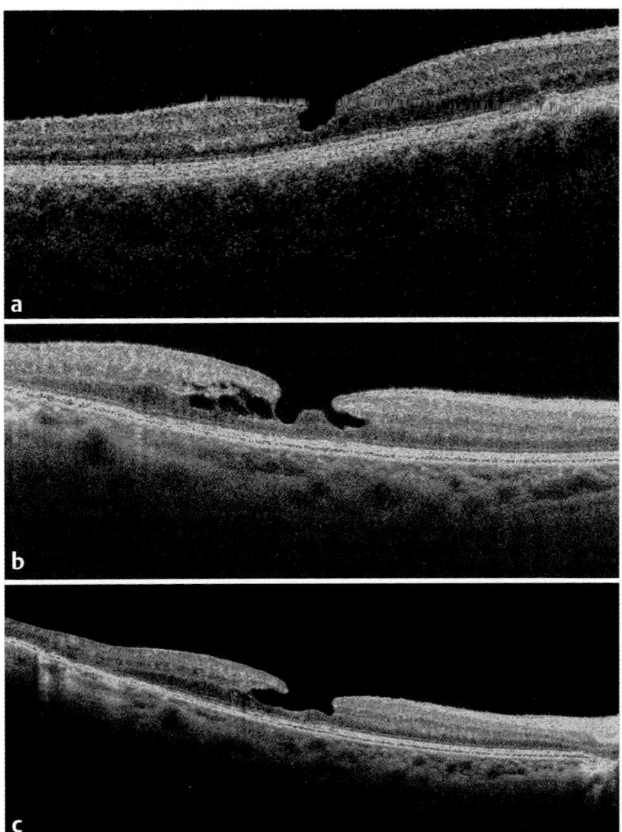

Fig. 21.9 (a-c) Three different cases of lamellar macular hole are observed in these spectral-domain optical coherence tomography (SD OCT) pictures. **(a)** A small lamellar hole is observed centrally. **(b)** Lamellar macular hole secondary to coalescence of intraretinal cysts in the inner nuclear layer is seen. The outer retina is intact. **(c)** Another case of classic lamellar macular hole is observed in this sSD OCT picture.

visual acuity deterioration during the follow-up of the natural course of the disease.

Recently, Lee et al[33] indicated that poor initial visual acuity, the presence of a disrupted inner segment/outer segment (IS/OS) junction (ellipsoid zone), or a thin fovea on preoperative spectral-domain (SD) OCT predicted poor vision outcome after LMH surgery. However, whether it is worthwhile to attempt surgical treatment for LMH remains a controversial issue.

21.1.3 Epiretinal Membranes

Epiretinal membrane is a disorder in which the vitreomacular interface induces a tangential tractional force on the retina, which can result in distortion of the macular architecture and development of vascular leakage with associated macular edema and vision loss. Visual symptoms range from mild to severe and usually are manifested by blurred vision or metamorphopsia.

Epiretinal membranes occur in 2.2% to 18.5%[34,35,36,37] of the population and can be either primary idiopathic, in which the incidence among elderly patients increases with age, or secondary to intraocular inflammatory conditions, retinal vascular disease, or surgical intervention. ERMs may also appear in otherwise healthy eyes as a result of incomplete vitreous detachment and mostly is characterized by the anatomical location of the ERM between the internal limiting membrane (ILM) and the vitreous body interface.[38]

Epiretinal membranes are caused by the migration of cells through small focal defects in the internal limiting membrane

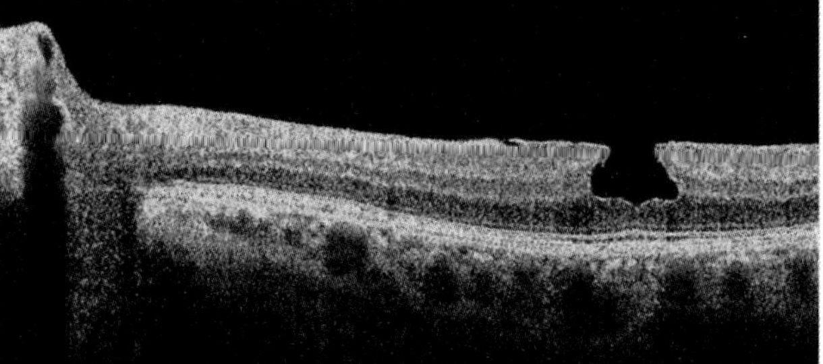

Fig. 21.10 Spectral-domain optical coherence tomography image of macular pseudohole is evident. Observe that the foveal contour is beneath the line representing the outer plexiform layer. The photoreceptor layer is intact. Visual acuity was 20/40 and remained stable during 12 months of follow-up.

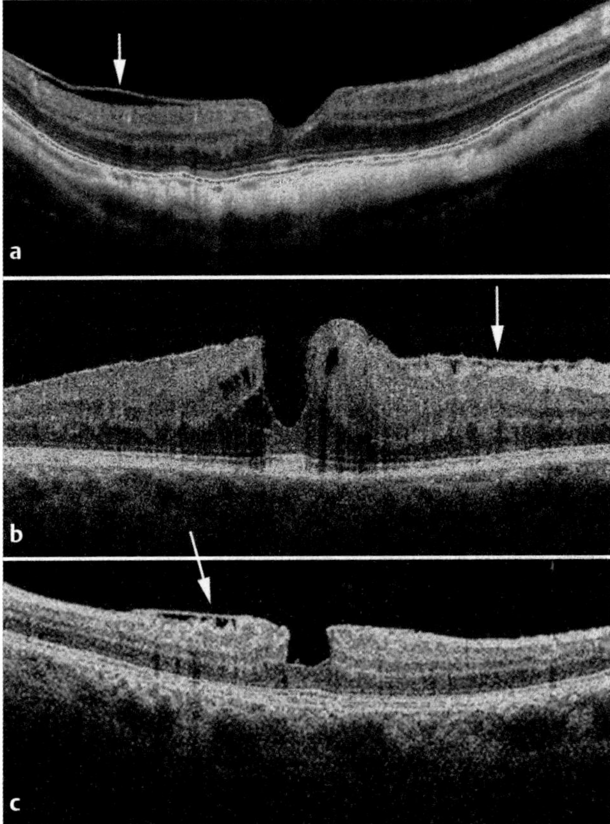

Fig. 21.11 Three examples of typical appearance of macular pseudohole with epiretinal membrane (arrows). **(a, c)** The most common form of macular pseudohole with thin epiretinal membrane is observed in these spectral-domain optical coherence tomography (SD OCT) pictures. **(b)** Pseudohole with cystoid spaces around the lesion but separated from the pseudohole by tissue is seen on this SD OCT picture. No photoreceptor layer damage is present.

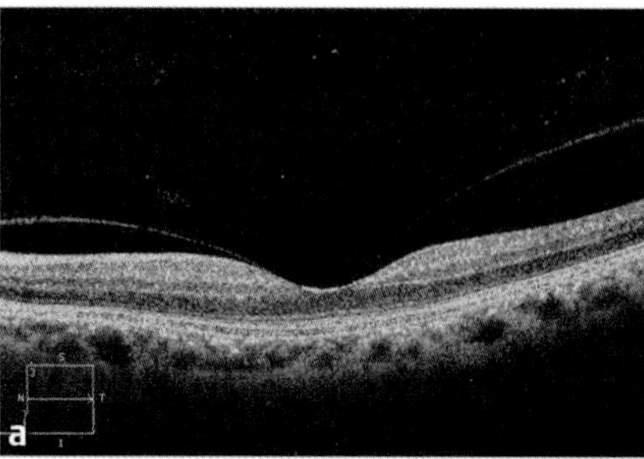
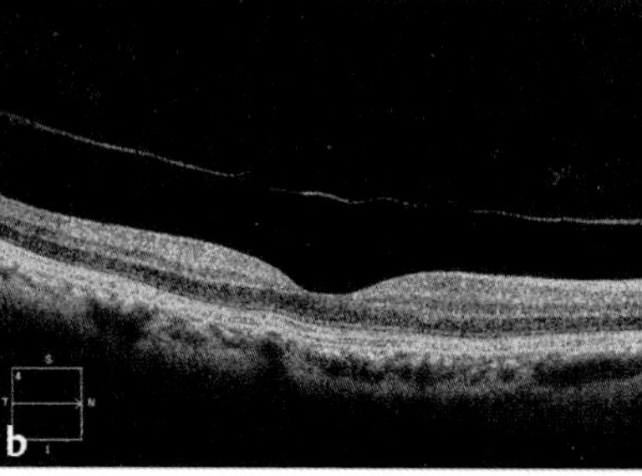

Fig. 21.12 **(a)** Partial posterior vitreous detachment is seen on this optical coherence tomography (OCT) image. **(b)** Complete posterior vitreous detachment is visible on the OCT image as a linear reflectivity suspended above the retinal surface.

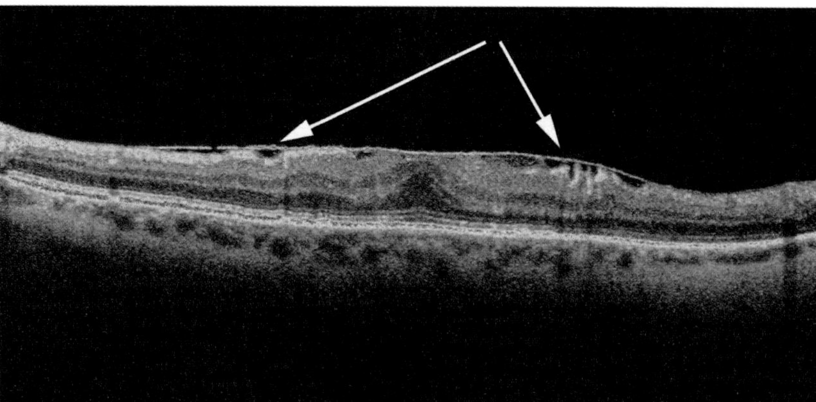

Fig. 21.13 The epiretinal membrane is delineated as a highly reflective band and is globally attached to the retina (arrows). There is a difference in reflectivity between the membrane and the underlying retina. The foveal depression was lost with intraretinal fluid accumulation.

after posterior vitreous detachment or by retinal breaks and detachments. These cells proliferate and create a thin veil of tissue at the retinal-vitreous interface. Purely glial cells are reported to occur in the earlier form of ERM, whereas a prominent fibrous, nonglial component has been reported in membranes, causing traction.

Gass[39] proposed grading the severity of ERMs on the following clinical scale: grade 0, translucent membranes unassociated with retinal distortion; grade 1, membranes causing irregular wrinkling of the inner retina; and grade 2, opaque membranes causing obscuration of the underlying vessels and marked full-thickness retinal distortion.

The early form of ERM, called cellophane macular reflex, is usually asymptomatic; therefore, most patients have normal or nearly normal vision with occasional metamorphopsia. However, the more severe form, known as *macular pucker*, can cause significant loss of visual acuity and visual symptoms such as distortion and metamorphopsia.[37] In severe cases, macular edema and retinal detachment have been known to occur.

Mori et al[40] and Wilkins et al[41] classified ERM based on a scale secondary to OCT findings. OCT images of ERMs may be classified into two broad categories: globally adherent membranes or partially nonadherent membranes. Both types of ERMs are usually visible on OCT images as a taut hyperreflective line contiguous with or anterior to the inner retinal surface. The secondary effects of the membrane, such as loss of the normal foveal contour, variable irregularity of the inner retinal layers, and macular thickening, are used to establish the presence of the membrane.

In addition, OCT provides a means to evaluate the cross-sectional characteristics of ERM, allowing a quantitative measurement of retinal thickness, membrane thickness, and the separation between the membrane and inner retina. Quantitative measurements of membrane thickness and reflectivity can be used to establish the degree of membrane opacity. The OCT tomogram can help to distinguish between membranes globally adherent to the retina and ERMs separated from the inner retina.[41]

The appearance of such an ERM might be mimicked by a partially detached posterior vitreous surface. However, ERMs tend to be thicker and more reflective than the posterior vitreous. The reflection from an ERM may measure up to 60 µm thick; this is rarely observed with a partially detached posterior vitreous. Complete posterior vitreous detachment (PVD) is visible on the OCT image as a linear reflectivity suspended above the retinal surface (▶ Fig. 21.12). On OCT, ERMs are visible as a highly reflective layer on the inner retinal surface (▶ Fig. 21.13, ▶ Fig. 21.14).

Characterization of the ERM with OCT may help in preoperative planning for membrane peeling.[36] In cases with separation between the membrane and retina, the surgeon may be directed to these areas to initiate membrane dissection. When the membrane is globally attached to the inner retina, the surgeon may anticipate more difficulty in peeling the membrane (▶ Fig. 21.15, ▶ Fig. 21.16, ▶ Fig. 21.17). The surgeon may also proceed with particular caution when extensive intraretinal edema leaves a thin, friable inner retinal layer beneath the membrane. In most ophthalmology centers, macular surgery for ERM removal is advocated if the best-corrected visual acuity falls below approximately 20/40, but there are no reports of objective indications for surgery, such as OCT findings.

Metamorphopsia induced by ERM may be related to the edematous areas of the inner nuclear layer (INL) detected with SD OCT. The classification of ERM based on INL thickness is a potentially useful indication for surgery.[35]

High-resolution OCT has several advantages for a detailed evaluation of vitreomacular traction (VMT) and ERM disease: raster scans provide a precise two- and three-dimensional

(3-D) image of the vitreomacular interface at each location. The high-resolution representation of all intraretinal layers identifies the level and location of alterations in functionally relevant structures, such as the neurosensory architecture and the photoreceptor layer.[34]

Several factors, such as preoperative visual acuity,[42] duration of symptoms before surgery,[43] and the presence or absence of cystoid macular edema,[44] have been suggested as prognostic factors influencing the postoperative visual acuity. Investigators have suggested that the macular microstructure, such as macular thickness and appearance of the photoreceptor layer, may be associated with postoperative visual acuity.[45,46] The introduction of SD OCT has improved the speed and sensitivity of the examination, allowing scanning at a higher resolution. Therefore, postoperative OCT imaging can be used to document surgical response. Usually, retinal thickness decreases after successful ERM peeling, visual acuity improves, and the distorted vascular pattern returns to its normal morphology.

The photoreceptor layer can be imaged with SD OCT as a hyperreflective line showing the IS/OS junction above the retinal pigment epithelium. An intact IS/OS junction can be defined as a continuous hyperreflective line, and the diagnosis of a disrupted IS/OS is made based on loss or irregularity of the hyperreflective line corresponding to the IS/OS junction. Existence of a correlation between photoreceptor IS/OS junction disruption and decreased postoperative visual acuity has been reported using time-domain (TD) OCT.[45,46] Macular edema resulting from the formation of ERM and some other artifacts may prevent a clear delineation of the IS/OS junction in TD OCT. However, SD OCT allows more precise visualization of the intraretinal morphologic features, such as the external limiting membrane and the photoreceptor layer, thereby enabling clear measurements of the IS/OS junction, even in the presence of a thickened retina caused by the presence of an ERM.[47,48]

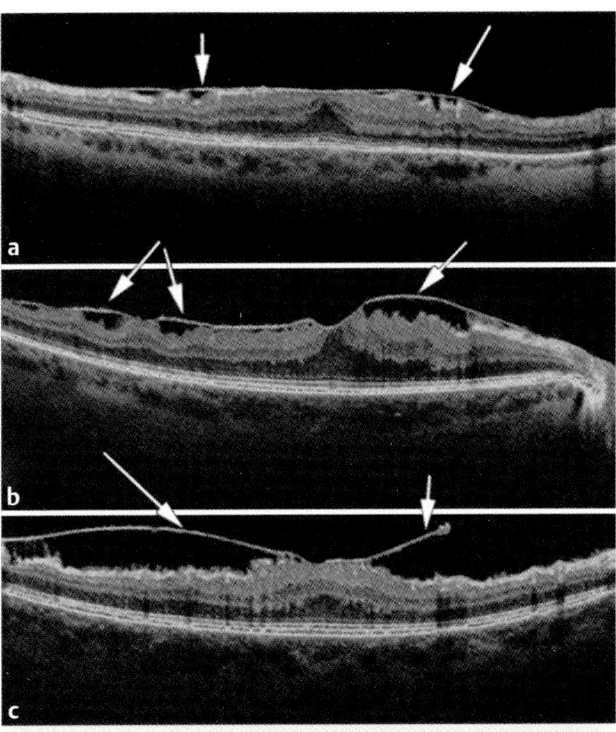

Fig. 21.14 (a-c) Epiretinal membranes are visible as a highly reflective layer on the inner retinal Surface (arrows) on these spectral-domain optical coherence tomography images.

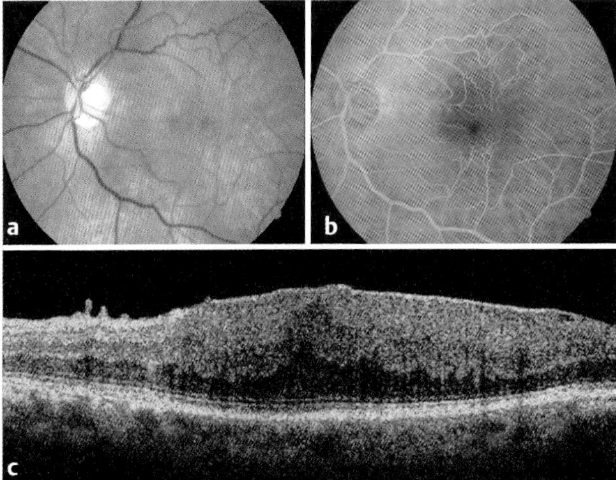

Fig. 21.16 (a) Color photograph of an epiretinal membrane. Vascular traction and loss of foveal reflex are observed. **(b)** Late fluorescein angiography demonstrates macular edema and vascular traction secondary to the epiretinal membrane. **(c)** Spectral-domain optical coherence tomography shows a continuous and adherent epiretinal membrane. Diverse and severe edematous changes in the inner nuclear layer, outer plexiform layer and outer nuclear layer are seen on this OCT. When the membrane is globally attached to the inner retina, the surgeon may anticipate more difficulty in peeling the membrane.

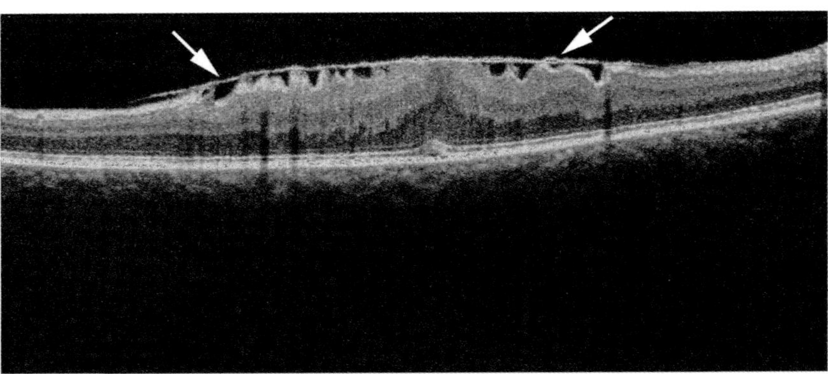

Fig. 21.15 When the surgeon observes a separation between the epiretinal membrane and the retina, surgery may be directed to these areas to initiate membrane dissection. Note the separated extreme of the epiretinal membrane from underlying retina.

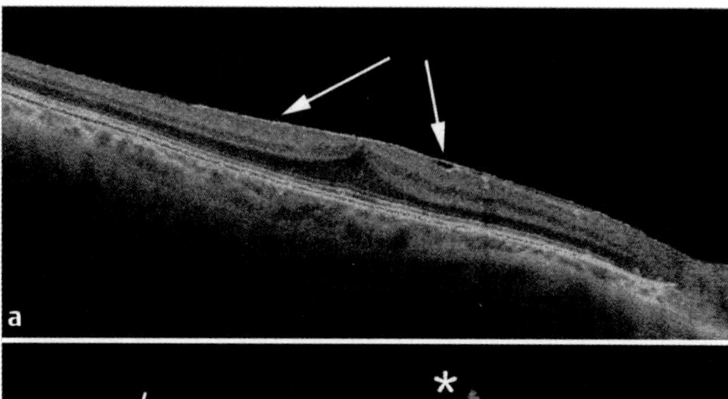

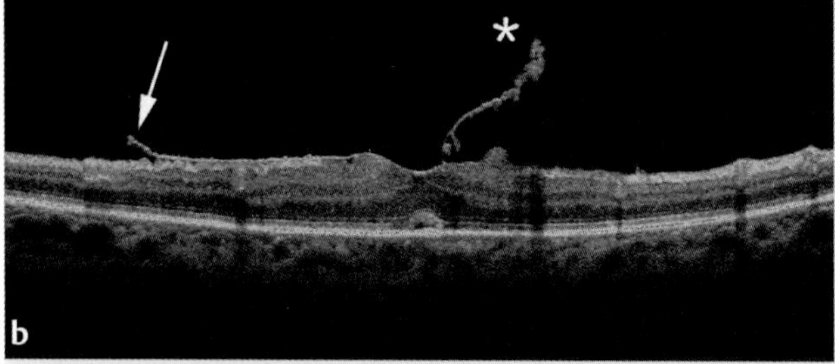

Fig. 21.17 (a) When epiretinal membrane is globally attached to the inner retina, the surgeon may anticipate more difficulty in peeling this type of membrane. **(b)** Partially adherent epiretinal membrane (arrow) and a total detachment of the ERM in the other extreme of the membrane (asterisk).

21.1.4 Vitreomacular Traction Syndrome

As the vitreous liquefies with age, it detaches from the macula; this natural progression has been demonstrated using OCT in normal eyes.[49] However, in some people, an abnormally strong adhesion is present between the vitreous cortex and the macula, and as the vitreous detaches peripherally, it continues to pull on focal areas of the macula. This configuration appears identical to the vitreous attachment identified in idiopathic macular hole and cystoid macular edema or submacular fluid. Macular thickening caused by continued pathologic adherence of the vitreous to the retina in the setting of a peripheral vitreous detachment has been termed *vitreomacular traction syndrome* (VMTS).[50]

First described in 1865 by Iwanoff,[51] VMTS refers to conditions in which retinal changes develop from incomplete posterior vitreous detachment with persistent vitreous adhesion to the macula leading to morphologic distortion of the retinal surface as a result of the proliferation of myofibroblasts and the contractile element of the ERM,[52] followed by functional changes such as metamorphopsia and visual deterioration. In a few of these eyes, the vitreous eventually separates from the macula on its own, leading to spontaneous resolution of vitreoretinal traction with normalization of the retinal contour and restoration of visual acuity. These changes have been documented with OCT.[53] However, in some eyes, vitreomacular traction persists and can lead to progressive retinal edema, metamorphopsia, and/or visual deterioration. In these cases, vitrectomy may be an effective treatment option for patients with persistent and symptomatic vitreomacular traction diagnosed biomicroscopically.[54] Although the vitreous attachment to the macula usually appears broad on clinical examination, OCT typically shows an incomplete v-shaped posterior vitreous detachment temporally and nasally to the fovea but with the fovea remaining attached (▶ Fig. 21.18). Early stages of PVD not detected biomicroscopically have been shown using OCT in normal subjects.[49] Therefore, in all cases with vitreoretinal interface abnormalities, OCT is extremely useful for diagnosis and follow-up after treatment of these diseases. OCT images of the interface between the macula and vitreous are very well defined because of the difference in reflectivity of the relatively acellular vitreous and parallel-fiber orientation of the inner retina.[9] PVD is visible on the OCT image as a thin, moderately reflective band suspended above the macular surface when it separates from the retina (▶ Fig. 21.19).[55]

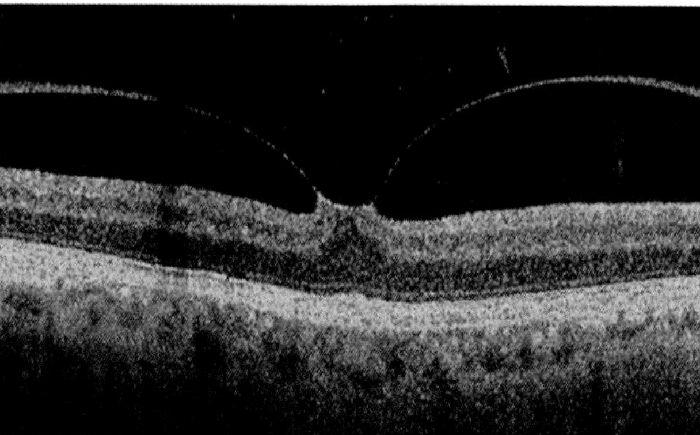

Fig. 21.18 Optical coherence tomography typically shows an incomplete v-shaped posterior vitreous detachment temporally and nasally to the fovea which remains attached to the posterior vitreous.

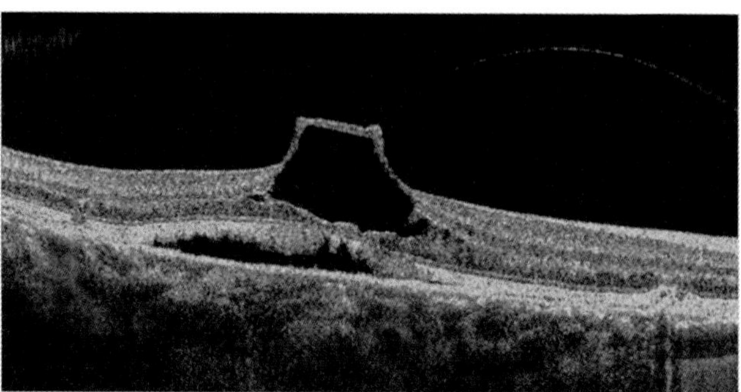

Fig. 21.19 An incomplete posterior vitreous detachment with vitreomacular traction and tractional foveal detachment is observed on this optical coherence tomography image.

Vitreomacular traction syndrome differs from idiopathic ERM in that the posterior hyaloid, rather than being totally detached from the posterior retina surface, remains attached to the perifoveal region. It is also frequently attached at the optic nerve or at multiple other points along or inside the vascular arcades. Sometimes the vitreous adherence can be difficult or impossible to identify directly on clinical examination (▶ Fig. 21.20). In VMTS, the PVD frequently is less reflective than ERMs (▶ Fig. 21.21) and is associated with substantial foveal traction, intraretinal cystoid changes, cystoid macular edema, and foveal detachment. These changes result in central vision loss and metamorphopsia.

Other VMTS cases can have a PVD temporally to the fovea but no posterior vitreous detachment nasal to it. In these cases,

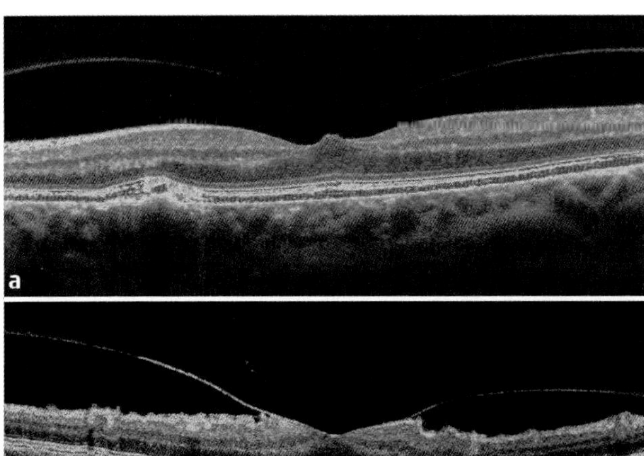

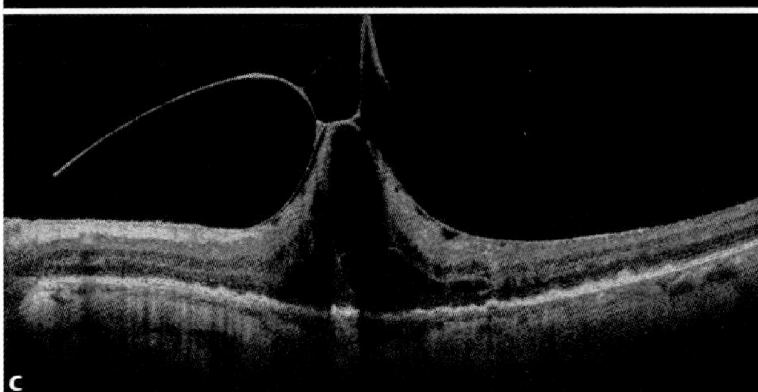

Fig. 21.20 **(a)** Spectral-domain optical coherence tomography demonstrating partial posterior vitreous detachment (PVD) with vitreofoveal traction and alteration of normal foveal architecture. **(b)** Partial PVD with a broad-based vitreous attachment to the fovea. **(c)** PVD with a macular detachment secondary to a large vitreous foveal traction is observed. A tent-like appearance of the tractional macular detachment is seen.

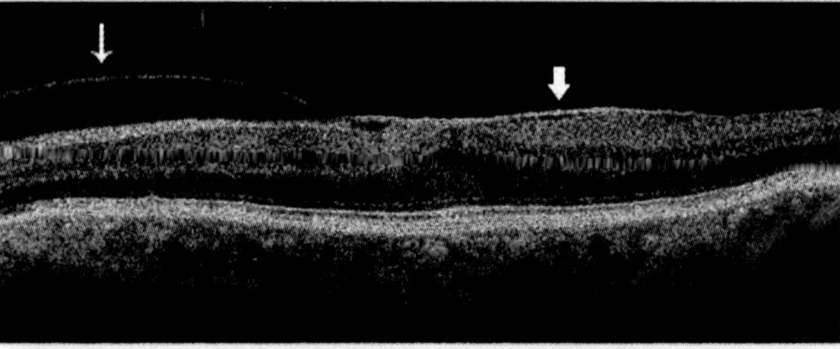

Fig. 21.21 Partial posterior vitreous detachment (thin arrow) is seen as a hyperreflective line above the retina and thinner than the epiretinal membrane (thick arrow). Epiretinal membranes are visible as a highly reflective layer on the inner retinal surface (thick arrow).

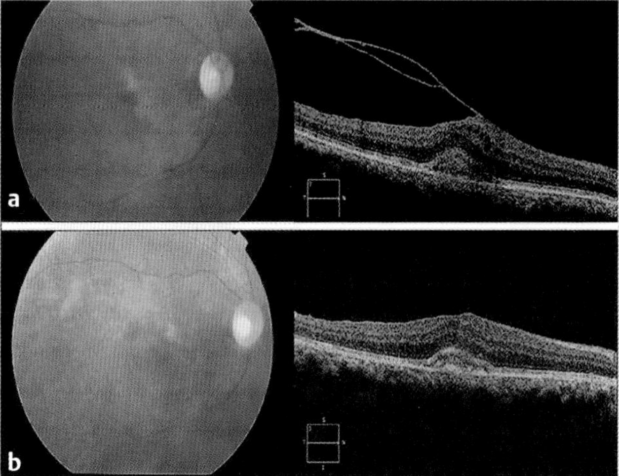

Fig. 21.22 **(a)** Preoperative optical coherence tomography (OCT) showed vitreomacular traction with attachment of the posterior hyaloid to the fovea. The tractional forces from the vitreous lead to the formation of macular edema and accumulation of subfoveal pseudovitelliform yellowish material. **(b)** Postoperative OCT demonstrates relief of the vitreomacular traction after surgery and a reduction on both macular edema and the subfoveal pseudovitelliform yellowish material.

prominent cystoid macular edema may develop, which may result in a macular hole or macular atrophy.[56] On the other hand, persistent traction can lead to progressive retinal edema and thickening. Quantifying such changes with OCT can be valuable in determining the need and timing of surgical intervention. As with ERMs, OCT can provide useful information in counseling VMTS patients preoperatively with regard to visual potential. Eyes demonstrating massive traction, distortion of retinal architecture, intraretinal edema, and foveal detachment may be anticipated to have a relatively poor ultimate outcome compared with eyes not exhibiting these features. After surgery, OCT can be used to evaluate the anatomic response (▶ Fig. 21.22). Case reports in the literature have documented improved retinal anatomy in association with increased visual acuity after vitrectomy surgery.[49,57]

High-resolution OCT has several advantages for a detailed evaluation of VMTS: raster scans provide a precise 2- and 3-D image of the vitreomacular interface at each location. The high-resolution representation of all intraretinal layers identifies the level and location of alteration in functionally relevant structures, such as the neurosensory architecture and the photoreceptor layer.[34,58] Other advantages of SD OCT are improved axial resolution, higher scan speed, and the possibility of scanning the entire macular area at each location using the raster mode. These improvements enable better reproducibility of the same area of interest at each visit and therefore enable superior results in a study aimed at evaluating distinct morphologic changes over time.

Recently, Sayegh et al[58] published a prospective analysis of the functional and morphologic parameters of retinal integrity over a 2-year follow-up of 30 patients undergoing vitreoretinal surgery for VMTS guided by high-resolution SD OCT imaging. They observed that the best-corrected visual acuity did not correlate significantly with central retinal thickness (CRT) or retinal volume (RV); thus, a specific reduction of CRT and RV has no significant effect on visual function. This result is consistent with the study by Haouchine et al,[22] who measured central foveal thickness and reported no correlation with best-corrected visual acuity (BCVA). Furthermore, no correlation was found between the shape of the foveal contour, the presence of foveal cysts, or other morphologic parameters with BCVA.

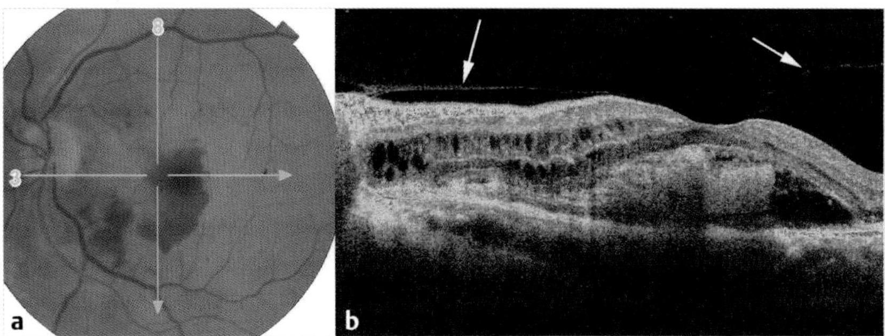

Fig. 21.23 (a) Color fundus photograph demonstrates retinal hemorrhages and macular edema secondary to exudative maculopathy. (b) Spectral-domain optical coherence tomography shows vitreomacular adhesion (arrow) with inner retinal changes in exudative age-related macular degeneration case.

The presence of the ERM induces folding and contraction of the retinal surface and surgical release, including the internal limiting membrane, results in a rapid and impressive restoration of the retinal surface with disappearance of folds and reformation of the foveal contour. These morphologic changes seem to precede functional recovery. Visual rehabilitation proceeds over several months, reaching significance as late as 6 months after surgery. The integrity of the inner and, most importantly, the outer retinal layer follows a prolonged pattern of recovery as well. Recovery of inner and outer retinal layer proceeds slowly, reaching significance at 12 months, and correlated strongly with visual function. Therefore, reconstitution of neurosensory layers may be the most relevant parameter for visual improvement.

Vitreomacular Traction and Age-Related Macular Degeneration

Vitreomacular traction alone is perhaps not able to induce AMD. However, it would seem sensible to consider vitreous changes when diagnosing and treating AMD patients because of the high coincidence of VMT and choroidal neovascularization (CNV) and the often successful treatment of other diseases of the vitreoretinal interface by vitrectomy. The concept of the pathogenesis of AMD should therefore be extended to include the influence of the vitreous, especially where therapeutic concepts such as pharmacologic vitreolysis and vitreous separation have been established as causative treatment of late forms of AMD.[59]

Krebs et al described the presence of vitreomacular adhesions in 36% of eyes with exudative AMD, significantly more frequently than in eyes with nonexudative AMD or control eyes (▶ Fig. 21.23).[60] These results were confirmed by Robison et al, who found vitreomacular adhesion (VMA) in 38% of eyes with exudative AMD[61] and by Lee et al,[62] who found VMA in 22.3% associated with neovascular AMD. These studies used primarily Stratus OCT examinations to verify VMA. Owing to the TD technology of Stratus OCT, differentiation between adhesion and traction was difficult, although traction was suspected in more than 50% of the cases. Signs of traction could clearly be identified in both SD OCT machines, the Spectralis and Cirrus OCT. Especially in the high-definition scans (five lines 6 mm long each in the Cirrus OCT and one single line 8 mm long each in the Spectralis OCT) the angulation of the posterior vitreous cortex was clearly visible. Furthermore, 3-D OCT shows splitting within the posterior vitreous cortex in the area of vitreopapillary adhesion and traction from different directions. 3-D OCT imaging was possible in most (83.3%) of the Cirrus OCT cube scans, but with Spectralis OCT volume scans, only 13.3% was sufficient scan density possible.

Krebs et al[63] identified traction with adhesions in 73.3% of cases with exudative AMD, and they showed that the location and the direction of the traction forces visualized by high-technology OCT and 3D-OCT correspond in 100% with the origin of the CNV.

21.1.5 Age-Related Macular Degeneration

Despite recent progress, AMD remains the leading cause of irreversible blindness among individuals older than 60 years in industrialized countries.[64] Cigarette smoking, genetic factors, aging, ischemia, and environmental characteristics are considered the main important etiologic factors of AMD.[64] Other additional factors influencing the development of exudative AMD include changes at the vitreomacular interface confirmed by OCT in several studies.[65,66] Early non-neovascular AMD is characterized by accumulation of macular drusen and changes in pigmentation, whereas late AMD progresses to geographic atrophy, neovascularization, and severe loss of central vision.

Diagnostic Methods

Fundus imaging provides an important contribution to the early and precise detection and diagnosis of AMD. Color fundus photographs and autofluorescence images document anatomical landmarks to monitor the progression of signs of AMD with its exudative and hemorrhagic complications. However, only angiographic methods can directly visualize CNV; fluorescein angiography (FA) demonstrates classic CNV, and indocyanine-green angiography can better demonstrate occult CNV.

Currently, determination of whether CNV is classic in type or an occult CNV is no longer necessary for the initiation of treatment because the management of AMD therapy with antiangiogenic agents now largely involves determining whether or not CNV exists, regardless of type.

Optical coherence tomography continues to evolve, with image resolution improving from 5 to 10 µm using TD techniques to less than 5 µm using SD techniques.[67] Most importantly, OCT is able to demonstrate the exudative component related to abnormal permeability of CNV. SD OCT techniques can also directly analyze the impact of CNV on outer retinal layers and evaluate alterations of photoreceptors and inner and outer segments.

For nearly every aspect of AMD management, OCT is critical. Although OCT can be useful in the diagnosis of non-neovascular

AMD, the true value of OCT is apparent in the management of neovascular AMD because OCT can help establish treatment and retreatment guidelines and help monitor treatment failure or success. This technology can identify indirect signs related to abnormal exudation, such as intraretinal fluid or increased retinal thickness, and it can be used to characterize drusen, geography atrophy, choroidal and subretinal neovascularization, neurosensory retinal detachment, and pigment epithelial detachments (PEDs) associated with AMD.[68] Therefore, OCT has become an essential part of the examination in routine follow-up for AMD to guide clinical practice and analyze the response to treatment.

Previously, when considering retreatment for AMD, FA was commonly used as an indicator of CNV activity; however, several reports have indicated poor agreement in the interpretation of FA in AMD, especially after intravitreal treatment.[69,70] Treatment of CNV with vascular endothelial growth factor inhibitors requires monthly evaluation of the activity of the lesion to support the decision for retreatment, and OCT can be quite useful.[71]

Recent studies have validated a good agreement in interpretation of Stratus (Carl Zeiss Meditech, Dublin, CA) TD OCT images between observers and good correlation between FA and TD OCT in terms of retinal thickness, subretinal fluid thickness, and CNV thickness.[69,72] According to several studies, OCT might partially replace FA in the follow-up of exudative AMD.[73,74]

Tomographic Characteristics in Age-Related Macular Degeneration

Geographic atrophy

Geographic atrophy is a significant cause of both moderate and severe central visual loss and is bilateral in most patients with advanced AMD. It represents the loss of photoreceptors, retinal pigment epithelium, and choriocapillaris within the macula. Geographic atrophy is highly distinctive on OCT because the overlying retina is thinned and the hypopigmented retinal pigment epithelium (RPE) causes increased penetration of the optical probe beam into the deeper choroid, significantly enhancing the reflections from this layer. The intense back shadowing in zones of atrophy, extending well into the choroid is the defining sign of atrophy. Another sign on OCT is thinning of the neurosensory retina over zones of atrophy, which is particularly serious when it involves the central zone. In addition, there are no exudative signs. Thinning and loss of the RPE are clearly visualized, but maintenance of the straight line representing Bruch membrane is an important sign (▶ Fig. 21.24, ▶ Fig. 21.25). In the most severe forms, the outer nuclear layer is no longer visible in the zones of atrophy. RPE atrophy is irreversible and causes death of almost all photoreceptors in the atrophic area, resulting in a corresponding scotoma.

Because of the current absence of effective treatment, dry AMD has a poor prognosis, despite the hopes raised by a recognized clinical trial (the Age-Related Eye Disease Study Research Group), which demonstrated the benefits of antioxidants, vitamin A, and vitamin C supplements. Dietary antioxidant supplementation reduced the risk of severe vision loss in intermediate forms of dry AMD and severe AMD, but it produced no conclusive effect on primary prevention of early AMD.[75,76]

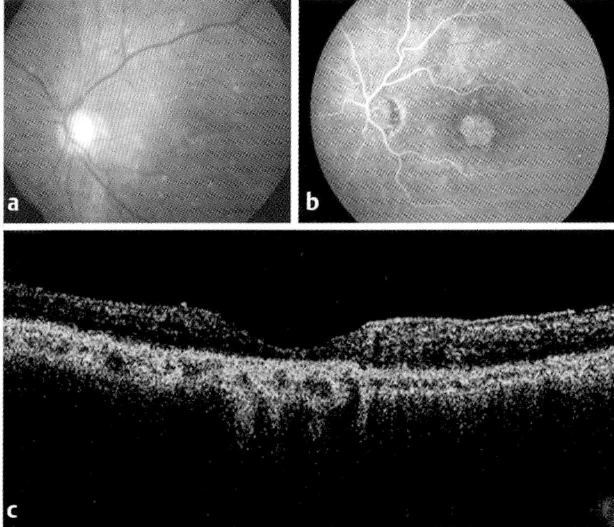

Fig. 21.24 **(a)** Color fundus photograph of geographic atrophy secondary to age-related macular degeneration showed a rounded, depigmented area with well-defined margins. **(b)** Fluorescein angiography demonstrated hyperfluorescence due to a window defect. **(c)** Stratus optical coherence tomography image. Note the backscatter in zones of atrophy with marked hyperreflectivity and retinal thinning in the entire zone of atrophy.

Drusen Analysis

Despite great advances in fundus image analysis in the past 20 years, with the development of various manual and automated

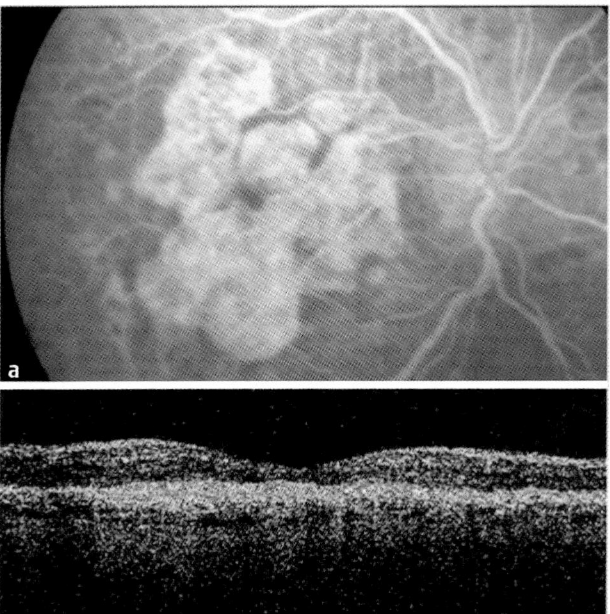

Fig. 21.25 Geographic atrophy. **(a)** Fluorescein angiography demonstrated hyperfluorescence resulting from a window defect and central sparing. **(b)** Stratus optical coherence tomography image shows a significant loss of the outer nuclear layer, photoreceptors, and retinal pigment epithelium, leading to significant hyperreflectivity and backscatter within the choroid.

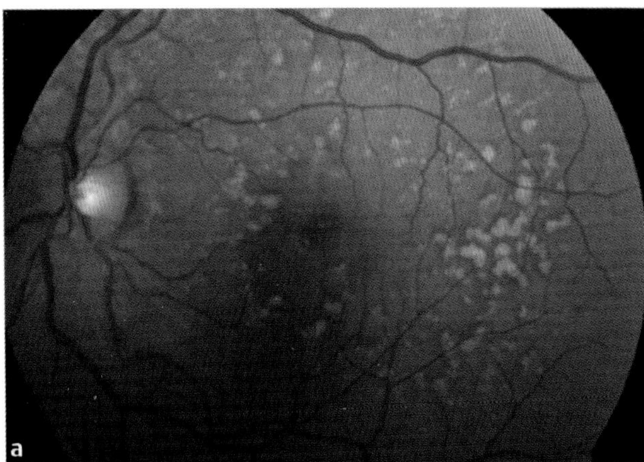

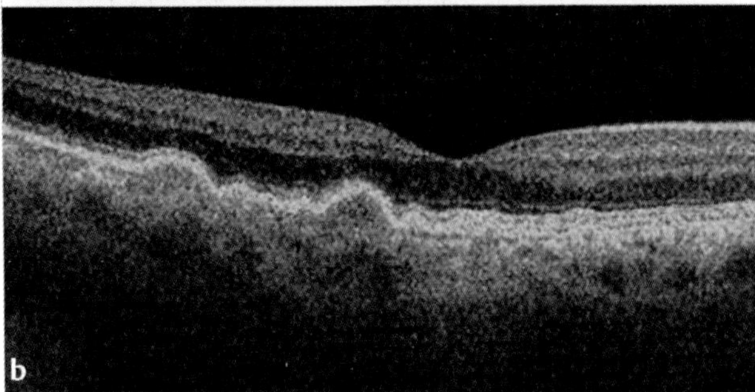

Fig. 21.26 (a) Color photograph. **(b)** Cirrus optical coherence tomography image. A drusenoid pigment epithelial detachment is a fairly well circumscribed, shallow and often multiple elevation of the reflective band corresponding to the retinal pigment epithelium/choriocapillaris complex, formed by one or more large drusen or as a result of the slow coalescence of soft drusen.

tools for drusen analysis, fundus photos have been the mainstay of drusen characterization until the introduction of OCT. These tools are capable of providing qualitative and quantitative analysis of drusen changes.

Gass noted that an increase in drusen area was associated with higher risk of progression to advanced AMD.[77] Several published studies have also shown that greater drusen diameter and area may be associated with a significant risk of progression to advanced AMD over 5 years.[78,79,80] Small, hard drusen are considered an early sign of AMD.[81] Large numbers of hard drusen have been shown to progress to geographic atrophy.[82] In the Blue Mountains Eye study, eyes with large soft drusen were 6 times more likely to develop advanced AMD compared with eyes without such drusen.[83,84,85] Approximately 25% of large drusen present at baseline may fade over the 10 years of follow-up in the absence of apparent clinical progression of AMD.[86,87]

Soft drusen are observed as focal elevations in the external highly reflective band (RPE-choriocapillaris complex), consistent with the accumulation of amorphous material within or beneath the Bruch membrane. SD OCT has been consistently able to identify morphologic parameters of drusen ultrastructure, which can be used to understand more clearly the natural history of drusen (▶ Fig. 21.26) and monitor drusen change in patients undergoing treatment.

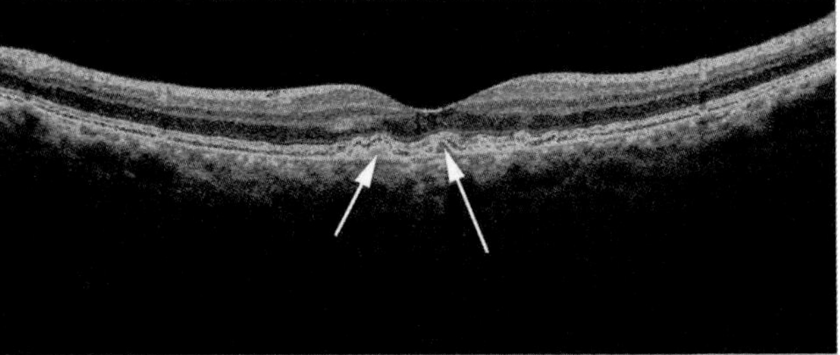

Fig. 21.27 Cirrus optical coherence tomography image. A drusenoid pigment epithelial detachment is a fairly well-circumscribed, shallow, and often multiple elevation of the reflective band (arrows) corresponding to the retinal pigment epithelium/choriocapillaris complex, formed by one or more large drusen or as a result of the slow coalescence of soft drusen.

Pigment Epithelial Detachment

A retinal pigment epithelial (RPE) detachment (PED) is formed by the separation of the RPE from the Bruch membrane as a result of the presence of sub-RPE fluid, blood, fibrovascular membrane, or drusenoid material.[88,89] PED is an important predictor of vision loss in patients with AMD. Around half of patients with a newly diagnosed PED will experience an average visual loss of more than three lines over 1-year of follow-up.[90] Four main types of PEDs are found in patients with AMD: drusenoid, serous, fibrovascular, and hemorrhagic. PEDs are a common presentation of neovascular AMD, seen in up to 62% of eyes with evidence of advanced AMD by FA.[65]

A drusenoid PED is a fairly well-circumscribed, shallow, and often multiple elevation of the reflective band corresponding to the RPE-choriocapillaris complex, formed by one or more large drusen or as a result of the slow coalescence of soft drusen[89,91] (▶ Fig. 21.27). It has been distinguished from the other types of PED by its relatively better prognosis.[92] However, the natural history usually follows progression to persistent drusenoid PED, geographic atrophy, and neovascularization (▶ Fig. 21.28, ▶ Fig. 21.29).[93,94]

Drusenoid PED has a particular evolution and potential risks for severe loss of visual acuity, and it should be considered a subgroup of AMD. Recently, antivascular endothelial growth factor therapy[95,96,97] has shown variable anatomical and visual outcomes in patients with symptomatic drusenoid PED without choroidal neovascularization in AMD (▶ Fig. 21.30).

Serous PEDs are sharply demarcated, smooth, dome-shaped elevations of the RPE.[98] By OCT, a serous PED is identified as a smooth, domed elevation of the RPE with a characteristic sharp angle of pigment epithelial layer detachment over an optically empty space bound inferiorly by a visible Bruch membrane (▶ Fig. 21.31).[91] Classically, the edges of the dome are sharply demarcated. An area of active neovascularization associated with a serous PED may lead to an associated smaller cuff of subretinal and intraretinal fluid that buttresses the serous PED, a characteristic finding on OCT cross-section (▶ Fig. 21.32, ▶ Fig. 21.33). With antivascular endothelial growth factor (anti-VEGF) therapy, this area of subretinal fluid will often improve despite persistence of the associated PED.

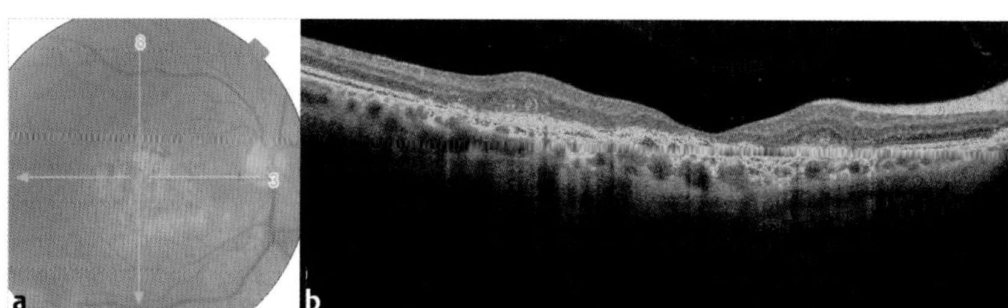

Fig. 21.28 **(a)** Color photograph shows macular atrophy secondary to persistent drusenoid pigment epithelial detachment. **(b)** Spectral-domain optical coherence tomography image demonstrates a band of hyperreflectivity and retinal thinning in the zone of atrophy.

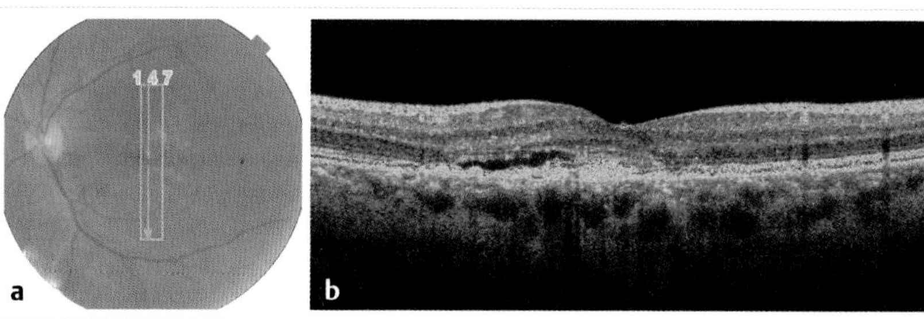

Fig. 21.29 **(a)** Color photograph of coalescence of soft drusen in the posterior pole. **(b)** Multiple drusenoid pigment epithelial detachments with subretinal fluid secondary to choroidal neovascularization.

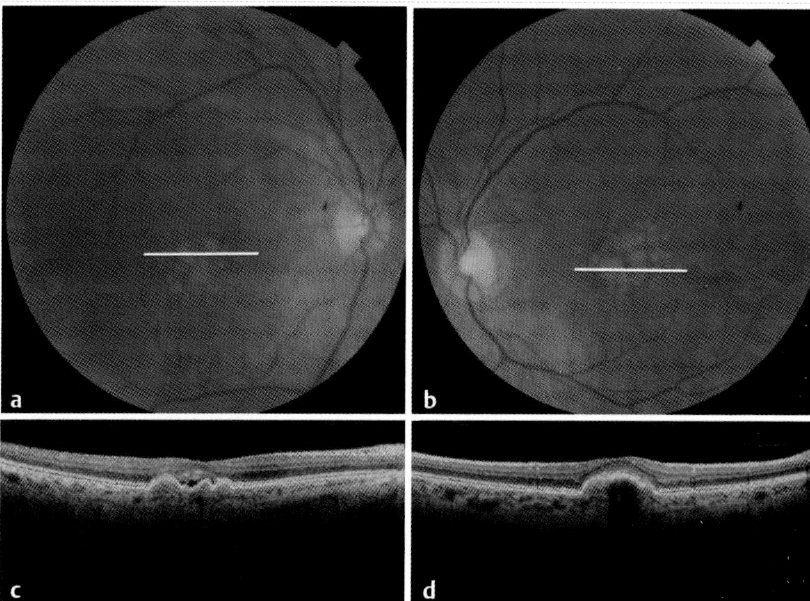

Fig. 21.30 **(a,b)** Color photograph of bilateral soft drussen in the macular area. **(c)** Spectral-domain optical coherence tomography (OCT) image shows a multiple drusenoid pigment epithelial detachmentswith the presence of subretinal fluid without choridal neovascularization. **(d)** A large subfoveal drusenoid pigment epithelial detachment is seen on this OCT image of the fellow eye.

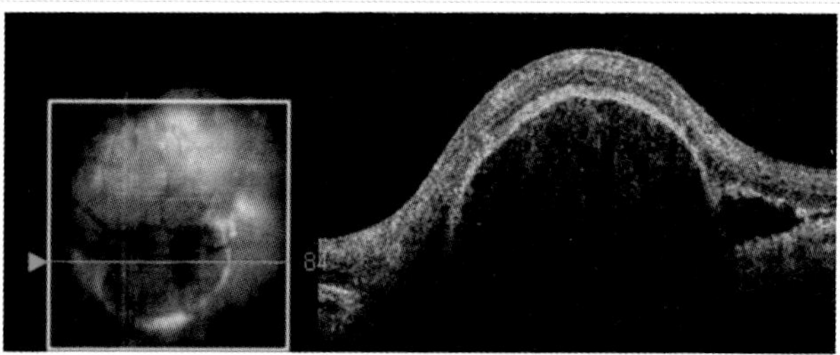

Fig. 21.31 In this Cirrus optical coherence tomography image, we can see the sharply demarcated classic edges of the dome on a serous pigment epithelial detachment.

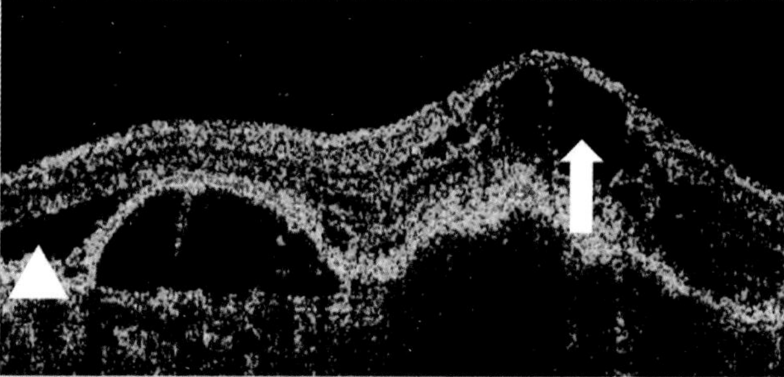

Fig. 21.32 An area of active neovascularization associated with a pigment epithelial detachment may lead to an associated smaller cuff of subretinal (arrowhead) and intraretinal (thin arrow) fluid.

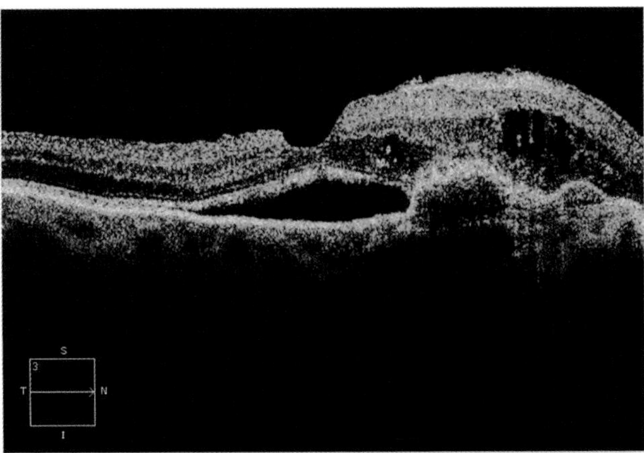

Fig. 21.33 The serous retinal detachment is an optically empty, black, spindle-shaped zone between the retinal pigment epithelium and the neurosensory retina. Anteriorly, the retina is thickened and infiltrated with several central cysts. Posteriorly, a pigment epithelium detachment can be seen, suggesting the presence of an occult choroidal neovascularization.

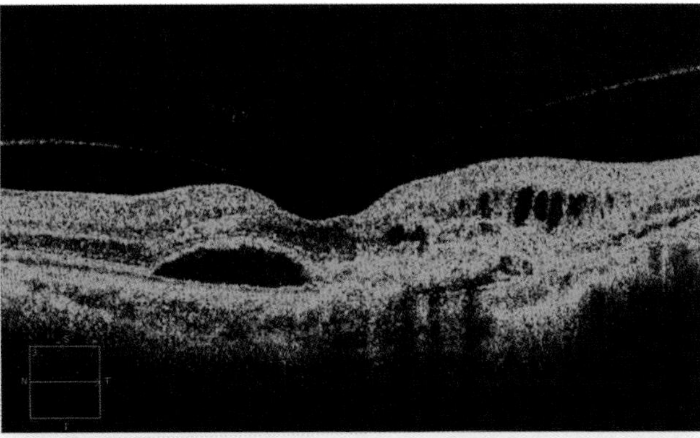

Fig. 21.34 The combination of a pigment epithelium detachment with accompanying subretinal fluid and intraretinal fluid may be a sign of choroidal neovascularization or retinal angiomatous proliferation in this Cirrus optical coherence tomography image.

Similarly, the combination of a PED with accompanying subretinal fluid and intraretinal fluid may be a sign of CNV or retinal angiomatous proliferation (RAP) (▶ Fig. 21.34). In distinction from CNV-associated serous PEDs, RAP-associated serous PEDs are almost always accompanied by overlying intraretinal cystic fluid.[99]

Certain OCT characteristics of serous PED may also help indicate whether the PED is related to AMD or to central serous chorioretinopathy (CSCR), another condition associated with serous RPE elevation and uncommonly associated with CNV. In a retrospective comparison of 100 eyes with either CSCR or neovascular AMD, Cho et al found that AMD eyes could be distinguished by the presence of intraretinal fluid ($P < 0.0001$), greater PED height (354 ± 35 µm in AMD vs 187 ± 39 µm in CSCR, $P < 0\ .002$), and alterations of the highly reflective line (irregularity, thickening, and attenuation) seen on TD OCT ($P < 0.0001$).[100]

Hemorrhagic PEDs occur when a CNV membrane bleeds into the sub-RPE space or as a result of an RPE tear. Hemorrhage may also invade the subretinal space, with sub-RPE blood having a typically darker appearance than subretinal blood. Hemorrhage associated with PED increases the suspicion for an occult CNV not seen on examination or OCT. The blood may also be located in both the subretinal and sub-RPE layers. The challenge in the treatment of hemorrhagic PEDs is that the CNV lesion cannot be directly visualized because of the presence of overlying hemorrhage. Hemorrhagic PEDs have a similar ophthalmoscopic character to serous PEDs, with a smooth, domed, and well-demarcated elevation, but with a dark gray or black color indicating the presence of blood.[92] In contrast to the other PEDs, imaging of hemorrhagic PEDs with FA will show blockage through all phases. If an associated CNV is located completely beneath the blood, it might not be visualized by FA because of blocking.

As with serous PEDs, hemorrhagic PEDs will often show a dome-shaped elevation of the RPE external reflective band; however, because of the optical opacification secondary to the highly pigmented and, therefore, reflective hemorrhage, the deepest posterior structures such as the choroid are blocked and not visualized. Therefore, subretinal hemorrhage leads to significant shadowing of posterior layers. Occult CNV is more commonly identified on OCT as a fibrovascular PED. The fibrovascular PED is not the typical dome-shaped elevation of the RPE/Bruch membrane/choriocapillaris external band with serous PED. The elevations are often irregular, and the interior of the detachment is often filled with backscattering material, consistent with the fibrous nature of the PED. Subretinal fluid appears as an optically transparent area geographically close to the CNV between the RPE/Bruch membrane/ choriocapillaris band and the posterior edge of the neurosensory retina.

Neovascular Age-Related Macular Degeneration

Although no definitive consensus exists for the histopathologic and clinical correlation of classic and occult CNV to the Gass classification of type I and type II membranes, some evidence exists that classic CNV is more commonly type I and that occult is more commonly type II (▶ Fig. 21.35).[101]

The advances in AMD treatment with anti-VEGF therapy have largely diminished the importance of the traditional fluorescein categories of CNV. OCT can be used to differentiate classic from occult CNV. Classic CNV membranes typically show a diffusely backscattering fusiform thickening in the RPE/Bruch membrane/choriocapillaris external band in the geographic area where the membrane is seen. It is characterized by increased optical reflectivity of the RPE or disruption of the highly reflective band layer RPE/choriocapillaris. Sometimes the parts of the external band may appear redundant or duplicated. Subretinal fluid and intraretinal fluid in the form of cystoid macular edema is often present (▶ Fig. 21.36, ▶ Fig. 21.37).[102] In contrast, occult subretinal neovascularization tends to show an irregular elevation of the RPE with a deeper area of mild backscattering corresponding to fibrous proliferation (▶ Fig. 21.38, ▶ Fig. 21.39, ▶ Fig. 21.40). *End-stage* means that the leaking or bleeding has stopped and has left a fibrous scar in the macula (▶ Fig. 21.41, ▶ Fig. 21.42).

Use of OCT is valuable in quantitatively evaluating the differences in macular morphology in eyes with polypoidal choroidal

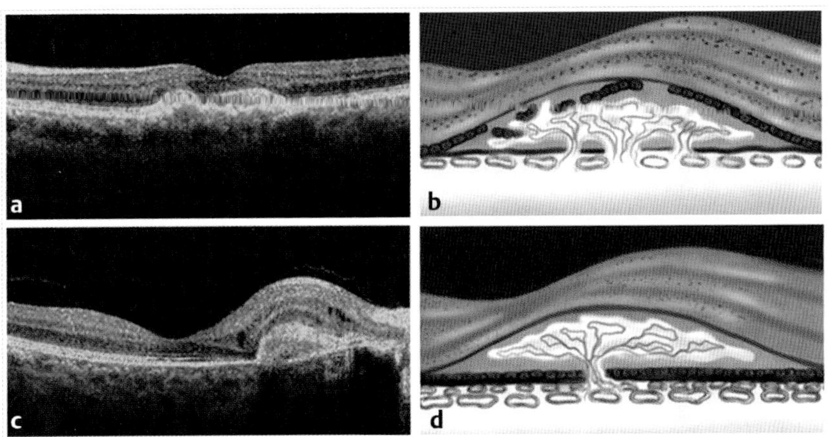

Fig. 21.35 The histopathologic (artist representation) and clinical correlation of occult and classic choroidal neovascularization to the Gass classification of type I **(a,b)** and type II membranes **(c,d)**.

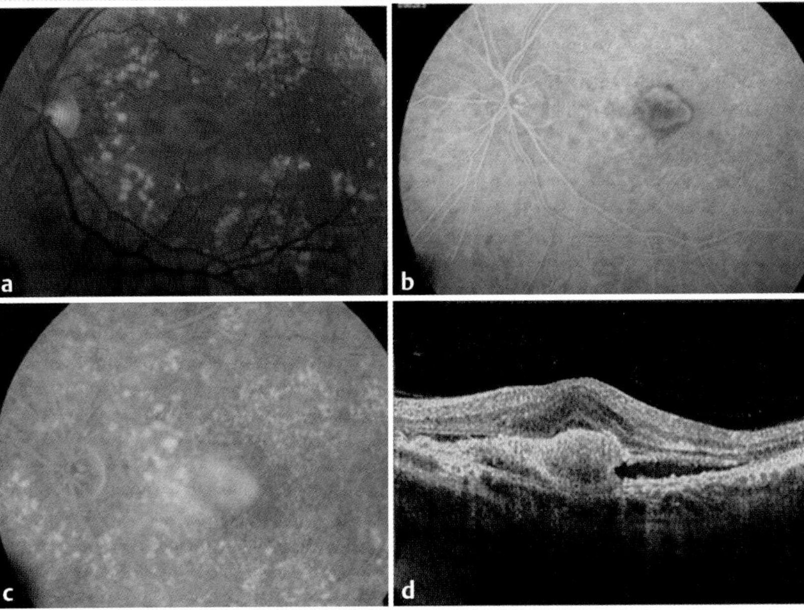

Fig. 21.36 **(a)** Fundus photography. **(b)** Fluorescein angiography at an early frame. **(c)** Fluorescein angiography at a late phase. **(d)** Cirrus optical coherence tomography image. Classic choroidal neovascular membranes typically show a diffuse backscatter and fusiform thickening in the retinal pigment epithelium/Bruch membrane/choriocapillaris external band in the area where the membrane is seen. Choroidal neovascularization induces a bulging cone-shaped zone of hyperreflectivity accompanied by posterior shadowing.

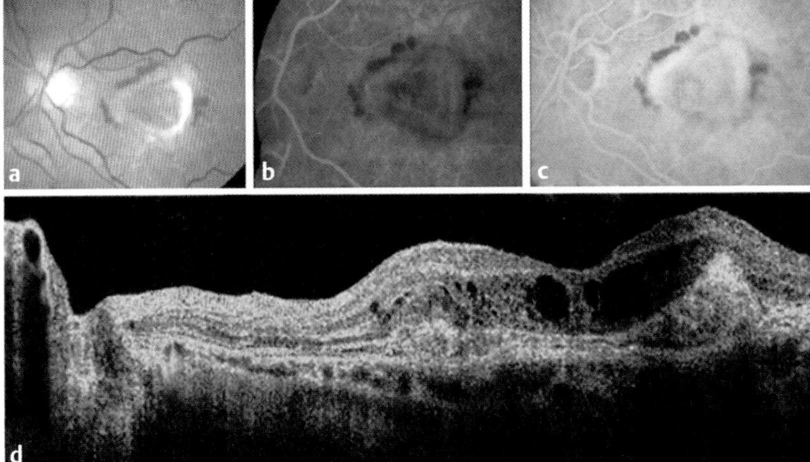

Fig. 21.37 **(a)** Fundus photography. **(b)** Fluorescein angiography at an early frame. **(c)** Fluorescein angiography at a late frame. **(d)** On Cirrus optical coherence tomography, the central retina is thickened by many well-delineated cysts, confluent in the center and associated with diffuse intraretinal fluid accumulation.

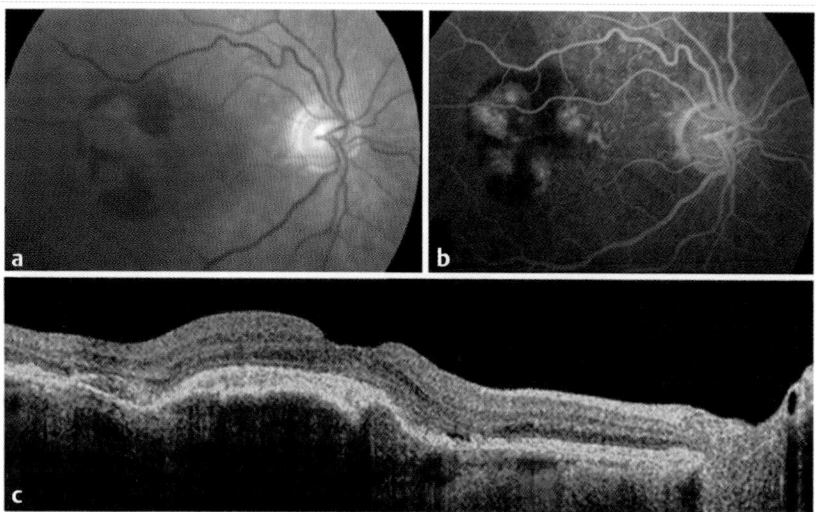

Fig. 21.38 (a) Fundus photography. (b) Fluorescein angiography at a late phase. (c) On Cirrus optical coherence tomography, occult subretinal neovascularization tends to show as an irregular elevation of the retinal pigment epithelium, with a deeper area of mild backscatter corresponding to fibrous proliferation.

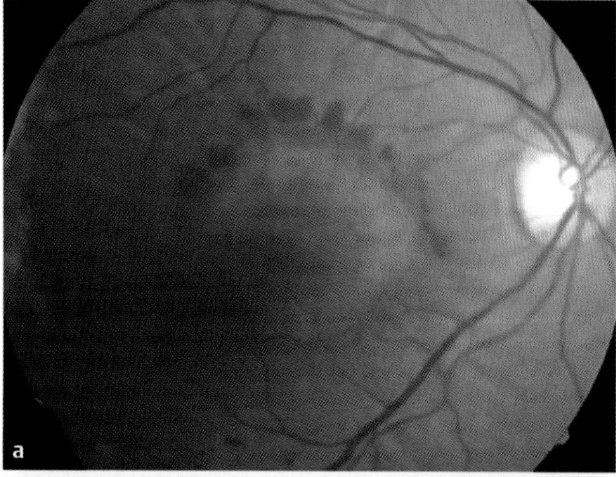

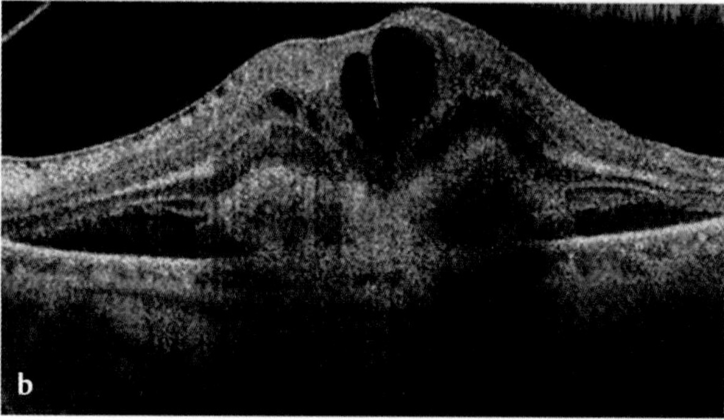

Fig. 21.39 (a) Fundus photography of subretinal neovascularization. (b) Cirrus optical coherence tomography reveals a large subretinal choroidal neovascularization with subretinal and intraretinal fluid in the macular area.

vasculopathy (PCV) from eyes with exudative AMD.[103] Ozawa et al reported that serous retinal detachments (SRDs) were observed in 53% (63/118) of eyes with exudative AMD and in 78% (69/89) of eyes with PCV ($P<0.001$). The height of the SRD was 21.9 ± 3.7 µm in eyes with exudative AMD and 56.3 ± 7.4 µm in eyes with PCV ($P<0.001$). The thickness of the neurosensory retina was 300.0 ± 5.2 µm in eyes with exudative AMD and 275.8 ± 4.7 µm in eyes with PCV ($P<0.001$). They concluded that eyes with PCV are characterized by a higher incidence of SRDs, greater SRD height, and less intraretinal edema than eyes with exudative AMD.[103]

Role of Abnormal Vitreomacular Adhesion in Age-Related Macular Degeneration

With OCT, the role of persistent vitreomacular adhesion (VMA) in the development of numerous macular pathologies— including idiopathic macular hole, vitreomacular traction syndrome, cystoid and diabetic macular edema, neovascularization in diabetic retinopathy and retinal vein occlusion, exudative AMD, and myopic traction maculopathy—has been established.

Although AMD primarily involves the outer retinal layers, several authors have suggested that the vitreous may possibly play a role in the pathogenesis and progression of AMD. A high incidence of posterior vitreous attachment was observed intraoperatively by different investigators.[104] Subsequent studies of the vitreous in AMD have been performed using ultrasound; the results of these studies suggest that complete posterior vitreous detachment occurs less frequently in AMD than in the age-matched elder normal population, and that a higher incidence of VMA is detected in both exudative and nonexudative AMD.[105,106] Hyaloid adhesion to the macula is associated with AMD and frequently causes VMT in eyes with CNV. These tractional forces may antagonize the effect of anti-VEGF treatment and cause pharmacologic resistance in a subpopulation of patients. OCT is an excellent method to allow careful diagnosis and follow-up in these cases.[107] Patients with a history of poorly responsive CNV despite aggressive anti-VEGF therapy and who show persistent attachment of hyaloid to the macula, with evidence of VMT on OCT, could be surgically treated (► Fig. 21.43, ► Fig. 21.44).

Mojana et al[107] showed that there is a higher incidence of tractional configuration of the attached posterior hyaloid in eyes with exudative AMD. Other investigators have also suggested a possible role of persistent VMA in eyes with exudative macular degeneration.[65,108]

VMTS could cause degeneration or breaks at the RPE and Bruch membrane, and the macula might be continuously exposed to free radicals and cytokines existing in the vitreous

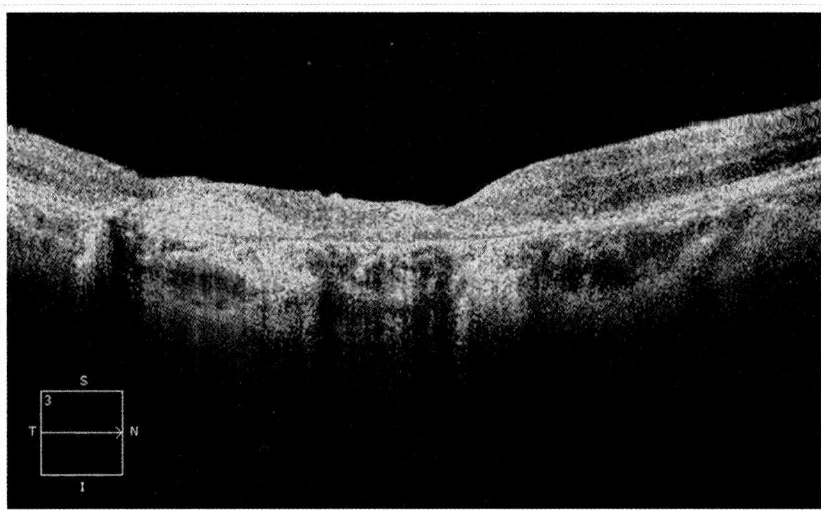

Fig. 21.40 Optical coherence tomographic image shows a hyperreflective band, suggesting residual fibrosis of classic choroidal neovascularization.

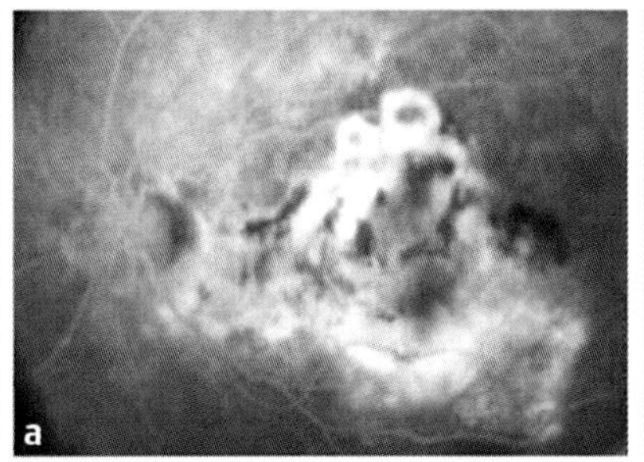

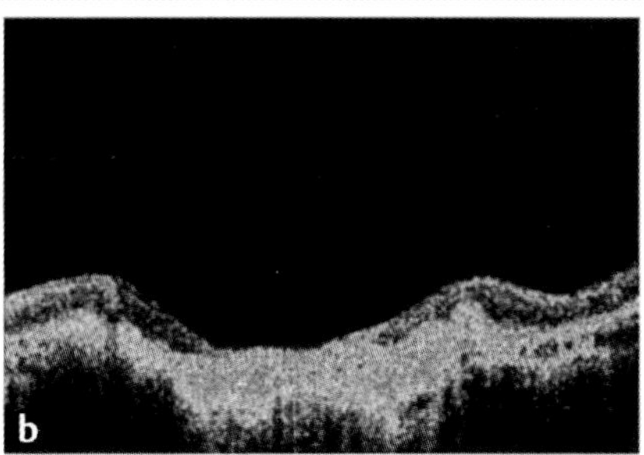

Fig. 21.41 **(a)** Angiography showed a scarred appearance of the lesion. **(b)** Stratus optical coherence tomography image showed an extensive fibrotic tissue with a complete atrophy of the outer and inner retinal layers in the macular area.

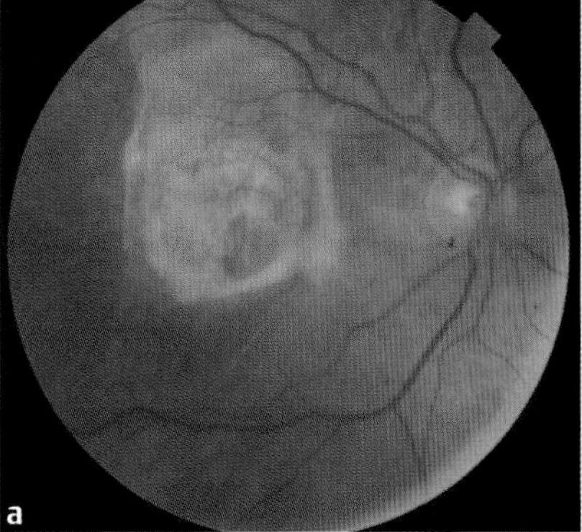

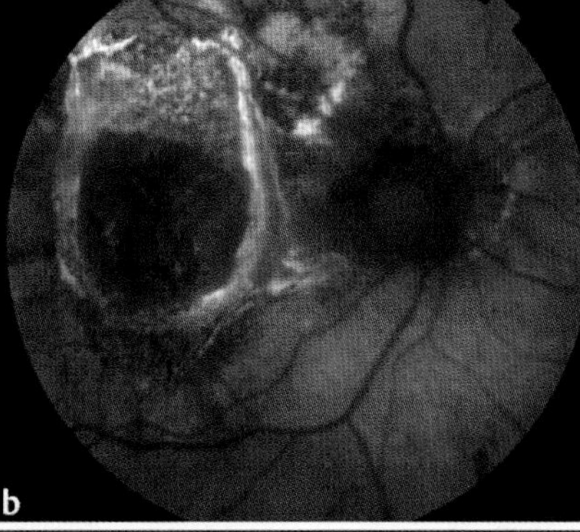

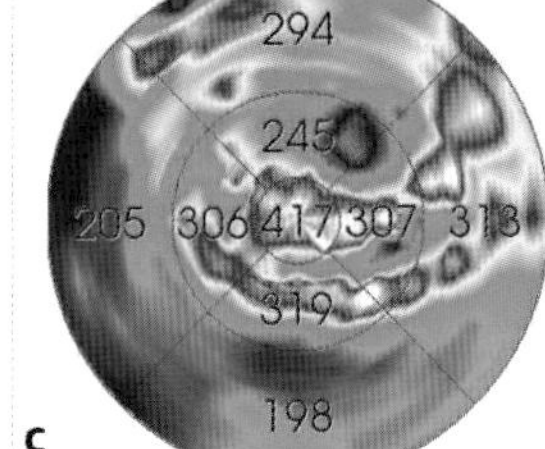

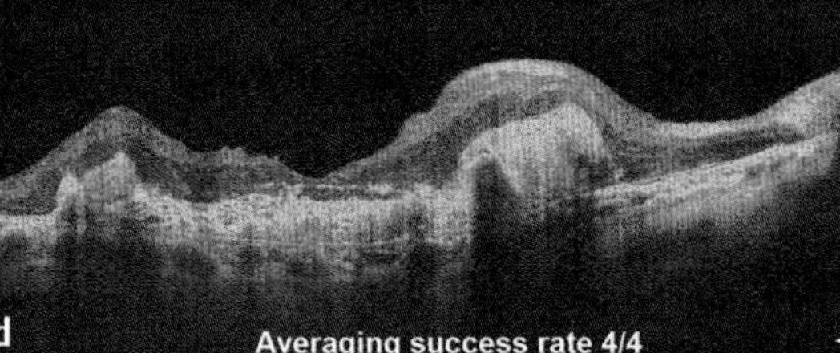

Fig. 21.42 **(a)** Fundus photography. **(b)** Fundus autofluorescence is severely decreased over the fibrotic area, which is surrounded by a rim of increased intensity. **(c)** Central macular thickness is thick. **(d)** Optical coherence tomographic image shows a hyperreflective band corresponding to subretinal residual fibrosis secondary to the end stage of age-related macular degeneration.

gel, resulting in the pathogenesis and/or progression of AMD. PVD may prevent continuous and direct exposure to these substances. It may increase the possibility of fluid circulating behind the vitreous gel over the macular area. The rapid fluid currents not only remove the waste products and toxic materials, but they also provide oxygenation and good perfusion.

Treatment of Age-Related Macular Degeneration and OCT

Laser treatment of subretinal neovascularization leads to atrophic scarring, which appears on OCT as highly reflective at the chorioretinal interface. Argon laser retinal lesions evaluated in vivo by OCT demonstrated relative high reflection in the middle of the lesion and relative low reflection around the lesion (▶ Fig. 21.45).[109]

In large multicenter studies dealing with the current treatment of exudative AMD with anti-vasoproliferative substances, a fixed treatment regimen with monthly injections was applied.[110,111] A flexible OCT-based retreatment regimen is used in new studies. Indication for retreatment is a decrease of visual acuity or an increase of retinal thickness as seen by OCT. Although new SD technology is available, Stratus OCT is still the most frequently used OCT machine in these studies. Therefore, newly planned studies will need to solve the problem of different machines with different software and different values for retinal thickness that comes with SD OCT technology.

Krebs et al[112] evaluated the repeatability and reproducibility of retinal thickness measurements in exudative AMD using Stratus OCT. A total of 200 eyes of 200 subjects with exudative AMD were examined. Macular thickness and fast macular thickness programs of Stratus OCT were performed twice by the same examiners or by two different examiners. The repeatability and reproducibility of retinal thickness measurements were high, presenting better results for the macular thickness program versus the fast macular thickness program. The reliability of retinal thickness measurement was most frequently affected by algorithm line failures and fixation problems.

Spectral-domain OCT has higher axial resolution and faster acquisition speeds compared with TD OCT that allow SD OCT to provide not only the detailed views of intraretinal microstructure but also 3-D images of the macula. Sayanagi et al[113] investigated the ability to delineate and detect the CNV activity in patients with exudative AMD treated with intravitreal injections of ranibizumab (Lucentis; Genentech, South San Francisco, CA) and found that SD OCT demonstrated a significantly better ability to delineate and detect CNV activity compared with TD OCT.[113]

Querques et al[114] studied the ability to appreciate qualitative features that indicate disease activity in patients with neovascular AMD and analyzed the differences in automated retinal thickness measurement using Stratus TD and two different SD OCT machines (Cirrus SD-OCT [Carl Zeiss Meditech, Dublin, CA] and Spectralis SD-OCT [Heidelberg Engineering, Carlsbad, CA]).

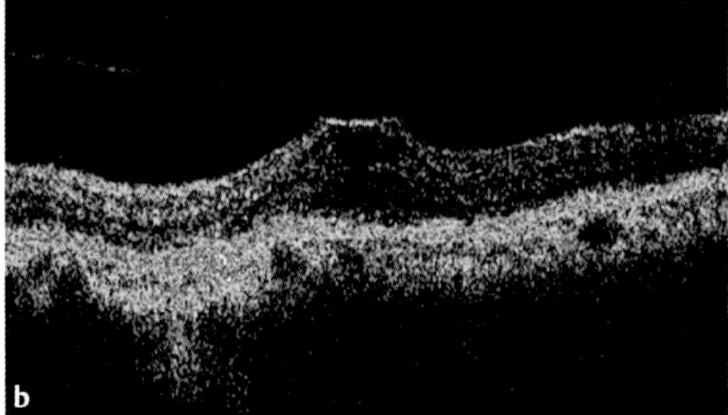

Fig. 21.43 (a) Fundus (black arrow) photography. **(b)** Persistent attachment of the hyaloid to the macula, with evidence of vitreomacular traction, on Stratus optical coherence tomography.

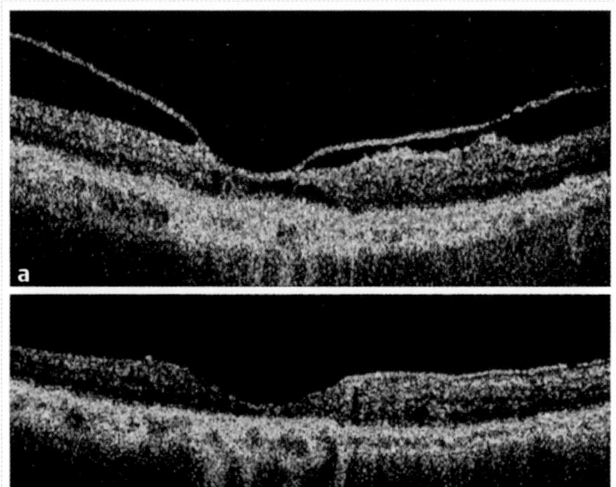

Fig. 21.44 Vitreomacular traction syndrome and geographic atrophy. **(a)** Preoperative Stratus optical coherence tomography showed vitreomacular traction with attachment of the posterior hyaloid to the fovea. **(b)** Postoperative Stratus optical coherence tomography demonstrates relief of the vitreomacular traction.

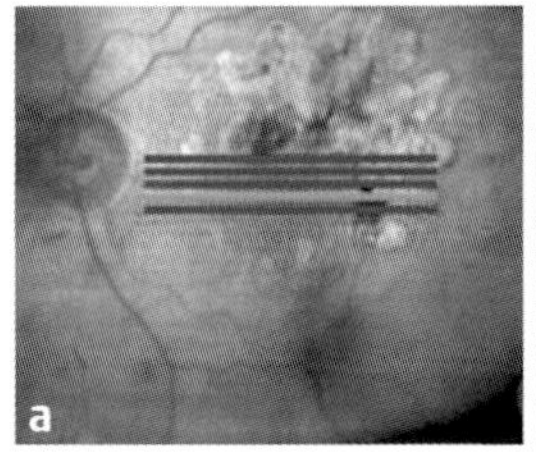

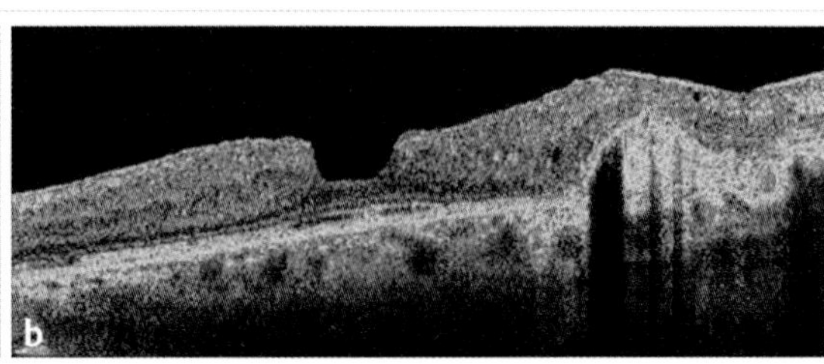

Fig. 21.45 Laser treatment of subretinal neovascularization leads to atrophic scarring, which appears, on Cirrus optical coherence tomography, as highly reflective at the chorioretinal interface.

The SD OCT showed a greater ability to evaluate qualitative features indicating disease activity and fewer errors in automated segmentation. However, differences in central macular thickness changes were similar between the TD OCT and SD OCT systems during follow-up.

Currently, 3-D scans allow visualization of the entire scanned area, resulting in a superior ability to detect CNV activity over linear scans and the TD OCT's radial line/fast macular thickness map scans.[113] All SD OCT devices had higher detection rates of CNV activity compared with TD OCT after ranibizumab injections for exudative AMD than TD OCT.[115]

21.2 Conclusion

One of the major advances with OCT has been the understanding of the pathophysiology of macular hole. Non-full-thickness macular holes have been renewed because high-resolution images can detect a lamellar macular defect that is not always visible clinically. In addition, OCT can be valuable in determining the need and timing of surgical intervention on vitreoretinal interface disorders. In ERM cases, characterization with OCT may help in preoperative planning for membrane peeling. OCT can also directly analyze the impact of CNV in AMD on outer retinal layers and evaluate alterations of photoreceptors and inner and outer segments being extremely useful for diagnostics and follow-up after treatment of these diseases. Therefore, we can use this technology to evaluate specific features that may serve as predictive factors in the prognosis, diagnosis, and follow-up after treatment of the most common posterior pole pathologies.

References

[1] Takahashi H, Kishi S. Tomographic features of a lamellar macular hole formation and a lamellar hole that progressed to a full-thickness macular hole. Am J Ophthalmol 2000; 130: 677–679

[2] Gass JDM. Idiopathic senile macular hole: its early stages and pathogenesis. Arch Ophthalmol 1988; 106: 629–639

[3] Johnson MW. Improvements in the understanding and treatment of macular hole. Curr Opin Ophthalmol 2002; 13: 152–160

[4] Gass JDM. Reappraisal of biomicroscopic classification of stages of development of a macular hole. Am J Ophthalmol 1995; 119: 752–759

[5] Avila MP, Jalkh AE, Murakami K, Trempe CL, Schepens CL. Biomicroscopic study of the vitreous in macular breaks. Ophthalmology 1983; 90: 1277–1283

[6] Gass JD, Joondeph BC. Observations concerning patients with suspected impending macular holes. Am J Ophthalmol 1990; 109: 638–646

[7] Gass JD. [Age-dependent idiopathic macular foramen: current concepts of the pathogenesis, diagnosis, and treatment] [in German] Ophthalmologe 1995; 92: 617–625

[8] Lewis ML, Cohen SM, Smiddy WE, Gass JD. Bilaterality of idiopathic macular holes. Graefes Arch Clin Exp Ophthalmol 1996; 234: 241–245

[9] Spiritus A, Dralands L, Stalmans P, Stalmans I, Spileers W. OCT study of fellow eyes of macular holes. Bull Soc Belge Ophtalmol 2000; 275: 81–84

[10] Kang SW, Ahn K, Ham D-I. Types of macular hole closure and their clinical implications. Br J Ophthalmol 2003; 87: 1015–1019

[11] Puliafito CA, Hee MR, Lin CP, et al. Imaging of macular diseases with optical coherence tomography. Ophthalmology 1995; 102: 217–229

[12] Duker JS, Puliafito CA, Wilkins JR, et al. Imaging fellow eyes in patients diagnosed with idiopathic macular holes using optical coherence tomography (OCT). Ophthalmology 1995; 102 (suppl): 118

[13] Benson SE, Schlottmann PG, Bunce C, Charteris DG. Comparison of macular hole size measured by optical coherence tomography, digital photography, and clinical examination. Eye (Lond) 2008; 22: 87–90

[14] Altaweel M, Ip M. Macular hole: improved understanding of pathogenesis, staging, and management based on optical coherence tomography. Semin Ophthalmol 2003; 18: 58–66

[15] Tilanus MA, Cuypers MH, Bemelmans NA, Pinckers AJ, Deutman AF. Predictive value of pattern VEP, pattern ERG and hole size in macular hole surgery. Graefes Arch Clin Exp Ophthalmol 1999; 237: 629–635

[16] Ullrich S, Haritoglou C, Gass C, Schaumberger M, Ulbig MW, Kampik A. Macular hole size as a prognostic factor in macular hole surgery. Br J Ophthalmol 2002; 86: 390–393

[17] Gass JD. Lamellar macular hole: a complication of cystoid macular edema after cataract extraction: a clinicopathologic case report. Trans Am Ophthalmol Soc 1975; 73: 231–250

[18] Allen AW Jr Gass JD. Contraction of a perifoveal epiretinal membrane simulating a macular hole. Am J Ophthalmol 1976; 82: 684–691

[19] Michalewska Z, Michalewski J, Odrobina D, et al. Surgical treatment of lamellar macular holes. Graefes Arch Clin Exp Ophthalmol 2010; 248: 1395–1400

[20] Haouchine B, Massin P, Gaudric A. Foveal pseudocyst as the first step in macular hole formation: a prospective study by optical coherence tomography. Ophthalmology 2001; 108: 15–22

[21] Witkin AJ, Ko TH, Fujimoto JG, et al. Redefining lamellar holes and the vitreomacular interface: an ultrahigh-resolution optical coherence tomography study. Ophthalmology 2006; 113: 388–397

[22] Haouchine B, Massin P, Tadayoni R, Erginay A, Gaudric A. Diagnosis of macular pseudoholes and lamellar macular holes by optical coherence tomography. Am J Ophthalmol 2004; 138: 732–739

[23] Michalewska Z, Michalewski J, Nawrocki J. [Can HRT be a useful tool in differentiating lamellar macular holes from full-thickness macular holes?] [in German] Ophthalmologe 2010; 107: 251–255

[24] Ophir A, Fatum S. Cystoid foveal oedema in symptomatic inner lamellar macular holes. Eye (Lond) 2009; 23: 1781–1785

[25] Michalewska Z, Michalewski J, Odrobina D, Nawrocki J. Non-full-thickness macular holes reassessed with spectral domain optical coherence tomography. Retina 2012; 32: 922–929

[26] Theodossiadis PG, Grigoropoulos VG, Emfietzoglou I, et al. Evolution of lamellar macular hole studied by optical coherence tomography. Graefes Arch Clin Exp Ophthalmol 2009; 247: 13–20

[27] Hirakawa M, Uemura A, Nakano T, Sakamoto T. Pars plana vitrectomy with gas tamponade for lamellar macular holes. Am J Ophthalmol 2005; 140: 1154–1155

[28] Witkin AJ, Castro LC, Reichel E, et al. Anatomic and visual outcomes of vitrectomy for lamellar macular holes. Ophthalmic Surg Lasers Imaging 2010; 41: 418–424

[29] Kokame GT, Tokuhara KG. Surgical management of inner lamellar macular hole. Ophthalmic Surg Lasers Imaging 2007; 38: 61–63

[30] Garretson BR, Pollack JS, Ruby AJ, Drenser KA, Williams GA, Sarrafizadeh R. Vitrectomy for a symptomatic lamellar macular hole. Ophthalmology 2008; 115: 884–886, e1

[31] Androudi S, Stangos A, Brazitikos PD. Lamellar macular holes: tomographic features and surgical outcome. Am J Ophthalmol 2009; 148: 420–426

[32] Bottoni F, Deiro AP, Giani A, Orini C, Cigada M, Staurenghi G. The natural history of lamellar macular holes: a spectral domain optical coherence tomography study. Graefes Arch Clin Exp Ophthalmol 2013; 251: 467–475

[33] Lee CS, Koh HJ, Lim HT, Lee KS, Lee SC. Prognostic factors in vitrectomy for lamellar macular hole assessed by spectral-domain optical coherence tomography. Acta Ophthalmol (Copenh) 2012; 90: e597–e602

[34] Legarreta JE, Gregori G, Knighton RW, Punjabi OS, Lalwani GA, Puliafito CA. Three-dimensional spectral-domain optical coherence tomography images of the retina in the presence of epiretinal membranes. Am J Ophthalmol 2008; 145: 1023–1030

[35] Ng CH, Cheung N, Wang JJ, et al. Prevalence and risk factors for epiretinal membranes in a multi-ethnic United States population. Ophthalmology 2011; 118: 694–699

[36] Klein R, Klein BE, Wang Q, Moss SE. The epidemiology of epiretinal membranes. Trans Am Ophthalmol Soc 1994; 92: 403–430

[37] Mitchell P, Smith W, Chey T, Wang JJ, Chang A. Prevalence and associations of epiretinal membranes. The Blue Mountains Eye Study, Australia. Ophthalmology 1997; 104: 1033–1040

[38] Koerner F, Garweg J. Vitrectomy for macular pucker and vitreomacular traction syndrome. Doc Ophthalmol 1999; 97: 449–458

[39] Gass JDM. Stereoscopic Atlas of Macular Diseases; Diagnosis and Treatment, 3rd ed. St. Louis, CV Mosby; 1987:716–717

[40] Mori K, Gehlbach PL, Sano A, Deguchi T, Yoneya S. Comparison of epiretinal membranes of differing pathogenesis using optical coherence tomography. Retina 2004; 24: 57–62

[41] Wilkins JR, Puliafito CA, Hee MR, et al. Characterization of epiretinal membranes using optical coherence tomography. Ophthalmology 1996; 103: 2142–2151

[42] Wong JG, Sachdev N, Beaumont PE, Chang AA. Visual outcomes following vitrectomy and peeling of epiretinal membrane. Clin Experiment Ophthalmol 2005; 33: 373–378

[43] Rice TA, De Bustros S, Michels RG, Thompson JT, Debanne SM, Rowland DY. Prognostic factors in vitrectomy for epiretinal membranes of the macula. Ophthalmology 1986; 93: 602–610

[44] Trese MT, Chandler DB, Machemer R. Macular pucker. I: prognostic criteria. Graefes Arch Clin Exp Ophthalmol 1983; 221: 12–15

[45] Suh MH, Seo JM, Park KH, Yu HG. Associations between macular findings by optical coherence tomography and visual outcomes after epiretinal membrane removal. Am J Ophthalmol 2009; 147: 473–480, e3

[46] Mitamura Y, Hirano K, Baba T, Yamamoto S. Correlation of visual recovery with presence of photoreceptor inner/outer segment junction in optical coherence images after epiretinal membrane surgery. Br J Ophthalmol 2009; 93: 171–175

[47] Michalewski J, Michalewska Z, Cisiecki S, Nawrocki J. Morphologically functional correlations of macular pathology connected with epiretinal membrane formation in spectral optical coherence tomography (SOCT). Graefes Arch Clin Exp Ophthalmol 2007; 245: 1623–1631

[48] Oster SF, Mojana F, Brar M, Yuson RM, Cheng L, Freeman WR. Disruption of the photoreceptor inner segment/outer segment layer on spectral domain-optical coherence tomography is a predictor of poor visual acuity in patients with epiretinal membranes. Retina 2010; 30: 713–718

[49] Uchino E, Uemura A, Ohba N. Initial stages of posterior vitreous detachment in healthy eyes of older persons evaluated by optical coherence tomography. Arch Ophthalmol 2001; 119: 1475–1479

[50] Gass JDM. Macular dysfunction caused by vitreous and vitreoretinal interface abnormalities. In: Gass JDM. Stereoscopic Atlas of Macular Diseases: Diagnosis and Treatment, 4th ed. St. Louis: Mosby-Year Book, Inc.; 1997: 903–914

[51] Iwanoff A. Beitrage zur normalen und pathologischen Anatomie des Auges. Graefes Arch Clin Exp Ophthalmol 1865; 11: 135–170

[52] Gandorfer A, Rohleder M, Kampik A. Epiretinal pathology of vitreomacular traction syndrome. Br J Ophthalmol 2002; 86: 902–909

[53] Hikichi T, Yoshida A, Trempe CL. Course of vitreomacular traction syndrome. Am J Ophthalmol 1995; 119: 55–61

[54] Smiddy WE, Michels RG, Glaser BM, deBustros S. Vitrectomy for macular traction caused by incomplete vitreous separation. Arch Ophthalmol 1988; 106: 624–628

[55] Gallemore RP, Jumper JM, McCuen BW II Jaffe GJ, Postel EA, Toth CA. Diagnosis of vitreoretinal adhesions in macular disease with optical coherence tomography. Retina 2000; 20: 115–120

[56] Yamada N, Kishi S. Tomographic features and surgical outcomes of vitreomacular traction syndrome. Am J Ophthalmol 2005; 139: 112–117

[57] Munuera JM, García-Layana A, Maldonado MJ, Aliseda D, Moreno-Montañés J. Optical coherence tomography in successful surgery of vitreomacular traction syndrome. Arch Ophthalmol 1998; 116: 1388–1389

[58] Sayegh RG, Georgopoulos M, Geitzenauer W, Simader C, Kiss C, Schmidt-Erfurth U. High-resolution optical coherence tomography after surgery for vitreomacular traction: a 2-year follow-up. Ophthalmology 2010; 117: 2010–2017, e1–e2

[59] Schulze S, Hoerle S, Mennel S, Kroll P. Vitreomacular traction and exudative age-related macular degeneration. Acta Ophthalmol (Copenh) 2008; 86: 470–481

[60] Krebs I, Brannath W, Glittenberg C, Zeiler F, Sebag J, Binder S. Posterior vitreomacular adhesion: a potential risk factor for exudative age-related macular degeneration? Am J Ophthalmol 2007; 144: 741–746

[61] Robison CD, Krebs I, Binder S, et al. Vitreomacular adhesion in active and end-stage age-related macular degeneration. Am J Ophthalmol 2009; 148: 79–82, e2

[62] Lee SJ, Lee CS, Koh HJ. Posterior vitreomacular adhesion and risk of exudative age-related macular degeneration: paired eye study. Am J Ophthalmol 2009; 147: 621–626, e1

[63] Krebs I, Glittenberg C, Zeiler F, Binder S. Spectral domain optical coherence tomography for higher precision in the evaluation of vitreoretinal adhesions in exudative age-related macular degeneration. Br J Ophthalmol 2011; 95: 1415–1418

[64] Klein R, Klein BE, Linton KL. Prevalence of age-related maculopathy. The Beaver Dam Eye Study. Ophthalmology 1992; 99: 933–943

[65] Krebs I, Brannath W, Glittenberg C, Zeiler F, Sebag J, Binder S. Posterior vitreomacular adhesion: a potential risk factor for exudative age-related macular degeneration? Am J Ophthalmol 2007; 144: 741–746

[66] Robison CD, Krebs I, Binder S, et al. Vitreomacular adhesion in active and end-stage age-related macular degeneration. Am J Ophthalmol 2009; 148: 79–82, e2

[67] Yi K, Mujat M, Park BH, et al. Spectral domain optical coherence tomography for quantitative evaluation of drusen and associated structural changes in non-neovascular age-related macular degeneration. Br J Ophthalmol 2009; 93: 176–181

[68] Hee MR, Baumal CR, Puliafito CA, et al. Optical coherence tomography of age-related macular degeneration and choroidal neovascularization. Ophthalmology 1996; 103: 1260–1270

[69] Friedman SM, Margo CE. Choroidal neovascular membranes: reproducibility of angiographic interpretation. Am J Ophthalmol 2000; 130: 839–841

[70] van Velthoven ME, de Smet MD, Schlingemann RO, Magnani M, Verbraak FD. Added value of OCT in evaluating the presence of leakage in patients with age-related macular degeneration treated with PDT. Graefes Arch Clin Exp Ophthalmol 2006; 244: 1119–1123

[71] Fung AE, Lalwani GA, Rosenfeld PJ, et al. An optical coherence tomography-guided, variable dosing regimen with intravitreal ranibizumab (Lucentis) for neovascular age-related macular degeneration. Am J Ophthalmol 2007; 143: 566–583

[72] Zhang N, Hoffmeyer GC, Young ES, et al. Optical coherence tomography reader agreement in neovascular age-related macular degeneration. Am J Ophthalmol 2007; 144: 37–44

[73] Krebs I, Ansari-Shahrezaei S, Goll A, Binder S. Activity of neovascular lesions treated with bevacizumab: comparison between optical coherence tomography and fluorescein angiography. Graefes Arch Clin Exp Ophthalmol 2008; 246: 811–815

[74] Malamos P, Sacu S, Georgopoulos M, Kiss C, Pruente C, Schmidt-Erfurth U. Correlation of high-definition optical coherence tomography and fluorescein angiography imaging in neovascular macular degeneration. Invest Ophthalmol Vis Sci 2009; 50: 4926–4933

[75] Chong EW, Wong TY, Kreis AJ, Simpson JA, Guymer RH. Dietary antioxidants and primary prevention of age related macular degeneration: systematic review and meta-analysis. BMJ 2007; 335: 755

[76] Age-Related Eye Disease Study Research Group. A randomized, placebo-controlled, clinical trial of high-dose supplementation with vitamins C and E, beta carotene, and zinc for age-related macular degeneration and vision loss: AREDS report no. 8. Arch Ophthalmol 2001; 119: 1417–1436

[77] Gass JD. Drusen and disciform macular detachment and degeneration. Arch Ophthalmol 1973; 90: 206–217

[78] Davis MD, Gangnon RE, Lee LY, et al. Age-Related Eye Disease Study Group. The Age-Related Eye Disease Study severity scale for age-related macular degeneration: AREDS Report No. 17. Arch Ophthalmol 2005; 123: 1484–1498

[79] Ferris FL, Davis MD, Clemons TE, et al. Age-Related Eye Disease Study (AREDS) Research Group. A simplified severity scale for age-related macular degeneration: AREDS Report No. 18. Arch Ophthalmol 2005; 123: 1570–1574

[80] Klein R, Klein BE, Knudtson MD, Meuer SM, Swift M, Gangnon RE. Fifteen-year cumulative incidence of age-related macular degeneration: the Beaver Dam Eye Study. Ophthalmology 2007; 114: 253–262

[81] Klein R, Peto T, Bird A, Vannewkirk MR. The epidemiology of age-related macular degeneration. Am J Ophthalmol 2004; 137: 486–495

[82] Sarks SH. Drusen patterns predisposing to geographic atrophy of the retinal pigment epithelium. Aust J Ophthalmol 1982; 10: 91–97

[83] Sebag M, Peli E, Lahav M. Image analysis of changes in drusen area. Acta Ophthalmol (Copenh) 1991; 69: 603–610

[84] Wang JJ, Foran S, Smith W, Mitchell P. Risk of age-related macular degeneration in eyes with macular drusen or hyperpigmentation: the Blue Mountains Eye Study cohort. Arch Ophthalmol 2003; 121: 658–663

[85] Green WR, Enger C. Age-related macular degeneration histopathologic studies. The 1992 Lorenz E. Zimmerman Lecture. Ophthalmology 1993; 100: 1519–1535

[86] Klein R, Klein BE, Tomany SC, Meuer SM, Huang GH. Ten-year incidence and progression of age-related maculopathy: the Beaver Dam eye study. Ophthalmology 2002; 109: 1767–1779

[87] Bressler NM, Munoz B, Maguire MG, et al. Five-year incidence and disappearance of drusen and retinal pigment epithelial abnormalities. Waterman study. Arch Ophthalmol 1995; 113: 301–308

[88] Casswell AG, Kohen D, Bird AC. Retinal pigment epithelial detachments in the elderly: classification and outcome. Br J Ophthalmol 1985; 69: 397–403

[89] Hartnett ME, Weiter JJ, Garsd A, Jalkh AE. Classification of retinal pigment epithelial detachments associated with drusen. Graefes Arch Clin Exp Ophthalmol 1992; 230: 11–19

[90] Pauleikhoff D, Löffert D, Spital G, et al. Pigment epithelial detachment in the elderly. Clinical differentiation, natural course and pathogenetic implications. Graefes Arch Clin Exp Ophthalmol 2002; 240: 533–538

[91] Age-Related Eye Disease Study Research Group. The Age-Related Eye Disease Study system for classifying age-related macular degeneration from stereoscopic color fundus photographs: the Age-Related Eye Disease Study Report Number 6. Am J Ophthalmol 2001; 132: 668–681

[92] Spraul CW, Grossniklaus HE. Characteristics of Drusen and Bruch's membrane in postmortem eyes with age-related macular degeneration. Arch Ophthalmol 1997; 115: 267–273

[93] Roquet W, Roudot-Thoraval F, Coscas G, Soubrane G. Clinical features of drusenoid pigment epithelial detachment in age related macular degeneration. Br J Ophthalmol 2004; 88: 638–642

[94] Cukras C, Agrón E, Klein ML, et al. Age-Related Eye Disease Study Research Group. Natural history of drusenoid pigment epithelial detachment in age-related macular degeneration: Age-Related Eye Disease Study Report No. 28. Ophthalmology 2010; 117: 489–499

[95] Querques G, Bux AV, Delle Noci N. Foveal geographic atrophy following intravitreal pegaptanib sodium (Macugen) for drusenoid pigment epithelium detachment. Eur J Ophthalmol 2009; 19: 890–893

[96] Krishnan R, Lochhead J. Regression of soft drusen and drusenoid pigment epithelial detachment following intravitreal anti-vascular endothelial growth factor therapy. Can J Ophthalmol 2010; 45: 83–84

[97] Gallego-Pinazo R, Marina A, Suelves-Cogollos, et al. Intravitreal ranibizumab for symptomatic drusenoid pigment epithelial detachment without choroidal neovascularization in age-related macular degeneration. Clin Ophthalmol 2011; 5: 161–165

[98] Yannuzzi LA, Hope-Ross M, Slakter JS, et al. Analysis of vascularized pigment epithelial detachments using indocyanine green videoangiography. Retina 1994; 14: 99–113

[99] Coscas F, Coscas G, Souied E, Tick S, Soubrane G. Optical coherence tomography identification of occult choroidal neovascularization in age-related macular degeneration. Am J Ophthalmol 2007; 144: 592–599

[100] Cho M, Athanikar A, Paccione J, Wald KJ. Optical coherence tomography features of acute central serous chorioretinopathy versus neovascular age-related macular degeneration. Br J Ophthalmol 2010; 94: 597–599

[101] Bressler SB, Silva JC, Bressler NM, Alexander J, Green WR. Clinicopathologic correlation of occult choroidal neovascularization in age-related macular degeneration. Arch Ophthalmol 1992; 110: 827–832

[102] Ting TD, Oh M, Cox TA, Meyer CH, Toth CA. Decreased visual acuity associated with cystoid macular edema in neovascular age-related macular degeneration. Arch Ophthalmol 2002; 120: 731–737

[103] Ozawa S, Ishikawa K, Ito Y, et al. Differences in macular morphology between polypoidal choroidal vasculopathy and exudative age-related macular degeneration detected by optical coherence tomography. Retina 2009; 29: 793–802

[104] Lambert HM, Capone A Jr Aaberg TM, Sternberg P Jr Mandell BA, Lopez PF. Surgical excision of subfoveal neovascular membranes in age-related macular degeneration. Am J Ophthalmol 1992; 113: 257–262

[105] Weber-Krause B, Eckardt U. [Incidence of posterior vitreous detachment in eyes with and without age-related macular degeneration: an ultrasonic study] (in German) Ophthalmologe 1996; 93: 660–665 German

[106] Ondeş F, Yilmaz G, Acar MA, Unlü N, Kocaoğlan H, Arsan AK. Role of the vitreous in age-related macular degeneration. Jpn J Ophthalmol 2000; 44: 91–93

[107] Mojana F, Cheng L, Bartsch DU, et al. The role of abnormal vitreomacular adhesion in age-related macular degeneration: spectral optical coherence tomography and surgical results. Am J Ophthalmol 2008; 146: 218–227

[108] Quaranta-El Maftouhi M, Mauget-Faÿsse M. Anomalous vitreoretinal adhesions in patients with exudative age-related macular degeneration: an OCT study. Eur J Ophthalmol 2006; 16: 134–137

[109] Toth CA, Birngruber R, Boppart SA, et al. Argon laser retinal lesions evaluated in vivo by optical coherence tomography. Am J Ophthalmol 1997; 123: 188–198

[110] Rosenfeld PJ, Brown DM, Heier JS, et al. MARINA Study Group. Ranibizumab for neovascular age-related macular degeneration. N Engl J Med 2006; 355: 1419–1431

[111] Kaiser PK, Brown DM, Zhang K, et al. Ranibizumab for predominantly classic neovascular age-related macular degeneration: subgroup analysis of first-year ANCHOR results. Am J Ophthalmol 2007; 144: 850–857

[112] Krebs I, Hagen S, Brannath W, et al. Repeatability and reproducibility of retinal thickness measurements by optical coherence tomography in age-related macular degeneration. Ophthalmology 2010; 117: 1577–1584

[113] Sayanagi K, Sharma S, Yamamoto T, Kaiser PK. Comparison of spectral-domain versus time-domain optical coherence tomography in management of age-related macular degeneration with ranibizumab. Ophthalmology 2009; 116: 947–955

[114] Querques G, Forte R, Berboucha E, et al. Spectral-domain versus time domain optical coherence tomography before and after ranibizumab for age-related macular degeneration. Ophthalmic Res 2011; 46: 152–159

[115] Spaide RF. Enhanced depth imaging optical coherence tomography of retinal pigment epithelial detachment in age-related macular degeneration. Am J Ophthalmol 2009; 147: 644–652

22 Optical Coherence Tomography and Anti-Vascular Endothelial Growth Factor Therapy

Mariana R. Thorell and Philip J. Rosenfeld

Vascular endothelial growth factor-A (VEGF) is the major cytokine responsible for physiologic and pathological angiogenesis. Retinal diseases characterized by pathologic neovascularization and exudation, such as neovascular age-related macular degeneration (AMD), diabetic retinopathy, and retinal vein occlusion (RVO) are associated with increased levels of VEGF. Their prognoses have significantly improved since the introduction of the anti-VEGF therapy. The initiation of treatment with anti-VEGF coincided with the development of a commercially viable optical coherence tomography (OCT) instrument. OCT imaging has improved the early diagnosis and appropriate management of these diseases by showing where the abnormal exudation resides. OCT imaging has greatly improved our understanding of how neovascularization and exudation in the macula interferes with visual acuity, and how anti-VEGF therapy improves outcomes. OCT imaging shows the response to therapy and helps guide the need for retreatment. OCT guidance is vital to our ability to identify when treatment should start and when treatment intervals can be extended. This chapter describes the use of anti-VEGF therapies in cases of neovascular AMD, diabetic retinopathy, and RVO. In addition, this chapter includes a broad overview of the clinical trials that have used OCT-guided therapy for exudative macular diseases and discusses future plans for this imaging strategy.

Significant vision loss is caused by pathological neovascularization and exudation in neovascular AMD, diabetic retinopathy, and RVO.[1] Diabetic retinopathy represents the main cause of legal blindness in 20- to 74-year olds in developed countries,[2] and macular edema is a frequent manifestation and an important cause of visual impairment in this disease.[3,4] AMD is the leading cause of abnormal neovascularization and exudation in the population over 50 years of age. If untreated, neovascular AMD leads to severe, irreversible vision loss.[5,6,7]

Over the years, imaging technologies have improved our ability to detect neovascular and exudative diseases, and these newer technologies have been incorporated into our evolving management strategies. Although fluorescein angiography was the gold standard for identifying neovascularization and exudation and remains an important imaging strategy in AMD, diabetic retinopathy, and vein occlusions, the new gold standard is OCT. OCT has emerged as the leading imaging modality for both diagnosis and the assessment of treatment. It provides a noninvasive, noncontact strategy for obtaining a three-dimensional anatomic image of the posterior pole, which includes the retina, retinal pigment epithelium (RPE), and choroid.[8,9] In the setting of macular edema and neovascularization, OCT now provides the essential information that is relevant in deciding when and how often to treat.

Since the introduction of therapy that inhibits VEGF-A (anti-VEGF therapy), the prognosis for these neovascular and exudative diseases has improved, especially when considering the diagnosis of neovascular AMD.[10,11] VEGF-A is the major cytokine responsible for the increased vascular permeability and growth of abnormal vessels.[12] The anatomical improvements seen with OCT after anti-VEGF therapy correlate well with visual acuity, and these improvements seen on OCT imaging are now expected whenever the results from clinical trials using anti-VEGF therapy are discussed. OCT is even useful in explaining why visual acuity does not improve as much as expected once the exudation has resolved. The anatomical integrity of the outer retina and RPE are often compromised whenever vision improvement fails to follow resolution of macular fluid. Thus, OCT imaging provides evidence of exudation and when treatment is needed, and it provides anatomical correlation for both vision improvement and loss. For any new drug undergoing clinical trials for the treatment of macular exudation, the need to show resolution of macular fluid by OCT imaging has become a requirement.

The current strategies for treating exudative macular diseases rely heavily on OCT. The only treatment strategy that does not require frequent OCT imaging is to treat monthly or every 2 months regardless of anatomical response. Although this strategy has been used successfully in clinical trials, most retina specialists have adopted a more personalized approach to therapy. The two most frequent OCT-based treatment strategies are referred to *as-needed* (pro re nata [PRN]) therapy and *treat-and-extend* therapy. OCT is integral to both strategies, but the number and frequency of visits as well as injections vary between the two approaches.

22.1 Anti-VEGF Therapies

22.1.1 Pegaptanib Sodium

In December 2004, pegaptanib sodium (Macugen, Eyetech Pharmaceuticals, San Francisco, CA) was the first VEGF-A inhibitor approved in the United States by the Food and Drug Administration (FDA) for the treatment of neovascular AMD. This RNA aptamer inhibited human $VEGF_{165}$, as well as longer isoforms of VEGF-A.[13] This intravitreal drug was shown to slow vision loss in neovascular AMD clinical studies[14,15,16,17] and was the first anti-VEGF reported in a clinical trial to have efficacy in the treatment of diabetic macular edema (DME).[18] In clinical use, this drug never demonstrated significant OCT or visual acuity benefits and was replaced by bevacizumab in May 2005.

22.1.2 Bevacizumab

The off-label use of bevacizumab (Avastin; Genentech Inc., South San Francisco, CA) for the treatment of exudative macular diseases was initiated after it was approved by the FDA in 2004 as an intravenous treatment for metastatic colorectal cancer.[19,20,21,22] This humanized immunoglobulin $(Ig)G_1$ monoclonal antibody selectively neutralizes the biologic activity of VEGF-A.[12] First used successfully as an intravenous treatment of neovascular AMD, a much smaller dose of bevacizumab was subsequently injected into the vitreous and shown to improve visual acuity and reduce exudation by OCT imaging without any apparent systemic side effects.[23,24,25] Subsequent studies confirmed its visual acuity and anatomical benefits for neovascular AMD[26,27,28,29,30,31,32,33,34,35,36,37,38,39,40] and other causes of macular edema.[25,41,42,43]

22.1.3 Ranibizumab

Ranibizumab (Lucentis; Genentech, Inc, South San Francisco, CA) is derived from the same murine monoclonal antibody against VEGF-A as bevacizumab. Whereas bevacizumab is the humanized full-length antibody, ranibizumab is a recombinant, humanized monoclonal antibody fragment that binds and inhibits all active forms identified of VEGF-A, just like bevacizumab.[44,45] Approved by the FDA in 2006 for the treatment of neovascular AMD, ranibizumab first showed benefits with monthly injections, demonstrating not only prevention of vision loss but also improvement of visual acuity.[10,46,47,48,49] Alternative dosing regimens were evaluated in subsequent studies,[50,51,52,53,54,55,56,57,58,59,60,61,62] and the Prospective OCT Imaging of Patients with Neovascular AMD Treated with IntraOcular Ranibizumab (PrONTO) study[63] (see *Clinical Trials*) was the first trial to use OCT imaging to monitor a PRN dosing strategy.

The FDA approved ranibizumab for the treatment of patients with macular edema owing to RVO in 2010 and, later, in 2012, the drug was approved for the treatment of DME based on two clinical trials, RISE and RIDE.[64]

22.1.4 Aflibercept

Aflibercept (Eylea; Regeneron, Tarrytown, NY) is a soluble receptor fusion-protein against all isoforms of VEGF-A, as well as VEGF-B and placental growth factor. It was approved in November 2011 for the treatment of neovascular AMD.[65,66,67] As with the other pan-VEGF inhibitors, macular exudation resolved as shown using OCT imaging and average visual acuity improved.[68,69] More recently, in September 2012, aflibercept was approved for macular edema owing to central retinal vein occlusion (CRVO) based on two randomized, multicenter, clinical trials, Investigation of Efficacy and Safety in Central Retinal Vein Occlusion (COPERNICUS)[70] and VEGF Trap-Eye for macular oedema secondary to central retinal vein occlusion (GALILEO).[71]

22.2 Role of OCT in Anti-VEGF Therapy

With OCT B-scan imaging, in vivo, high-resolution optical cross-sections of the retina can be made in which the major cellular layers can be identified.[9,72] Since the release of the first OCT instruments, we now have a much better understanding of the structural alterations associated with the diagnosis, natural history, and treatment of macular exudative diseases such as neovascular AMD, DME, and RVO. The time-domain (TD) OCT instrument known as the Stratus OCT (Carl Zeiss Meditec, Dublin, CA) was the first successfully commercialized OCT instrument launched in 2002,[73,74] and the first instrument used to demonstrate the utility of OCT monitoring to detect a treatment response to anti-VEGF drugs.[75,76,77] Compared with this TD OCT, the current commercially available spectral domain (SD) OCT instruments provide a significant improvement in speed, sensitivity, axial resolution, and imaging depth.[78,79]

Optical coherence tomography is used to identify the integrity of the retinal layers, the RPE, and the choroid. This evaluation provides qualitative and quantitative information that is important to guide therapy, including the decision to initiate, continue, and withhold treatment with intravitreal anti-VEGF drugs. In exudative diseases such as neovascular AMD, the examination is used to identify and localize the macular fluid or blood in the macula. This fluid can be found in the retina, under the retina, or under the RPE.[80] The presence, persistent, or recurrence of fluid determines when treatment with anti-VEGF dugs is needed. In addition, OCT imaging identifies other potential anatomical causes of vision loss, such as atrophy of photoreceptors in the outer retina, vitreomacular traction, epiretinal membranes, or macular holes.

22.3 Qualitative Analysis

Optical coherence tomography depends on illuminating the tissue with a defined light source and capturing the light that is reflected back to the detector. The scattering and time delay of the reflected light from each tissue layer and interface provide the information that is used to reconstruct an anatomical image using different colors or shades of gray for different layers according to its reflectivity.[9] With advances in OCT technology, retinal structures and the changes in the appearance of the macular anatomy have become easier to identify, and more sophisticated algorithms have been developed to measure the changes identified in the anatomical layers.[74]

Optical coherence tomography is most frequently used to identify fluid in the macula, which arises from vitreomacular interface abnormalities, exudative diseases, and retinal detachment. In addition to fluid, visual acuity is associated with the integrity of the retinal layers, with abnormalities in the photoreceptor layer and the continuity of the inner segment-outer segment (IS/OS) junction often associated with decreased vision. OCT can also identify the presence of both vascularized and nonvascularized PEDs. It is the vascularized pigment epithelial detachment (PED) that is often associated with the risk of rapid, severe vision loss.[81] In these cases, OCT can provide detailed anatomical and morphologic assessment of the PED area and volume that proves when following these lesions during anti-VEGF therapy (▸ Fig. 22.1).[82]

22.4 Quantitative Analysis

Central retinal thickness (CRT) is the parameter used to quantitate retinal morphology and is a distance calculated in microns from the internal limiting membrane (ILM) to the RPE. Small thickness changes and elevations of individual retinal layers have been correlated with clinical findings. Increased CRT measurements are often correlated with the accumulation of macular fluid, and studies in a variety of macular diseases have shown that OCT is useful in quantifying retinal thickness in eyes with macular edema.[83,84,85,86] By following the CRT, the retina specialist can evaluate the effects of treatment.

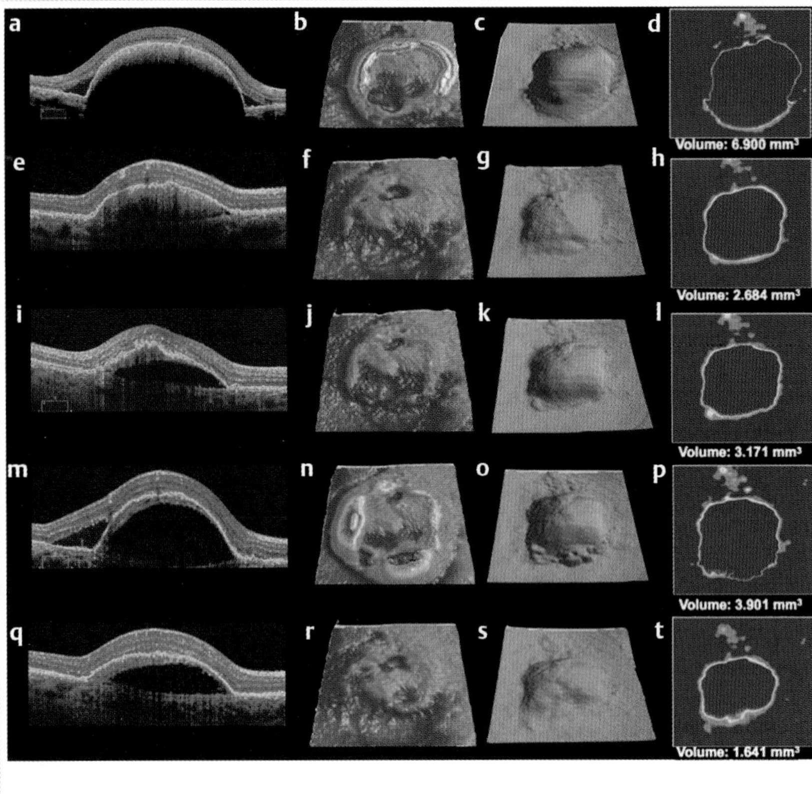

Fig. 22.1 a–t Spectral-domain optical coherence tomography imaging of a 65-year-old woman with a hemorrhagic pigment epithelial detachment (PED) at baseline treated with intravitreal injections of ranibizumab. In each row, the first column shows the B-scan at the center of the PED, retinal thickness (RT) map, retinal pigment epithelium (RPE) elevation map, and RPE difference map with the PED volume below. **(a)** Baseline visit with the best-corrected visual acuity (BCVA) of 20/32, B-scan showing an elevation of the RPE with subretinal fluid. **(b)** The RT map illustrates the ring of subretinal fluid in red surrounding the PED. **(c)** The RPE elevation map shows the PED itself. **(d)** The RPE difference map shows the PED with an area of 14 mm^2 and a volume of 6.9 mm^3. At this visit, the first injection of ranibizumab was given, followed by one additional injection, resulting in the absence of intraretinal and subretinal fluid. **(e)** Six weeks after the second injection, there is no fluid on the B-scan or **(f)** the RT map. **(g)** The RPE elevation map seems to show a smaller PED. **(h)** The RPE difference map shows a decrease in the PED area (11.35 mm^2) and volume (2.68 mm^3). At this visit, the patient was observed. Eight weeks after the second injection, there is still no fluid on the **(i)** B-scan or **(j)** the RT map. **(l)** The RPE difference map shows that the PED is larger with an area of 11.54 mm^2 and a volume of 3.17 mm^3. At this time, the patient was observed because of the absence of fluid on the B-scans. Ten weeks after the second injection, the fluid has returned and is observed on the **(m)** B-scan and the **(n)** RT map. **(o)** The RPE elevation map and the **(p)** RPE difference map show a larger PED with an area of 13.04 mm^2 and a volume of 3.9 mm^3. At this visit, the patient receives the third injection. Four weeks after the third injection, there is no fluid on the **(q)** B-scan or the **(r)** RT map. **(s)** On the RPE elevation map, the PED seems smaller. **(t)** The RPE difference map shows a decrease in the PED area (10.13 mm^2) and volume (1.64 mm^3). At this visit, the patient was observed. ((From Penha F, Gregori G, Garcia Filho C, Yehoshua Z, Feuer W, Rosenfeld P. Quantitative changes in retinal pigment epithelial detachments as a predictor for retreatment with anti-VEGF therapy. Retina. Mar 2013;33(3):459–466.))

Because of its three-dimensional characteristics, the volume of PEDs can be measured using SD-OCT. The development of an algorithm using SD-OCT, which was first used to measure drusen volume,[87] was shown to be highly reproducible strategy for monitoring disease progression and response to anti-VEGF therapy.[88] In contrast, volumetric assessment is not possible with more traditional imaging strategies used to monitor PEDs, such as color fundus photography, fluorescein angiography, and indocyanine green angiography.

Limitations of OCT scans may include a low signal strength that can compromise the correct interpretation of the images. Signal strength corresponds to the averaged intensity value of the signal pixels in the OCT image and is represented in a scale of 0 to 10. The higher the signal strength, the more reliable the interpretation of the scans.[89,90] Errors in automated segmentation algorithms and thickness measurements are well known and are not rare when assessing macular anatomy with complex morphologies such as neovascular AMD and macular edema. Theses anatomical changes can interfere with the ability of segmentation algorithms to detect normal anatomic boundaries.[91,92,93,94,95] However, manual editing can be performed and the scan corrected when an inaccurate segmentation is identified.

A more recent advance in OCT technology is the ability to use ultrahigh-speed swept-source OCT to evaluate the retinal, choriocapillaris, and choroidal microvasculature without the need for intravenous injection of contrast agents. OCT angiography has been shown to reproducibly image the three-dimensional vascular structures of the retina and choroid, and

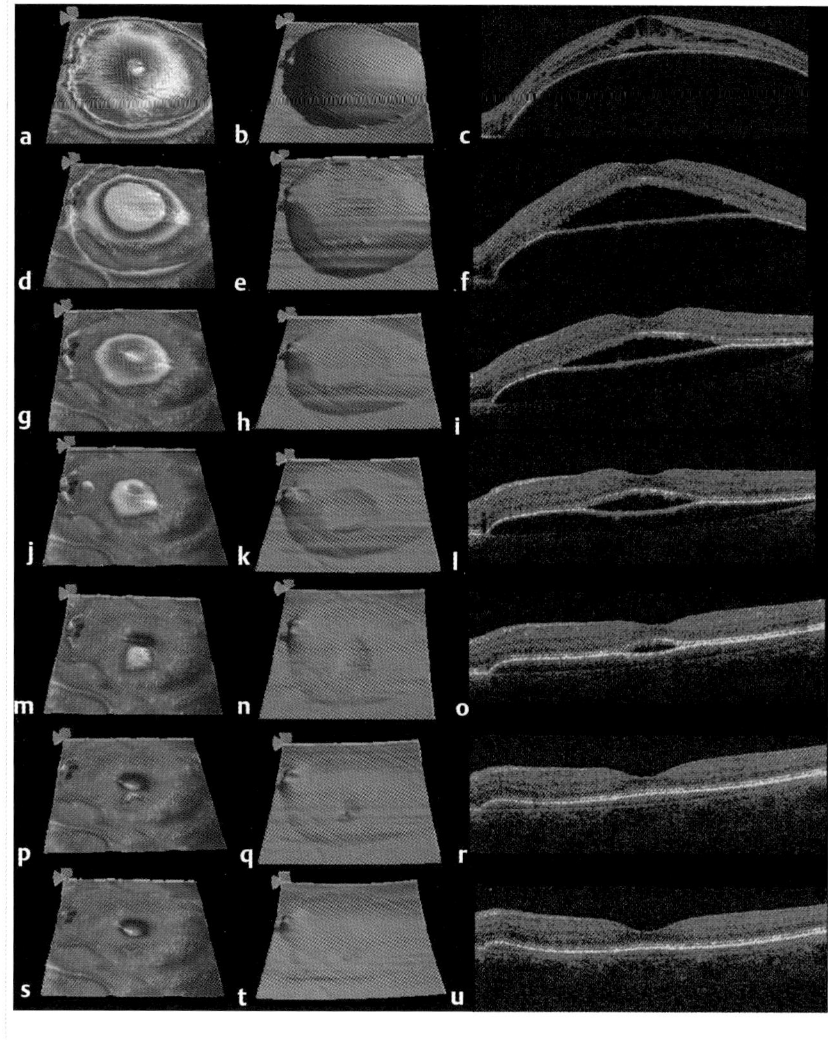

Fig. 22.2 a-u Spectral-domain optical coherence tomography (OCT) images of an eye with worsening neovascular age-related macular degeneration (AMD) undergoing biweekly treatment with ranibizumab alternating with bevacizumab. Spectral-domain OCT retinal thickness maps **(a,d,g,j,m,p,s)**, retinal pigment epithelium segmentation maps **(b,e,h,k,n,q,t)**, and horizontal spectral-domain OCT B-scans through the foveal center **(c,f,l,l,o,r,u)** are shown during the period of biweekly injections. **(a–c)** A hemorrhagic retinal pigment epithelial detachment (PED) with overly subretinal and intraretinal fluid is shown at baseline with a visual acuity of 20/200. **(d–f)** A dose of intravitreal ranibizumab (0.5 mg) was given at baseline, and after 2 weeks, the intraretinal fluid resolved, the subretinal fluid increased, the PED decreased, and visual acuity improved to 20/40. **(g–i)** A dose of intravitreal bevacizumab (1.25 mg) was given, and after 2 weeks, there was less subretinal fluid, the size of the PED had decreased further, and visual acuity had improved to 20/30. **(j–l)** Another ranibizumab (0.5 mg) injection was given, and the patient returned 2 weeks later with stable visual acuity at 20/30 with further improvement in the OCT appearance of her lesion. **(m–o)** Another bevacizumab injection was given, and 2 weeks later, the OCT image revealed continued improvement associated with stable visual acuity. **(p–r)** Another intravitreal dose of ranibizumab was given, and 2 weeks later, the subretinal fluid had resolved and visual acuity was stable at 20/30. **(s–u)** Intravitreal bevacizumab was again given, and 2 weeks later, there was no evidence of macular fluid except for a small PED adjacent to the peripapillary area, where the choroidal neovascularization (CNV) was visualized on angiography; visual acuity was 20/30. Another injection of ranibizumab was given, and with this last injection, a total of seven injections were given over 12 weeks at 2-week intervals: four ranibizumab injections and three bevacizumab injections. The next follow-up visit was extended to 4 weeks. ((From Stewart M, Rosenfeld PJ, Penha F, Wang F, Yehoshua Z, Bueno-Lopez E, Lopez P. Pharmacokinetic rationale for dosing every 2 weeks versus 4 weeks with intravitreal Ranibizumab, bevacizumab, and aflibercept (vascular endothelial growth factor trap-eye). Retina 2012; 32(3):434–457.))

the resulting images are consistent with histologic and electron micrographic images.[96]

22.5 Initiation and Maintenance of Anti-VEGF Therapy

With OCT imaging, the fluid associated with macular neovascularization can be identified. The fluid can accumulate in the retina, under the retina, and under the RPE.[97] As more fluid accumulates and the longer the fluid persists, there is a greater chance of irreversible damage to the retina. A delay in treatment of newly diagnosed patients is associated with an increasing risk of vision loss.[98] OCT is now the gold standard for the early diagnosis of macular fluid in exudative retinal diseases. OCT was shown to be very sensitive in detecting changes in retinal morphology over time and is a valuable tool for following up on patients with AMD (▶ Fig. 22.2, ▶ Fig. 22.3).[99] The visit-to-visit changes in the appearance of the OCT images play an increasingly important clinical role in deciding when to treat and when to monitor patients with exudative eye diseases, and this retreatment and follow-up schedule has a profound impact on the visual acuity outcomes of patients with neovascular AMD.[100,101] Studies have focused on retreatment decisions based on OCT imaging, and OCT imaging has been confirmed as an appropriate strategy for managing patients with anti-VEGF

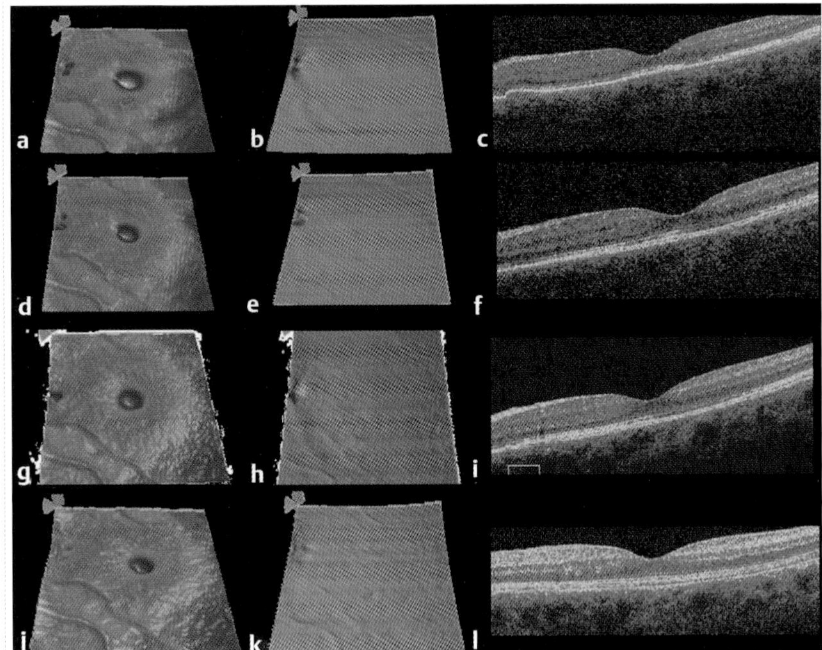

Fig. 22.3 a-l Spectral-domain optical coherence tomography (OCT) images of an eye with resolution of macular fluid after biweekly injections of ranibizumab alternating with bevacizumab now followed using a treat-and-extend strategy. Spectral-domain (SD) OCT retinal thickness maps **(a,d,g,j)**, retinal pigment epithelium segmentation maps **(b,e,h,k)**, and horizontal SD OCT B-scans through the foveal center **(c,f,i,l)** are shown during the period when treatment intervals were extended 4 weeks after her last injection of ranibizumab. **(a–c)** The SD OCT images remained stable. Another injection of bevacizumab was given followed by another injection of ranibizumab 4 weeks later, followed by another injection of ranibizumab 6 weeks later. **(d–f)** At this 6-week follow-up visit, visual acuity was stable at 20/30, and she received a dose of bevacizumab. **(g–i)** Her treatment intervals were then extended to every 8 weeks, then every 10 weeks, and then every 12 weeks. Because of the presence of a symptomatic steroid-induced subcapsular cataract, an injection of ranibizumab was given just before cataract extraction and lens implantation. **(j–l)** The last follow-up was 27 weeks after the cataract surgery, and visual acuity was 20/20 vision and there was no evidence of recurrent choroidal neovascularization. ((From Stewart M, Rosenfeld PJ, Penha F, Wang F, Yehoshua Z, Bueno-Lopez E, Lopez P. Pharmacokinetic rationale for dosing every 2 weeks versus 4 weeks with intravitreal ranibizumab, bevacizumab, and aflibercept (vascular endothelial growth factor trap-eye). Retina 2012;32(3):434–457.))

therapy.[102,103] However, for the OCT-guided retreatment strategy to be successful, it is imperative that the clinician carefully review the entire OCT scan to determine whether fluid is present. In clinical practice, the retina specialist needs to consider the risks, benefits, and cost of the treatment, and the OCT appearance of the retina is crucial to minimizing the need for retreatment and the cost associated with therapy.

22.6 Clinical Trials

Both qualitative and quantitative OCT imaging has been used as endpoints in major clinical studies.[63,102,103]

22.6.1 Age-Related Macular Degeneration

The usefulness of an OCT-based management strategy for the treatment in patients with neovascular AMD was first demonstrated in the Prospective OCT Study with Lucentis for Neovascular AMD (PrONTO). PrONTO was a 2-year trial based on a PRN dosing regimen followed according to the assessment of the OCT B-scans. The study resulted in visual acuity outcomes comparable to the outcomes from the monthly dosing in the phase III clinical studies (MARINA[10,49] and ANCHOR[46,48]), but the PrONTO study achieved those outcomes by requiring treatment whenever fluid appeared or persisted at monthly visits. In PrONTO, fewer intravitreal injections of ranibizumab were needed to achieve these similar visual acuity outcomes compared with Minimally Classic/Occult Trial of the Anti-VEGF Antibody Ranibizumab in the Treatment of Neovascular AMD (MARINA) trial and Anti-VEGF Antibody for the Treatment of Predominantly Classic Choroidal Neovascularization in AMD (ANCHOR) trial over a two-year period. The PrONTO results demonstrated that the OCT could be used to successfully guide treatment with anti-angiogenic drugs.[63]

The HARBOR study randomly assigned 1097 participants with subfoveal neovascular AMD to receive 2.0 or 0.5 mg ranibizumab dosed monthly or PRN after three loading doses. At month 12, all 4 treatment groups demonstrated similar improvement in visual acuity and anatomic outcomes.[61] The 2-year HARBOR trial results showed the maintenance of visual acuity gains and improvements in central foveal thickness measurements between the different treatment groups.[60] The noninferiority of the PRN strategy suggests that an individualized approach can be effective in patients with neovascular AMD treated with ranibizumab.

An OCT-based re-treatment strategy was also shown to be effective in managing patients with neovascular AMD undergoing treatment with bevacizumab.[102] The re-treatment criteria in this study were based on the second year re-treatment criteria of the PrONTO study. A total of 102 eyes of 102 patients with a follow-up of at least 6 months after the first intravitreal injection of bevacizumab were analyzed. Compared with baseline, visual acuity remained stable at 6 months and 12 months, whereas the OCT retinal thickness decreased in the same periods.

Two large, multicenter, randomized, clinical trials compared ranibizumab and bevacizumab using monthly and an PRNs dosing regimen that was dependent on the presence of macular fluid based on OCT imaging.[50,52,53,103] The Comparison of Age-Related Macular Degeneration Treatment Trial (CATT) was a prospective clinical trial of patients with neovascular AMD randomized at enrollment into four groups defined by drug (0.5 mg ranibizumab or 1.25 mg bevacizumab) and dosing regimen (monthly or PRN). After 1 year of treatment, patients initially assigned to monthly groups were randomly reassigned to monthly versus as-needed treatment. When administered in the same dosing regimen (monthly or PRN), bevacizumab and ranibizumab demonstrated similar beneficial effects on visual acuity at both 1 and 2 years.[52,104]

Performed in the United Kingdom, the Inhibition of VEGF in Age-Related Choroidal Neovascularization (IVAN) trial was a prospective, noninferiority clinical trial in patients with previously untreated neovascular AMD comparing ranibizumab and bevacizumab and using different dosing strategies (continuous and discontinuous regimens). Patients were randomly assigned to intravitreal injections of 1.25 mg bevacizumab or 0.5 mg ranibizumab monthly or PRN with monthly follow-up visits. The discontinuous treatment group received three loading injections before starting the PRN treatment, which was based on clinical and OCT re-treatment criteria. When re-treatment was required, injections were performed with another cycle of three monthly doses. The 2-year IVAN results showed similar efficacy for both drugs and the two different dosing regimens.[50]

Two multicenter, prospective, clinical trials from Europe also compared the safety and efficacy of intravitreal injections of bevacizumab and ranibizumab in the treatment of neovascular AMD. Both studies randomly assigned patients to one of the two drug groups, and three monthly injections were followed up by monthly visits with PRN treatment over 9 months. In the Groupe d'Evaluation Français Avastin versus Lucentis (GEFAL) Study,[105] thirty-eight French centers participated and in the Treatment With Ranibizumab or Bevacizumab in Patients With Neovascular Age-related Macular Degeneration Multicenter Anti VEGF Trial in Austria (MANTA) Study,[106,107] and 10 Austrian centers enrolled patients. Results from these studies were consistent with the other studies and demonstrated that bevacizumab was noninferior to ranibizumab when OCT-guided therapy was used. Visual acuity and CRT improved in the two groups with a rapid improvement observed during the three initial monthly injections. The vision in the two groups then remained stable using an OCT-guided PRN re-treatment regimen.

22.6.2 Diabetic Macular Edema

The identification of macular edema and the ability to compare qualitative and quantitative retinal changes between visits are extremely important in deciding when to reinject with antiangiogenic drugs. OCT-based strategies to determine re-treatment with intravitreal injections have been shown to be effective in clinical trials. The prospective randomized controlled trial of Intravitreal Bevacizumab or Laser Therapy in the Management of Diabetic Macular Edema (BOLT) study, performed in a single-center, randomized patients to either bevacizumab or macular laser therapy. In the bevacizumab arm, after three loading doses, patients were injected every 6 weeks using an OCT-guided re-treatment protocol. Patients in the laser arm were re-treated every 4 months based on clinical ETDRS guidelines. After 2 years, the results showed that the improvements in visual acuity and retinal thickness observed at 1 year were maintained in the bevacizumab group.[108,109]

The Ranibizumab for the Edema of the Macula in Diabetes (READ-2) study randomized patients to either ranibizumab 0.5 mg every 2 months, laser every 3 months, or a combined therapy at baseline and at month three for the first six months.[110] After 6 months, patients in the ranibizumab and laser group were seen every 2 months, and patients in the combination treatment group were seen every 3 months until month 24. During this second period, patients received treatment based on OCT guidelines (CRT 250 µm or greater) and could cross over to the ranibizumab group.[111] In the subsequent 12 months, patients from the three groups returned monthly and received 0.5 mg of anibizumab if the CRT was 250 µm or greater on OCT. Anatomically, all three groups showed improvement on OCT macular thickness. The greatest improvement in vision was seen in the ranibizumab group. The final mean improvements in letters compared with baseline were 10.3 for the ranibizumab group, 1.4 for the laser group, and 8.9 for the ranibizumab + laser group.[112]

The READ-3 study enrolled 152 eyes and randomized these eyes to either 0.5 mg or 2.0 mg dose of ranibizumab given monthly for 6 months and then PRN through 12 months based on the presence of DME as documented by OCT imaging (CRT > 275 µm on TD OCT or any fluid on SD OCT). The OCT results were similar at 12 months of follow-up, and visual acuity gains favored the 0.5 mg of ranibizumab dose (mean BCVA gain of 10.88 letters) over the 2.0 mg dose (mean best-corrected visual acuity (BCVA) gain of 7.39 letters).[113,114,115]

Two randomized, multicenter, phase III clinical trials, RISE and RIDE, using fixed dosing of ranibizumab at two different doses showed an improvement in retinal anatomy at month 24, and this was sustained through month 36.[116] The RISE and RIDE led to the FDA approval of the anti-VEGF treatment for diabetic macular edema.

Macular Edema from Retinal Vein Occlusion

Macular edema is the major contributor to vision loss in patients with RVO.[117] OCT identifies macular edema and has been used to monitor treatments.[86,118,119,120,121,122,123] The efficacy of anti-VEGF drugs was evaluated in published studies based on the reduction in CRT,[71,124,125] once again showing that this parameter is useful for monitoring the treatment of patients with macular edema.

The BRAVO[128,127] and CRUISE[119,128] studies evaluated the safety and efficacy of treatment with ranibizumab in patients with macular edema after branch retinal vein occlusion (BRVO) or central retinal vein occlusion (CRVO), respectively. With the same design, patients in these clinical trials were randomized on a 1:1:1 ratio to monthly treatment with 0.3 mg or 0.5 mg of ranibizumab or sham injection for 6 months. Patients with BRVO could have laser rescue therapy. In the subsequent 6 months, all patients in both studies were eligible for ranibizumab PRN therapy based on OCT imaging (CRT ≥ 250 µm on TD OCT) or visual acuity (Early Treatment Diabetic Retinopathy Study [ETDRS] BCVA ≤ 40 letters) criteria. Results of these clinical trials demonstrated improvements in visual acuity and macular edema with reduction of CRT after 6 months of therapy in the ranibizumab groups compared with the sham. Subsequent treatment with ranibizumab PRN maintained the visual and anatomical benefits during the 12-month period in these patients. An extension of BRAVO and CRUISE, a multicenter, open-label, single-arm study known as the Ranibizumab for macular edema due to retinal vein occlusions (HORIZON)[129] trial, included patients from both clinical trials and continued treatment with ranibizumab 0.5 mg at PRN intervals (between 1 and 3 months) during an additional 12 months. Patients with BRVO were eligible for the laser rescue therapy. After the second year of treatment, results demonstrated that visual acuity and OCT changes were maintained in the BRVO group using a PRN strategy. However, the fewer number of ranibizumab injections in the CRVO group was associated with a decline in vision and a moderate increase in CRT. This suggests the need of an individualized approach for patients with CRVO and BRVO.

The use of intravitreal aflibercept for macular edema caused by CRVO was evaluated in the COPERNICUS study.[70,130] During 24 weeks, patients received 2 mg of aflibercept or sham injection every 4 weeks. From week 24 to week 52, all patients were evaluated monthly and received 2 mg of aflibercept PRN. Between weeks 52 and 100, patients received 2 mg of aflibercept PRN and were evaluated at least quarterly. Two-year results demonstrated that visual and anatomical improvements observed during the first two periods using fixed dosing and monthly visits with PRN dosing were not maintained from week 52 to week 100, when a reduced monitoring schedule was established for the PRN dosing treatment. This outcome suggests that PRN OCT-guided dosing is successful only when close follow-up is continued.

The GALILEO study[71,124] randomized patients with CRVO to receive either 2 mg of intravitreal aflibercept or sham injected every 4 weeks for 20 weeks. From week 24 to week 48, patients were evaluated monthly, and the aflibercept group received aflibercept PRN or sham injection if the criteria for treatment were not present. The sham group was maintained with the sham injections. All patients were eligible to receive laser photocoagulation if necessary. One-year results revealed that intravitreal injections of aflibercept provided significant functional and anatomical benefits compared with sham after 6 monthly doses, and these results were maintained until week 52 with PRN dosing. From week 52 to week 76, all patients were evaluated every 8 weeks using a PRN strategy. However, during this period of PRN dosing and less frequent monitoring, visual acuity gains were diminished.

22.7 Conclusions and Future Directions

OCT has revolutionized our ability to detect, diagnose, and manage vitreoretinal diseases. It has become an essential tool in the diagnosis and management of patients with exudative diseases, such as neovascular AMD. By monitoring exudative diseases with OCT imaging, we have been able to tailor treatments to the patient and reduce the number of injections compared with monthly dosing. In addition, OCT imaging has dramatically decreased the need for invasive, time-consuming imaging strategies such as fluorescein and indocyanine green angiography, which also are associated with some risks. As the technology advances over the next few years, we will be able to scan larger areas faster, with higher resolution, with better choroidal resolution, and with the ability to visualize retinal and choroidal blood flow in the absence of any fluorescent dyes. Improvements in the algorithms, along with the axial, lateral, and depth resolution, are expected to help with monitoring diseases and their response to the therapy. Ultrahigh-speed swept-source OCTs are under development to better visualize the microstructural details of the vitreous, retina and choroid. As long as anti-VEGF therapy remains the standard of care for the treatment of exudative retinal diseases, OCT imaging will be needed to achieve the maximum benefit from these drugs with the least risk and cost.

References

[1] Ciulla TA, Rosenfeld PJ. Anti-vascular endothelial growth factor therapy for neovascular ocular diseases other than age-related macular degeneration. Curr Opin Ophthalmol 2009; 20: 166–174

[2] Semeraro F, Parrinello G, Cancarini A, et al. Predicting the risk of diabetic retinopathy in type 2 diabetic patients. J Diabetes Complications 2011; 25: 292–297

[3] Klein R, Klein BE, Moss SE, Davis MD, DeMets DL. The Wisconsin epidemiologic study of diabetic retinopathy. IV: diabetic macular edema. Ophthalmology 1984; 91: 1464–1474

[4] Moss SE, Klein R, Klein BE. Ten-year incidence of visual loss in a diabetic population. Ophthalmology 1994; 101: 1061–1070

[5] Veritti D, Sarao V, Lanzetta P. Neovascular age-related macular degeneration. Ophthalmologica 2012; 227 Suppl 1: 11–20

[6] Bressler NM. Age-related macular degeneration is the leading cause of blindness... JAMA 2004; 291: 1900–1901

[7] Do DV. Detection of new-onset choroidal neovascularization. Curr Opin Ophthalmol 2013; 24: 244–247

[8] Regatieri CV, Branchini L, Duker JS. The Role of Spectral-Domain OCT in the Diagnosis and Management of Neovascular Age-Related Macular Degeneration. Ophthalmic Surg Lasers Imaging 2011; 42: S56–S66

[9] Keane PA, Patel PJ, Liakopoulos S, Heussen FM, Sadda SR, Tufail A. Evaluation of age-related macular degeneration with optical coherence tomography. Surv Ophthalmol 2012; 57: 389–414

[10] Rosenfeld PJ, Brown DM, Heier JS, et al. MARINA Study Group. Ranibizumab for neovascular age-related macular degeneration. N Engl J Med 2006; 355: 1419–1431

[11] Kovach JL, Schwartz SG, Flynn HW, Jr, Scott IU. Anti-VEGF Treatment Strategies for Wet AMD. J Ophthalmol 2012; 2012: 786870

[12] Ferrara N. Vascular endothelial growth factor: basic science and clinical progress. Endocr Rev 2004; 25: 581–611

[13] Stewart MW. Pharmacokinetics, pharmacodynamics and pre-clinical characteristics of ophthalmic drugs that bind VEGF. Expert Rep Clin Pharmacol 2014;7(2):167–180

[14] D'Amico DJ, Masonson HN, Patel M, et al. VEGF Inhibition Study in Ocular Neovascularization (V.I.S.I.O.N.) Clinical Trial Group. Pegaptanib sodium for neovascular age-related macular degeneration: two-year safety results of the two prospective, multicenter, controlled clinical trials. Ophthalmology 2006; 113: 992–1001, e6

[15] Gragoudas ES, Adamis AP, Cunningham ET, Jr, Feinsod M, Guyer DR VEGF Inhibition Study in Ocular Neovascularization Clinical Trial Group. Pegaptanib for neovascular age-related macular degeneration. N Engl J Med 2004; 351: 2805–2816

[16] Chakravarthy U, Adamis AP, Cunningham ET, Jr, et al. VEGF Inhibition Study in Ocular Neovascularization (V.I.S.I.O.N.) Clinical Trial Group. Year 2 efficacy results of 2 randomized controlled clinical trials of pegaptanib for neovascular age-related macular degeneration. Ophthalmology 2006; 113: e1–e25

[17] Doggrell SA. Pegaptanib: the first antiangiogenic agent approved for neovascular macular degeneration. Expert Opin Pharmacother 2005; 6: 1421–1423

[18] Sultan MB, Zhou D, Loftus J, Dombi T, Ice KS Macugen 1013 Study Group. A phase 2/3, multicenter, randomized, double-masked, 2-year trial of pegaptanib sodium for the treatment of diabetic macular edema. Ophthalmology 2011; 118: 1107–1118

[19] Yancopoulos GD. Clinical application of therapies targeting VEGF. Cell 2010; 143: 13–16

[20] Hurwitz H, Fehrenbacher L, Novotny W, et al. Bevacizumab plus irinotecan, fluorouracil, and leucovorin for metastatic colorectal cancer. N Engl J Med 2004; 350: 2335–2342

[21] D'Orazio A, Lee D, Ellis L, Chu E. Adding a humanized antibody to vascular endothelial growth factor (bevacizumab, Avastin) to chemotherapy improves survival in metastatic colorectal cancer. Clin Colorectal Cancer 2003; 3: 85–88

[22] Dirican A, Kucukzeybek Y, Alacacioglu A, et al. Impact of pre-angiogenic factors on the treatment effect of bevacizumab in patients with metastatic colorectal cancer. Med Oncol 2014; 31: 905

[23] Michels S, Rosenfeld PJ, Puliafito CA, Marcus EN, Venkatraman AS. Systemic bevacizumab (Avastin) therapy for neovascular age-related macular degeneration twelve-week results of an uncontrolled open-label clinical study. Ophthalmology 2005; 112: 1035–1047

[24] Rosenfeld PJ, Moshfeghi AA, Puliafito CA. Optical coherence tomography findings after an intravitreal injection of bevacizumab (avastin) for neovascular age-related macular degeneration. Ophthalmic Surg Lasers Imaging 2005; 36: 331–335

[25] Rosenfeld PJ, Fung AE, Puliafito CA. Optical coherence tomography findings after an intravitreal injection of bevacizumab (avastin) for macular edema from central retinal vein occlusion. Ophthalmic Surg Lasers Imaging 2005; 36: 336–339

[26] Lynch SS, Cheng CM. Bevacizumab for neovascular ocular diseases. Ann Pharmacother 2007; 41: 614–625

[27] Rich RM, Rosenfeld PJ, Puliafito CA, et al. Short-term safety and efficacy of intravitreal bevacizumab (Avastin) for neovascular age-related macular degeneration. Retina 2006; 26: 495–511

[28] Spaide RF, Laud K, Fine HF, et al. Intravitreal bevacizumab treatment of choroidal neovascularization secondary to age-related macular degeneration. Retina 2006; 26: 383–390

[29] Avery RL, Pieramici DJ, Rabena MD, Castellarin AA, Nasir MA, Giust MJ. Intravitreal bevacizumab (Avastin) for neovascular age-related macular degeneration. Ophthalmology 2006; 113: 363–372, e5

[30] Bashshur ZF, Bazarbachi A, Schakal A, Haddad ZA, El Haibi CP, Noureddin BN. Intravitreal bevacizumab for the management of choroidal neovascularization in age-related macular degeneration. Am J Ophthalmol 2006; 142: 1–9

[31] Geitzenauer W, Michels S, Prager F, et al. [Early effects of systemic and intravitreal bevacizumab (avastin) therapy for neovascular age-related macular degeneration] Klin Monatsbl Augenheilkd 2006; 223: 822–827

[32] Ladewig MS, Ziemssen F, Jaissle G, et al. [Intravitreal bevacizumab for neovascular age-related macular degeneration]. Ophthalmologe 2006; 103: 463–470

[33] Costa RA, Jorge R, Calucci D, Cardillo JA, Melo LA, Jr, Scott IU. Intravitreal bevacizumab for choroidal neovascularization caused by AMD (IBeNA Study): results of a phase 1 dose-escalation study. Invest Ophthalmol Vis Sci 2006; 47: 4569–4578

[34] Yoganathan P, Deramo VA, Lai JC, Tibrewala RK, Fastenberg DM. Visual improvement following intravitreal bevacizumab (Avastin) in exudative age-related macular degeneration. Retina 2006; 26: 994–998

[35] Hughes MS, Sang DN. Safety and efficacy of intravitreal bevacizumab followed by pegaptanib maintenance as a treatment regimen for age-related macular degeneration. Ophthalmic Surg Lasers Imaging 2006; 37: 446–454

[36] Aggio FB, Farah ME, Silva WC, Melo GB. Intravitreal bevacizumab for exudative age-related macular degeneration after multiple treatments. Graefes Arch Clin Exp Ophthalmol 2007; 245: 215–220

[37] Chen CY, Wong TY, Heriot WJ. Intravitreal bevacizumab (Avastin) for neovascular age-related macular degeneration: a short-term study. Am J Ophthalmol 2007; 143: 510–512

[38] Chen E, Kaiser RS, Vander JF. Intravitreal bevacizumab for refractory pigment epithelial detachment with occult choroidal neovascularization in age-related macular degeneration. Retina 2007; 27: 445–450

[39] Giansanti F, Virgili G, Bini A, et al. Intravitreal bevacizumab therapy for choroidal neovascularization secondary to age-related macular degeneration: 6-month results of an open-label uncontrolled clinical study. Eur J Ophthalmol 2007; 17: 230–237

[40] Tufail A, Patel PJ, Egan C, et al. ABC Trial Investigators. Bevacizumab for neovascular age related macular degeneration (ABC Trial): multicentre randomised double masked study. BMJ 2010; 340: c2459

[41] Roh MI, Kim JH, Kwon OW. Features of optical coherence tomography are predictive of visual outcomes after intravitreal bevacizumab injection for diabetic macular edema. Ophthalmologica 2010; 224: 374–380

[42] Scott IU, Edwards AR, Beck RW, et al. Diabetic Retinopathy Clinical Research Network. A phase II randomized clinical trial of intravitreal bevacizumab for diabetic macular edema. Ophthalmology 2007; 114: 1860–1867

[43] Tareen IU, Rahman A, Mahar PS, Memon MS. Primary effects of intravitreal bevacizumab in patients with diabetic macular edema. Pak J Med Sci 2013; 29: 1018–1022

[44] Osaadon P, Fagan XJ, Lifshitz T, Levy J. A review of anti-VEGF agents for proliferative diabetic retinopathy. Eye (Lond) 2014; 28: 510–520

[45] Pieramici DJ, Rabena MD. Anti-VEGF therapy: comparison of current and future agents. Eye (Lond) 2008; 22: 1330–1336

[46] Brown DM, Michels M, Kaiser PK, Heier JS, Sy JP, Ianchulev T ANCHOR Study Group. Ranibizumab versus verteporfin photodynamic therapy for neovascular age-related macular degeneration: Two-year results of the ANCHOR study. Ophthalmology 2009; 116: 57–65, e5

[47] Brown DM, Kaiser PK, Michels M, et al. ANCHOR Study Group. Ranibizumab versus verteporfin for neovascular age-related macular degeneration. N Engl J Med 2006; 355: 1432–1444

[48] Kaiser PK, Brown DM, Zhang K, et al. Ranibizumab for predominantly classic neovascular age-related macular degeneration: subgroup analysis of first-year ANCHOR results. Am J Ophthalmol 2007; 144: 850–857

[49] Kaiser PK, Blodi BA, Shapiro H, Acharya NR. MARINA Study Group. Angiographic and optical coherence tomographic results of the MARINA study of ranibizumab in neovascular age-related macular degeneration. Ophthalmology 2007; 114: 1868–1875

[50] Chakravarthy U, Harding SP, Rogers CA, et al. IVAN study investigators. Alternative treatments to inhibit VEGF in age-related choroidal neovascularisation: 2-year findings of the IVAN randomised controlled trial. Lancet 2013; 382: 1258–1267

[51] Abraham P, Yue H, Wilson L. Randomized, double-masked, sham-controlled trial of ranibizumab for neovascular age-related macular degeneration: PIER study year 2. Am J Ophthalmol 2010; 150: 315–324, e1

[52] Martin DF, Maguire MG, Fine SL, et al. Comparison of Age-related Macular Degeneration Treatments Trials (CATT) Research Group. Ranibizumab and bevacizumab for treatment of neovascular age-related macular degeneration: two-year results. Ophthalmology 2012; 119: 1388–1398

[53] Chakravarthy U, Harding SP, Rogers CA, et al. IVAN Study Investigators. Ranibizumab versus bevacizumab to treat neovascular age-related macular degeneration: one-year findings from the IVAN randomized trial. Ophthalmology 2012; 119: 1399–1411

[54] Singer MA, Awh CC, Sadda S, et al. HORIZON: an open-label extension trial of ranibizumab for choroidal neovascularization secondary to age-related macular degeneration. Ophthalmology 2012; 119: 1175–1183

[55] Regillo CD, Brown DM, Abraham P, et al. Randomized, double-masked, sham-controlled trial of ranibizumab for neovascular age-related macular degeneration: PIER Study year 1. Am J Ophthalmol 2008; 145: 239–248

[56] Mitchell P, Korobelnik JF, Lanzetta P, et al. Ranibizumab (Lucentis) in neovascular age-related macular degeneration: evidence from clinical trials. Br J Ophthalmol 2010; 94: 2–13

[57] Silva R, Axer-Siegel R, Eldem B, et al. SECURE Study Group. The SECURE study: long-term safety of ranibizumab 0.5 mg in neovascular age-related macular degeneration. Ophthalmology 2013; 120: 130–139

[58] Schmidt-Erfurth U, Eldem B, Guymer R, et al. EXCITE Study Group. Efficacy and safety of monthly versus quarterly ranibizumab treatment in neovascular age-related macular degeneration: the EXCITE study. Ophthalmology 2011; 118: 831–839

[59] Holz FG, Amoaku W, Donate J, et al. SUSTAIN Study Group. Safety and efficacy of a flexible dosing regimen of ranibizumab in neovascular age-related macular degeneration: the SUSTAIN study. Ophthalmology 2011; 118: 663–671

[60] Ho AC, Busbee BG, Regillo CD, et al. HARBOR 2-Year Results Support Individualized Dosing in Patients With Wet Age-Related Macular Degeneration. PRESENTED AT the 31st Annual Meeting of the American Society of Retina Specialists (ASRS), August 2013, Toronto, Canada

[61] Busbee BG, Ho AC, Brown DM, et al. HARBOR Study Group. Twelve-month efficacy and safety of 0.5 mg or 2.0 mg ranibizumab in patients with subfoveal neovascular age-related macular degeneration. Ophthalmology 2013; 120: 1046–1056

[62] Boyer DS, Heier JS, Brown DM, Francom SF, Ianchulev T, Rubio RG. A Phase IIIb study to evaluate the safety of ranibizumab in subjects with neovascular age-related macular degeneration. Ophthalmology 2009; 116: 1731–1739
[63] Lalwani GA, Rosenfeld PJ, Fung AE, et al. A variable-dosing regimen with intravitreal ranibizumab for neovascular age-related macular degeneration: year 2 of the PrONTO Study. Am J Ophthalmol 2009; 148: 43–58, e1
[64] Nguyen QD, Brown DM, Marcus DM, et al. RISE and RIDE Research Group. Ranibizumab for diabetic macular edema: results from 2 phase III randomized trials: RISE and RIDE. Ophthalmology 2012; 119: 789–801
[65] Xu D, Kaiser PK. Intravitreal aflibercept for neovascular age-related macular degeneration. Immunotherapy 2013; 5: 121–130
[66] Heier JS, Boyer D, Nguyen QD, et al. CLEAR-IT 2 Investigators. The 1-year results of CLEAR-IT 2, a phase 2 study of vascular endothelial growth factor trap-eye dosed as-needed after 12-week fixed dosing. Ophthalmology 2011; 118: 1098–1106
[67] Hanout M, Ferraz D, Ansari M, et al. Therapies for neovascular age-related macular degeneration: current approaches and pharmacologic agents in development. Biomed Res Int 2013; 2013: 830–837
[68] Heier JS, Brown DM, Chong V, et al. VIEW 1 and VIEW 2 Study Groups. Intravitreal aflibercept (VEGF trap-eye) in wet age-related macular degeneration. Ophthalmology 2012; 119: 2537–2548
[69] Schmidt-Erfurth U, Kaiser PK, Korobelnik JF, et al. Intravitreal aflibercept injection for neovascular age-related macular degeneration: ninety-six-week results of the VIEW studies. Ophthalmology 2014; 121: 193–201
[70] Brown DM, Heier JS, Clark WL, et al. Intravitreal aflibercept injection for macular edema secondary to central retinal vein occlusion: 1-year results from the phase 3 COPERNICUS study. Am J Ophthalmol 2013; 155: 429–437, e7
[71] Korobelnik JF, Holz FG, Roider J, et al. GALILEO Study Group. Intravitreal Aflibercept Injection for Macular Edema Resulting from Central Retinal Vein Occlusion: one-year results of the Phase 3 GALILEO study. Ophthalmology 2014; 121: 202–208
[72] You JY, Chung H, Kim HC. Evaluation of changes in choroidal neovascularization secondary to age-related macular degeneration after anti-VEGF therapy using spectral domain optical coherence tomography. Curr Eye Res 2012; 37: 438–445
[73] Drexler W, Fujimoto JG. State-of-the-art retinal optical coherence tomography. Prog Retin Eye Res 2008; 27: 45–88
[74] Srinivasan VJ, Wojtkowski M, Witkin AJ, et al. High-definition and 3-dimensional imaging of macular pathologies with high-speed ultrahigh-resolution optical coherence tomography. Ophthalmology 2006; 113: e1–e14
[75] Kanagasingam Y, Bhuiyan A, Abràmoff MD, Smith RT, Goldschmidt L, Wong TY. Progress on retinal image analysis for age related macular degeneration. Prog Retin Eye Res 2014; 38: 20–42
[76] Keane PA, Bhatti RA, Brubaker JW, Liakopoulos S, Sadda SR, Walsh AC. Comparison of clinically relevant findings from high-speed fourier-domain and conventional time-domain optical coherence tomography. Am J Ophthalmol 2009; 148: 242–248, e1
[77] Sayanagi K, Sharma S, Yamamoto T, Kaiser PK. Comparison of spectral-domain versus time-domain optical coherence tomography in management of age-related macular degeneration with ranibizumab. Ophthalmology 2009; 116: 947–955
[78] Schimel AM, Fisher YL, Flynn HW, Jr. Optical coherence tomography in the diagnosis and management of diabetic macular edema: time-domain versus spectral-domain. Ophthalmic Surg Lasers Imaging 2011; 42: 41–45
[79] Potsaid B, Baumann B, Huang D, et al. Ultrahigh speed 1050 nm swept source/Fourier domain OCT retinal and anterior segment imaging at 100,000 to 400,000 axial scans per second. Opt Express 2010; 18: 20029–20048
[80] Hee MR, Baumal CR, Puliafito CA, et al. Optical coherence tomography of age-related macular degeneration and choroidal neovascularization. Ophthalmology 1996; 103: 1260–1270
[81] Gass JD. Pathogenesis of tears of the retinal pigment epithelium. Br J Ophthalmol 1984; 68: 513–519
[82] Coscas F, Coscas G, Souied E, Tick S, Soubrane G. Optical coherence tomography identification of occult choroidal neovascularization in age-related macular degeneration. Am J Ophthalmol 2007; 144: 592–599
[83] Puliafito CA, Hee MR, Lin CP, et al. Imaging of macular diseases with optical coherence tomography. Ophthalmology 1995; 102: 217–229
[84] Sánchez-Tocino H, Alvarez-Vidal A, Maldonado MJ, Moreno-Montañés J, García-Layana A. Retinal thickness study with optical coherence tomography in patients with diabetes. Invest Ophthalmol Vis Sci 2002; 43: 1588–1594
[85] Massin P, Vicaut E, Haouchine B, Erginay A, Paques M, Gaudric A. Reproducibility of retinal mapping using optical coherence tomography. Arch Ophthalmol 2001; 119: 1135–1142
[86] Hee MR, Puliafito CA, Wong C, et al. Quantitative assessment of macular edema with optical coherence tomography. Arch Ophthalmol 1995; 113: 1019–1029
[87] Gregori G, Wang F, Rosenfeld PJ, et al. Spectral domain optical coherence tomography imaging of drusen in nonexudative age-related macular degeneration. Ophthalmology 2011; 118: 1373–1379
[88] Penha FM, Rosenfeld PJ, Gregori G, et al. Quantitative imaging of retinal pigment epithelial detachments using spectral-domain optical coherence tomography. Am J Ophthalmol 2012; 153: 515–523
[89] Balasubramanian M, Bowd C, Vizzeri G, Weinreb RN, Zangwill LM. Effect of image quality on tissue thickness measurements obtained with spectral domain-optical coherence tomography. Opt Express 2009; 17: 4019–4036
[90] Liu S, Paranjape AS, Elmaanaoui B, et al. Quality assessment for spectral domain optical coherence tomography (OCT) images. Proc SPIE 2009; 7171: 71710X
[91] Ghazi NG, Kirk T, Allam S, Yan G. Quantification of error in optical coherence tomography central macular thickness measurement in wet age-related macular degeneration. Am J Ophthalmol 2009; 148: 90–96, e2
[92] Keane PA, Liakopoulos S, Jivrajka RV, et al. Evaluation of optical coherence tomography retinal thickness parameters for use in clinical trials for neovascular age-related macular degeneration. Invest Ophthalmol Vis Sci 2009; 50: 3378–3385
[93] Keane PA, Liakopoulos S, Walsh AC, Sadda SR. Limits of the retinal-mapping program in age-related macular degeneration. Br J Ophthalmol 2009; 93: 274–275
[94] Krebs I, Falkner-Radler C, Hagen S, et al. Quality of the threshold algorithm in age-related macular degeneration: Stratus versus Cirrus OCT. Invest Ophthalmol Vis Sci 2009; 50: 995–1000
[95] Keane PA, Mand PS, Liakopoulos S, Walsh AC, Sadda SR. Accuracy of retinal thickness measurements obtained with Cirrus optical coherence tomography. Br J Ophthalmol 2009; 93: 1461–1467
[96] Choi W, Mohler KJ, Potsaid B, et al. Choriocapillaris and choroidal microvasculature imaging with ultrahigh speed OCT angiography. PLoS ONE 2013; 8: e81499
[97] Chen Y, Vuong LN, Liu J, et al. Three-dimensional ultrahigh resolution optical coherence tomography imaging of age-related macular degeneration. Opt Express 2009; 17: 4046–4060
[98] Arias L, Armadá F, Donate J, et al. Delay in treating age-related macular degeneration in Spain is associated with progressive vision loss. Eye (Lond) 2009; 23: 326–333
[99] Manousaridis K, Manjunath V, Talks J. Information used to decide on retreatment of exudative age-related macular degeneration with anti-VEGF in clinical practice. Eur J Ophthalmol 2012; 4: 0
[100] Emerson MV, Lauer AK, Flaxel CJ, et al. Intravitreal bevacizumab (Avastin) treatment of neovascular age-related macular degeneration. Retina 2007; 27: 439–444
[101] Sayed KM, Naito T, Nagasawa T, Katome T, Mitamura Y. Early visual impacts of optical coherence tomographic parameters in patients with age-related macular degeneration following the first versus repeated ranibizumab injection. Graefes Arch Clin Exp Ophthalmol 2011; 249: 1449–1458
[102] Leydolt C, Michels S, Prager F, et al. Effect of intravitreal bevacizumab (Avastin) in neovascular age-related macular degeneration using a treatment regimen based on optical coherence tomography: 6- and 12-month results. Acta Ophthalmol (Copenh) 2010; 88: 594–600
[103] Fung AE, Lalwani GA, Rosenfeld PJ, et al. An optical coherence tomography-guided, variable dosing regimen with intravitreal ranibizumab (Lucentis) for neovascular age-related macular degeneration. Am J Ophthalmol 2007; 143: 566–583
[104] Martin DF, Maguire MG, Ying GS, Grunwald JE, Fine SL, Jaffe GJ CATT Research Group. Ranibizumab and bevacizumab for neovascular age-related macular degeneration. N Engl J Med 2011; 364: 1897–1908
[105] Kodjikian L, Souied EH, Mimoun G, et al. GEFAL Study Group. Ranibizumab versus Bevacizumab for Neovascular Age-related Macular Degeneration: results from the GEFAL Noninferiority Randomized Trial. Ophthalmology 2013; 120: 2300–2309
[106] Krebs I, Schmetterer L, Boltz A, et al. MANTA Research Group. A randomised double-masked trial comparing the visual outcome after treatment with ranibizumab or bevacizumab in patients with neovascular age-related macular degeneration. Br J Ophthalmol 2013; 97: 266–271
[107] Ehlers JP. The MANTA 1-year results: the anti-VEGF debate continues. Br J Ophthalmol 2013; 97: 248–250
[108] Michaelides M, Kaines A, Hamilton RD, et al. A prospective randomized trial of intravitreal bevacizumab or laser therapy in the management of diabetic

macular edema (BOLT study) 12-month data: report 2. Ophthalmology 2010; 117: 1078–1086, e2

[109] Rajendram R, Fraser-Bell S, Kaines A, et al. A 2-year prospective randomized controlled trial of intravitreal bevacizumab or laser therapy (BOLT) in the management of diabetic macular edema: 24 month data: report 3. Arch Ophthalmol 2012; 130: 972–979

[110] Nguyen QD, Shah SM, Heier JS, et al. READ-2 Study Group. Primary end point (six months) results of the anibizumab for Edema of the mAcula in Diabetes (READ-2) study. Ophthalmology 2009; 116: 2175–2181, e1

[111] Nguyen QD, Shah SM, Khwaja AA, et al. READ-2 Study Group. Two-year outcomes of the ranibizumab for edema of the macula in diabetes (READ-2) study. Ophthalmology 2010; 117: 2146–2151

[112] Do DV, Nguyen QD, Khwaja AA, et al. READ-2 Study Group. Ranibizumab for edema of the macula in diabetes study: 3-year outcomes and the need for prolonged frequent treatment. JAMA Ophthalmol 2013; 131: 139–145

[113] Do DV, Campochiaro PA, Boyer DS, et al. Six-month and one-year interim results of the READ 3 study: Ranibizumab for Edema of the Macula in Diabetes. Abstract presented at: 2012 Annual Meeting of the Association for Research in Vision and Ophthalmology (ARVO); 2012; Fort Lauderdale, FL

[114] Thomas BJ, Shienbaum G, Boyer DS, Flynn HW, Jr. Evolving strategies in the management of diabetic macular edema: clinical trials and current management. Can J Ophthalmol 2013; 48: 22–30

[115] Stewart MW. Critical appraisal of ranibizumab in the treatment of diabetic macular edema. Clin Ophthalmol 2013; 7: 1257–1267

[116] Brown DM, Nguyen QD, Marcus DM, et al. RIDE and RISE Research Group. Long-term outcomes of ranibizumab therapy for diabetic macular edema: the 36-month results from two phase III trials: RISE and RIDE. Ophthalmology 2013; 120: 2013–2022

[117] Decroos FC, Stinnett SS, Heydary CS, Burns RE, Jaffe GJ. Reading center characterization of central retinal vein occlusion using optical coherence tomography during the COPERNICUS trial. Transl Vis Sci Technol 2013; 2: 7–9

[118] Lerche RC, Schaudig U, Scholz F, Walter A, Richard G. Structural changes of the retina in retinal vein occlusion—imaging and quantification with optical coherence tomography. Ophthalmic Surg Lasers 2001; 32: 272–280

[119] Brown DM, Campochiaro PA, Singh RP, et al. CRUISE Investigators. Ranibizumab for macular edema following central retinal vein occlusion: six-month primary end point results of a phase III study. Ophthalmology 2010; 117: 1124–1133, e1

[120] Domalpally A, Blodi BA, Scott IU, et al. SCORE Study Investigator Group. The Standard Care vs Corticosteroid for Retinal Vein Occlusion (SCORE) study system for evaluation of optical coherence tomograms: SCORE study report 4. Arch Ophthalmol 2009; 127: 1461–1467

[121] Haller JA, Bandello F, Belfort R, Jr, et al. OZURDEX GENEVA Study Group. Randomized, sham-controlled trial of dexamethasone intravitreal implant in patients with macular edema due to retinal vein occlusion. Ophthalmology 2010; 117: 1134–1146, e3

[122] Prager F, Michels S, Kriechbaum K, et al. Intravitreal bevacizumab (Avastin) for macular oedema secondary to retinal vein occlusion: 12-month results of a prospective clinical trial. Br J Ophthalmol 2009; 93: 452–456

[123] Priglinger SG, Wolf AH, Kreutzer TC, et al. Intravitreal bevacizumab injections for treatment of central retinal vein occlusion: six-month results of a prospective trial. Retina 2007; 27: 1004–1012

[124] Holz FG, Roider J, Ogura Y, et al. VEGF Trap-Eye for macular oedema secondary to central retinal vein occlusion: 6-month results of the phase III GALILEO study. Br J Ophthalmol 2013; 97: 278–284

[125] Singer MA, Cohen SR, Groth SL, Porbandarwalla S. Comparing bevacizumab and ranibizumab for initial reduction of central macular thickness in patients with retinal vein occlusions. Clin Ophthalmol 2013; 7: 1377–1383

[126] Campochiaro PA, Heier JS, Feiner L, et al. BRAVO Investigators. Ranibizumab for macular edema following branch retinal vein occlusion: six-month primary end point results of a phase III study. Ophthalmology 2010; 117: 1102–1112, e1

[127] Brown DM, Campochiaro PA, Bhisitkul RB, et al. Sustained benefits from ranibizumab for macular edema following branch retinal vein occlusion: 12-month outcomes of a phase III study. Ophthalmology 2011; 118: 1594–1602

[128] Campochiaro PA, Brown DM, Awh CC, et al. Sustained benefits from ranibizumab for macular edema following central retinal vein occlusion: twelve-month outcomes of a phase III study. Ophthalmology 2011; 118: 2041–2049

[129] Heier JS, Campochiaro PA, Yau L, et al. Ranibizumab for macular edema due to retinal vein occlusions: long-term follow-up in the HORIZON trial. Ophthalmology 2012; 119: 802–809

[130] Heier JS, Clark WL, Boyer DS, et al. Intravitreal Aflibercept injection for macular edema due to central retinal vein occlusion: two-year results from the COPERNICUS Study. Ophthalmology 2014: 26

Part 5

Miscellaneous

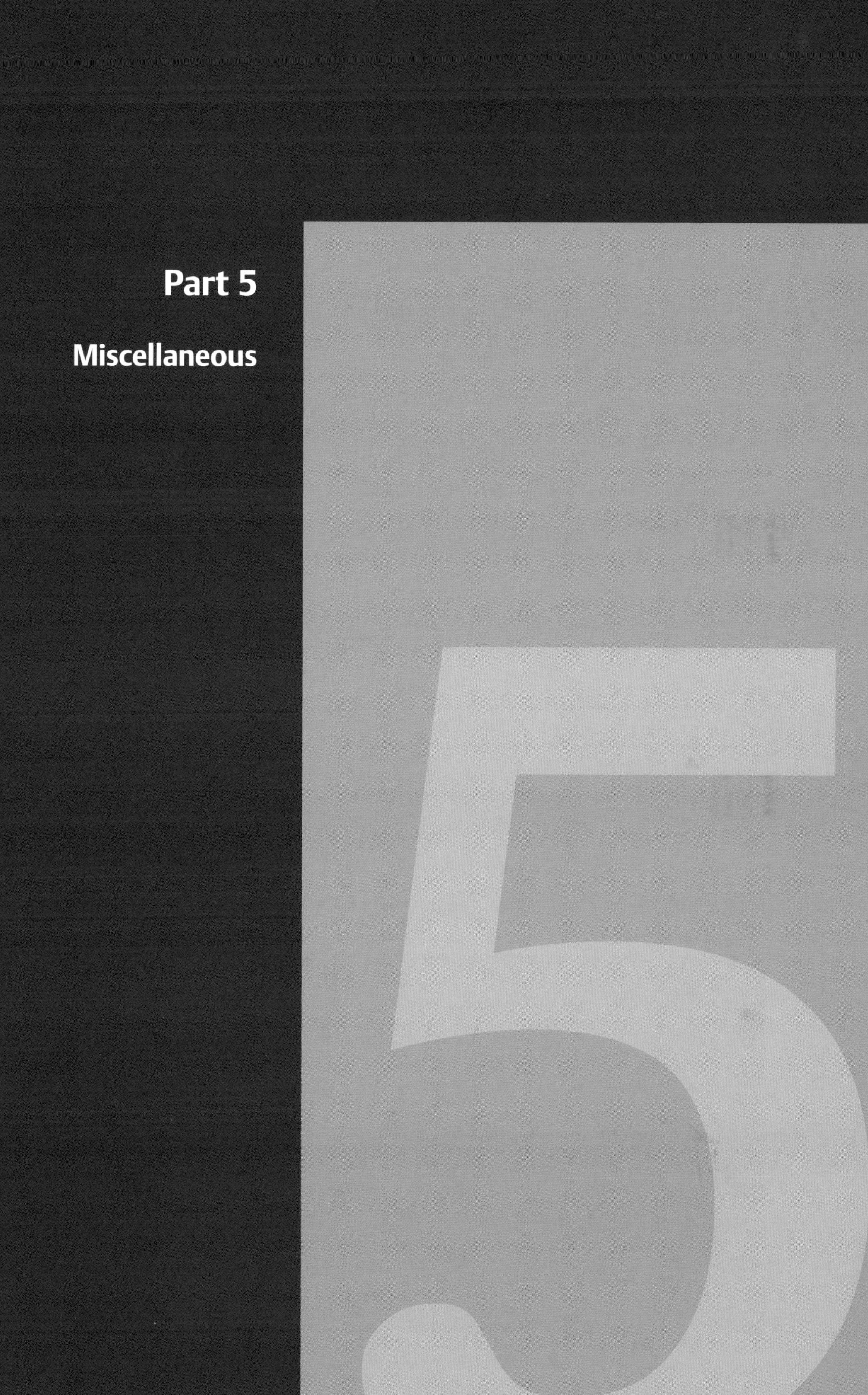

23 Optical Coherence Tomography for Imaging Anterior-Chamber Inflammatory Reaction in Uveitis

Dhivya Ashok Kumar and Amar Agarwal

Anterior chamber (AC) cellular reaction is often clinically observed by slit-lamp biomicroscopy.[1] However, it cannot be performed in eyes with postoperative corneal edema or haze, and the grading ability is also dependent on the experience of the examiner. The existing objective method for AC reaction grading is the flare meter, which is based on the principle of laser photometry. Counting cells by laser flare meter is effective and linear in controlled laboratory situations, but it appears to be less accurate than flare measurements in vivo.[2] Moreover, its reliability in edematous cornea has not been proved so far. Laser flare photometry has been known to be affected by the aqueous humor protein concentration, the mydriatic agent used, and the presence of red blood cells.[2]

Optical coherence tomography (OCT) has evolved as a widely used imaging modality in ophthalmology in the last decade. Earlier, we reported a case series on the objective method of diagnosing the AC cells in anterior uveitis with time-domain (TD) anterior-segment OCT.[3] Recently, OCT machines with sophisticated optics with spectral (SD) or Fourier domain (FD), which enabled examination of both the anterior and posterior segment in a single setup, have been developed.[4,5,6,7,8,9] This development has enabled high-definition scanning of the AC. In this chapter, we discuss the use of OCT, both TD and the FD, in grading AC reaction and the methods of evaluation in uveitis.

23.1 Time-Domain OCT in Anterior-Chamber Cell Detection

Various causes of uveitis, including acute and chronic idiopathic anterior uveitis, postoperative uveitis, panuveitis, herpetic keratouveitis, interstitial keratitis, corneal ulcer, posterior corneal abscess, and endophthalmitis were included in the study. Sixty-two eyes of 45 patients referred to the uvea clinic were studied. Patients not willing to undergo follow-up were excluded. A detailed slit-lamp examination was performed in all patients, and the AC reaction was graded clinically from 0 to 4 using the Standardization of the Uveitis Nomenclature (SUN).[10] Cross-sectional imaging of AC with anterior-segment OCT (Carl Zeiss Meditec, Dublin, CA) was used. Corneal high-resolution single-scan mode (▶ Fig. 23.1) was used. Four images were taken in one axis. The single capture image of the AC included the central cornea to the anterior surface of the lens.

23.1.1 Automated Cell Analysis

The hyperreflective spots detected in the AC were counted in nonenhanced image manually and using an automated computer algorithm. The mean numbers of cells were determined by counting the hyperreflective spots from the OCT image (▶ Fig. 23.1). In the automated method, hyperreflective spots were segmented (▶ Fig. 23.2) from the OCT image by a pixel-based candidate object extraction and counted with a connected component-labeling technique using custom MATLAB software version 7.1 (MathWorks, Natick, MA).[3]

23.2 Comparison between Manual and Automated Cell-Counting Methods

23.2.1 Anterior Chamber Cells

In the manual counting method, mean hyperreflective spots were 3 ± 1.8 in grade 1, 12 ± 3.5 in grade 2, 33.8 ± 10.2 in grade 3, and 61.4 ± 9.6 in grade 4. The automated method showed mean 3 ± 1.9 hyperreflective spots in grade 1, 12.4 ± 3.6 in grade 2, 33.2 ± 9.6 in grade 3, and 74.8 ± 17 in grade 4. We observed good correlation (Pearson coefficient for grade 1: 0.995, grade 2: 0.948, grade 3: 0.985, and grade 4: 0.893) between automated and manual methods. Except for grade 4

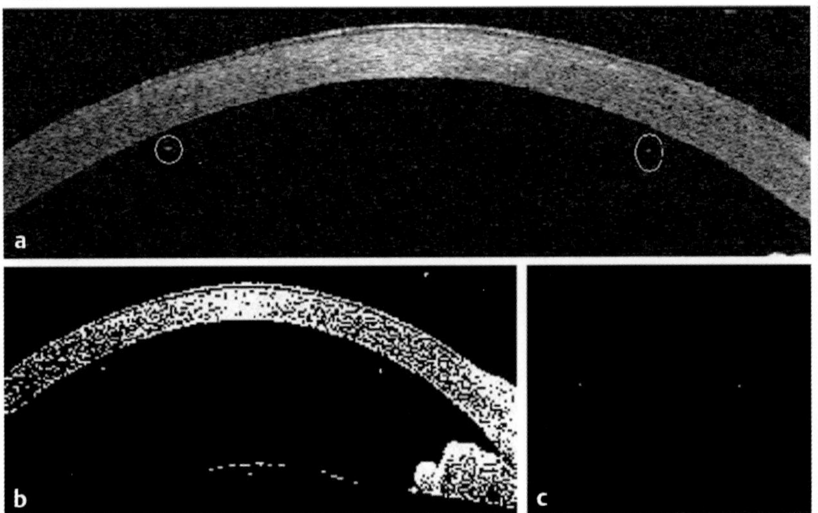

Fig. 23.1 Cross-sectional image of a subject's anterior chamber (AC) in clinical grade 1 uveitis. **(a)** Anterior segment time domain optical coherence tomographic (OCT) image showing hyperreflective spots and **(b)** picture showing the hyperreflective spots as detected in pixel-based candidate object extraction algorithm and **(c)** picture of the hyperreflective spots counted by the connected component labeling technique using custom MATLAB software (MathWorks, Natick, MA).

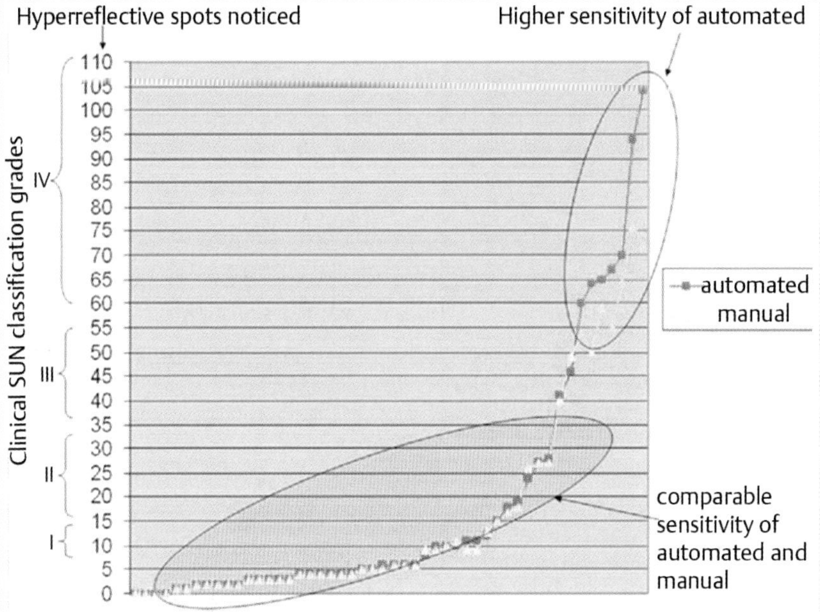

Fig. 23.2 Graph showing the results of manual and automated method of cell counting in time domain optical coherence tomography, suggesting higher sensitivity of the automated method at higher grades of uveitis.

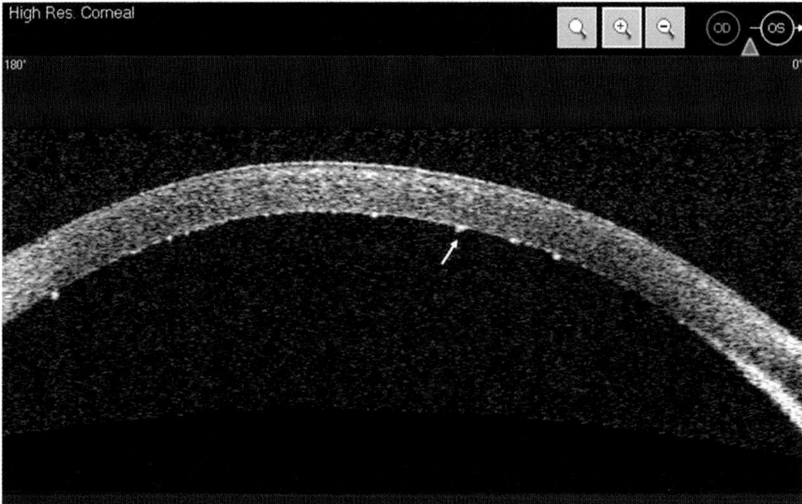

Fig. 23.3 Keratic precipitates (arrow) seen on the endothelium of the cornea in anterior uveitis in time-domain optical coherence tomography. OD, right eye; OS, left eye.

($P = 0.009$), there were no significant differences in mean values between the manual and automated method in lower grades. The automated method was more sensitive in grade 4 uveitis and detected a greater number of cells (▶ Fig. 23.2).

23.2.2 Aqueous Flare

Aqueous flare up to grade 3 was not detected in anterior-segment OCT. However, grade 4 aqueous flare, which was characterized by intense fibrinous reaction, was seen by OCT in seven (11.2%) eyes.

23.2.3 Keratic Precipitates

Keratic precipitates were seen as discrete hyperreflective spots attached to the endothelium of the cornea (▶ Fig. 23.3). They were counted similar to AC cells. Keratic precipitates were noted in 12 eyes in the study.

23.2.4 Membrane

Fibrinous membrane was seen in three eyes in the pupillary area and in one eye on the endothelium of the cornea (▶ Fig. 23.4).

23.2.5 Corneal Edema and OCT Cell Counting

Of the 12 eyes with corneal edema, anterior-segment OCT was also able to detect AC cells (▶ Fig. 23.5) in 11 (91.6%) eyes in which slit-lamp grading was not possible because of corneal edema. The central corneal thickness ranged from 702 to 1020 µm (mean, 843± 109 µm). The eyes with postoperative uveitis, endophthalmitis, and corneal infection had corneal edema. The mean number of hyperreflective spots detected in eyes with corneal edema using the manual method was 12.27 ± 12.1 and 12.9 ± 13 using the automated method.

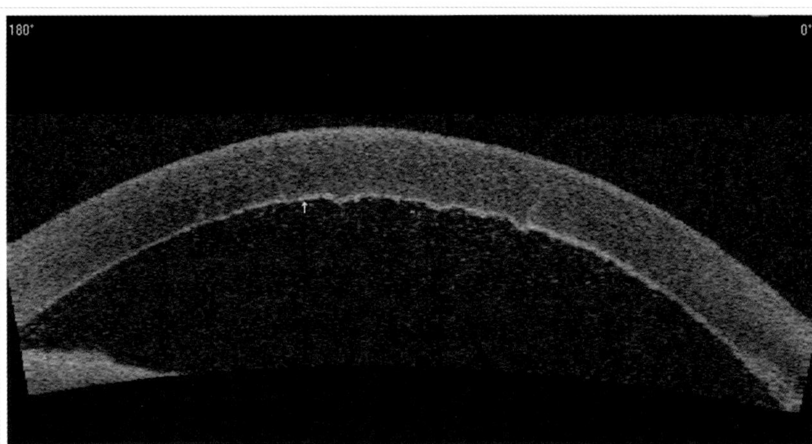

Fig. 23.4 Thick fibrinous membrane (arrow) seen on the endothelium of cornea in anterior uveitis in time-domain optical coherence tomography.

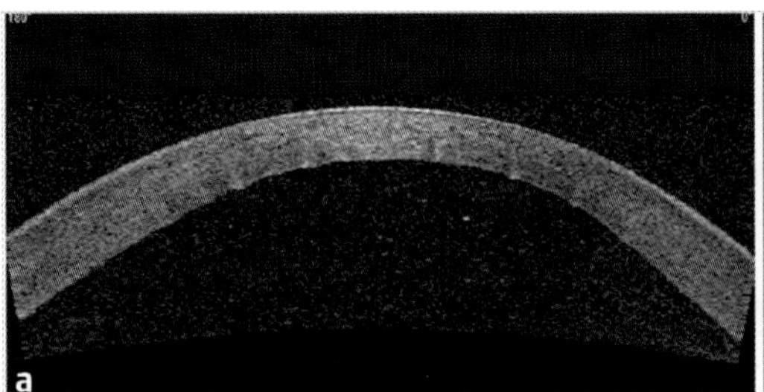

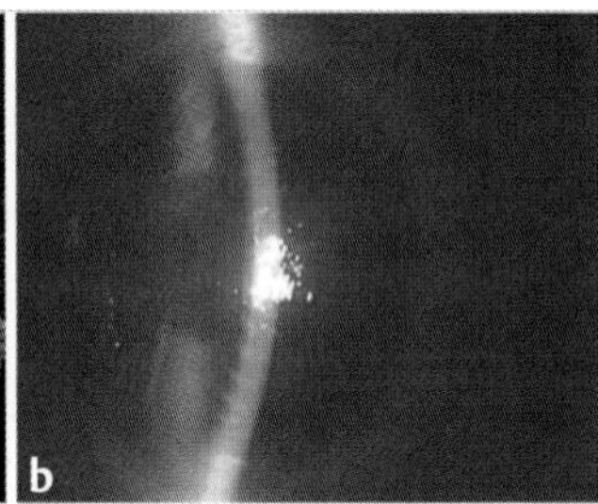

Fig. 23.5 Postoperative uveitis with corneal edema. **(a)** Slit-lamp picture of an eye with corneal edema and **(b)** the anterior-segment time-domain optical coherence tomography image of the same eye showing the AC cells and edematous cornea.

23.3 Fourier-Domain OCT in AC Cell Detection

The FD OCT prototype system (Cirrus HD OCT, model 4000, Carl Zeiss Meditec Inc., Dublin, CA) with anterior-segment module used in this study has been previously described and used for posterior-segment examination.[11,12,13] This FD OCT system consisted of an inbuilt anterior-segment focus adjustment lens. It had the 840-nm wavelength superluminescent laser diode as the optical source. The axial resolution was 5 µm, and transverse resolution was 25 µm in tissue. It had a scanning speed of up to 27,000 A-scans/s.[5,11] Other features included the scanning depth in tissue (2 mm) and the optical power at the cornea < 725 µW. After adjusting the three-dimensional motorized patient alignment unit and the table heights, the cornea was focused. Anterior-segment five-line raster pattern in a horizontal axis of 0 to 180 degrees was used for AC cell grading. The raster scan had five lines (length 3 mm; 250 µm distance between the lines) (▶ Fig. 23.6). The line-scanning quasi-confocal ophthalmoscope illumination of the retina mode was turned off, and the internal fixation target was centered. There is a "click" as the internal lens is brought into position.

The scan was centered at the corneal vertex, and two scans in three positions (inferior, central, and superior) in the AC were taken for each eye at an interval of 15 minutes. Raster lines overlapped the pupillary zone (▶ Fig. 23.7) for central AC while straddling the lower and upper pupillary margins for the inferior and superior AC quadrant grading, respectively. A single examiner took all the images, and the location of scan acquisition was strictly followed. AC cells were seen as hyperreflective particles in the AC.

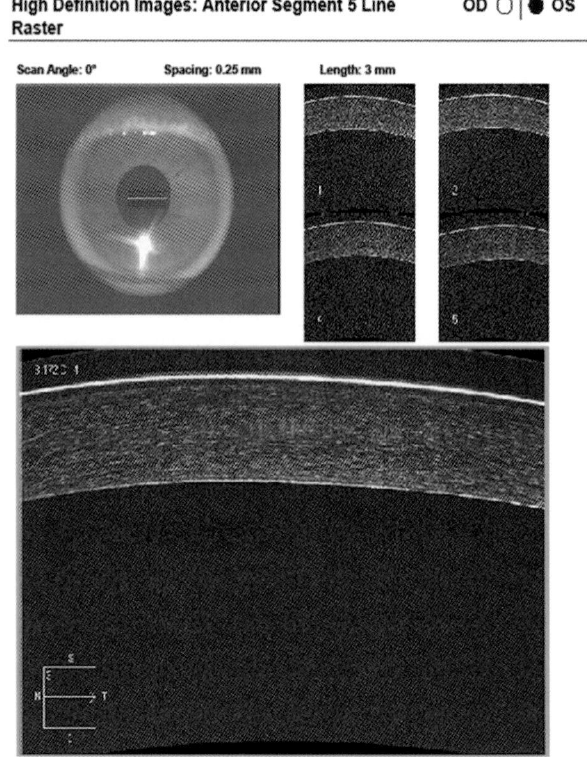

Fig. 23.6 Fourier-domain OCT (Cirrus HD OCT, model 4000, Carl Zeiss Meditec Inc., Dublin, CA) with anterior-segment module of raster line scan used for cell count analysis.

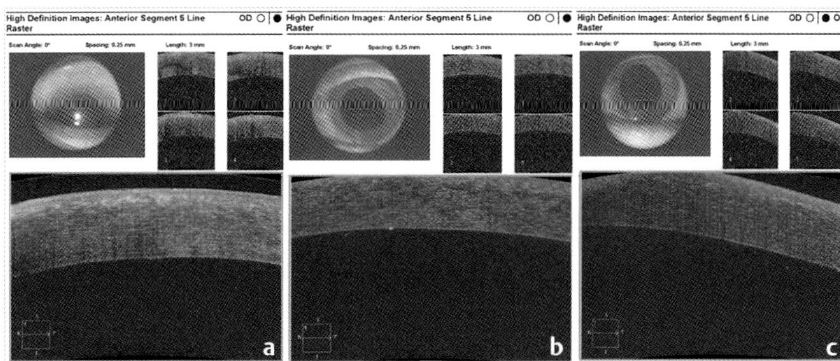

Fig. 23.7 Anterior chamber being scanned for **(a)** superior, **(b)** central, and **(c)** inferior cell distributions using raster line scan in Fourier domain optical coherence tomography.

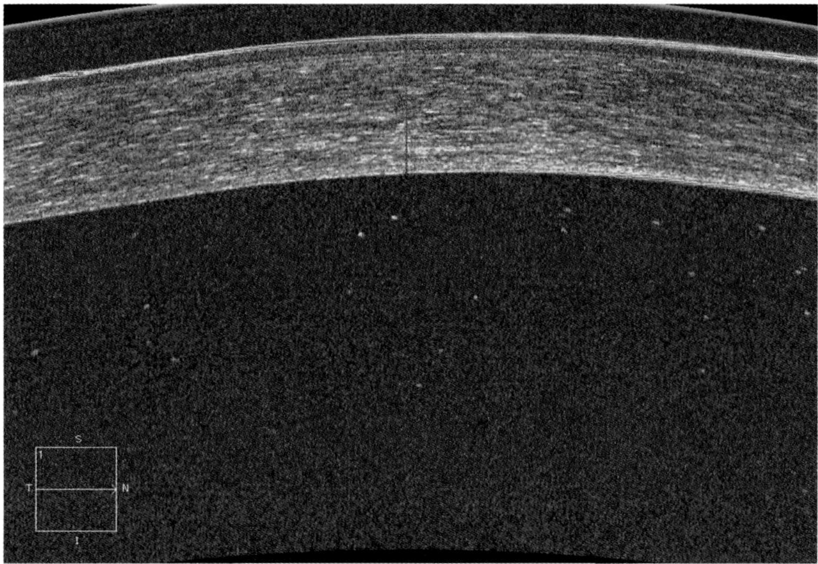

Fig. 23.8 Ordinal scale for Fourier-domain optical coherence tomography (OCT) is made depending on the number of hyperreflective spots per OCT field seen in the anterior chamber.

23.3.1 Ordinal Scale for Fourier-Domain OCT Cell Count

Eighty-three eyes in the control group were evaluated for AC cells using OCT. The control group included the known uveitis patients (with AC reaction graded by slit lamp) with a clear cornea. The results are shown in ▶ Table 23.1. Patients with grade 0.5 + AC cell count by slit lamp showed the least number of cell counts by OCT. However, in increasing reactions, OCT was able to delineate the cells up to 180 counts. Ordinal scale for FD OCT was made depending on the number of hyperreflective spots per OCT field (▶ Fig. 23.8). Coefficient of repeatability (CoR) is the value under which the difference between any two repeat measurements in the same patient acquired under identical conditions, should fall with 95% probability. The CoR values in control eyes were calculated using cell count numbers and are shown in ▶ Table 23.1. We divided the OCT ordinal scale as grade 0.5 (1 cell), grade 1 (2 cells), grade 2 (4–7 cells), grade 3 (8–14 cells), grade 4 (more than or equal to 15 cells).

Table 23.1 Evaluation of Fourier-domain optical coherence tomography (OCT) cell count in control group (N = 83) with clear cornea

Slit-lamp grade	*n*	OCT count mean	OCT count SD	OCT count CoR
0.5 +	11	0.81	0.4	0.2
1 +	21	2.1	0.8	0.6
2 +	11	4.4	0.9	0.8
3 +	17	8.9	1.6	3
4 +	23	52.5	45.2	4.4

Abbreviations: CoR, coefficient of repeatability; SD, standard deviation.

23.3.2 Anterior-Chamber Cell Distribution

Lowder et al initially reported the objective method of quantifying the AC reaction with TD OCT.[11] A significant difference was found in the cell count in the central, superior, and inferior parts of the AC (▶ Table 23.2). The mean count was higher in the inferior quadrant compared with that in the superior quadrant. Li et al, in an in vivo study, noted that particles in the inferior AC that were missed by slit-lamp were detected by OCT.[12] The uneven distribution of cells in the AC was caused by the thermal-driven aqueous humor circulation inside the AC. The gentle aqueous current may not be strong enough to circulate the large and relatively heavy cells. Hence the larger cells were held in the inferior quadrant of the AC. The average size of the neutrophils, monocytes, and lymphocytes usually ranges from

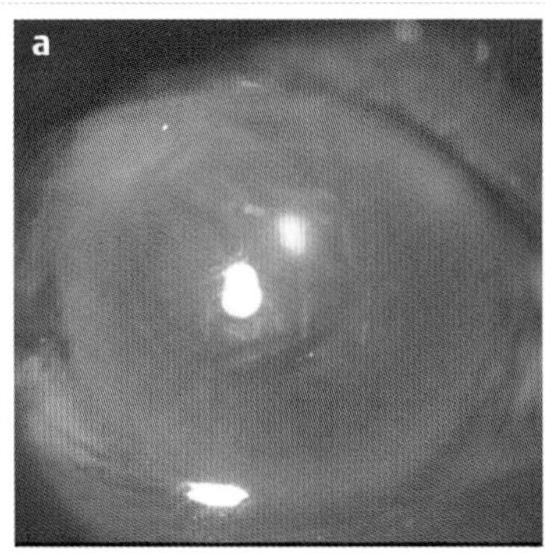

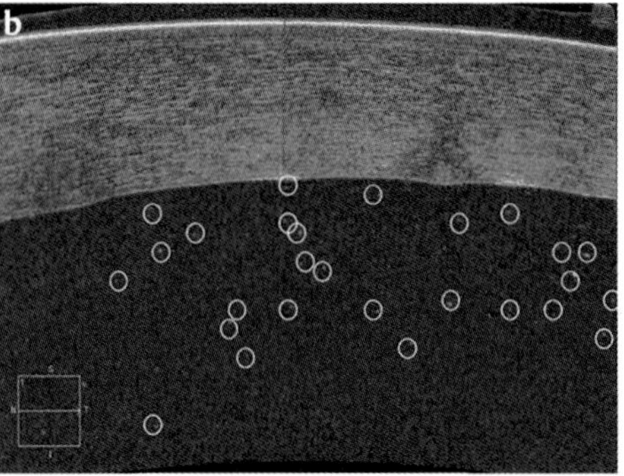

Fig. 23.9 **(a)** Clinical picture and **(b)** Fourier-domain (FD) optical coherence tomography (OCT) image of an eye with postoperative corneal edema. It had slit-lamp grade 4 + and FD OCT cell count 27 (OCT grade 4).

Table 23.2 Test-retest repeatability in Fourier-domain optical coherence tomography (OCT) cell count

	Grade 0.5 +	Grade 1 +	Grade 2 +	Grade 3 +	Grade 4 +
AC superior	$r = 0.5$	$r = 0.93$	$r = 0.76$	$r = 0.74$	$r = 0.99$
AC central	$r = 0.67$	$r = 0.94$	$r = 0.98$	$r = 0.87$	$r = 0.99$
AC inferior	$r = 0.90$	$r = 0.96$	$r = 0.79$	$r = 0.61$	$r = 0.99$

Abbreviations: AC, anterior chamber; r, Pearson correlation coefficient.

10 to 20 µm.[13] Such small inflammatory cells, which are not visible by slit lamp, may be observed through the higher-resolution of FD OCT; however, when the cellular reaction is sparse, it might not be detected by OCT, given that OCT scans cover a far smaller area compared with slit lamp.

23.4 Time versus Fourier-Domain OCT

Cells that are smaller than the resolution size of TD OCT may also be detected by FD OCT. This is because the axial (5 µm) and transverse (25 µm) resolution of the FD OCT is better than the axial (18 µm) and transverse resolution (60 µm) of TD OCT.[14] FD OCT has greater sensitivity than TD OCT[15,16,17] because it uses a higher-bandwidth light source, which provides a finer axial resolution of 5 µm.

23.4.1 Advantage of Fourier-Domain OCT Compared with Existing Methods

The first and foremost advantage of FD OCT is the objective nature of the technique and the sensitivity. Second is the affordability, as it may not be affordable for all ophthalmic centers to have a single dedicated instrument like laser flare meter for aqueous cell count. Ophthalmic centers having only posterior-segment FD OCT system can also use this objective method by opting for the anterior-segment scan mode. A separate instrument dedicated to the cell counting alone might not be mandatory. Third, OCT cell counts correlate well with the slit-lamp biomicroscopic cell grades and are unaffected by corneal edema (▶ Fig. 23.9). Thus, OCT can be a valuable tool for objective quantification and documentation of AC reaction in the treatment and prognosis of postoperative uveitis or graft-rejection uveitis with corneal edema.

References

[1] Whitcup SM. Examination of patient with uveitis. In: Nussenblatt RB, Whitcup SM, eds. Uveitis: Fundamentals and Clinical Practice, 3rd ed. Philadelphia, PA: Mosby, 2004:54–65

[2] Ladas JG, Wheeler NC, Morhun PJ, Rimmer SO, Holland GN. Laser flare-cell photometry: methodology and clinical applications. Surv Ophthalmol 2005; 50: 27–47

[3] Agarwal A, Ashokkumar D, Jacob S, Agarwal A, Saravanan Y. High-speed optical coherence tomography for imaging anterior chamber inflammatory reaction in uveitis: clinical correlation and grading. Am J Ophthalmol 2009; 147: 413–416, e3

[4] Prakash G, Agarwal A, Jacob S, Kumar DA, Agarwal A, Banerjee R. Comparison of fourier-domain and time-domain optical coherence tomography for assessment of corneal thickness and intersession repeatability. Am J Ophthalmol 2009; 148: 282–290, e2

[5] Cirrus TMHD-OCT. Details Define your Decisions. Dublin, CA: Carl Zeiss Meditec. CIR. 1595 DS-Nr. 0–1487–872

[6] Lim JI, Tan O, Fawzi AA, Hopkins JJ, Gil-Flamer JH, Huang D. A pilot study of Fourier-domain optical coherence tomography of retinal dystrophy patients. Am J Ophthalmol 2008; 146: 417–426

[7] Li Y, Shekhar R, Huang D. Corneal pachymetry mapping with high-speed optical coherence tomography. Ophthalmology 2006; 113: 792–, e2

[8] Yi K, Mujat M, Park BH, et al. Spectral domain optical coherence tomography for quantitative evaluation of drusen and associated structural changes in non-neovascular age-related macular degeneration. Br J Ophthalmol 2009; 93: 176–181

[9] Potsaid B, Gorczynska I, Srinivasan VJ, et al. Ultrahigh speed spectral /Fourier domain OCT ophthalmic imaging at 70,000 to 312,500 axial scans per second. Opt Express 2008; 16: 15149–15169

[10] Jabs DA, Nussenblatt RB, Rosenbaum JT. Standardization of Uveitis Nomenclature (SUN) Working Group. Standardization of uveitis nomenclature for reporting clinical data. Results of the First International Workshop. Am J Ophthalmol 2005; 140: 509–516

[11] Lowder CY, Li Y, Perez VL, Huang D. Anterior chamber cell grading with high-speed optical coherence tomography. IOVS 2004; 45:ARVO E-abstract 3372. Available at: http://abstracts.iovs.org/cgi/content/abstract/45/5/3372. Accessed July 12, 2014

[12] Li Y, Lowder C, Zhang X, Huang D. Anterior chamber cell grading by optical coherence tomography. Invest Ophthalmol Vis Sci 2013; 54: 258–265

[13] Williams WJ. Clinical evaluation of patient: approach to the patient. In: Williams WJ, Beutler E, Ersler AJ, Litchman MA, eds. Book of Hematology, 3rd ed. New York, NY: McGraw Hill 1983:11–19

[14] Radhakrishnan S, Rollins AM, Roth JE, et al. Real-time optical coherence tomography of the anterior segment at 1310 nm. Arch Ophthalmol 2001; 119: 1179–1185

[15] Moreno-Montañés J, Olmo N, Alvarez A, García N, Zarranz-Ventura J. Cirrus high-definition optical coherence tomography compared with Stratus optical coherence tomography in glaucoma diagnosis. Invest Ophthalmol Vis Sci 2010; 51: 335–343

[16] Gupta V, Gupta P, Singh R, Dogra MR, Gupta A. Spectral-domain Cirrus high-definition optical coherence tomography is better than time-domain Stratus optical coherence tomography for evaluation of macular pathologic features in uveitis. Am J Ophthalmol 2008; 145: 1018–1022

[17] Kumar DA, Agarwal A, Sivangnanam S, et al. Aqueous reaction quantification after phacoemulsification: Fourier-domain optical coherence tomography versus slitlamp biomicroscopy. J Cataract Refract Surg. 2014 Dec;40 (12):2082-90

24 Optical Coherence Tomography for Imaging the Sub-Tenon Space, Sclera, and Choroid

Soundari Sivagnanam, Dhivya Ashok Kumar, Amar Agarwal, and Rekha S. Bainchincholemath

Optical coherence tomography (OCT) has been extensively used for cornea and angle evaluation in anterior-segment (AS) and macula and retinal examination in posterior segment. With advancements in OCT image-processing software, more refined details of the posterior segment can be appreciated and characterized in vivo. Newer-generation OCT devices like spectral-domain (SD) OCT and enhanced depth imaging (EDI) OCT have revolutionized ocular imaging of posterior segments like the choroid. In this chapter, we discuss the imaging of structures like the sub-Tenon space, sclera, and choroid. We analyze the applications and use of OCT in imaging these structures.

24.1 OCT for Imaging the Sub-Tenon Space

The Tenon capsule is a tenuous tissue layer composed of dense collagen that lies between the episclera and the substantia propria. It extends forward from the rectus muscle insertions, becoming thinner as it moves anteriorly. Sub-Tenon injections have been used for decades for drug delivery in uveitis or macular edema.[1,2,3] The sub-Tenon space is preferred for drug administration because of its prolonged effect and minimal systemic side effects.[4,5] Although sub-Tenon injections have been given by various methods, the position of the cannula or the drug has not been imaged in vivo until now.[4,5] We (idea conceived by D. A.K.) have used high-speed AS OCT (Carl Zeiss Meditec, Dublin, CA) for imaging the sub-Tenon space in vivo.

24.2 OCT-Assisted Sub-Tenon Injection

The periocular skin is cleaned with povidone iodine 5%, and a few drops are instilled into the conjunctiva. A drop of proparacaine 0.5% is then instilled in the eye. A sterile cotton-tipped applicator soaked in 4% lidocaine is placed over the superotemporal quadrant for 2 minutes as the patient looks inferonasally. The patient is made to sit in a comfortable position in a sliding chair and asked to fixate on an inferonasal target. The eyelids are retracted. Under sterile conditions, the superotemporal conjunctiva is lifted with a forceps and an intravenous polytetrafluoroethylene (PFTE) cannula of 22 G, 0.8/25-mm size, is introduced superotemporally 10 mm from the limbus. The needle is then removed, and the cannula alone is pushed 3 mm into the sub-Tenon space. The patient's head is positioned on the chin rest in the AS OCT machine, and the patient is asked to fixate on the inferonasal target. Then the tuberculin syringe with 1 mL of triamcinolone acetonide (Kenalog-40, Bristol-Myers-Squibb, NJ) suspension is injected into the cannula. Cross-sectional (180–0 axis) images centered on the cannula are taken with AS OCT (▶ Fig. 24.1). Corneal high-resolution single-scan mode is used. Scan is taken at the posteriormost cannula visible on the OCT screen (▶ Fig. 24.1).

24.3 OCT Features in Subtenon Injection

The mean conjunctiva-Tenon complex is 0.38 ± 0.08 mm. The mean thickness of the Tenon layer is 0.21 ± 0.07 mm. The drug is tracked behind the Tenon capsule as bright white fluid during the injection (▶ Fig. 24.2). There is no conjunctival chemosis or scleral perforation during the procedure (▶ Fig. 24.3). The drug is localized in 100% of the eyes. Sub-Tenon space of about 10 to 13 mm from the limbus is visualized. Because the underlying sclera is always visualized in OCT-assisted posterior sub-Tenon triamcinolone in vivo, the risk of scleral perforation is decreased. OCT has been shown to have significant role in various clinical situations.[6,7,8] This noncontact and noninvasive imaging method gives an axial resolution of 18 µm and a transverse resolution of 60 µm. The 1310-nm wavelength reduces the amount of signal scattering, which allows better penetration into turbid tissue, such as the sclera. Because of its high speed, it minimizes patient motion artifacts and improves the quality of captured images. Thus, high-speed anterior segment OCT can be used to visualize the sub-Tenon space, and clinically it can be used for imaging the periocular or depot delivery of drugs in the potential space.

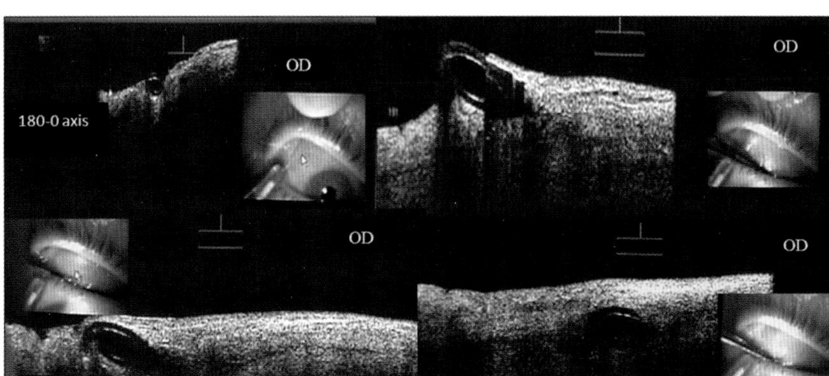

Fig. 24.1 Real-time sub-Tenon injection given with optical coherence tomography visualization.

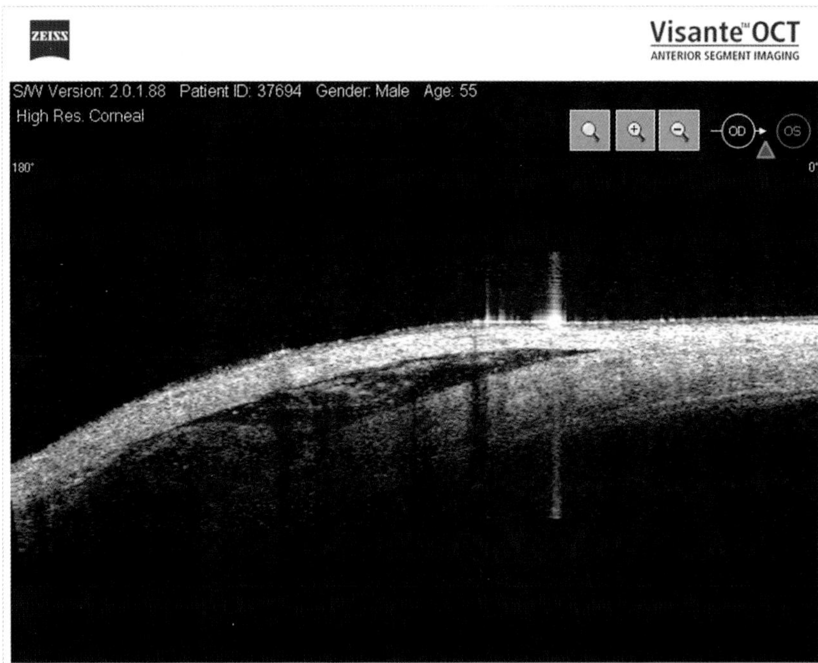

Fig. 24.2 Anterior-segment optical coherence tomography taken after posterior sub-Tenon injection. Note the drug below the Tenon space. OD, right eye; OS, left eye.

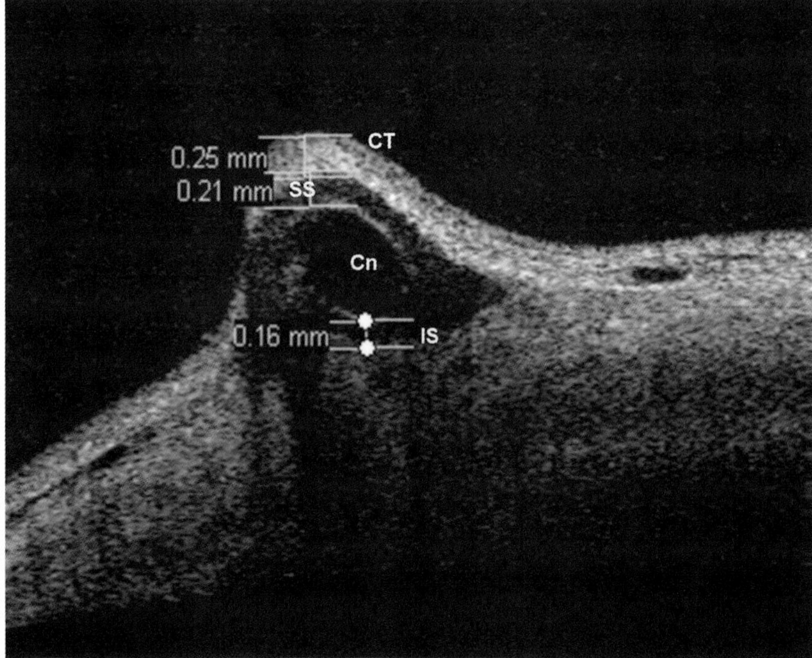

Fig. 24.3 Optical coherence tomography–guided sub-Tenon injection. Cn, cannula; CT, conjunctival thickness; IS, inferior space; SS, superior space.

24.4 OCT for Imaging Sclera

Sclera is not routinely seen in time-domain or SD OCT. However, swept-source OCT can image scleral tissue. Sclera has the tendency of scattering light, and hence lower wavelength may be suboptimal in delineating sclera. OCT imaging of the AS with a longer wavelength of 1310 nm had the advantages of better penetration through sclera. Recent advances in OCT have enabled investigators to image the tissues deeper than the neural retina, such as the choroid and sclera. Especially in eyes with pathological myopia, the retina and choroid of which are very thin, it is possible to observe the entire thickness of the sclera. Normal sclera in OCT is observed as a relatively uniform, hyperreflective structure exterior to the thin choroid on swept-source OCT images. Grulkowski et al has imaged scleral and limbal vasculature in swept-source OCT with 1050-nm wavelength and 100-kHz A-scan rate.[9]

24.4.1 High Myopia

Imamura et al applied EDI OCT for imaging sclera in myopic eyes.[10] Patients with dome-shaped macula, a condition defined as convex elevation of the macula compared with the surrounding staphylomatous region in a highly myopic eye, were

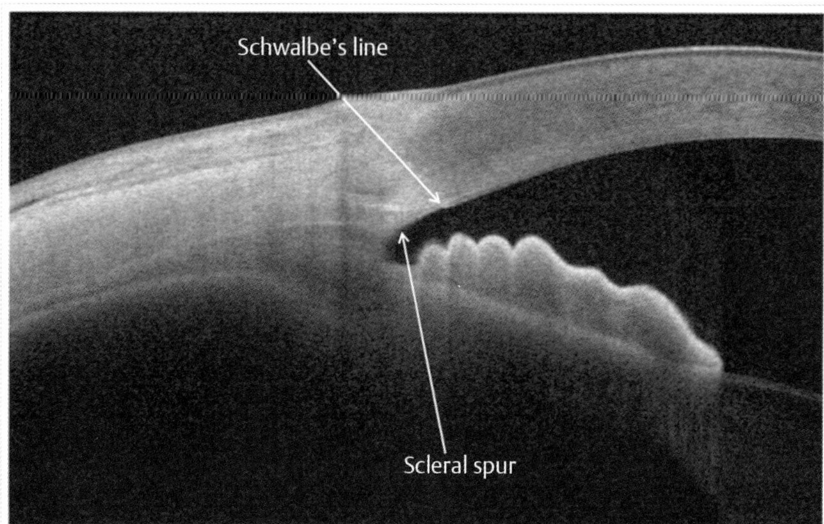

Fig. 24.4 Scleral spur and Schwalbe's line as seen with swept-source optical coherence tomography.

identified through routine examinations using OCT.[9] The scleral thickness was measured from the outer border of the choroid to the outer scleral border under the fovea and 3000 µm temporal to the fovea. The mean subfoveal scleral thickness reported by the study in 23 eyes with dome-shaped macula was 570 (± 221) µm.[10] These investigators concluded that the dome-shaped macula was the result of localized thickness variation in the sclera.

The mean subfoveal scleral thickness as noted by Ohno-Matusi et al was 227.9 ± 82.0 µm in highly myopic eyes.[11] The sclera was thickest at 3000 µm nasal to the fovea. They were able to divide the curvatures of the inner scleral surface of highly myopic eyes into curvatures that sloped toward the optic nerve, those that were symmetrical and centered on the fovea, those that were asymmetrical, and those that were irregular.[11]

24.4.2 Scleral Spur

Scleral spur location represents an important anatomical landmark in imaging the anterior-chamber angle because it is a reference point for the relative position of the trabecular meshwork. The probability of time-domain anterior-segment OCT showing the scleral spur is 70%.[12] Swept-source OCT can be used for visualizing scleral spur (▸ Fig. 24.4).[13]

24.4.3 Spectral-Domain OCT

Optical coherence tomography can be used to assess the prognosis and pathophysiology of scleral inflammation. In a study conducted in our center, cross-sectional imaging of the eye centered on the nodular lesion was taken with a high-speed AS OCT (Visante, Carl Zeiss Meditec) in nodular scleritis. In chronic cases, there was apparent nodular elevation seen from the limbus. There was thickening of the anterior sclera with hyperreflectivity compared with the sclera of the normal fellow eye (▸ Fig. 24.5). A few spaces of hyporeflective spots and focal thinning were seen in the deep sclera (▸ Fig. 24.6). In early cases, the anterior AS OCT showed marked thickening of conjunctiva, episcleral, and sclera over the nodule. A prominent elevation was noted starting from the limbus (▸ Fig. 24.7), and there was a prominent line or hyporeflective zone seen longitudinally in the scleral surface, which is suggestive of the cleavage seen between the scleral lamellae in acute inflammation (▸ Fig. 24.7); this is due to inflammatory fluid accumulation.

Miura et al showed that polarization-sensitive OCT is useful as a contrast engine of the anterior eye segment and for the evaluation of pathological change in the sclera.[14] Neema et al (http://www.abstractsonline.com/plan/ViewAbstract.aspx, ARVO2011 ABSTRACT) has used AS OCT in scleral inflammation. Transcleral high-speed OCT for imaging intraocular structures has been tried ex vivo in cadaveric eyes.[15]

In inflammation, tissue edema is seen as thickening of the involved sclera, and the hyperreflectivity is due to tissue infiltration. Focal hyporeflective spots seen in deep sclera may represent the tissue damage, which can lead to scleral thinning in later stages. One can also see the prominent line or hyporeflective zone seen longitudinally in the sclera, which is suggestive of the cleavage seen between the scleral lamellae in acute inflammation and may be due to fluid accumulation in the acute stage. Resolution of the scleral edema, increase in homogeneous reflectivity of the sclera, and disappearance of the cleavage line or fluid accumulation are the OCT indicators of the response to treatment.

24.5 Role of OCT in Choroid Evaluation

The choroid plays a vital role in the pathophysiology of many diseases affecting the retina, like age-related macular degeneration (AMD) or pathologic myopic degeneration. Previously, the full thickness of the choroid could not be seen in most eyes because of scattering and insufficient light penetration beyond the retinal pigment epithelium (RPE). With the introduction of advances in optics of OCT and ED imaging OCT, the issues of visualizing the choroid has been solved. The choroid is not imaged well in current clinical SD OCT devices for several reasons: decreasing sensitivity and resolution with increasing displacement from zero delay, decreased maximal dynamic range inherent in Fourier-domain systems, wavelength-dependent light scattering and signal loss in the image path, and the lateral width of the defocused imaging beam.

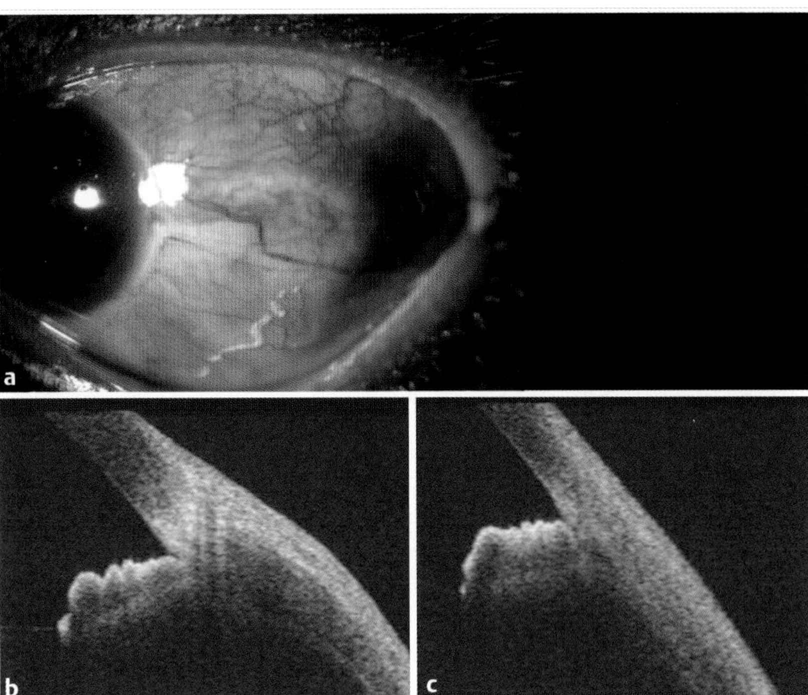

Fig. 24.5 Clinical photograph (a) of an eye showing the nodular scleritis and inferior areas of scleral thinning. Anterior-segment optical coherence tomography showing prominent elevation at the limbus and hyper reflective sclera (b) compared with normal fellow eye (c).

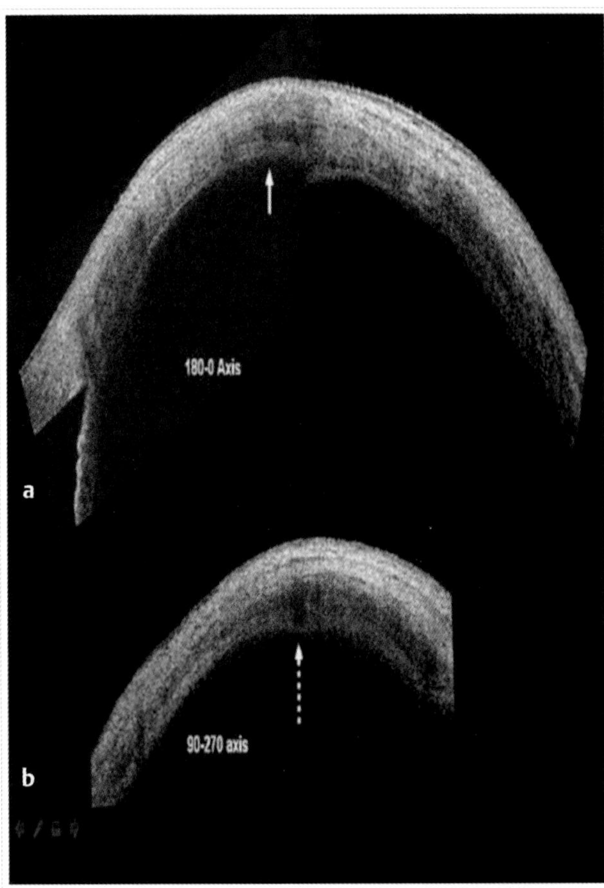

Fig. 24.6 Montage image of anterior-segment optical coherence tomography of case 1 showing focal hyporeflective spots (arrows) along the horizontal (a) and vertical axis (b).

24.5.1 Closer Imaging for Posterior Structures

Spaide demonstrated the ability of the SD OCT systems to show an inverted OCT image by moving the device close to the patient's eye.[16,17,18,19,20,21] SD detection has the highest sensitivity and near zero-delay, and sensitivity decreases for larger delays. The choroid is closer to the zero-delay line, providing enhanced sensitivity and increased imaging depth.

24.5.2 Enhanced Depth Imaging OCT

Enhanced depth imaging optical coherence tomography images are obtained by positioning the SD OCT device close enough to the eye to acquire an enhanced signal of the choroidal layer. Choroidal depth is measured as the distance between the outer reflective RPE layer and the inner sclera border. Heidelberg Spectralis (Heidelberg Engineering, Heidelberg, Germany) has been used for enhanced-depth OCT.[18] Line raster scan from SD OCT (Cirrus OCT) has also been used (▶ Fig. 24.8) for imaging the choroid.[22] One study with Cirrus OCT has shown the average cross-sectional area of the choroid in the central 1-mm region in 34 eyes as 0.27 mm^2 and choroidal thickness beneath the fovea as 272 ± 81 µm.[22]

24.5.3 High Myopia

The mean subfoveal choroid thickness in myopic eyes as studied by Fujiwara et al was 93.2 ± 62.5 µm by EDI OCT.[18] The choroid in highly myopic eyes was very thin (▶ Fig. 24.9) and undergoes further thinning with increasing age and degree of myopia. Abnormalities of the choroid may play a role in the pathogenesis of myopic degeneration. The choroid in normal eyes is thickest at the fovea and becomes thinner both temporally and nasally.

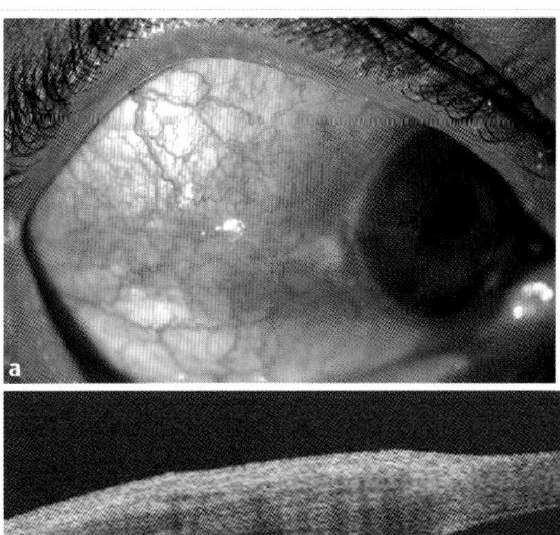

Fig. 24.7 Clinical photograph (a) of an eye showing acute inflammatory nodular scleritis with surrounding congestion of superficial and deep vessels. Anterior-segment optical coherence tomography showing scleral edema (b) and cleavage line resulting from fluid accumulation in the scleral lamellae (c, arrow).

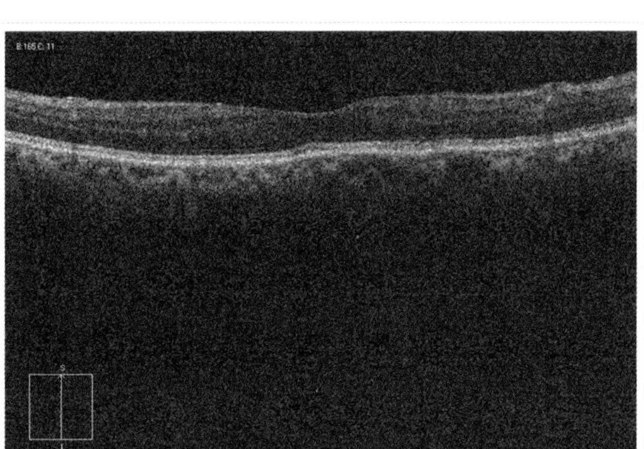

Fig. 24.8 Spectral-domain enhanced depth imaging for visualization of choroid in normal eye.

24.6 Age-Related Macular Degeneration and Choroidal Neovascularization

Spectral-domain OCT, which gives 5-µm resolution, has been used for evaluating the pathophysiology of AMD, especially classic choroidal neovascularization (▶ Fig. 24.10) and underlying changes in the choroid (▶ Fig. 24.11). EDI OCT helps in the detection of early neovascularization and changes in the choroid, which might not be detectable in regular SD OCT.[16] It can be used to understand the pathophysiology of pigment epithelial detachment and AMD. EDI OCT can be applied for the follow-up of patients with intravitreal anti-vascular endothelial growth factor agents.[21] SD OCT can identify indirect signs related to abnormal exudation as intraretinal fluid or increased retinal thickness, and it can be used to characterize drusen,

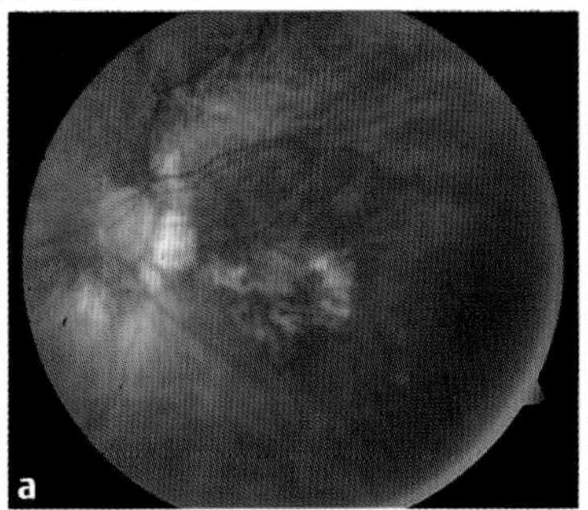

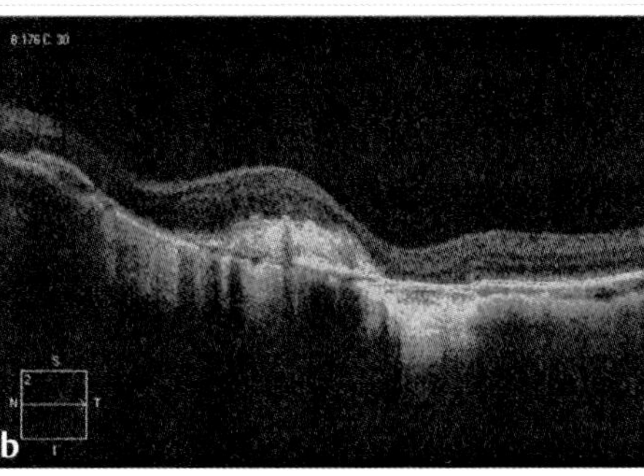

Fig. 24.9 Fundus picture (a); spectral-domain optical coherence tomography (b) for visualization of choroid in high myopia.

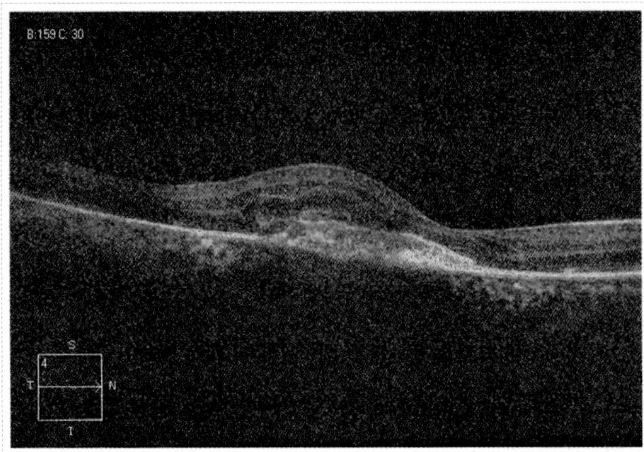

Fig. 24.10 Spectral-domain optical coherence tomography showing the classic choroidal neovascular membrane.

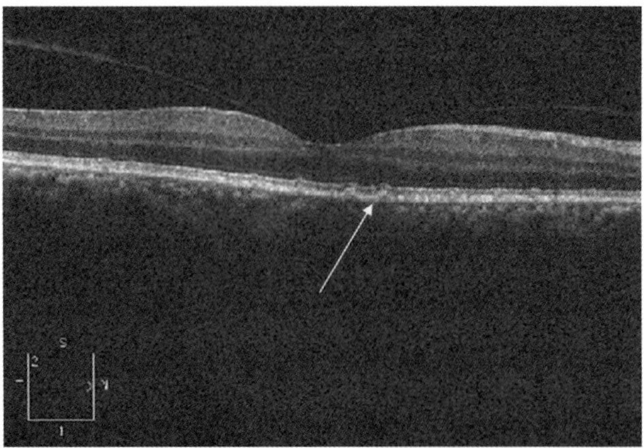

Fig. 24.13 Spectral-domain optical coherence domain of early pigment epithelial changes (arrow) in age-related macular degeneration.

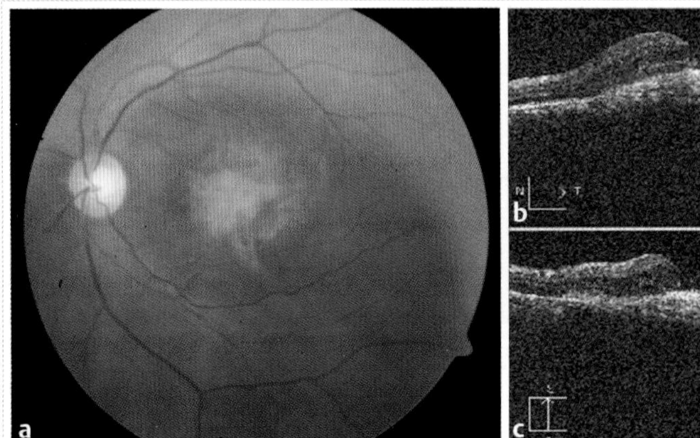

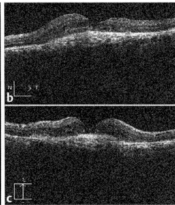

Fig. 24.11 (a) Clinical picture and (b,c) spectral-domain optical coherence tomography of an eye with choroidal neovascular membrane.

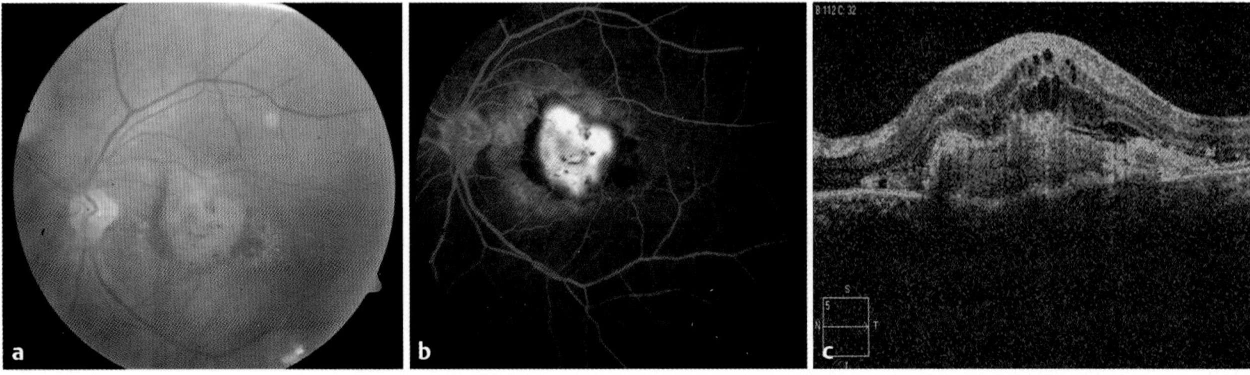

Fig. 24.12 (a) Fundus photograph, (b) fundus fluoresin angiography, and (c) spectral-domain optical coherence tomography of chronic choroidal neovascularization with macular edema and sub retinal fluid.

geography atrophy, choroidal and subretinal neovascularization (▶ Fig. 24.12), neurosensory retinal detachment, and pigment epithelial detachments (▶ Fig. 24.13) associated with AMD. OCT images can be used for assessing the regression of neovascularization after specific treatment lines.

24.6.1 Choroidal Rupture

Indirect choroidal ruptures (ICRs), which result from concussional force transmitted through the wall of the globe, are discontinuities in the choroid, Bruch membrane, and the RPE. Nair

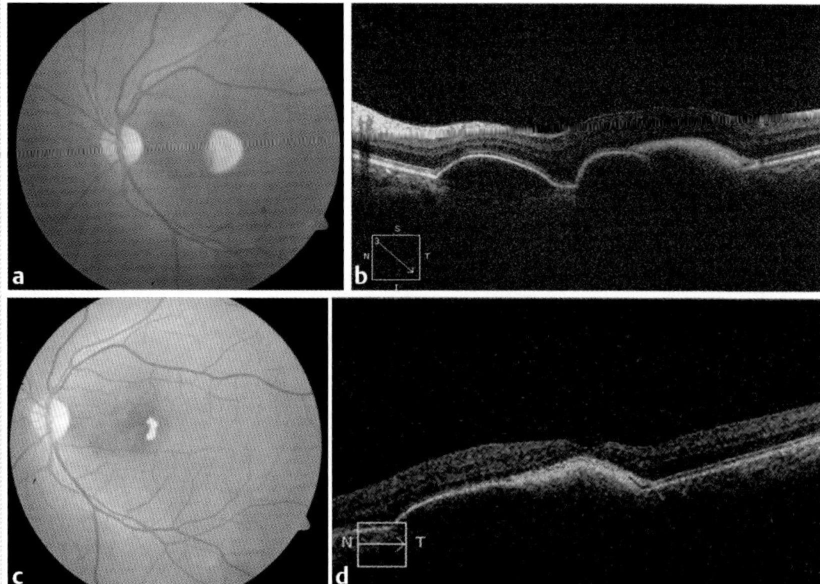

Fig. 24.14 (a) Fundus photograph and (b) spectral-domain optical coherence tomography of an idiopathic polypoidal choroidal vasculopathy showing the polypoidal subretinal lesions. (c,d) The regression noted after treatment with intravitreal ranibizumab.

et al reported two patterns of choroidal rupture seen on SD OCT. The first pattern (type 1 ICR) was a forward protrusion of the RPE-choriocapillaris (CC) layer with an acute pyramid or dome shape[23] associated with either a small loss of continuity of the RPE layer or a break in the wall of the elevated RPE-CC herniation, along with a variable quantity of subretinal hemorrhage. Reflectivity under the dome seemed variable. The second type (type 2 ICR) comprised a posteriorly concave area of disruption of the RPE-CC associated with a loss of photoreceptor inner segment/outer segment and external limiting membrane reflectivity. There was apparent sliding down of the overlying retinal layers into the defect. Eyes with a type 2 ICR need close monitoring with serial SD OCT for early detection of CNV.

24.6.2 Age-Related Choroidal Atrophy

Age-related choroidal atrophy affects older individuals in whom posterior pole abnormalities develop; these abnormalities may mimic and also be associated with findings typical for AMD. The features seen in OCT include decreased choroidal thickness, obliterated choroid before the demarcation of the zone of peripapillary atrophy, pigmentary changes, and rarefaction of small vessels of choroid. Spaide and colleagues showed the loss of choroidal thickness to be associated with loss of visible vessels, implying that age-related choroidal atrophy is a manifestation of small-vessel disease affecting the choroid.[20] Patients with age-related choroidal atrophy may be at higher risk for glaucoma.

Eyes with choroidal atrophy to the point of peripapillary atrophy formation are likely to have profound decreases in the choroidal contribution of blood supply to the prelaminar optic nerve. It is also possible that patients with marked choroidal thinning also have concurrent small-vessel disease to the prelaminar optic nerve arising from other sources. To the extent that optic nerve perfusion influences the development of glaucomatous damage, it is likely that patients with age-related choroidal atrophy have lesser amounts of perfusion than do people with normal choroidal configurations.[20] The present method of EDI OCT measurement of the choroidal thickness offers the possibility of objective quantification of the choroid and its relationship to glaucoma.

24.6.3 Idiopathic Polypoidal Choroidal Vasculopathy

Idiopathic polypoidal choroidal vasculopathy (IPCV) appears to represent a distinct entity that differs clinically and demographically from AMD and other macular diseases associated with subretinal neovascularization. Polypoidal, subretinal, and vascular lesions may be seen associated with serous and hemorrhagic detachments of the RPE (▶ Fig. 24.14). OCT will show the RPE detachment with attenuation of internal reflectivity corresponding to the polypoidal structure, and it is highly sensitive and specific for IPCV.[24]

24.6.4 Choroiditis

Chronic choroiditis can predispose for choroidal neovascularization. Especially in eyes with multifocal choroiditis, the risk of neovascularization can be assessed by follow-up OCT scan (▶ Fig. 24.15).

24.6.5 Choroidal Coloboma

Ocular coloboma results from incomplete closure of the embryonic fissure of the neuroectodermal optic cup at around 5 to 8 weeks of gestation. If the fissure fails to close posteriorly, then a coloboma affecting the RPE, neurosensory retina, or choroid occurs. In choroidal coloboma, the defect is clinically seen as visible sclera with the overlying RPE, retina, or choroid missing. The OCT study of the margin of coloboma of the choroid revealed several interesting features, including variability in

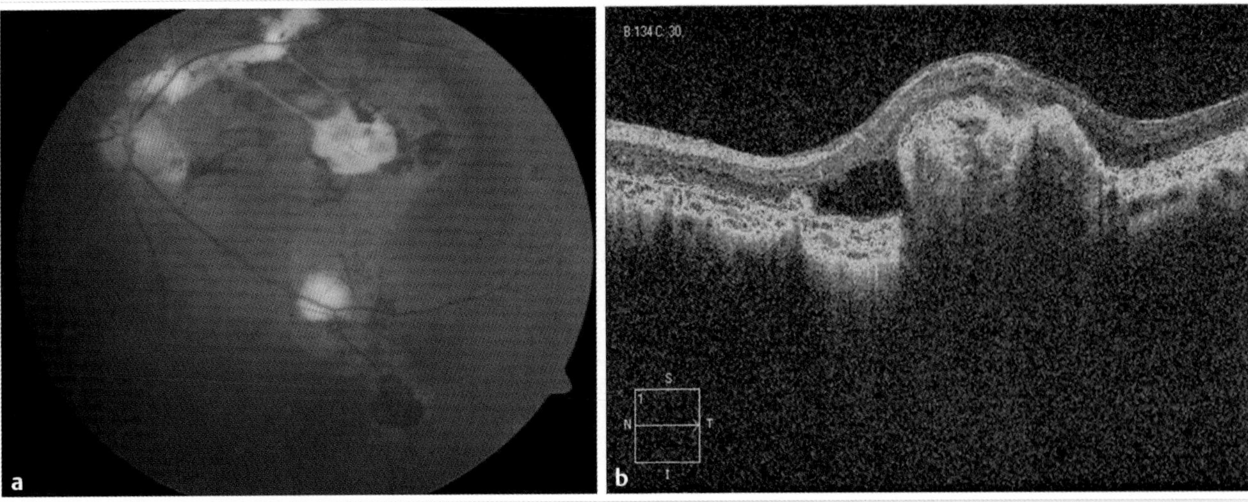

Fig. 24.15 (a) Fundus photograph and (b) spectral-domain optical coherence tomography of multifocal choroiditis with choroidal neovascular membrane.

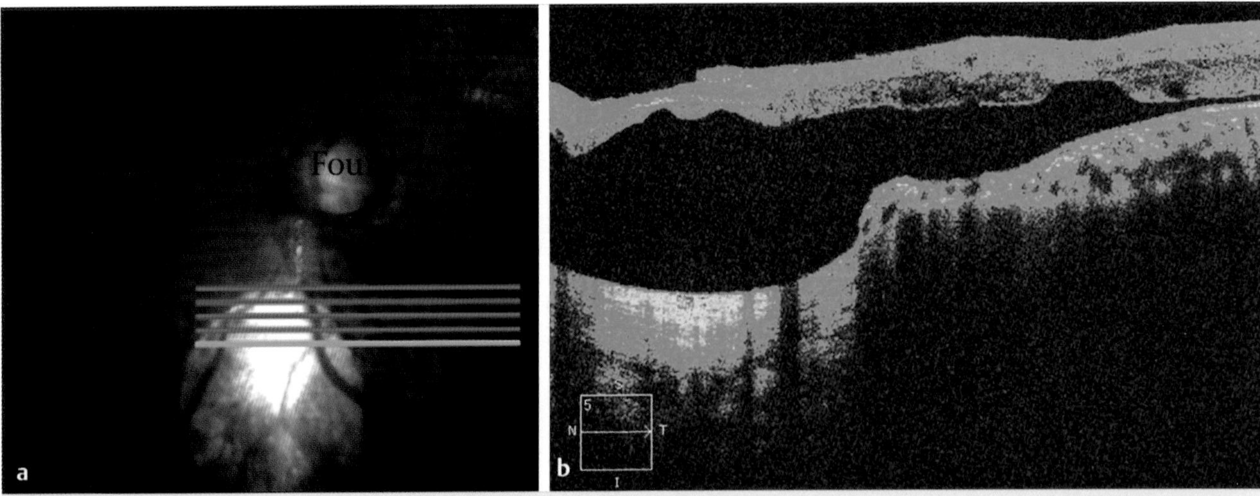

Fig. 24.16 (a,b) Spectral-domain optical coherence tomography of choroidal coloboma.

transition from normal retina to intercalary membrane (gradual or abrupt), the presence of subclinical retinal detachments, focal communications between the subretinal space and the subintercalary membrane space in eyes with extra-colobomatous retinal detachments, and inward humping of the eye wall[25] (▶ Fig. 24.16).

24.7 Conclusion

To summarize, OCT with its high resolution has proven to be a widely accepted modality for imaging structures like the sclera and choroid. However, improvised techniques like EDI OCT and ultrahigh-resolution OCT might provide more detailed evaluations. The noninvasive and noncontact nature of OCT has aided in the determination of prognosis in scleritis or choroidal neovascularization.

References

[1] Cardillo JA, Melo LA Jr Costa RA, et al. Comparison of intravitreal versus posterior sub-Tenon's capsule injection of triamcinolone acetonide for diffuse diabetic macular edema. Ophthalmology 2005; 112: 1557–1563

[2] Helm CJ, Holland GN. The effects of posterior subtenon injection of triamcinolone acetonide in patients with intermediate uveitis. Am J Ophthalmol 1995; 120: 55–64

[3] Thach AB, Dugel PU, Flindall RJ, Sipperley JO, Sneed SR. A comparison of retrobulbar versus sub-Tenon's corticosteroid therapy for cystoid macular edema refractory to topical medications. Ophthalmology 1997; 104: 2003–2008

[4] Venkatesh P, Garg SP, Verma L, Lakshmaiah NC, Tewari HK. Posterior subtenon injection of corticosteroids using polytetrafluoroethylene (PTFE) intravenous cannula. Clin Experiment Ophthalmol 2002; 30: 55–57

[5] Venkatesh P, Kumar CS, Abbas Z, Garg S. Comparison of the efficacy and safety of different methods of posterior subtenon injection. Ocul Immunol Inflamm 2008; 16: 217–223

[6] Bakri SJ, Singh AD, Lowder CY, et al. Imaging of iris lesions with high-speed optical coherence tomography. Ophthalmic Surg Lasers Imaging 2007; 38: 27–34

[7] Kumar DA, Agarwal A, Prakash G, Jacob S, Saravanan Y, Agarwal A. Evaluation of intraocular lens tilt with anterior segment optical coherence tomography. Am J Ophthalmol 2011; 151: 406–412, e2

[8] Francoz M, Karamoko I, Baudouin C, Labbé A. Ocular surface epithelial thickness evaluation with spectral-domain optical coherence tomography. Invest Ophthalmol Vis Sci 2011; 52: 9110–9123

[9] Grulkowski I, Liu JJ, Baumann B, Potsaid B, Lu C, Fujimoto JG. Imaging limbal and scleral vasculature using swept source optical coherence tomography. Photonics Lett Pol 2011; 3: 132–134

[10] Imamura Y, Iida T, Maruko I, Zweifel SA, Spaide RF. Enhanced depth imaging optical coherence tomography of the sclera in dome-shaped macula. Am J Ophthalmol 2011; 151: 297–302

[11] Ohno-Matsui K, Akiba M, Modegi T, et al. Association between shape of sclera and myopic retinochoroidal lesions in patients with pathologic myopia. Invest Ophthalmol Vis Sci 2012; 53: 6046–6061

[12] Sakata LM, Lavanya R, Friedman DS, et al. Assessment of the scleral spur in anterior segment optical coherence tomography images. Arch Ophthalmol 2008; 126: 181–185

[13] McKee H, Ye C, Yu M, Liu S, Lam DS, Leung CK. Anterior chamber angle imaging with swept-source optical coherence tomography: detecting the scleral spur, Schwalbe's Line, and Schlemm's Canal. J Glaucoma 2013; 22: 468–472

[14] Miura M, Yamanari M, Iwasaki T, Itoh M, Yatagai T, Yasuno Y. Polarization-sensitive optical coherence tomography of necrotizing scleritis. Ophthalmic Surg Lasers Imaging 2009; 40: 607–610

[15] Hoerauf H, Winkler J, Scholz C, et al. Transscleral optical coherence tomography—an experimental study in ex-vivo human eyes. Lasers Surg Med 2002; 30: 209–215

[16] Spaide RF, Koizumi H, Pozzoni MC. Enhanced depth imaging spectral-domain optical coherence tomography. Am J Ophthalmol 2008; 146: 496–500

[17] Margolis R, Spaide RF. A pilot study of enhanced depth imaging optical coherence tomography of the choroid in normal eyes. Am J Ophthalmol 2009; 147: 811–815

[18] Fujiwara T, Imamura Y, Margolis R, Slakter JS, Spaide RF. Enhanced depth imaging optical coherence tomography of the choroid in highly myopic eyes. Am J Ophthalmol 2009; 148: 445–450

[19] Imamura Y, Fujiwara T, Margolis R, Spaide RF. Enhanced depth imaging optical coherence tomography of the choroid in central serous chorioretinopathy. Retina 2009; 29: 1469–1473

[20] Spaide RF. Age-related choroidal atrophy. Am J Ophthalmol 2009; 147: 801–810

[21] Spaide RF. Enhanced depth imaging optical coherence tomography of retinal pigment epithelial detachment in age-related macular degeneration. Am J Ophthalmol 2009; 147: 644–652

[22] Manjunath V, Taha M, Fujimoto JG, Duker JS. Choroidal thickness in normal eyes measured using Cirrus HD optical coherence tomography. Am J Ophthalmol 2010; 150: 325–329, e1

[23] Nair U, Soman M, Ganekal S, Batmanabane V, Nair K. Morphological patterns of indirect choroidal rupture on spectral domain optical coherence tomography. Clin Ophthalmol 2013; 7: 1503–1509

[24] Sa HS, Cho HY, Kang SW. Optical coherence tomography of idiopathic polypoidal choroidal vasculopathy. Korean J Ophthalmol 2005; 19: 275–280

[25] Gopal L. A clinical and optical coherence tomography study of choroidal colobomas. Curr Opin Ophthalmol 2008; 19: 248–254

25 Optical Coherence Tomography and Glaucoma

Jullia Ann Rosdahl and Sanjay Asrani

Glaucoma is characterized by optic-nerve cupping with associated visual-field defects. Diagnosing glaucoma by visualizing the optic nerve is something eye doctors have done for the past century, either with the use of a direct ophthalmoscope or indirectly with the slit lamp. However, measurement of the optic nerve or the polarization of the retinal nerve-fiber layer (RNFL) using various instruments was unable to give physicians an objective and reliable measure of a patient's glaucoma status. Additionally, early glaucoma was difficult to diagnose because of the overlap between structural measures of normal and early glaucoma. Diagnosing glaucoma early enables treatment at its early stages, thus preventing patients from reaching advanced stages of the disease. Optical coherence tomography (OCT) provides a direct objective measurement of tissues such as the optic nerve and the peripapillary circumferential RNFL. Whereas imaging the RNFL in glaucoma patients and in patients suspected to have glaucoma is currently the most common use for OCT,[1] OCT imaging of the macula and anterior segment have important roles as well. Time-domain OCT has been replaced currently by spectral-domain OCT because it provides an ability to capture measurements over larger areas in a much quicker and reproducible manner.[2,3,4]

25.1 OCT of the Retinal Nerve-Fiber Layer

The hallmark of glaucomatous vision loss is progressive loss of RNFL manifested by loss of the neuroretinal rim and seen as cupping of the optic nerve head.[5,6,7] However, computerized imaging of the optic nerve head has been limited in its adoption because of the significant variability among both normal and glaucomatous individuals. Imaging the circumferential RNFL, however, is reproducible and reliable[8,9] and allows for comparison with normative databases, giving doctors valuable diagnostic information, especially for suspected glaucoma and ocular hypertension. In patients with already diagnosed glaucoma, RNFL measurements provide an objective measure of tissue loss, as well as an objective way to confirm clinical findings such as loss of the neuroretinal rim.[10]

Abnormal thinning of the RNFL, particularly in the inferior and superior quadrants, is supportive of the diagnosis of glaucoma. RNFL defects seen on OCT scans have corresponding nerve-fiber defects on clinical examination, often seen best with the red-free filter, and corresponding visual-field defects on automated perimetry. Given the high resolution of OCT imaging, especially using spectral-domain OCT, abnormalities on OCT can precede clinical findings and visual-field abnormalities, making OCT of the RNFL particularly helpful for patients with normal visual field or for patients with poorly reliable visual fields or who are unable to perform them (for example, pediatric patients or patients with significant cognitive impairment).

In addition, OCT of the RNFL can be used to assess cup:disc asymmetry, another hallmark of glaucoma. A patient's RNFL OCT is compared with the normative database, as well as to the patient's other eye (▶ Fig. 25.1). This analysis is particularly helpful for patients who are not represented in the normative database, such as those with myopia, and patients with early focal defects that are missed by the quadrant analysis.

Optical coherence tomography of the RNFL is also useful in monitoring for progression (▶ Fig. 25.2). This imaging test takes only a few minutes and requires minimal patient participation; thus, it is a well-tolerated adjunct to automated visual-field testing in monitoring patients. Using eye-tracking capabilities of the high-resolution OCT devices, small changes in the RNFL thickness can be assessed, enabling the doctor to consider advancing treatment or monitoring more closely to prevent vision loss from glaucoma.

Computerized analysis is useful to doctors by highlighting abnormally thin and thick regions compared with the normative database. However, abnormally thin areas (red) and areas of normal or thick RNFL (green) can be misleading. Some common diagnostic masqueraders are listed in ▶ Table 25.1.

Also, OCT can be used for cross-sectional imaging of the optic nerve head. This type of imaging of the optic nerve head can be useful clinically for differentiating other optic nerve head findings from glaucoma, for example, visual-field defect in the setting of buried optic nerve head drusen.[11] In addition, cross-sectional imaging of the optic nerve head can allow for visualization of the lamina cribrosa (▶ Fig. 25.5). Although generally not used clinically at present, imaging the lamina cribrosa is of interest in understanding the pathophysiology of glaucomatous cupping.

Whereas OCT imaging of the RNFL is the most common use for this technology in glaucoma patients, OCT of the macula and of the anterior segment can also be quite useful both for the diagnosis of glaucoma and its management.

25.2 OCT of the Macula

Glaucoma is characterized by cupping of the optic nerve head; however, the macular region of the retina is also affected by glaucoma. Retinal ganglion cells and the RNFL constitute 40% of the macular thickness. Using OCT, retinal thickness can be measured, and losses of retinal ganglion cells and axons can be mapped. Because the numbers of retinal ganglion cells in the macula are relatively constant in healthy eyes, this structural measurement is quite useful for the diagnosis of glaucoma. It is estimated that 40 to 50% of retinal ganglion cells are lost before visual-field defects can be measured by automated perimetry,[12] making this technology particularly useful in finding early glaucoma.

Glaucomatous defects in the retina[13] are best seen using thickness maps that are larger in area than for other retinal pathologies: 10-mm square for glaucoma compared with 6-mm circle for retinal pathologies. In addition, thickness maps with a modified color scale to reveal retinal thickness differences of 10 to 15 µm are helpful in locating glaucomatous defects. Glaucomatous retinal defects are frequently arcuate in nature, extending superotemporally or inferotemporally from the optic

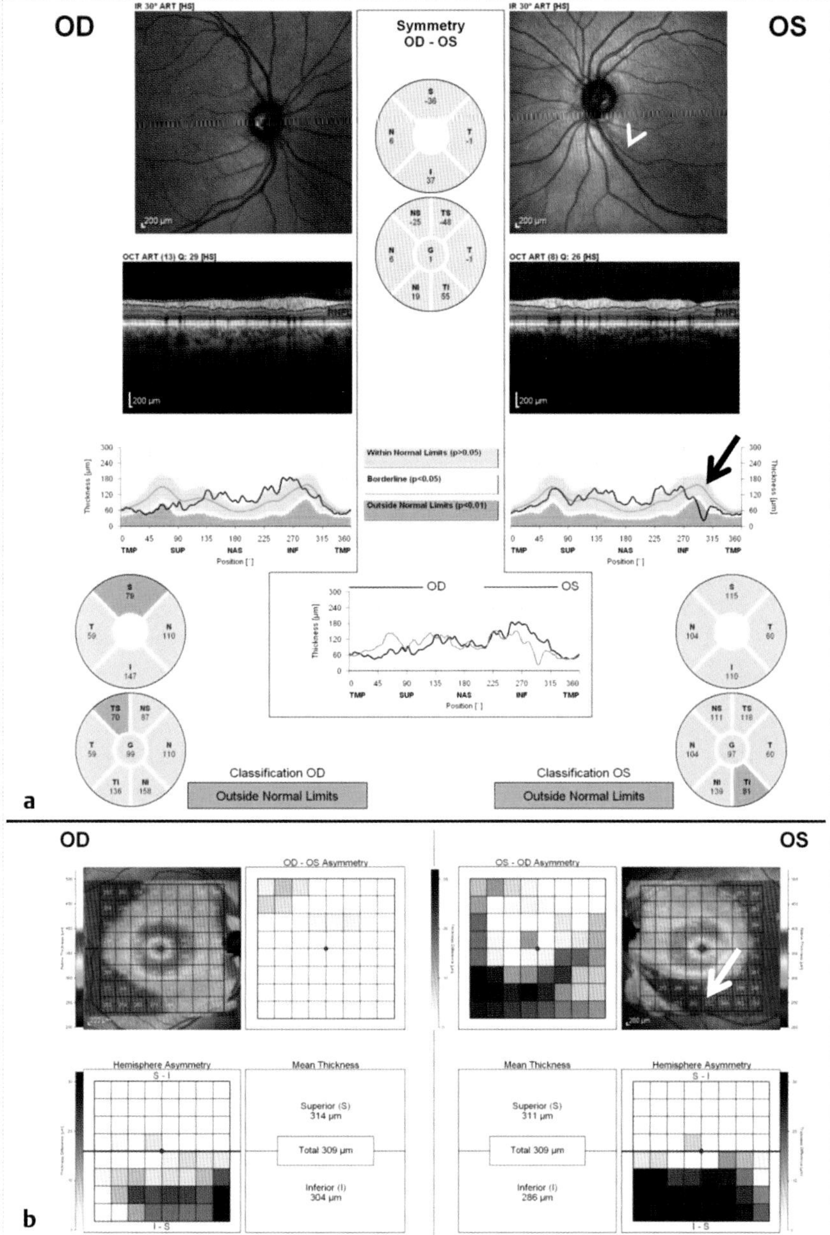

Fig. 25.1 Optical coherence tomography (OCT) asymmetry analysis. (a) The retinal nerve-fiber layer (RNFL) asymmetry analysis includes the image of the optic nerve head and the circumferential OCT of the RNFL. The RNFL is identified and measured by the software and then compared both with the normative database (red-yellow-green) and between the two eyes (OD, right eye in black; OS, left eye, in gray). The colored diagrams highlight the thin quadrants. In this patient with glaucoma, flattening of the superior bundle is seen in the right eye and focal inferior thinning in the left eye (black arrow). The nerve-fiber layer defect can be visualized on the scout image (white arrowhead). **(b)** The macular asymmetry analysis includes the color thickness map overlying the image of the posterior pole, with cooler colors (purple-blue) denoting thinner areas and warmer colors (red) denoting thicker areas. The OD-OS asymmetry plots compare the macular thickness of corresponding areas between the right and left eyes. The grayscale denotes comparative thinning, with black representing a 30-µm difference between the eyes. The hemisphere asymmetry plots compare the macular thickness of corresponding areas between the superior and inferior hemimaculae, within each eye. The average thicknesses of the total macula, the superior hemimacula, and the inferior hemimacula are noted for each eye. In this patient, the focal inferior thinning seen on the RNFL has a corresponding wedge-shaped defect in the inferior macula (white arrow). This area of inferior thinning is highlighted in both the OS-OD asymmetry plot and the hemisphere asymmetry plot.

nerve into the macula. Parafoveal thinning can also be seen in glaucoma, corresponding to paracentral losses on the visual field.

Macular retinal thickness measurements, as well as RNFL measurements, using spectral-domain OCT show high reproducibility for both glaucoma and suspected glaucoma.[14] In the eyes of both adults and children, the intravisit and intervisit intraclass correlation coefficients for macular thickness measurements (both central macular and perimacular thicknesses) and the average RNFL measurements were greater than 0.8 in all cases, indicating excellent reproducibility.

As with the analysis of the RNFL, asymmetry analyses of the macular thickness maps can reveal or highlight early or subtle defects (▶ Fig. 25.1b). Comparing the superior and inferior hemimaculae within each eye can reveal clinically significant asymmetry, analogous to the glaucoma hemifield analysis of automated perimetry. Asymmetry of the maculae between the eyes, similar to the asymmetry analysis of the RNFL, can reveal clinically significant thinning.

Asymmetry of the macular thickness correlates with defects in the visual field.[15] Asymmetry within each eye, determined by comparing the macular thickness measurements of the superior and inferior hemimaculae, correlates with the pattern standard deviation score of the automated visual field: A greater difference in macular thickness between the hemimaculae correlated with a higher pattern standard deviation score. Asymmetry between the two eyes, determined by comparing the average total macular thickness of the right and left eyes, correlates with the mean deviation score of the automated visual field, showing that glaucoma patients with greater visual-field defects in one eye also had thinner macular thickness in that eye.

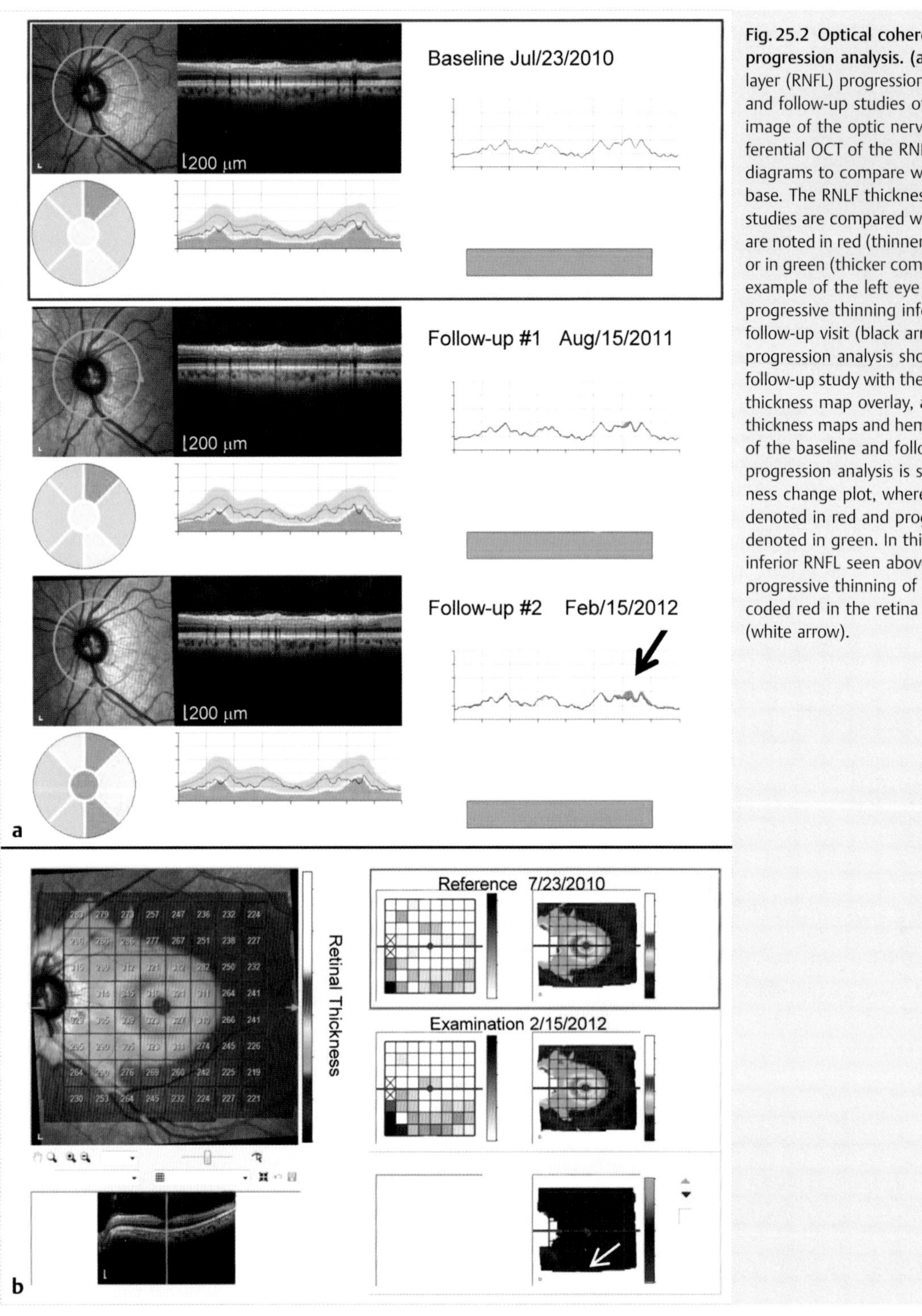

Fig. 25.2 Optical coherence tomography (OCT) progression analysis. (a) The retinal nerve-fiber layer (RNFL) progression analysis shows baseline and follow-up studies of each eye, including the image of the optic nerve head and circumferential OCT of the RNFL, as well as the colored diagrams to compare with the normative database. The RNLF thickness plots of the follow-up studies are compared with baseline, and changes are noted in red (thinner compared with baseline) or in green (thicker compared to baseline). In this example of the left eye of a glaucoma patient, progressive thinning inferiorly is seen at the follow-up visit (black arrow). **(b)** The macular progression analysis shows a larger view of the follow-up study with the posterior pole and color-thickness map overlay, as well as the color thickness maps and hemisphere asymmetry plots of the baseline and follow-up studies. The progression analysis is shown in the retina thickness change plot, where progressive thinning is denoted in red and progressive thickening is denoted in green. In this example, the change in inferior RNFL seen above corresponds to the progressive thinning of the inferior macula, coded red in the retina thickness change plot (white arrow).

25.3 Glaucoma Masqueraders

Optical coherence tomography of the RNFL and macula can also be helpful in differentiating glaucoma from nonglaucomatous optic neuropathies and retinopathies.[16] With regard to the RNFL measurements, patients with nonglaucomatous optic nerve cupping (from optic neuritis, nonarteritic anterior ischemic optic neuropathy, and others) had a pattern of more diffuse RNFL loss, particularly in the nasal and temporal quadrants, compared with the more typical pattern seen in glaucoma patients with RNFL losses in the superior and inferior quadrants.[17] Nonglaucomatous retinal pathologies can also mimic the macular thinning seen in some patients with glaucoma[11]: For example, hemiretinal vein occlusion can result in profound hemimacular thinning and corresponding arcuate visual field defects (▸ Fig. 25.6). This highlights the importance of clinical examination of the patient.

Table 25.1 "Red" and "green" disease

"Red" disease (false positives). The OCT RNFL analysis shows abnormally thin RNFL, giving the false impression in favor of glaucoma.	
Artifacts	Examples: Segmentation artifact, where the segmentation software has not properly identified the RNFL borders (▶ Fig. 25.3) Alignment artifact, where the technician has performed the analysis using an image with a corner or edge cut off
Nonglaucomatous optic neuropathies	Examples: Ischemic optic neuropathies can result in segmental superior or inferior thinning. Inflammatory optic neuropathies, such as optic neuritis, can result in subsequent RNFL thinning, often diffuse or of the temporal quadrant.
"Green" disease (false negatives). The OCT RNFL analysis shows normal or thick RNFL, giving the false impression against the diagnosis of glaucoma	
Active uveitis	The RNFL may not be abnormally thin despite loss of retinal ganglion cell axons if the tissue is edematous due to inflammation
Vitreoretinal disease	Example: Epiretinal membrane pulling anteriorly, giving the appearance of normal thickness despite loss of retinal ganglion cell axons
Artifacts	Segmentation artifact example, where the segmentation software has misidentified a prominent inner limiting membrane (▶ Fig. 25.4)
Some solutions: Review the OCT scans themselves, in addition to reviewing the computerized analysis Use the computerized analyses with caution in patients with ocular comorbidities Clinical correlation of OCT findings is key[20]	

Abbreviations: OCT, optical coherence tomography; RNFL, retinal nerve-fiber layer.

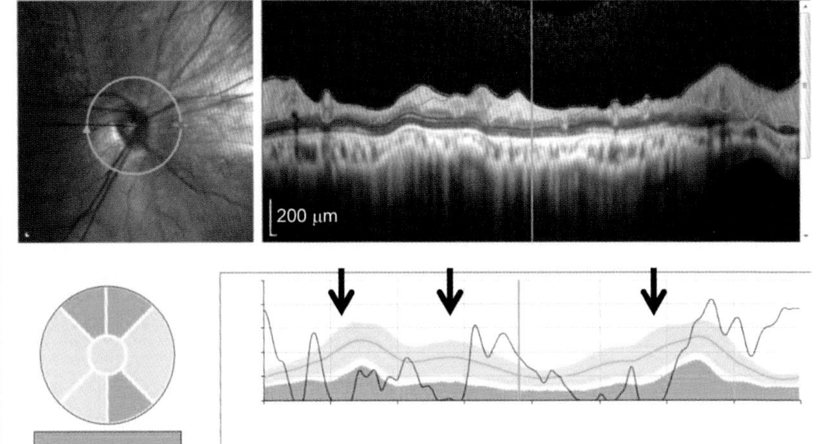

Fig. 25.3 Segmentation artifact "red disease." This is an example of a segmentation artifact resulting from myopia. The software is unable to assign the posterior and anterior borders of the retinal-nerve-fiber layer (RNFL) properly, resulting in erroneous RNFL defects on the analysis. Thickness measurements of 0 µm (black arrows) are not physiologic and are helpful prompts to review the optical coherence tomography scan itself.

25.4 OCT of the Anterior Segment

There are several useful indications for anterior segment OCT in the glaucoma patient[18,19]:

- Evaluation of the angle: OCT of the anterior segment can be used to study the angle without incident light. Gonioscopy requires the placement of a contact lens and light from the slit lamp, which can constrict the pupil, causing the angle to appear open. OCT uses light in the infrared spectrum, which does not affect the pupil. In addition, it is noncontact and can provide an objective evaluation of the angle. Differentiating between open-angle glaucoma and narrow angles is essential for the diagnosis and management of glaucoma (▶ Fig. 25.7).
- Evaluation of a filtering bleb: A cross-sectional image of a filtering bleb using anterior-segment OCT (▶ Fig. 25.8) allows for evaluation of scarring and fibrosis. This information can impact postoperative management.
- Imaging the trabecular meshwork and Schlemm canal: OCT imaging of the angle structures allows for both a better understanding of the pathophysiology of glaucoma, as well as the status of newer glaucoma surgical procedures such as canaloplasty, Trabectome, iStent, and others. For example,

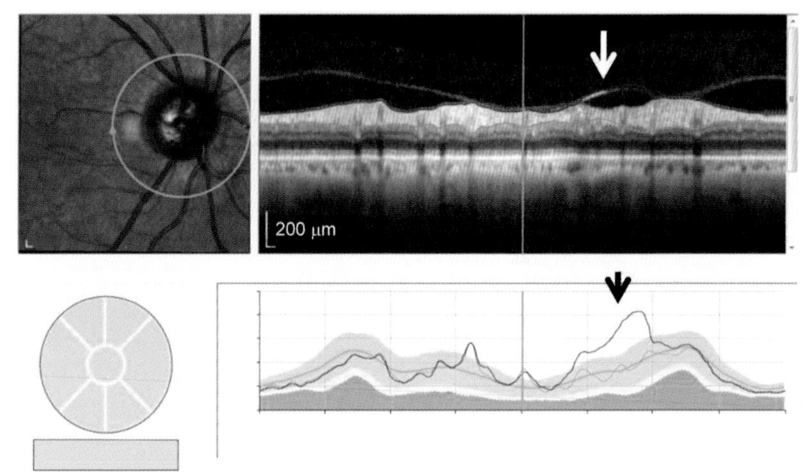

Fig. 25.4 Segmentation artifact "green disease." This is an example of a segmentation artifact from a prominent inner limiting membrane. The software has erroneously assigned the anterior border of the retinal nerve-fiber layer at the inner limiting membrane (white arrow), resulting in a falsely thick measurement (black arrow).

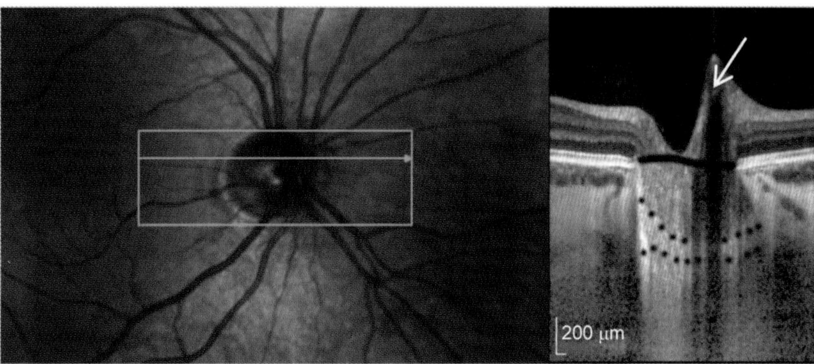

Fig. 25.5 Optical coherence tomography of the lamina cribrosa. A cross-sectional scan of the optic nerve head is shown on the right. The location is indicated by the green arrow on the left image. The borders of the lamina cribrosa are marked with the black dots. Shadowing from the central retinal vessels is marked with the white arrow.

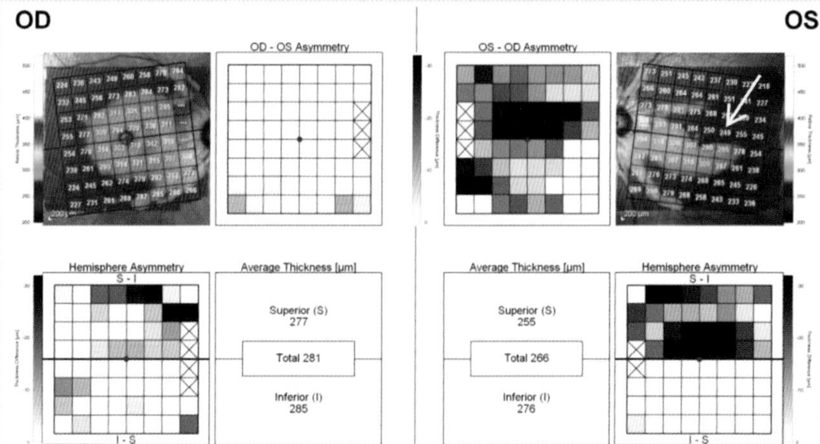

Fig. 25.6 Glaucoma masquerader. Profound thinning of the superior macula in the left eye (OS, white arrow) with respect to the horizontal meridian was due to hemiretinal vein occlusion, not to glaucoma. OD, right eye.

OCT imaging of the angle after failure of a Trabectome procedure could reveal iris blocking to allow for determining the appropriate next step in management, such as pilocarpine in this case.

- Evaluation of the iris: OCT imaging of the peripheral anterior segment allows for evaluation of the iris; for example, it is useful for monitoring plateau iris (▶ Fig. 25.9) and peripheral synechiae (▶ Fig. 25.10).

25.5 Conclusion

In summary, computerized imaging of the optic nerve tissues is commonly used for glaucoma management, both at diagnosis and to monitor for progression. OCT of the RNFL is a reliable and reproducible method for evaluating the optic nerve changes seen in glaucoma patients. OCT of the macula is a useful adjunct, both to detect early defects and later in disease.

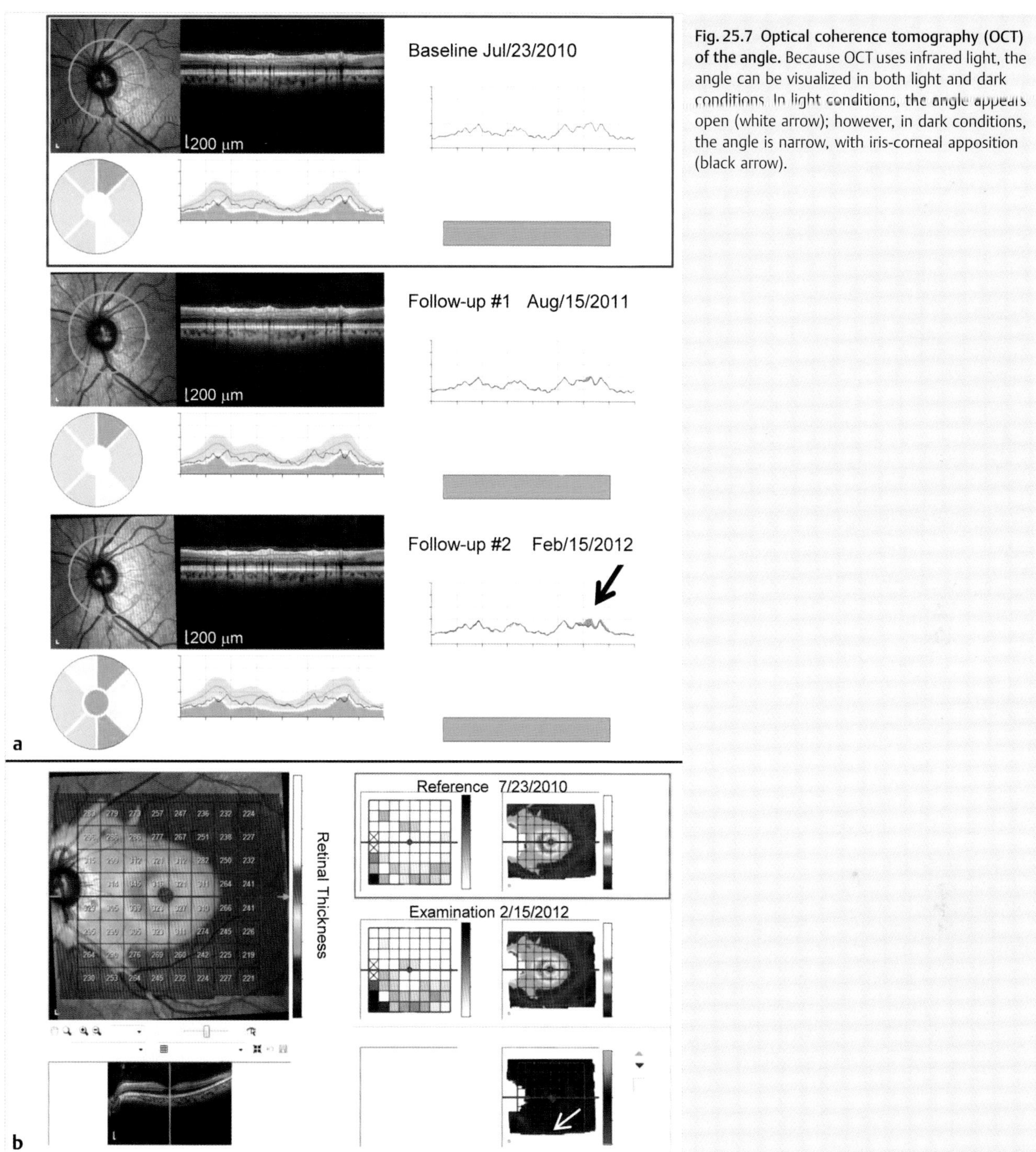

Fig. 25.7 Optical coherence tomography (OCT) of the angle. Because OCT uses infrared light, the angle can be visualized in both light and dark conditions. In light conditions, the angle appears open (white arrow); however, in dark conditions, the angle is narrow, with iris-corneal apposition (black arrow).

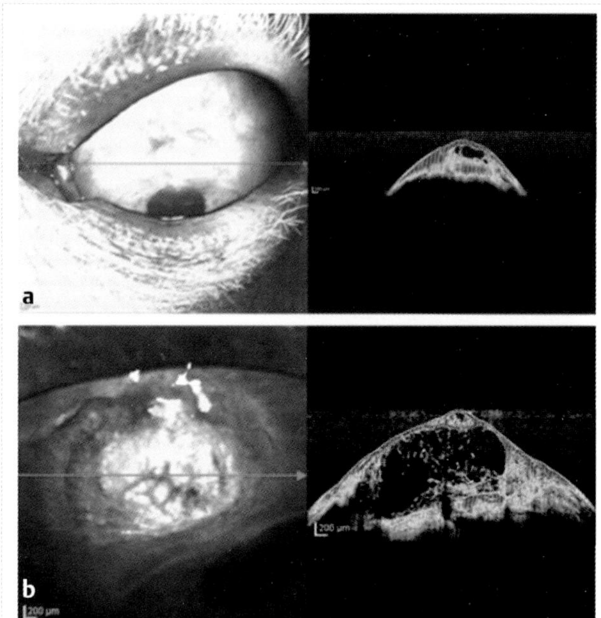

Fig. 25.8 **Optical coherence tomography (OCT) of filtering blebs.** Anterior-segment OCT images of two blebs are shown: **(a)** an encapsulated bleb and **(b)** a diffuse bleb.

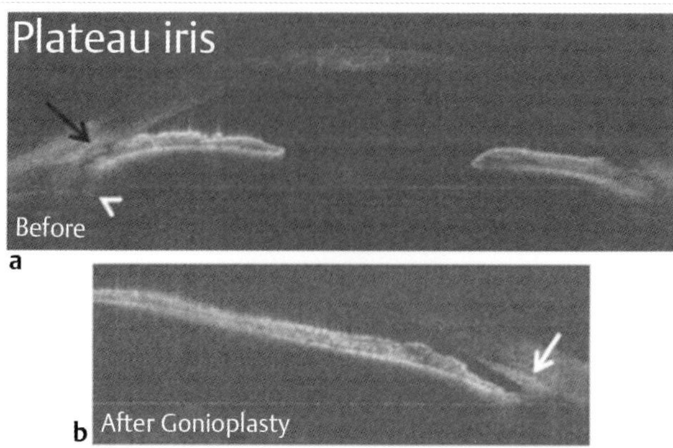

Fig. 25.9 **Optical coherence tomography (OCT) of plateau iris, before and after gonioplasty.** Anterior-segment OCT images of a patient with plateau iris configuration are shown, **(a)** before and **(b)** after gonioplasty. The peripheral narrowing of the angle (black arrow) and anteriorly rotated ciliary body (white arrowhead) are visualized with this technology. After gonioplasty, thinning of the iris tissue and more open configuration of the angle are seen (white arrow).

OCT of the anterior segment is helpful for evaluating the configuration of the angle and the angle structures, as well as for postoperative assessment of filtering blebs. The ability to see the structures affected by glaucoma, the optic nerve, and drainage angle is changing how we care for patients and helping us to understand better the pathophysiology of glaucoma.

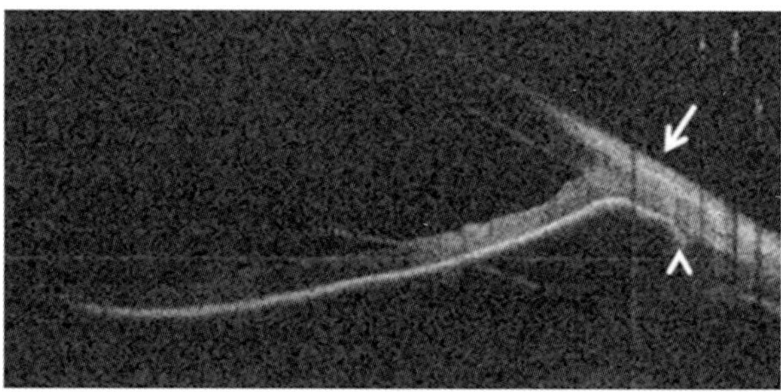

Fig. 25.10 **Optical coherence tomography (OCT) of the angle with peripheral anterior synechiae.** Anterior-segment OCT image of a patient with synechial closure of the angle (white arrow) is shown. The approximate location of the physiologic insertion of the iris is noted with the white arrowhead.

References

[1] Greenfield DS, Weinreb RN. Role of optic nerve imaging in glaucoma clinical practice and clinical trials. Am J Ophthalmol 2008; 145: 598–603

[2] Chen TC, Cense B, Pierce MC, et al. Spectral domain optical coherence tomography: ultra-high speed, ultra-high resolution ophthalmic imaging. Arch Ophthalmol 2005; 123: 1715–1720

[3] de Boer JF, Cense B, Park BH, Pierce MC, Tearney GJ, Bouma BE. Improved signal-to-noise ratio in spectral-domain compared with time-domain optical coherence tomography. Opt Lett 2003; 28: 2067–2069

[4] Yaqoob Z, Wu J, Yang C. Spectral domain optical coherence tomography: a better OCT imaging strategy. Biotechniques 2005; 39 Suppl: S6–S13

[5] Quigley HA, Addicks EM. Quantitative studies of retinal nerve fiber layer defects. Arch Ophthalmol 1982; 100: 807–814

[6] Quigley HA, Addicks EM, Green WR. Optic nerve damage in human glaucoma. III. Quantitative correlation of nerve fiber loss and visual field defect in glaucoma, ischemic neuropathy, papilledema, and toxic neuropathy. Arch Ophthalmol 1982; 100: 135–146

[7] Quigley HA, Miller NR, George T. Clinical evaluation of nerve fiber layer atrophy as an indicator of glaucomatous optic nerve damage. Arch Ophthalmol 1980; 98: 1564–1571

[8] Langenegger SJ, Funk J, Töteberg-Harms M. Reproducibility of retinal nerve fiber layer thickness measurements using the eye tracker and the retest function of Spectralis SD-OCT in glaucomatous and healthy control eyes. Invest Ophthalmol Vis Sci 2011; 52: 3338–3344

[9] Wu H, de Boer JF, Chen TC. Reproducibility of retinal nerve fiber layer thickness measurements using spectral domain optical coherence tomography. J Glaucoma 2011; 20: 470–476

[10] Savini G, Carbonelli M, Barboni P. Spectral-domain optical coherence tomography for the diagnosis and follow-up of glaucoma. Curr Opin Ophthalmol 2011; 22: 115–123

[11] Rosdahl JA, Asrani S. Glaucoma masqueraders: diagnosis by spectral domain optical coherence tomography. Saudi J Ophthalmol 2012; 26: 433–440

[12] Harwerth RS, Quigley HA. Visual field defects and retinal ganglion cell losses in patients with glaucoma. Arch Ophthalmol 2006; 124: 853–859

[13] Asrani S, Rosdahl JA, Allingham RR. Novel software strategy for glaucoma diagnosis: asymmetry analysis of retinal thickness. Arch Ophthalmol 2011; 129: 1205–1211

[14] Ghasia FF, El-Dairi M, Freedman SF, Rajani A, Asrani S. Reproducibility of spectral-domain optical coherence tomography measurements in adult and pediatric glaucoma. J Glaucoma 2013 May 29. [Epub ahead of print]

[15] Mathers K, Rosdahl JA, Asrani S. Correlation of macular thickness with visual fields in glaucoma patients and suspects. J Glaucoma 2014; 23: e98–e104

[16] Pasol J. Neuro-ophthalmic disease and optical coherence tomography: glaucoma look-alikes. Curr Opin Ophthalmol 2011; 22: 124–132

[17] Gupta PK, Asrani S, Freedman SF, El-Dairi M, Bhatti MT. Differentiating glaucomatous from non-glaucomatous optic nerve cupping by optical coherence tomography. Open Neurol J 2011; 5: 1–7

[18] Asrani S, Sarunic M, Santiago C, Izatt J. Detailed visualization of the anterior segment using fourier-domain optical coherence tomography. Arch Ophthalmol 2008; 126: 765–771

[19] Sarunic MV, Asrani S, Izatt JA. Imaging the ocular anterior segment with real-time, full-range Fourier-domain optical coherence tomography. Arch Ophthalmol 2008; 126: 537–542

[20] Asrani S, Essaid L, Alder BD, Santiago-Turla C. Artifacts in spectral-domain optical coherence tomography measurements in glaucoma. JAMA Ophthalmol 2014; 132: 396–402

26 Optical Coherence Tomography in Intraocular Tumors

Santosh G. Honavar, Tika Siburt, and Carol L. Shields

A wide spectrum of benign and malignant intraocular tumors occurs in the eye. Appropriate diagnosis and management of these tumors can help save the life, salvage the eye, and optimize visual potential. Accurate clinical diagnosis and objective assessment of anatomical and functional alterations are the basic prerequisites to successful management. Most intraocular tumors are diagnosed by a thorough clinical evaluation and good indirect ophthalmoscopy. Fundus fluorescein angiography (FFA) and indocyanine green angiography (ICG-A), ultrasonography, color Doppler imaging, computed tomography scan, magnetic resonance imaging, and positron-emission tomography are the useful adjunctive diagnostic tools that often help make a clinical diagnosis and an appropriate management strategy.

Introduced by Huang in 1991 and popularized as a sensitive and an objective tool for macular imaging for retina specialists, optical coherence tomography (OCT) has rapidly evolved.[1] The improvement in resolution, sensitivity, depth of imaging, speed, and portability, and the more recent introduction of ultrahigh-resolution OCT and enhanced depth imaging OCT (EDI OCT) have resulted in a better understanding of the alterations in the retina and the choroid, and thereby expanding clinical applications.[2,3,4] OCT helps assess the effects of intraocular tumors on the retinal architecture such as retinal edema, subretinal fluid, retinal atrophy, photoreceptor loss, outer retinal thinning, and retinal pigment epithelial (RPE) detachment.[2,3,4] EDI OCT is specifically useful in the evaluation of small choroidal tumors.[2,3,4,5,6] OCT is currently one of the favored tools for the diagnosis and management of intraocular tumors, assessment of secondary changes, identification of complications, and accurate monitoring of the response to treatment. In this chapter, we discuss the typical OCT features of common intraocular tumors.

26.1 Choroidal Tumors

26.1.1 Melanocytic Choroidal Tumors

Choroidal Nevus

Choroidal nevus is a common benign melanocytic tumor with an incidence in the general population that ranges from 1 to 3% and is found mostly in the postpubertal age group.[7] More than 90% of choroidal nevi occur posterior to the equator and therefore are likely to be detected on routine ophthalmic examination. A choroidal nevus characteristically appears as a placoid or minimally elevated lesion (< 2 mm) ranging in diameter from

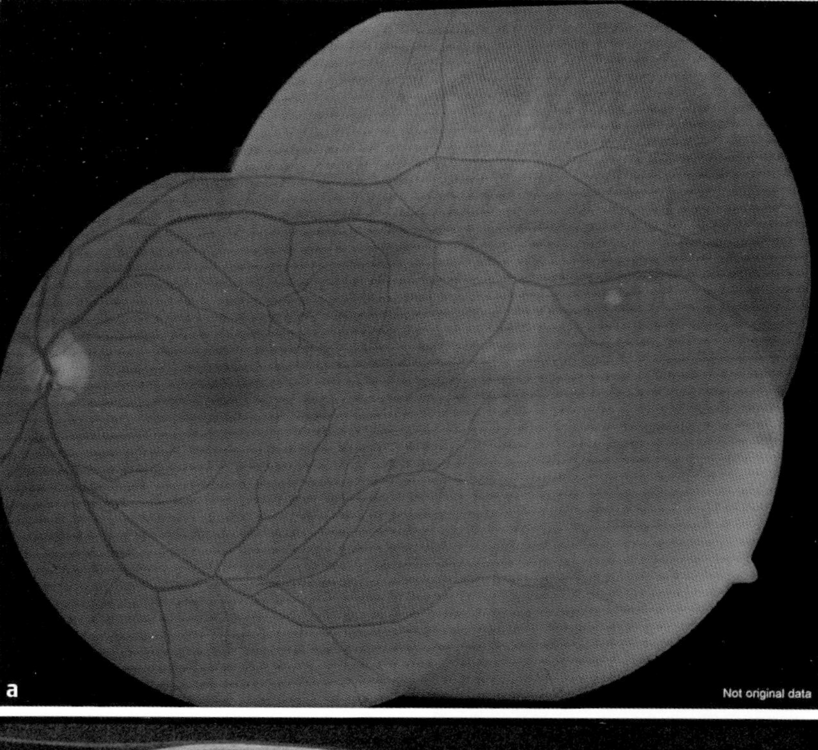

Fig. 26.1 Choroidal nevus. (a) Color fundus photograph shows pigmented choroidal nevus with overlying drusen. **(b)** Enhanced depth imaging optical coherence tomography confirming drusen, retinal pigment epithelial thinning, and thinning of choriocapillaris.

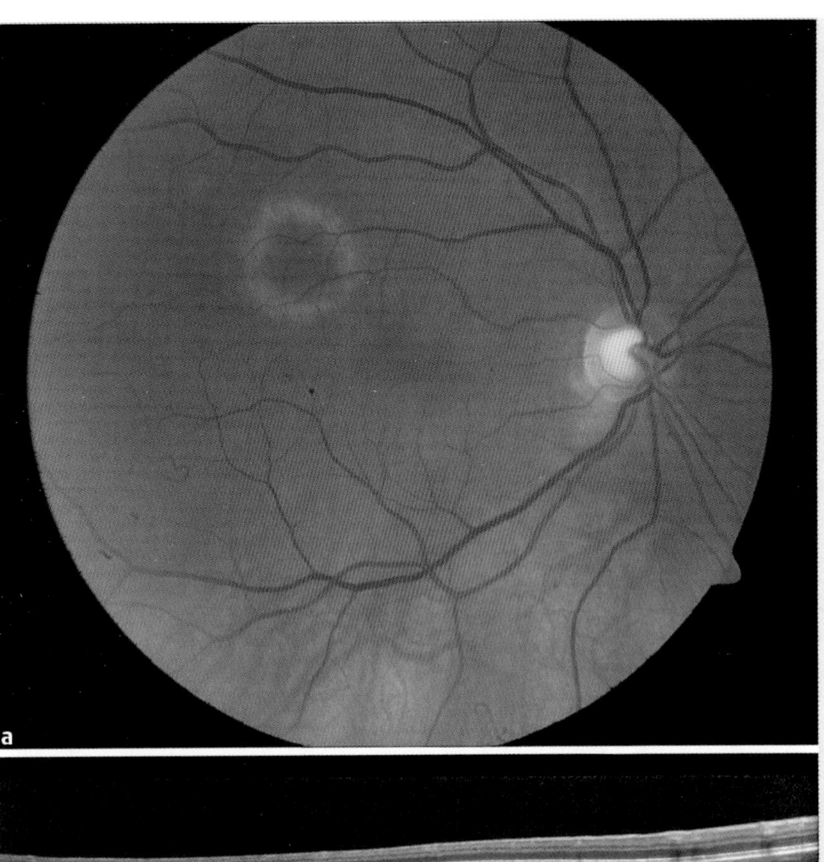

Fig. 26.2 Halo choroidal nevus. (a) Color fundus photograph shows halo nevus of choroid. **(b)** Enhanced depth imaging optical coherence tomography of the nevus showing drusen, retinal pigment epithelial thinning, and thinning of choriocapillaris.

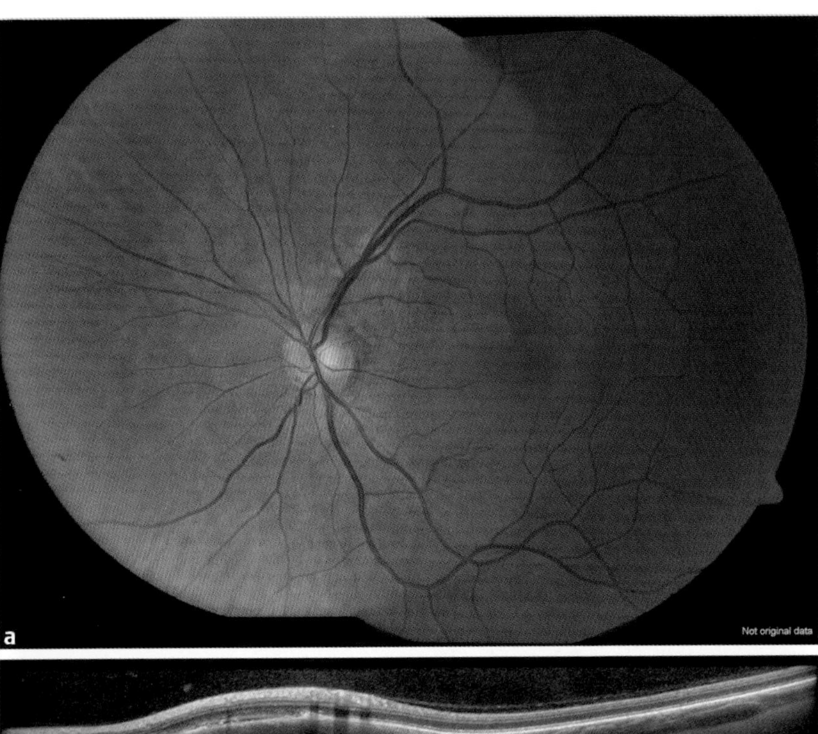

Fig. 26.3 Choroidal melanoma. (a) Color fundus photograph shows a small juxtapapillary choroidal melanoma with overlying orange pigment. **(b)** The enhanced depth optical coherence tomography shows shaggy photoreceptors, shallow subretinal fluid (which could have been easily missed on clinical examination), and subretinal deposits (orange pigment) overlying the melanoma.

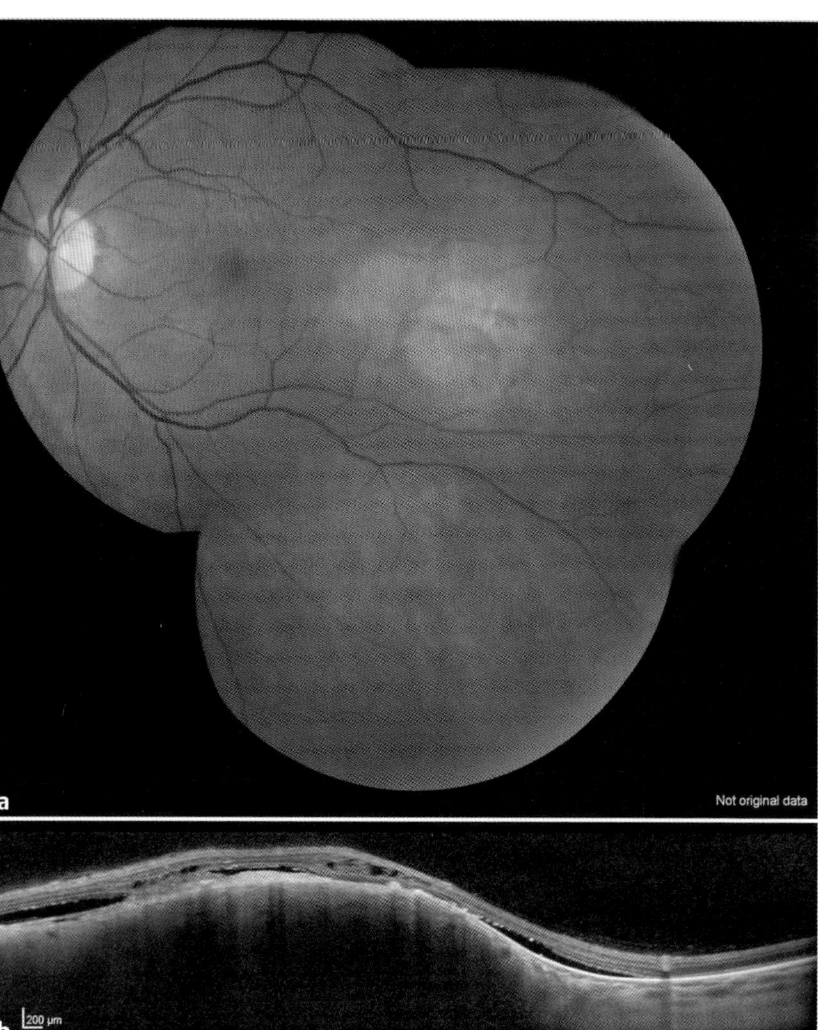

Fig. 26.4 Choroidal melanoma. (a) Color fundus photograph shows a medium-sized choroidal melanoma with orange pigment and subretinal fluid. The enhanced depth imaging optical coherence tomography shows shaggy photoreceptors, shallow subretinal fluid, and subretinal deposits (orange pigment) overlying the melanoma. **(b)** Overlying the dome-shaped elevation of the choroid is a thickened, irregular retinal pigment epithelium and thickening of the outer retinal layers.

1.5 to 5 mm, with variable pigmentation: brown to slate gray to amelanotic.[7] The clinical picture is often altered by secondary changes such as surface drusen, RPE clumping, atrophy, fibrous metaplasia or detachment, subretinal neovascular membrane, and serous retinal detachment.[7] It is estimated that 1 in 8845 choroidal nevi undergoes malignant transformation into melanoma.[8] Despite the rarity, careful evaluation and follow-up of all choroidal nevi are advised. Factors predictive of nevus transformation into melanoma include thickness greater than 2 mm, the presence of subretinal fluid, orange pigment, juxtapapillary location, and symptoms of blurred vision or photopsia.[9,10] In the setting of a suspicious nevus, OCT is useful in identifying some of these differentiating signs.

Although time-domain OCT (TD OCT) features of choroidal nevus are extensively documented, limited visualization of the deeper layers of the choroid and sclera secondary to light scattering from the RPE and choroid had limited the early descriptions to the retina and anterior choroid.[4] In an assessment of 120 eyes with choroidal nevus using OCT, Shields et al described secondary retinal alterations that included overlying retinal edema (15%), subretinal fluid (26%), retinal thinning (22%), drusen (41%), and RPE detachment (12%).[11] The overlying retinal edema could be further classified as focal cystoid (3%), diffuse cystoid (8%), coalescent cystoid (3%), and noncystoid (1%), which may have value in deciding on treatment in patients who have visual loss and in prognosticating the outcome. By OCT, the overlying retina was of normal thickness (32%), thin (22%), or thick (45%) and photoreceptor loss or attenuation present in 51% of cases. The choroidal findings in nevi were limited to the anterior surface and included hyporeflectivity in 62%, isoreflectivity in 29%, and hyperreflectivity in 9%. Anterior choroidal reflectivity is affected by overlying RPE alterations and the amount of pigmentation. Nevi with dense pigment tend to show posterior shadowing, whereas those with minimal pigment allow some light transmission. The OCT findings rather reflect pigment within the mass and do not correlate to internal reflectivity and acoustic quality as elicited by ultrasonography (which implies density of cellularity).[11]

Compared with the clinical examination, OCT is more sensitive in detecting the secondary changes: retinal edema, subretinal fluid, retinal thinning, photoreceptor attenuation, and RPE detachment.[11] Retinal edema, RPE alterations, photoreceptor loss, and RPE detachment are related to chronic retinal degeneration and suggest a stable, chronic choroidal nevus.[11] In contrast, the presence of subretinal fluid and photoreceptor preservation suggests a relatively acute process with risk for growth into a melanoma or even a small melanoma.[12] Serial OCT in a suspicious nevus can demonstrate subtle clinically

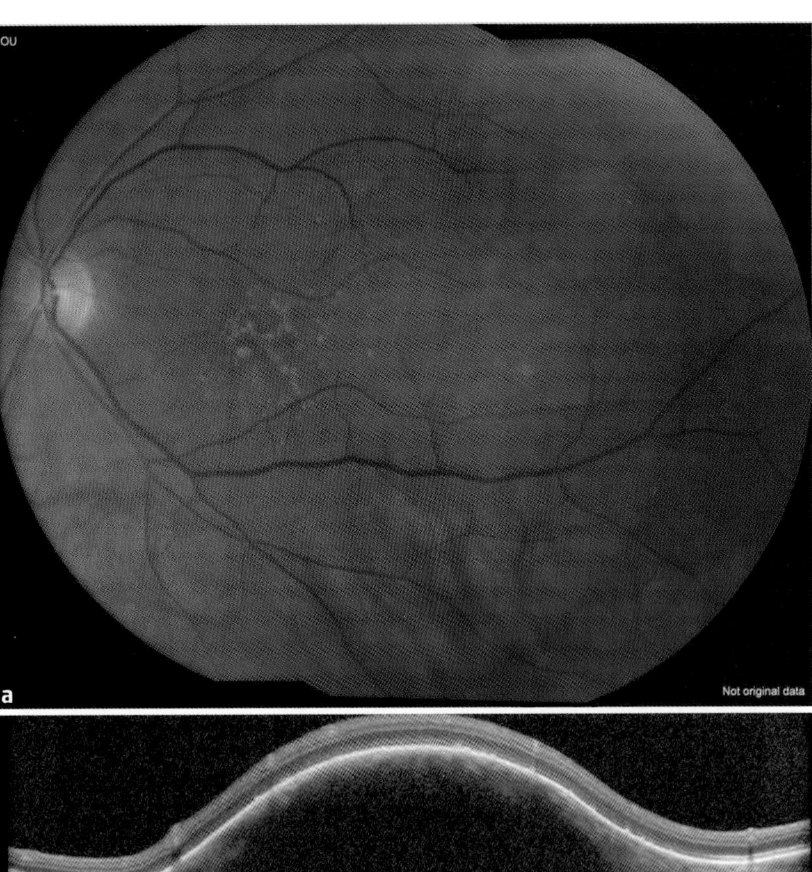

Fig. 26.5 Choroidal hemangioma. (a) Color fundus photograph shows a choroidal hemangioma on the temporal aspect with intraretinal exudates. **(b)** The enhanced depth imaging optical coherence tomography shows a regular dome-shaped choroidal mass with overlying subtle retinal edema and exudates.

undetectable changes that may help in making a treatment decision.

The more recent descriptions have used high-resolution spectral-domain (SD) EDI OCT, which allows detailed study of the internal architecture of the tumor and its precise measurement (▸ Fig. 26.1, ▸ Fig. 26.2).[5,12] EDI OCT is sensitive in identifying drusen and photoreceptor loss. Subretinal fluid, a predictor of activity of a melanocytic choroidal lesion, can be detected by EDI OCT when it has been overlooked clinically and ultrasonographically. Visualization of explicit alterations specifically within the various layers of the retina allows characterization of subtle alterations such as RPE atrophy (43%), RPE loss (14%), RPE nodularity (8%), inner segment/outer segment (IS/OS) junction irregularity (37%), IS/OS junction loss (6%), external limiting membrane irregularity (18%), outer nuclear and outer plexiform layer irregularity (8%), and inner nuclear layer irregularity (6%).[5] Choroidal shadowing deep to the nevus (partial 59%, complete 35%) and choriocapillary thinning overlying the nevus (94%) can be reliably demonstrated on EDI OCT. Although EDI OCT provides much useful information, its inability to acquire images of good quality in about half the cases remains a barrier. Ideal candidates with choroidal nevus for EDI OCT imaging include younger (i.e., < 60 years) patients with nevus located in the posterior pole and < 3 mm tumor thickness.[5]

Choroidal Melanoma

Choroidal melanoma is the most common primary intraocular malignant tumor. It is relatively rare in pigmented races and has known association with oculocutaneous melanocytosis. Choroidal melanomas manifest a range of growth patterns. Clinical appearances often change with the increasing size of the tumor. A small choroidal melanoma appears as a placoid, dome-shaped, or nodular well-circumscribed choroidal mass. As it grows, it may break through the Bruch membrane, assume a collar-button shape, and infiltrate the retina. A rare variant is a diffuse choroidal melanoma where the tumor thickness is < 20% of its overall basal diameter. Degree of pigmentation varies from characteristic deep brown to rare pale white. Secondary changes associated with choroidal melanoma include RPE mottling and localized detachment, orange pigment, subretinal neovascular membrane, overlying retinal phototoreceptor degeneration, retinoschisis, exudative retinal detachment, vitreous hemorrhage, vitreous pigment and tumor seeding, and scleral invasion and extraocular extension.[13] A good indirect

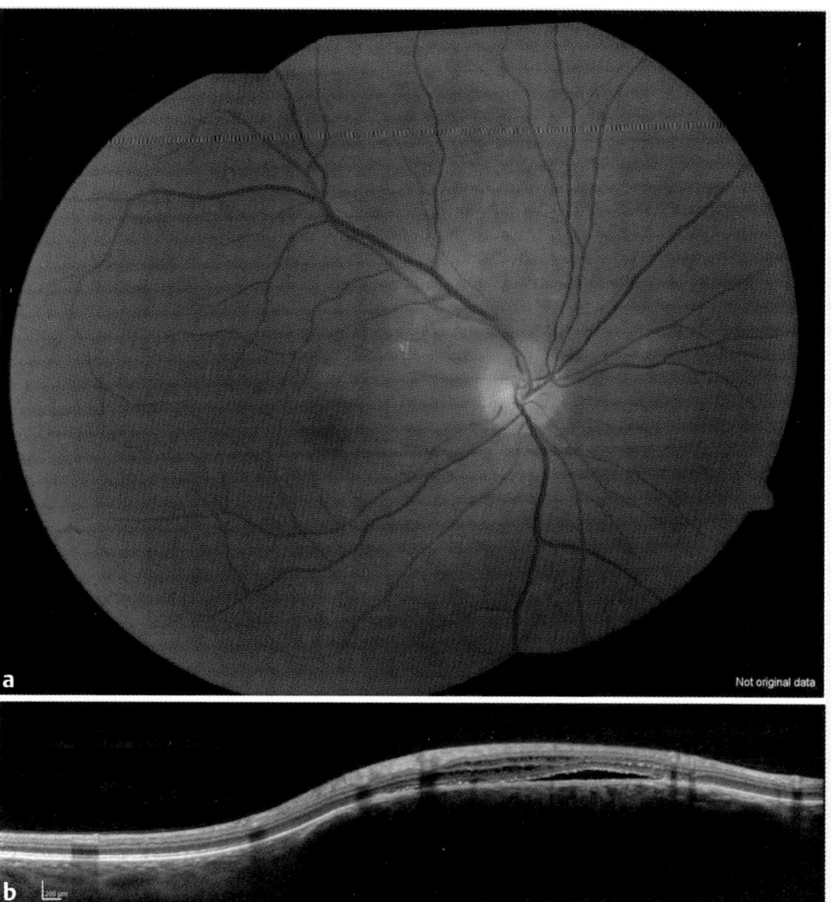

Fig. 26.6 Choroidal hemangioma. (a) Color fundus photograph shows a superior juxtapapillary choroidal hemangioma. **(b)** The enhanced depth imaging OCT shows a placoid choroidal mass with overlying retinal edema and subretinal fluid.

ophthalmoscopy and ultrasound B-scan often aided by FFA and ICG are generally adequate to diagnose a typical melanoma.[13]

Although TD OCT is not helpful in imaging the tumor itself, it can elucidate secondary retinal changes. Detection of overlying subretinal fluid by OCT could be important in confirming the suspicion of melanoma in eyes with borderline tumors.[12] Muscat et al studied 20 untreated choroidal melanomas and detected subretinal fluid using TD OCT in all cases.[14] Espinoza et al showed that localized serous retinal detachment associated with retina of normal thickness was highly associated with documented tumor growth and future treatment.[12] In contrast, a chronic OCT pattern with a thin retina, intraretinal cysts, and RPE thickening was associated with a long-standing dormant lesion.[12] Sayanagi, using three-dimensional SD OCT, found subretinal fluid, retinal edema, and subretinal deposits in choroidal melanoma.[15] Singh and colleagues used SD OCT to describe dispersed subretinal deposits corresponding to orange pigment over a small choroidal melanoma that was missed with TD OCT.[16]

Choroidal melanomas showed a highly reflective band in the anterior choroid by EDI OCT with lack of visibility of either the choroidal vessels or inner sclera.[17] Shields used EDI OCT to compare the features of small choroidal melanomas (≤ 3 mm thick on ultrasonography) with similarly sized choroidal nevi.[6] Of 37 eyes with small choroidal melanoma imaged using EDI OCT, the mean tumor thickness was 55% less by EDI OCT compared with ultrasonography.[6] Choroidal features included optical shadowing in and overlying choriocapillary thinning in all. Outer retinal features included shaggy photoreceptors in 49%, an absence of photoreceptors in 24%, IS/OS junction in 65%, external limiting membrane in 43%, outer nuclear layer in 6%, and outer plexiform layer in 11% (▶ Fig. 26.3, ▶ Fig. 26.4).[6] Inner retinal features were irregularity of the inner nuclear layer, inner plexiform layer, and ganglion cell layer in 8% each, nerve fiber layer in 5%. Secondary changes were subretinal fluid in 92%, subretinal lipofuscin in 95%, and intraretinal edema in 16%. Using EDI OCT, a comparison with similar-sized choroidal nevus revealed that small choroidal melanoma showed increased tumor thickness, subretinal fluid, subretinal lipofuscin, RPE atrophy, and retinal irregularities, including shaggy photoreceptors.[6] The difficulty of imaging the overlying retina for large melanomas and the inability to characterize the tumor itself beyond its anterior surface limit the routine use of OCT in the diagnosis of melanoma.[3]

After radiotherapy, OCT has been used to monitor treatment response and complications of choroidal melanoma. Horgan et al performed pre- and post-plaque radiotherapy OCT and found that the mean time to onset of radiation maculopathy was 12 months.[18] They reported macular edema in 17% by OCT at 6 months, in 40% at 12 months, and in 61% at 24 months, much

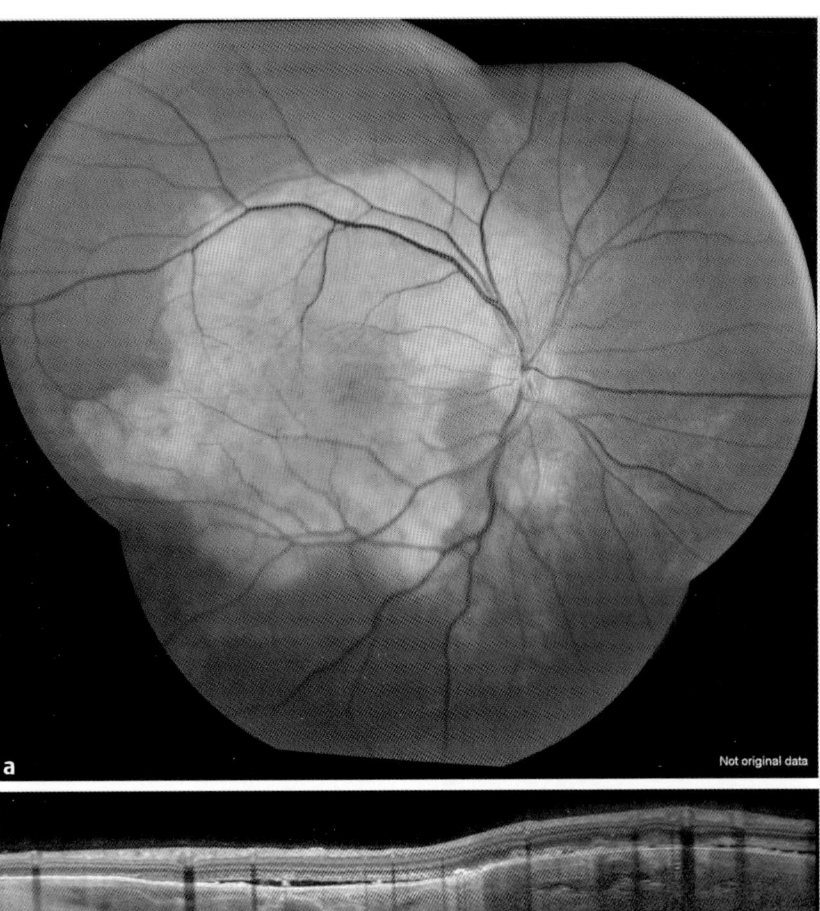

Fig. 26.7 Choroidal osteoma. **(a)** Partially decalcified choroidal osteoma with associated retinal pigment epithelial atrophy. **(b)** Enhanced depth imaging optical coherence tomography demonstrates replacement of the normal choriocapillaris with a dense hyperreflective mass. The lesion is almost continuous with the overlying retinal pigment epithelium. Overlying neurosensory retina is thinned with the loss of the outer layers.

higher than by clinical evaluation: 1% at 6 months, 12% at 12 months, and 29% at 24 months.[18] Further, they were able to classify macular edema into extrafoveolar noncystoid (grade 1), extrafoveolar cystoid (grade 2), foveolar noncystoid (grade 3), mild-to-moderate foveolar cystoid (grade 4), and severe foveolar cystoid (grade 5).[18] This qualitative classification correlated with quantification of central foveolar thickness. OCT can therefore be used to diagnose and monitor radiation macular edema.

26.1.2 Choroidal Vascular Tumors: Circumscribed and Diffuse Choroidal Hemangioma

Circumscribed choroidal hemangioma is a common benign vascular tumor that manifests in middle-aged individuals with sudden-onset blurred vision or metamorphopsia.[19,20] It is generally unifocal and unilateral, with no systemic association. Ophthalmoscopically, circumscribed choroidal hemangioma appears as a subtle reddish orange mass posterior to the equator. It is usually dome shaped, ranging in size from 3 to 10 mm in diameter and 2 to 4 mm thick.[19,20] Whereas FFA features might not be diagnostic of circumscribed choroidal hemangioma, ICG angiography is characteristic: bright early filling and a characteristic late washout.

The diffuse choroidal hemangioma involves the entire choroid but with maximal thickness in the posterior pole. It is associated with facial hemangioma as part of the Sturge-Weber syndrome. Secondary changes in both circumscribed and diffuse choroidal hemangioma include subretinal fluid, overlying RPE atrophy, hyperplasia or fibrous metaplasia, retinal cystoid degeneration, and intraretinal macrocysts.[19,20] On ultrasonography, choroidal hemangiomas have a high internal reflectivity and acoustic solidity matching that of the surrounding choroid, which helps to differentiate choroidal hemangiomas from other choroidal tumors, such as melanoma.[20]

On TD OCT, choroidal hemangioma shows poor resolution. The tumor appears to be hyperreflective at its anterior surface but with little deeper detail. On EDI OCT, circumscribed choroidal hemangiomas appear to have a medium-to-low reflective band with a homogeneous signal and intrinsic spaces (▶ Fig. 26.5).[17] EDI OCT allows quantifying choroidal thickness in the posterior pole, even in diffuse choroidal hemangioma. It can detect choroidal thickness in eyes with subclinical choroidal abnormalities in patients with Sturge-Weber syndrome.[21]

Optical coherence tomography helps image the overlying retina and elucidate the reason for visual loss, such as subretinal fluid, intraretinal edema, chronic photoreceptor loss, and tilt of the fovea (▶ Fig. 26.6). OCT findings in circumscribed choroidal hemangioma include subretinal fluid (19%), retinal edema (42%), retinal schisis (12%), macular edema (24%), and localized

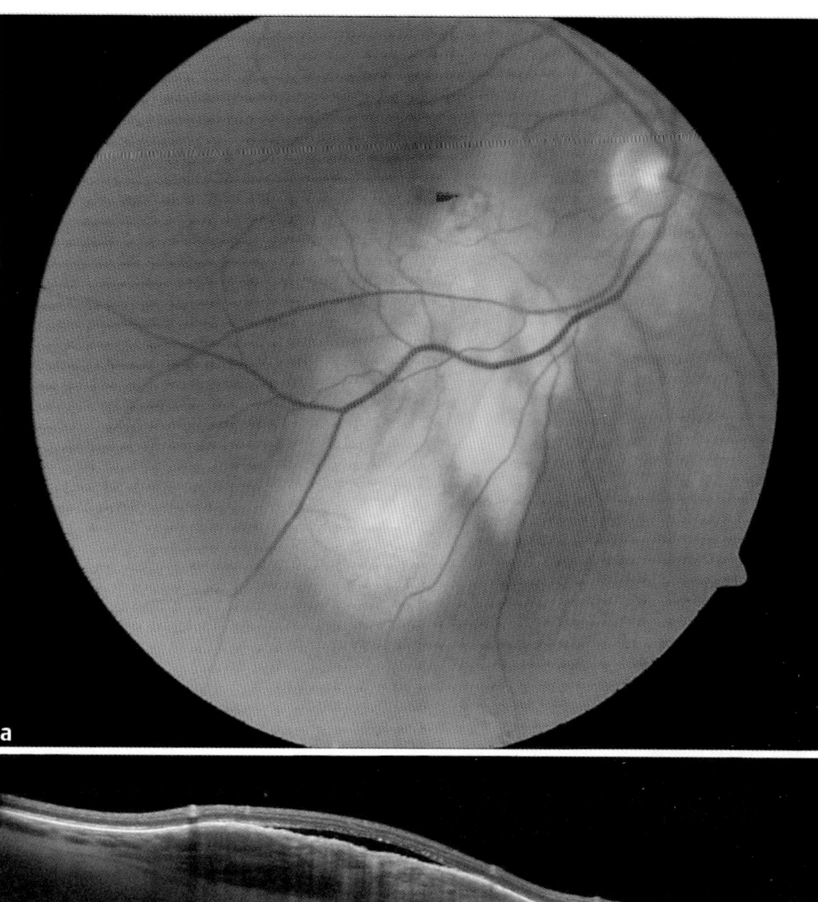

Fig. 26.8 Choroidal metastasis. (a) Color fundus photograph shows choroidal metastasis as an irregular placoid amelanotic choroidal mass. **(b)** Enhanced depth imaging optical coherence tomography demonstrates both the anterior and posterior margins of the metastasis. Overlying subretinal fluid is evident.

photoreceptor loss (35%).[3,22] OCT findings in diffuse choroidal hemangioma are subretinal fluid (28%), retinal edema (14%), and photoreceptor loss (43%).[3,22] Newly active choroidal hemangioma shows subretinal fluid and preserved photoreceptor layer with minimal intraretinal edema.[2] Chronically leaking choroidal hemangioma displays photoreceptor attenuation and overlying intraretinal edema and bullous retinoschisis.[2] Together with the evaluation of the IS/OS photoreceptor line and the integrity of the RPE layer, this information may be useful when considering treatment options and predicting the potential outcome.[23] Preservation of outer retinal thickness and integrity of the IS/OS photoreceptor line are important prognostic factors for visual recovery after treatment.[24] When the tumor causes visual loss, treatment is advised. Options for treatment include laser photocoagulation, transpupillary thermotherapy, plaque brachytherapy, and photodynamic therapy. OCT is an important tool in depicting resolution of subretinal fluid and foveal edema after treatment.[2] Recurrent subretinal fluid after therapy can be detected before the vision deteriorates and before this fluid becomes apparent clinically.[25,26]

26.1.3 Choroidal Osseous Tumors: Choroidal Osteoma

Choroidal osteoma is a rare benign tumor that comprises mature bone in various stages of calcification, mostly unilateral, and typically is found in healthy females in the second or third decades of life.[27] Most patients are asymptomatic, but a few have mild visual symptoms, metamorphopsia, and localized scotoma. Ophthalmoscopically, it appears as a rather well-defined yellow-orange placoid choroidal mass with scalloped margins in juxtapapillary or peripapillary location, with overlying clumping of brown, orange, or gray pigment.[27] It ranges in size from 2 to 22 mm in basal diameter and 0.5 to 2.5 mm thick. Secondary changes include growth, decalcification, subretinal fluid, subretinal neovascular membrane, and subretinal hemorrhage.[27] Shields et al have reported that the 10-year probability for tumor growth was 51%, tumor decalcification 46%, and related choroidal neovascularization 31%.[27]

The anterior tumor surface is hyperreflective in 48% and isoreflective in 52% if calcified but mostly hyperreflective (90%) when decalcified.[28] The internal structure of choroidal osteoma is difficult to evaluate using OCT.[2] Abrupt elevation of the choroidal tumor at its margin, dense optical reflectivity, and complete shadowing are characteristic of the choroidal osteoma.[2] The overlying inner retina is often preserved while changes in the outer retinal layers are often observed.[2] The RPE can be continuous with the inner surface of the underlying tumor, and the degree of calcification affects the amount of light transmission.[8,29,30] Shields et al reported heterogeneity that largely depends on the amount of calcification.[28] Calcified portions of the tumor reveal mostly intact inner (100%) and outer (95%)

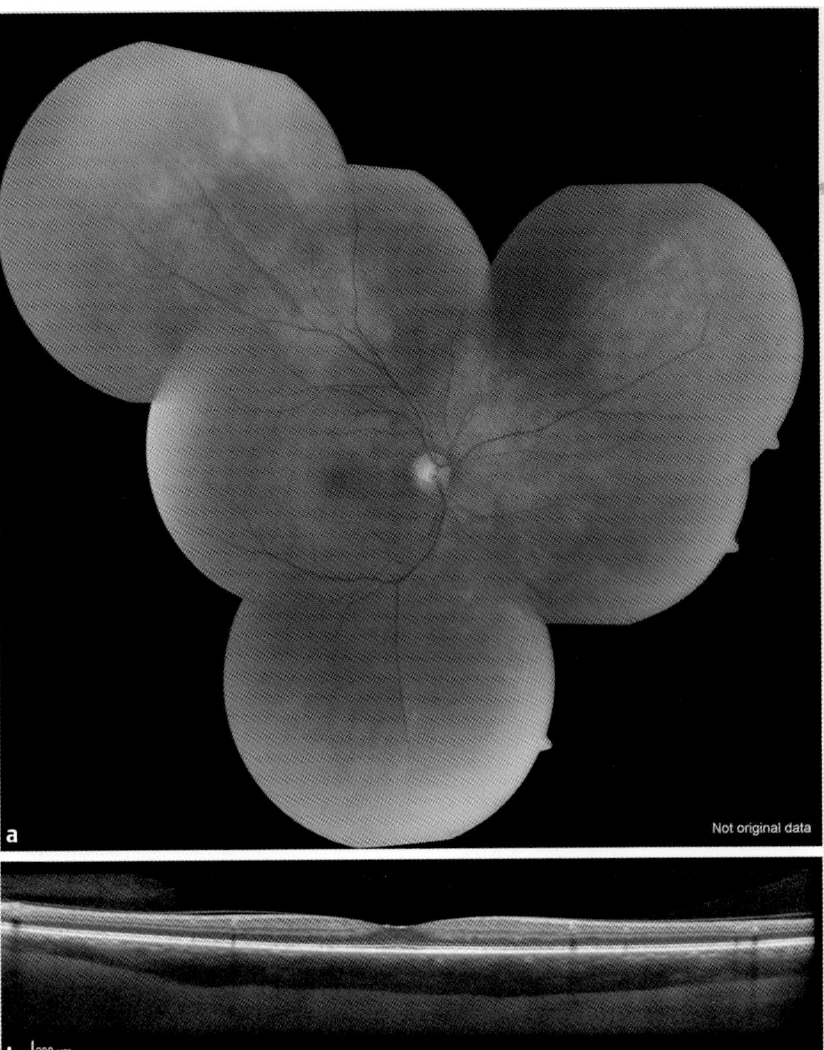

Fig. 26.9 Choroidal lymphoma. (a) Color fundus photograph shows a placoid choroidal mass. **(b)** Enhanced depth imaging optical coherence tomography shows regular placoid choroidal thickening and loss of choriocapillaris. The overlying retinal pigment epithelium and neurosensory retina are unaffected and retain the normal contour.

retinal layers, a distinct RPE (57%), and mild transmission of light (95%). In contrast, decalcified portions of the tumor reveal intact inner retinal layers (90%), thinned outer retinal layers (100%), an indistinct RPE (90%), and marked light transmission into the tumor (70%).[28] EDI OCT in choroidal osteoma revealed a characteristic sponge-like tumor appearance with the presence of multiple intralesional layers (▶ Fig. 26.7). The lesion showed a typical transparency with visibility of sclerochoroidal junction.[31]

Choroidal Metastasis

Choroidal metastasis is considered the most common form of intraocular malignancy.[32] Breast and lung cancers account for most choroidal metastases. It is important to note that a substantial number of patients with choroidal metastasis have an undiagnosed primary malignancy and consult an ophthalmologist first with visual symptoms. Ophthalmoscopic examination of choroidal metastasis shows a creamy yellow placoid or a dome-shaped choroidal mass posterior to the equator. Choroidal metastasis could be multifocal and bilateral. Exudative retinal detachment is a common secondary change along with pronounced RPE alterations.[32]

Optical coherence tomography of choroidal metastasis demonstrates a dome-shaped elevation of the neurosensory retina and RPE and subretinal fluid. It can also be associated with retinal edema, intraretinal cysts, and thickening and detachment of the RPE (▶ Fig. 26.8).[3] Highly reflective subretinal deposits corresponding to RPE clumping overlying the tumor[33] and highly reflective points within neurosensory detachment that may correspond to tumor cells or macrophages containing lipofuscin and melanin granules have been described.[34] Choroidal features in TD OCT are limited to the anterior surface, which shows variable reflectivity.[15] OCT is valuable in gauging treatment response by resolution of subretinal fluid and return of normal retinal architecture.[34,35]

The EDI OCT features of the metastasis include anterior compression or obliteration of the overlying choriocapillaris (93%), an irregular (lumpy bumpy) anterior contour (64%), and posterior shadowing (86%). Overlying RPE abnormalities were noted (78%). Outer retinal features have included structural loss of the interdigitation of the cone outer segment tips (64%), the ellipsoid portion of photoreceptors (57%), external limiting membrane (29%), outer nuclear layer (7%), and outer plexiform layer (7%). The inner retinal layers (inner nuclear layer to nerve fiber layer) were normal. Subretinal fluid (79%), subretinal lipofuscin

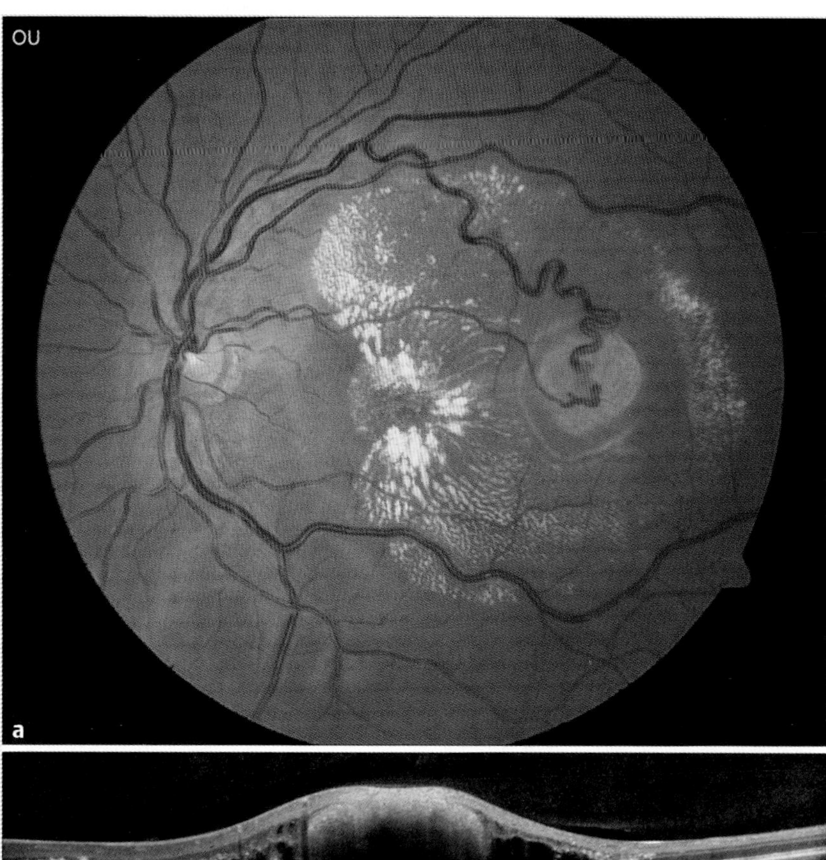

Fig. 26.10 Retinal hemangioblastoma. (a) Retinal hemangioblastoma with exudation and subretinal fluid. **(b)** Enhanced depth imaging optical coherence tomography demonstrates a dome-shaped elevation of the inner retina with abrupt transition to the adjacent normal tissue and complete shadowing of the posterior layers. Note the subretinal fluid and intraretinal exudates.

pigment (7%), and intraretinal edema (14%) were also identified.[36]

26.1.4 Lymphoma

Intraocular lymphoid has two basic types: vitreoretinal and choroidal. Vitreoretinal lymphoma is primarily diffuse large B-cell lymphomas.[37] The vitreoretinal form is aggressive and highly associated with central nervous system lymphoma,[37] Patients are often elderly and immunocompetent or young and immunocompromised. Clinically, this condition manifests as bilateral multifocal yellowish deposits in the retina, subretina, or sub-RPE with overlying vitreous opacities. Pigment migration and RPE clumping are sometimes visible overlying the tumor as brown "leopard spots." The choroidal form of lymphoid tumors is usually unilateral. This condition presents as multifocal yellow choroidal infiltrates or unifocal placoid or dome-shaped lesions causing a diffuse thickening of the uvea on ultrasonography.[38] The overlying retina and vitreous remain clear.[37] Compared with vitreoretinal lymphoma, choroidal lymphoma is more indolent, but an association with systemic lymphoma exists.

In vitreoretinal lymphomas, OCT may show dome-shaped elevations of the RPE or small nodular RPE irregularities from sub-RPE tumor deposits, retinal elevation or thickening from tumor infiltration, and cystoid macular edema.[38,39,40] EDI OCT shows subretinal deposits and outer retinal atrophy.[41] OCT in choroidal lymphoma shows choroidal thickening and loss of choriocapillaris layer (▶ Fig. 26.9).[42] Shields et al found that thin infiltration has a smooth topography on EDI OCT, whereas thicker lymphoid infiltration shows a rippled effect, and the thickest has a "seasick," undulating topography.[43] The overlying RPE and neurosensory retina are unaffected and retain regular, smooth contour.[42]

26.2 Retinal Tumors

26.2.1 Retinal Vascular Tumors

Retinal vascular tumors can be classified into four distinct clinical entities—retinal hemangioblastoma, retinal cavernous hemangioma, retinal arteriovenous communications (Wyburn-Mason syndrome), and retinal vasoproliferative tumor.[44]

Retinal Hemangioblastoma

Retinal hemangioblastoma (RH) is a benign vascular tumor of the retina that has a specific association with von Hippel-Lindau (vHL) disease. RH is often bilateral and multifocal and is clinically diagnosed at a mean of age of about 25 years.[44] Ophthalmoscopically, RH appears as a well-circumscribed round retinal lesion with an intense orange-red color and prominent feeder

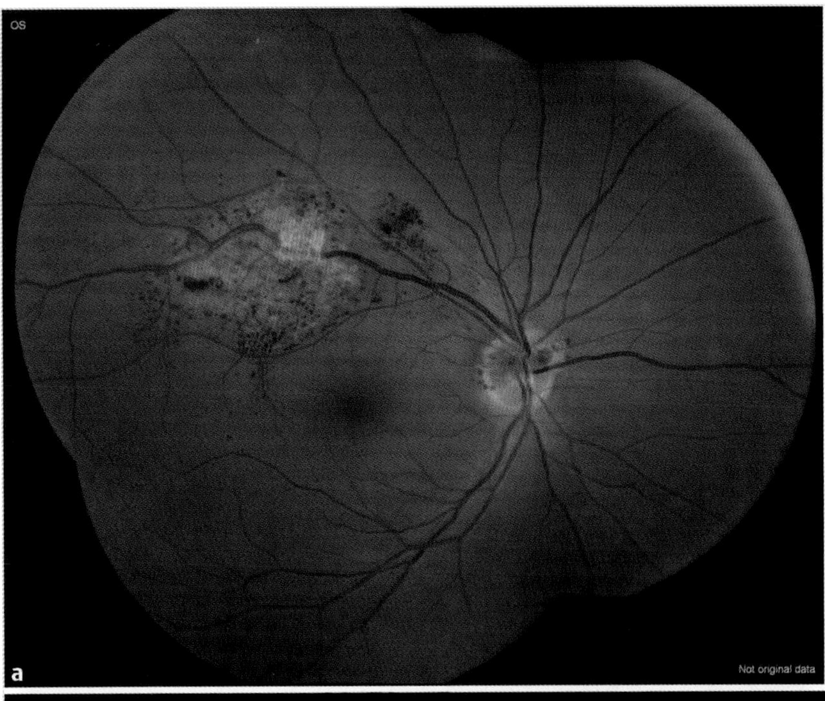

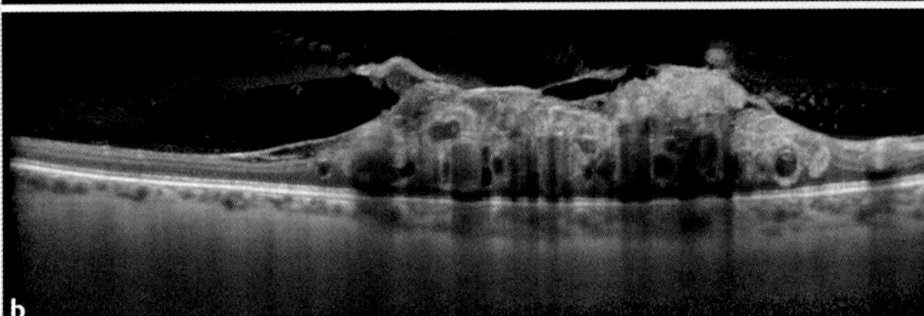

Fig. 26.11 Retinal cavernous hemangioma. (a) Saccular discrete and confluent lesions along the superotemporal arcade with associated preretinal fibrosis. Note similar lesions over the optic disc. **(b)** Enhanced depth imaging optical coherence tomography shows a lobulated inner retina with optically clear spaces representing the saccular aneurysms. The underlying retinal pigment epithelium is intact.

and drainage vessels. It is typically located in the temporal peripheral retina, although it can also occur in a juxtapapillary location or over the optic nerve head. Secondary changes include intraretinal and subretinal exudation around the tumor and remotely at the macula, subretinal fluid, and vitreoretinal fibrovascular proliferation.[44]

The use of OCT in the treatment of patients with RH relates to the identification and monitoring of associated secondary retinal changes such as macular edema, retinal atrophy, retinal detachment, and epiretinal or subretinal membrane formation, which are not always as well demonstrated clinically.[2] Early identification and treatment of these effects may have a greater influence on visual outcome. RH appears as an optically dense, inner-retinal mass with posterior shadowing or thickening and disorganization of the retinal layers on OCT (▶ Fig. 26.10).[2,3,4]

Retinal Cavernous Hemangioma

Retinal cavernous hemangioma can be sporadic, or it may have autosomal dominant neuro-oculo-cutaneous syndromic association.[44] It is a congenital hamartoma that is often recognized later in life, when the patient may become symptomatic with reduced vision. Clinically, it shows grape-like clusters of blood-filled saccular spaces in the inner retinal layers or on the optic disc surface. Secondary changes include spontaneous thrombosis, epiretinal membrane, intraretinal hemorrhage, and vitreous hemorrhage.[44] Features of retinal cavernous hemangioma on OCT include lobulated, hyperreflective lesions in the inner retina that correspond to the aneurysms (▶ Fig. 26.11). Optically clear cystic spaces may represent larger aneurysms.[45,46] A preretinal membrane with traction on the adjacent retina may also be found; subretinal fluid is typically absent.[3]

Retinal Arteriovenous Malformation

Congenital retinal arteriovenous malformation is a dramatic feature of Wyburn Mason syndrome.[44] The diagnosis is made later in childhood as an incidental finding in an asymptomatic individual or in a child with poor visual acuity. Typically, there are three specific configurations: group 1, with an abnormal capillary plexus between the major vessels and arteriovenous malformation, manifesting small lesion in an asymptomatic patient; group 2, with absent capillary network with consequent high flow, retinal edema, hemorrhage, and moderate visual impairment; and group 3, with the most severe from, with no apparent distinction between the artery and the vein and

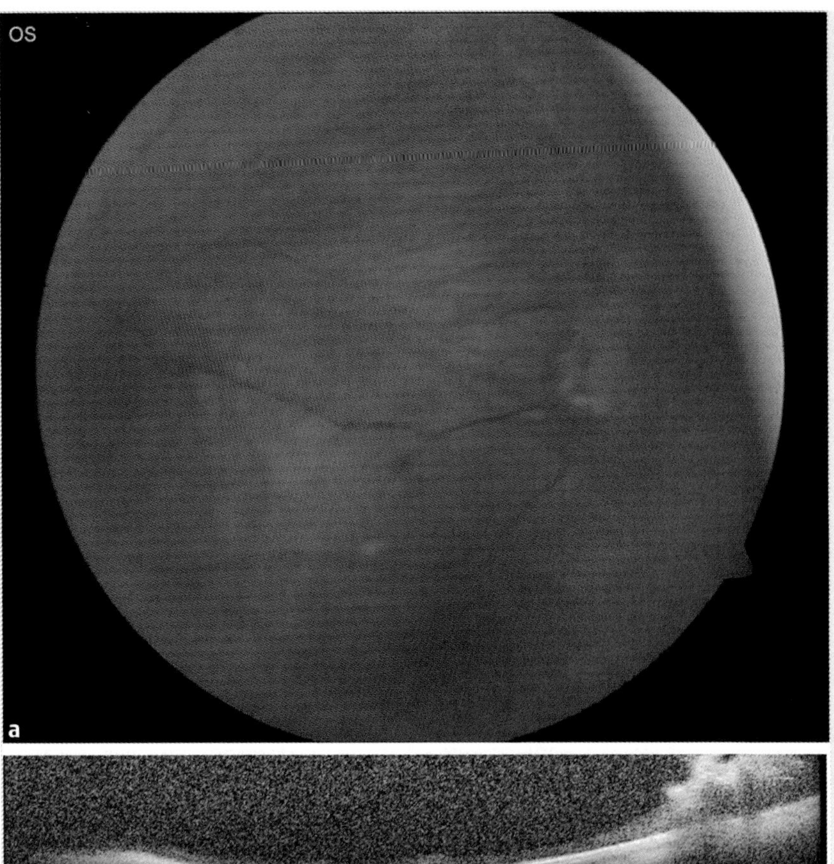

Fig. 26.12 Vasoproliferative tumor. (a) Vasoproliferative tumor located at the periphery. **(b)** Optical coherence tomography reveals a hyperreflective, disorganized inner retina with some shadowing of the posterior layers, including the retinal pigment epithelium.

severe visual loss.[44] However, the there is no distinct mass, retinal exudation, or retinal detachment. With OCT, retinal arteriovenous malformation appears as a relatively large intraretinal cystic mass owing to the dilated vessels.[2] Rarely, surrounding retinal changes of retinal atrophy, edema, and hemorrhage can be found.[2]

Retinal Vasoproliferative Tumor

Retinal vasoproliferative tumor is a distinct entity that is mostly idiopathic (74%) or secondary (24%) to intermediate uveitis, retinitis pigmentosa, or toxoplasmosis.[45] The lesion is generally solitary if idiopathic and multiple if secondary and occurs mostly in the inferotemporal peripheral fundus as a raised globular reddish vascular mass. Associated retinal vascular abnormality is conspicuous by its absence. Secondary changes include subretinal exudation, exudative retinal detachment, vitreous hemorrhage, epiretinal membrane, and macular edema. Retinal vasoproliferative tumors are too peripheral to be imaged by standard OCT. Posterior lesions demonstrate inner retinal layer disorganization and posterior shadowing.[47] Visual loss caused by retinal vasoproliferative tumors is related to retinal changes in the macular region: epiretinal membrane formation and macular edema (▶ Fig. 26.12, ▶ Fig. 26.13). OCT is used to monitor treatment response and complications.

26.2.2 Tumors of the Retinal Pigment Epithelium

Congenital Hypertrophy of Retinal Pigment Epithelium

Congenital hypertrophy of retinal pigment epithelium (CHRPE) is usually observed in an asymptomatic individual during routine screening; it appears as a deeply pigmented, flat, well-circumscribed retinal lesion measuring 1 to 6 mm in diameter, with characteristic halo and lacunae of depigmentation.[48] It may be solitary with systemic association with neurofibromatosis type 1 or multifocal and bilateral, having a specific association with Gardner syndrome.

Because of the peripheral location of CHRPEs, OCT imaging can be difficult. Shields and colleagues described overlying retinal thinning and photoreceptor loss in all patients with CHRPE, which likely account for the visual-field defects.[49] The neurosensory retina overlying CHRPE is attenuated.[49] Pigmented CHRPE has thicker RPE than adjacent normal retina, which prevents light transmission and shadows the underlying choroid (▶ Fig. 26.14).[49] Nonpigmented CHRPE has large areas of lacunae with thinner RPE that allow transmission of light and partial visualization of the choroid.[49] On EDI OCT, CHRPE seems flat with thickened, irregular RPE and absent RPE within lacunae. A

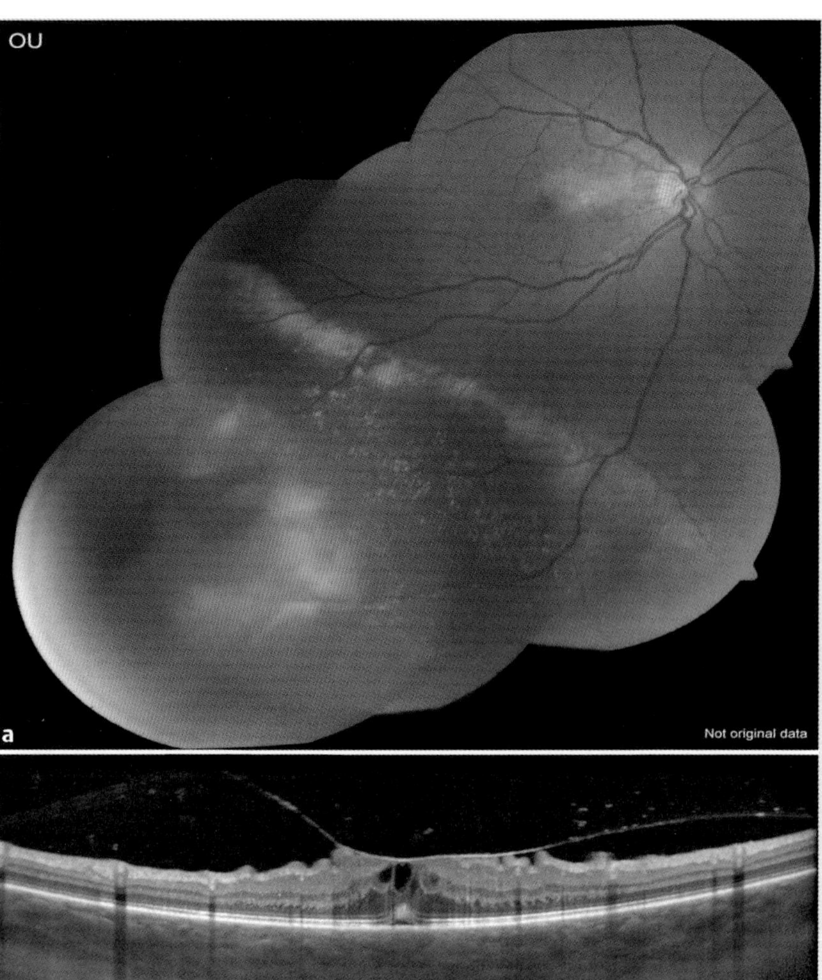

Fig. 26.13 Vasoproliferative tumor. (a) Vasoproliferative tumor located at the inferotemporal periphery with epiretinal membrane at the macula. **(b)** Enhanced depth imaging optical coherence tomography (OCT) reveals vitreomacular traction with cystoids macula edema. OCT helps in assessing the secondary retinal and specifically macular morphological changes and thus plan treatment.

prominent feature is outer retinal loss, generally involving the outer nuclear layer to photoreceptors, occasionally with a characteristic subretinal cleft.[50]

26.2.3 Combined Hamartoma

Combined hamartoma of the RPE and sensory retina is a unique condition manifesting with a gray-white juxtapapillary solitary placoid lesion with varying amount of pigmentation and intrinsic vascularity with known systemic association with neurofibromatosis type 1.[51] Retinal vessels related to the lesion are often straightened, stretched, or tortuous and are obscured by fibroglial tissue. There may be contraction of fibroglial tissue leading to retinal striae, chronic vitreoretinal traction, rhegmatogenous retinal detachment, and vitreous hemorrhage. The peripheral variant appears as an elevated ridge concentric to the margin of the optic disc with dragging of the large retinal vessels toward the lesion and normal vasculature posterior to it. Schachat et al reported that vascular tortuosity was present in 93%, vitreoretinal surface abnormalities in 78%, pigmentation in 87%, and associated lipid exudation in 7%.[52] Shields and colleagues described anatomical disorganization with loss of identifiable retinal layers by TD OCT in all cases in their series.[53] OCT evidence of epiretinal membrane was found in 91%, and mean retinal thickness was 766 µm.[53] OCT images showed intact RPE in cases without significant posterior shadowing. SD OCT has been reported recently but did not add significantly to the findings (► Fig. 26.15).[54]

26.2.4 Retinal Astrocytic Hamartoma

Retinal astrocytic hamartoma (astrocytoma) is a congenital or an acquired benign glial tumor of the retina. Congenital astrocytic hamartomas are seen in younger patients, often calcified, and associated with central nervous system astrocytomas as part of tuberous sclerosis.[3] Acquired astrocytic hamartomas appear as yellow-white acalcific lesions of the inner retina with associated retinal traction, cystoid macular edema, exudation, and nondilated feeder vessels.[3] Astrocytic hamartomas show inner retinal thickening and disorganization with a gradual transition to the adjacent normal retina.[55,56] Calcified tumors have higher reflectivity and greater posterior shadowing, whereas noncalcified tumors allow some light transmission to demonstrate intact outer retinal layers.[56,57] There may be

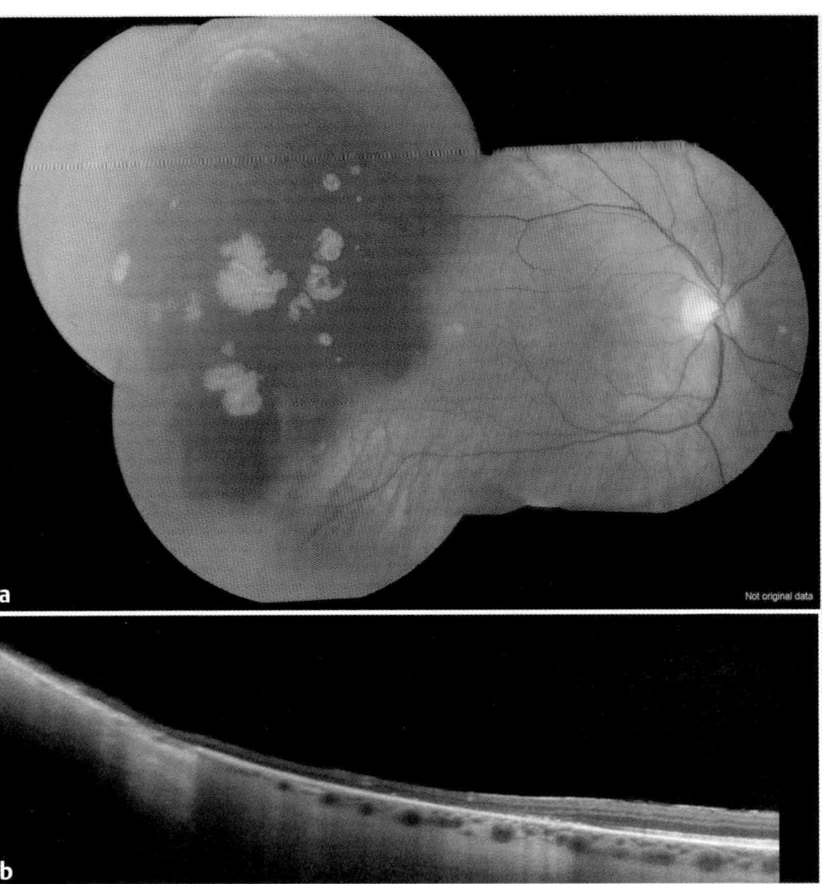

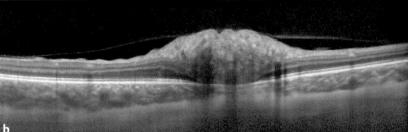

Fig. 26.14 Congenital hypertrophy of the retinal pigment epithelium (CHRPE). (a) Large, peripheral CHRPE with centrally located lacunae. **(b)** Optical coherence tomography shows thinning of the overlying retina and loss of photoreceptors, posterior shadowing of the choroid in pigmented regions, and light transmission to the underlying choroid in scans along lacunae.

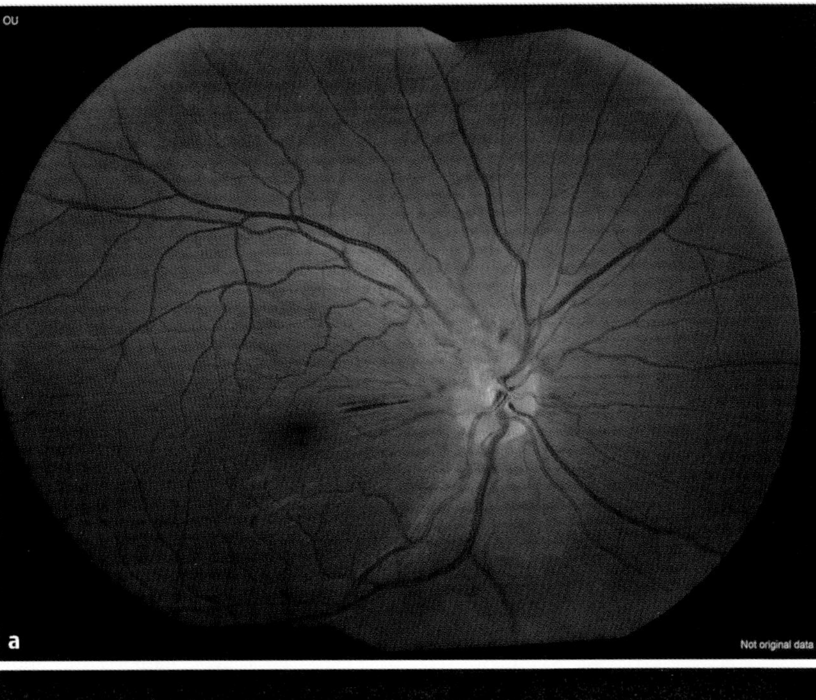

Fig. 26.15 Combined hamartoma of the retina and retinal pigment pithelium. (a) Juxtapapillary combined hamartoma with preretinal fibrosis. **(b)** Enhanced depth imaging optical coherence tomography demonstrates gradual transition from the normal adjacent inner retinal layers to a disorganized mass with overlying preretinal fibrosis.

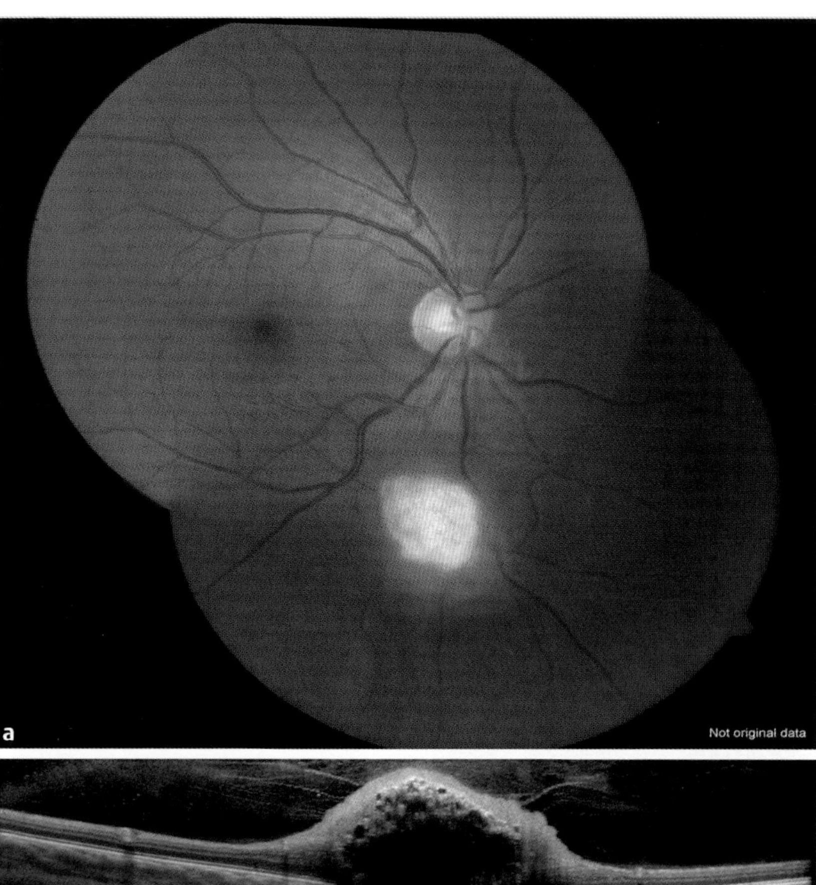

Fig. 26.16 Retinal astrocytic hamartoma. (a) Retinal astrocytic hamartoma located inferior to the optic disc, with preretinal fibrosis. **(b)** Enhanced depth imaging optical coherence tomography image exhibits disorganization of the inner retinal layers and an intact retinal pigment epithelium underlying the tumor. Trabecular internal architecture mimics the "mulberry" appearance of the lesion seen clinically. There is posterior shadowing from calcification of the tumor.

associated retinal traction in 27%, intratumoral cysts in 67%, and retinal or macular edema in 47%.[56] OCT may be used to detect and document secondary changes and follow resolution of subretinal fluid or release of macular traction after treatment.[58,59] SD OCT confirms the intact outer retinal structures, as well as the underlying choriocapillaris (▶ Fig. 26.16).[60] Three-dimensional reconstruction demonstrates tumor architecture and its relationship to the adjacent retina in a single image.[60]

26.2.5 Retinoblastoma

Retinoblastoma is the most common malignant intraocular tumor in children. It may be unifocal or multifocal, unilateral or bilateral, and sporadic or hereditary. Common clinical manifestations include leucocoria, strabismus, or visual loss. Ophthalmoscopically, retinoblastoma appears as an endophytic, exophytic, diffuse infiltrative or mixed, yellow-white vascular retinal mass and may be associated with vitreous seeds (endophytic tumors) subretinal seeds (exophytic tumors), or subretinal fluid (exophytic tumors). A thorough clinical evaluation using indirect ophthalmoscopy, aided by ultrasonography B-scan, helps in the diagnosis.

It is difficult to obtain conventional OCT images in children. With the advent of SD OCT in the hand-held mode, OCT can be easily performed in supine children under anesthesia. Imaging features of retinoblastoma vary with the lesion size. It appears on OCT as homogeneous thickening and disorganization of the neurosensory retina with posterior shadowing from calcification.[55,61] The small lesions show a distinctive intraretinal appearance (▶ Fig. 26.17).[61] These spherical lesions appear isodense, with smooth, distinct borders centered on the inner nuclear layer, and they appear to involve the middle layers.[61] This classic appearance may help detect early tumors and edge recurrence.[61] Associated subretinal fluid or intraretinal cysts are demonstrated by OCT.[55,61]

The role of OCT lies in its ability to image the macula, specifically the fovea, to assess restoration of normal foveal anatomy after treatment.[62] Further, differentiation from an organic (i.e., macular edema and loss of photoreceptors) versus a nonorganic (i.e., amblyopia) cause of vision loss is essential to plan for long-term visual rehabilitation and maximizing outcome in all patients.[3]

26.3 Conclusion

The role of OCT in the diagnosis, prognostication, management, and follow-up of intraocular tumors continues to rapidly evolve. Typical OCT features of intraocular tumors may help in clinical diagnosis and detection of clinically subtle secondary

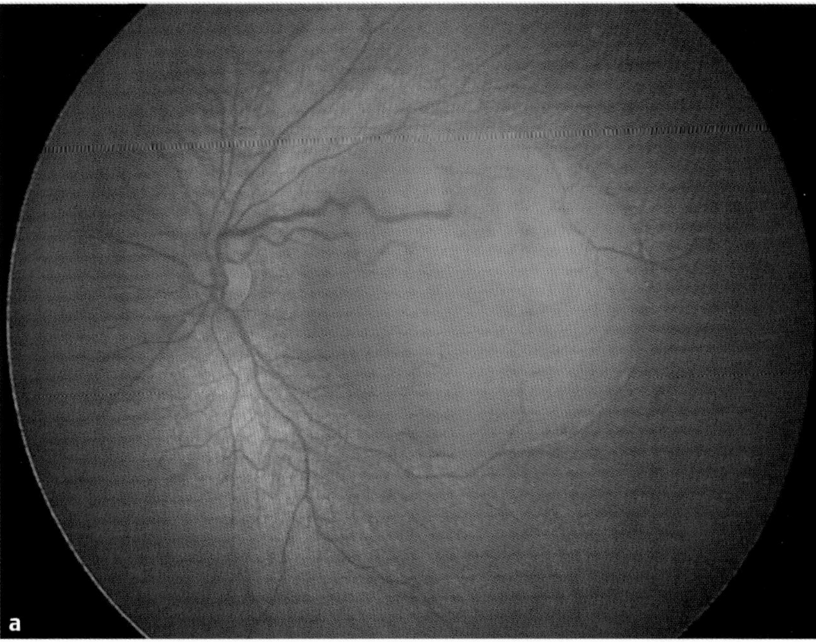

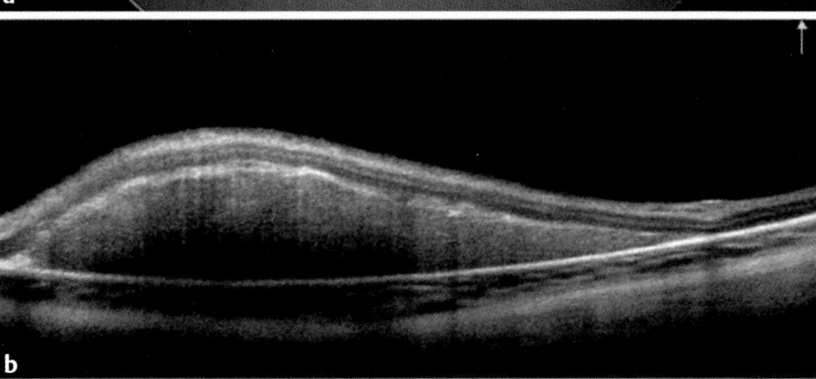

Fig. 26.17 Retinoblastoma. (a) An early macular retinoblastoma. **(b)** Optical coherence tomography shows a distinctive intraretinal appearance of an isodense lesion with smooth, distinct borders centered on the inner nuclear layer that appears to involve the middle layers.

changes of functional (visual) consequence. The clinical application of OCT has immensely expanded with the ability to image the choroid in high-resolution by EDI OCT and image children by handheld SD OCT. With the recent advancements in the technology of OCT and the understanding of the clinical significance of OCT findings, this imaging modality has become a routine part of the clinical evaluation of a patient in an ocular oncology practice.

References

[1] Huang D, Swanson EA, Lin CP, et al. Optical coherence tomography. Science 1991; 254: 1178–1181

[2] Shields CL, Pellegrini M, Ferenczy SR, Shields JA. Enhanced depth imaging optical coherence tomography (EDI-OCT) of intraocular tumors: from placid to seasick to rock and rolling topography. The 2013 Francesco Orzalesi Lecture. Retina 2014 Aug; 34: 1495–512

[3] Say EA, Shah SU, Ferenczy S, Shields CL. Optical coherence tomography of retinal and choroidal tumors. J Ophthalmol 2012; 2012: 385058

[4] Medina CA, Plesec T, Singh AD. Optical coherence tomography imaging of ocular and periocular tumours. Br J Ophthalmol 2014; 98 Suppl 2: ii40–ii46

[5] Shah SU, Kaliki S, Shields CL, Ferenczy SR, Harmon SA, Shields JA. Enhanced depth imaging optical coherence tomography of choroidal nevus in 104 cases. Ophthalmology 2012; 119: 1066–1072

[6] Shields CL, Kaliki S, Rojanaporn D, Ferenczy SR, Shields JA. Enhanced depth imaging optical coherence tomography of small choroidal melanoma: comparison with choroidal nevus. Arch Ophthalmol 2012; 130: 850–856

[7] Shields JA, Shields CL. Chroidal nevus. In: Intraocular Tumors: A Text and Atlas. Philadelphia: WB Saunders; 1992:85–100

[8] Singh AD, Kalyani P, Topham A. Estimating the risk of malignant transformation of a choroidal nevus. Ophthalmology 2005; 112: 1784–1789

[9] Shields CL, Shields JA, Kiratli H, De Potter P, Cater JR. Risk factors for growth and metastasis of small choroidal melanocytic lesions. Ophthalmology 1995; 102: 1351–1361

[10] Shields CL, Cater J, Shields JA, Singh AD, Santos MC, Carvalho C. Combination of clinical factors predictive of growth of small choroidal melanocytic tumors. Arch Ophthalmol 2000; 118: 360–364

[11] Shields CL, Mashayekhi A, Materin MA, et al. Optical coherence tomography of choroidal nevus in 120 patients. Retina 2005; 25: 243–252

[12] Espinoza G, Rosenblatt B, Harbour JW. Optical coherence tomography in the evaluation of retinal changes associated with suspicious choroidal melanocytic tumors. Am J Ophthalmol 2004; 137: 90–95

[13] Shields JA, Shields CL. Diagnostic approaches to posterior uveal melanoma. In: Intraocular Tumors: A Text and Atlas. Philadelphia: WB Saunders; 1992:155–169

[14] Muscat S, Parks S, Kemp E, Keating D. Secondary retinal changes associated with choroidal naevi and melanomas documented by optical coherence tomography. Br J Ophthalmol 2004; 88: 120–124

[15] Sayanagi K, Pelayes DE, Kaiser PK, Singh AD. 3D Spectral domain optical coherence tomography findings in choroidal tumors. Eur J Ophthalmol 2011; 21: 271–275

[16] Singh AD, Belfort RN, Sayanagi K, Kaiser PK. Fourier domain optical coherence tomographic and auto-fluorescence findings in indeterminate choroidal melanocytic lesions. Br J Ophthalmol 2010; 94: 474–478

[17] Torres VL, Brugnoni N, Kaiser PK, Singh AD. Optical coherence tomography enhanced depth imaging of choroidal tumors. Am J Ophthalmol 2011; 151: 586–593, e2

[18] Horgan N, Shields CL, Mashayekhi A, Teixeira LF, Materin MA, Shields JA. Early macular morphological changes following plaque radiotherapy for uveal melanoma. Retina 2008; 28: 263–273

[19] Singh AD, Kaiser PK, Sears JE. Choroidal hemangioma. Ophthalmol Clin North Am 2005; 18: 151–161, ix

[20] Shields CL, Honavar SG, Shields JA, Cater J, Demirci H. Circumscribed choroidal hemangioma: clinical manifestations and factors predictive of visual outcome in 200 consecutive cases. Ophthalmology 2001; 108: 2237–2248

[21] Arora KS, Quigley HA, Comi AM, Miller RB, Jampel HD. Increased choroidal thickness in patients with Sturge-Weber syndrome. JAMA Ophthalmol 2013; 131: 1216–1219

[22] Ramasubramanian A, Shields CL, Harmon SA, Shields JA. Autofluorescence of choroidal hemangioma in 34 consecutive eyes. Retina 2010; 30: 16–22

[23] Heimann H, Jmor F, Damato B. Imaging of retinal and choroidal vascular tumours. Eye (Lond) 2013; 27: 208–216

[24] Liu W, Zhang Y, Xu G, Qian J, Jiang C, Li L. Optical coherence tomography for evaluation of photodynamic therapy in symptomatic circumscribed choroidal hemangioma. Retina 2011; 31: 336–343

[25] Kwon HJ, Kim M, Lee CS, Lee SC. Treatment of serous macular detachment associated with circumscribed choroidal hemangioma. Am J Ophthalmol 2012; 154: 137–145, e1

[26] Zhang Y, Liu W, Fang Y, et al. Photodynamic therapy for symptomatic circumscribed macular choroidal hemangioma in Chinese patients. Am J Ophthalmol 2010; 150: 710–715, e1

[27] Shields CL, Sun H, Demirci H, Shields JA. Factors predictive of tumor growth, tumor decalcification, choroidal neovascularization, and visual outcome in 74 eyes with choroidal osteoma. Arch Ophthalmol 2005; 123: 1658–1666

[28] Shields CL, Perez B, Materin MA, Mehta S, Shields JA. Optical coherence tomography of choroidal osteoma in 22 cases: evidence for photoreceptor atrophy over the decalcified portion of the tumor. Ophthalmology 2007; 114: e53–e58

[29] Ide T, Ohguro N, Hayashi A, et al. Optical coherence tomography patterns of choroidal osteoma. Am J Ophthalmol 2000; 130: 131–134

[30] Fukasawa A, Iijima H. Optical coherence tomography of choroidal osteoma. Am J Ophthalmol 2002; 133: 419–421

[31] Pellegrini M, Invernizzi A, Giani A, Staurenghi G. Enhanced depth imaging optical coherence tomography features of choroidal osteoma. Retina 2014; 34: 958–963

[32] Shields JA, Shields CL. Metastatic tumors of the intraocular structures. In: Intraocular Tumors: A Text and Atlas. Philadelphia: WB Saunders; 1992:207–238

[33] Natesh S, Chin KJ, Finger PT. Choroidal metastases fundus autofluorescence imaging: correlation to clinical, OCT, and fluorescein angiographic findings. Ophthalmic Surg Lasers Imaging 2010; 41: 406–412

[34] Arevalo JF, Fernandez CF, Garcia RA. Optical coherence tomography characteristics of choroidal metastasis. Ophthalmology 2005; 112: 1612–1619

[35] Manquez ME, Shields CL, Karatza EC, Shields JA. Regression of choroidal metastases from breast carcinoma using aromatase inhibitors. Br J Ophthalmol 2005; 89: 776–777

[36] Al-Dahmash SA, Shields CL, Kaliki S, Johnson T, Shields JA. Enhanced depth imaging optical coherence tomography of choroidal metastasis in 14 eyes. Retina 2014 Aug; 34: 1588–93

[37] Coupland SE, Damato B. Understanding intraocular lymphomas. Clin Experiment Ophthalmol 2008; 36: 564–578

[38] Chang TS, Byrne SF, Gass JDM, Hughes JR, Johnson RN, Murray TG. Echographic findings in benign reactive lymphoid hyperplasia of the choroid. Arch Ophthalmol 1996; 114: 669–675

[39] Ishida T, Ohno-Matsui K, Kaneko Y, et al. Fundus autofluorescence patterns in eyes with primary intraocular lymphoma. Retina 2010; 30: 23–32

[40] Fardeau C, Lee CPL, Merle-Béral H, et al. Retinal fluorescein, indocyanine green angiography, and optic coherence tomography in non-Hodgkin primary intraocular lymphoma. Am J Ophthalmol 2009; 147: 886–894, e1

[41] Forooghian F, Merkur AB, White VA, Shen D, Chan CC. High-definition optical coherence tomography features of primary vitreoretinal lymphoma. Ophthalmic Surg Lasers Imaging 2011; 42 Online: e97–e99

[42] Williams BK Jr Tsui I, McCannel TA. Spectral-domain optical coherence tomography of conjunctival mucosa-associated lymphoid tissue lymphoma with presumed choroidal involvement. Graefes Arch Clin Exp Ophthalmol 2010; 248: 1837–1840

[43] Shields CL, Arepalli S, Pellegrini M, Mashayekhi A, Shields JA. Choroidal lymphoma shows calm, rippled, or undulating topography on enhanced depth imaging optical coherence tomography in 14 eyes. Retina 2014; 34: 1347–1353

[44] Singh AD, Rundle PA, Rennie I. Retinal vascular tumors. Ophthalmol Clin North Am 2005; 18: 167–176, x

[45] Spaide RF, Koizumi H, Pozzoni MC. Enhanced depth imaging spectral-domain optical coherence tomography. Am J Ophthalmol 2008; 146: 496–500

[46] Andrade RE, Farah ME, Costa RA, Belfort R Jr. Optical coherence tomography findings in macular cavernous haemangioma. Acta Ophthalmol Scand 2005; 83: 267–269

[47] Turell ME, Singh AD. Vascular tumors of the retina and choroid: diagnosis and treatment. Middle East Afr J Ophthalmol 2010; 17: 191–200

[48] Shields CL, Mashayekhi A, Ho T, Cater J, Shields JA. Solitary congenital hypertrophy of the retinal pigment epithelium: clinical features and frequency of enlargement in 330 patients. Ophthalmology 2003; 110: 1968–1976

[49] Shields CL, Materin MA, Walker C, Marr BP, Shields JA. Photoreceptor loss overlying congenital hypertrophy of the retinal pigment epithelium by optical coherence tomography. Ophthalmology 2006; 113: 661–665

[50] Fung AT, Pellegrini M, Shields CL. Congenital hypertrophy of the retinal pigment epithelium: enhanced-depth imaging optical coherence tomography in 18 cases. Ophthalmology 2014; 121: 251–256

[51] Vianna RN, Pacheco DF, Vasconcelos MM, de Laey JJ. Combined hamartoma of the retina and retinal pigment epithelium associated with neurofibromatosis type-1. Int Ophthalmol 2001; 24: 63–66

[52] Schachat AP, Shields JA, Fine SL, et al. Combined hamartomas of the retina and retinal pigment epithelium. Ophthalmology 1984; 91: 1609–1615

[53] Shields CL, Mashayekhi A, Dai VV, Materin MA, Shields JA. Optical coherence tomographic findings of combined hamartoma of the retina and retinal pigment epithelium in 11 patients. Arch Ophthalmol 2005; 123: 1746–1750

[54] Huot CS, Desai KB, Shah VA. Spectral domain optical coherence tomography of combined hamartoma of the retina and retinal pigment epithelium. Ophthalmic Surg Lasers Imaging 2009; 40: 322–324

[55] Shields CL, Mashayekhi A, Luo CK, Materin MA, Shields JA. Optical coherence tomography in children: analysis of 44 eyes with intraocular tumors and simulating conditions. J Pediatr Ophthalmol Strabismus 2004; 41: 338–344

[56] Shields CL, Benevides R, Materin MA, Shields JA. Optical coherence tomography of retinal astrocytic hamartoma in 15 cases. Ophthalmology 2006; 113: 1553–1557

[57] Soliman W, Larsen M, Sander B, Wegener M, Milea D. Optical coherence tomography of astrocytic hamartomas in tuberous sclerosis. Acta Ophthalmol Scand 2007; 85: 454–455

[58] Eskelin S, Tommila P, Palosaari T, Kivelä T. Photodynamic therapy with verteporfin to induce regression of aggressive retinal astrocytomas. Acta Ophthalmol (Copenh) 2008; 86: 794–799

[59] Inoue M, Hirakarta A, Iizuka N, Futagami S, Hida T. Tractional macular detachment associated with optic disc astrocytic hamartoma. Acta Ophthalmol (Copenh) 2009; 87: 239–240

[60] Kimoto K, Kishi D, Kono H, Ikewaki J, Shinoda K, Nakatsuka K. Diagnosis of an isolated retinal astrocytic hamartoma aided by optical coherence tomography. Acta Ophthalmol (Copenh) 2008; 86: 921–922

[61] Rootman DB, Gonzalez E, Mallipatna A, et al. Hand-held high-resolution spectral domain optical coherence tomography in retinoblastoma: clinical and morphologic considerations. Br J Ophthalmol 2013; 97: 59–65

[62] Shields CL, Materin MA, Shields JA. Restoration of foveal anatomy and function following chemoreduction for bilateral advanced retinoblastoma with total retinal detachment. Arch Ophthalmol 2005; 123: 1610–1612

27 Optical Coherence Tomography–Assisted Anterior-Segment Surgery

Gabor B. Scharioth

Femtosecond laser–assisted cataract surgery has been used to create the main corneal incision, side-port incision, capsulorhexis, and precutting of the nucleus.[1] The aim of this technology is to increase precision. Incision size and shape become more predictable. Capsulorhexis size, shape, and centration reach previously unknown accuracy.[2] Initially, femtosecond laser technology was used without additional control with intraoperative optical coherence tomography (OCT). Today, all available femtosecond-assisted cataract machines take advantage of increased control using intraoperative OCT monitoring (▶ Fig. 27.1).

27.1 Intraoperative OCT in Cataract Surgery

Future perspectives on the intraoperative use of OCT technology in cataract surgery (▶ Fig. 27.2) could include continuous monitoring of the anterior-chamber depth or volume to prevent surge phenomenon. An automated posterior-capsule recognition modes could be used to prevent phaco-tip contact to the posterior capsule and capsular breaks, which would increase dramatically the safety of cataract surgery, as capsular breaks with vitreous loss are still the most common complication of phacoemulsification.[3] OCT-assisted grading of hardness of the crystalline lens with automated selection of machine settings could optimize applied energy and fluidics and increase the effectiveness and safety of cataract surgery. Intraoperative control of intraocular lens (IOL) position could help to prevent refractive surprises. Once capsular bag refilling becomes available, intraoperative OCT control could be an option.

Besides cataract surgery, OCT technology seems quite useful in other anterior-segment surgeries.[4] Mounting an OCT to a microscope makes it possible to create intraoperative images or videos. With future developments, high-speed OCT (swept-source technology) and three-dimensional (3-D) calculations could be used. If the images are mirrored into a head-up display into the surgeon's microscope view, the surgeon is enabled to continue surgery while moving his or her attention from the surgical area. Furthermore, both hands remain free and able to continue bimanual surgery. As technology improves, OCT might be added to view areas (like the anterior-chamber angle) that were previously difficult to observe. Microscope-mounted OCTs (Zeiss Meditec, Oberkochen, Germany) have intraoperative settings that monitor images using 3-D anterior-segment OCT reconstruction of the anterior-chamber angle region (Tomey Corporation, Tokyo, Japan) (▶ Fig. 27.3).

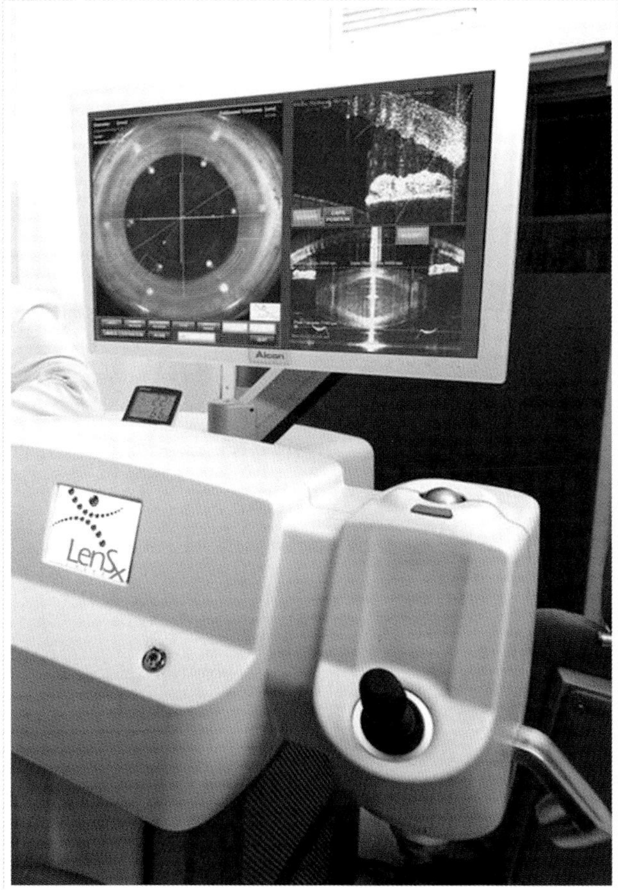

Fig. 27.1 LensEx (Alcon, Inc., Irvine, CA) system for femtosecond laser–asissted cataract surgery. Note the monitor with online optical coherence tomography images of the cornea and anterior segment with crystalline lens before surgery.

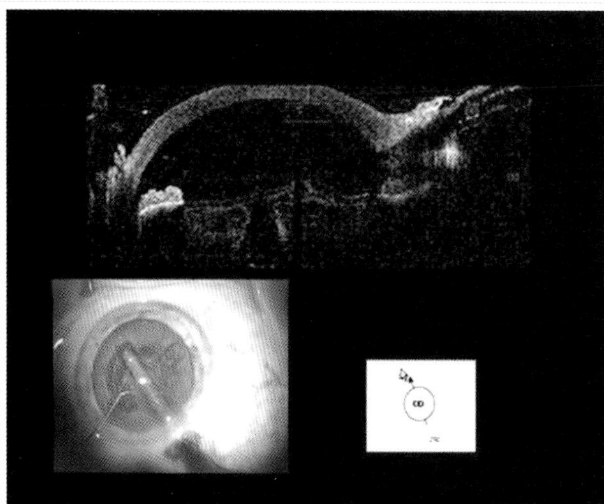

Fig. 27.2 Intraoperative optical coherence tomography during phacoemulsification. Note the phaco tip in the main incision and the horizontal groove after initial sculpting. The scan direction is indicated in the right inferior corner; scan direction could be changed. OD, right eye.

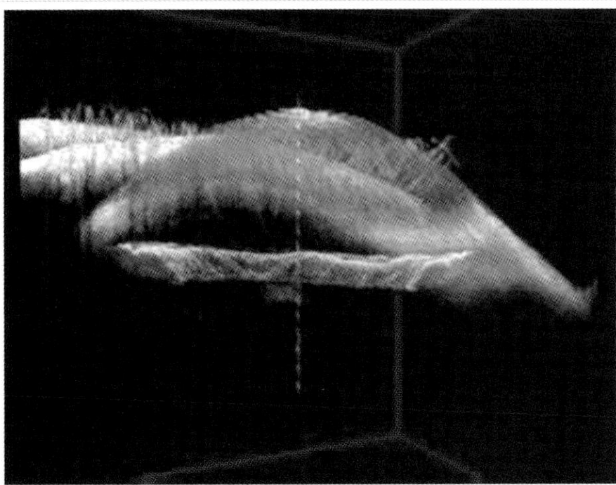

Fig. 27.3 Image of three-dimensional optical coherence tomography (OCT) reconstruction of the anterior-chamber angle region with anterior-segment OCT.

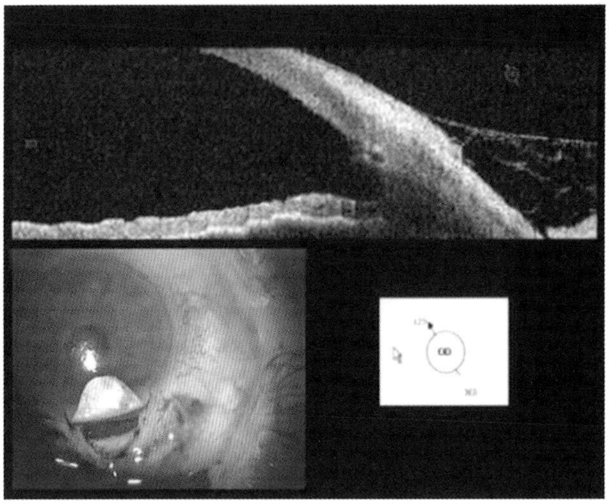

Fig. 27.4 Schlemm canal scan during canaloplasty, lumen of the Schlemm canal, distension of trabecular meshwork, and tensioning suture are clearly visible. OD, right eye.

27.2 Intraoperative OCT in Glaucoma Surgery

Glaucoma surgery is moving from trabeculectomy toward microinvasive glaucoma surgery and canaloplasty. Today, in canaloplasty, a deep sclerectomy is performed manually. Currently, lasers are investigated to create this step, but in the future, this step could be controlled by OCT. Then, with the help of a microcatheter, a suture can be placed into the Schlemm canal and tightened under tension to open it (▶ Fig. 27.4). This effect could be controlled directly during the surgery with the help of a microscope-mounted OCT. Distension of the trabecular meshwork could be estimated and, if necessary, suture tension increased.

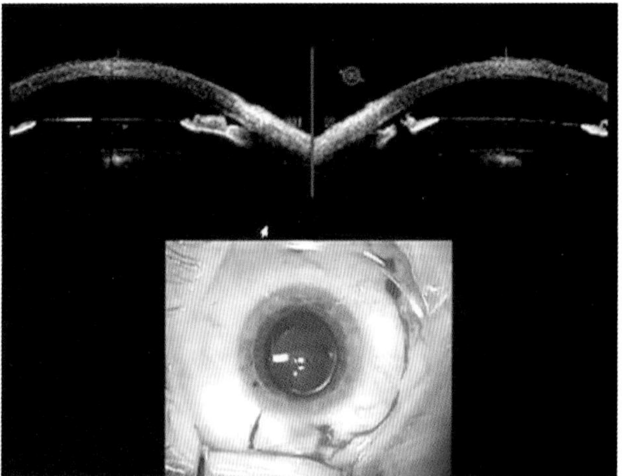

Fig. 27.5 Cross-scan after implantation of Implantable Collamer lens (ICL). Note proper vaulting without contact between the ICL and the anterior surface of the crystalline lens.

27.3 Intraoperative OCT in Refractive Surgery

Refractive surgeries with corneal laser surgery or phakic IOL implantation are other fields for application of intraoperative OCT technology. Essential for uncomplicated implantation of phakic IOL are sizing and correct vaulting. Direct contact to the crystalline lens should be prevented with the use of posterior-chamber phakic IOL, which could be controlled intraoperatively, and the distance between the intracorneal lens and the anterior surface of the crystalline lens could be documented. If anterior-chamber phakic IOL is used, the sufficient safety distance to the corneal endothelium is mandatory to prevent excessive endothelial cell loss with corneal decompensation (▶ Fig. 27.5). Intraoperative control of phakic IOL position will decrease the complication rates of these techniques.

For laser refractive corneal surgeries like femtolaser-assisted flap preparation in LASIK (laser-assisted in situ keratomileusis), the use of OCT is already well established. Calculations and settings are based on intraoperative corneal-thickness measurements and detection. These technologies created an unknown precision of laser refractive corneal surgery, ultrathin corneal flaps, and reduced risk for corneal ectasia with an increased therapeutic window.

27.4 Intraoperative OCT in Corneal Surgery

Besides perforating corneal transplantation, modern cornea surgery includes techniques like deep anterior lamellar keratoplasty and Descemet membrane endothelium keratoplasty. The dissection plane could be controlled with the help of an OCT. Finally, adaptation of transplant to the corneal bed could be controlled intraoperatively with the chance of immediate intervention. This could reduce the postoperative failure rate and postoperative astigmatism, thus leading to improved outcome.

References

[1] Palanker DV, Blumenkranz MS, Andersen D, et al. Femtosecond laser-assisted cataract surgery with integrated optical coherence tomography. Sci Transl Med 2010; 2: 58ra85

[2] He L, Sheehy K, Culbertson W. Femtosecond laser-assisted cataract surgery. Curr Opin Ophthalmol 2011; 22: 43–52

[3] Nguyen P, Chopra V. Applications of optical coherence tomography in cataract surgery. Curr Opin Ophthalmol 2013; 24: 47–52

[4] Hatch KM, Talamo JH. Laser-assisted cataract surgery: benefits and barriers. Curr Opin Ophthalmol 2014; 25: 54–61

28 Optical Coherence Tomography in Neurophthalmology

Dhivya Ashok Kumar and Amar Agarwal

Optical coherence tomography (OCT) is a rapid noncontact method that allows in vivo imaging of the optic nerve head (ONH) and retinal nerve fiber layer (RNFL). Since its introduction in early 1990s, the technology has deeply disseminated into clinical practice.[1,2,3,4] High acquisition speed and high resolution have made it better than any available imaging methods. Although OCT had been used for diagnosis and prognosis in varied ophthalmologic conditions, to start with it, was used for ONH and retinal evaluation.[2,3,4] In ONH, it was initially used for the determination of thickness of the retinal nerve fiber layer (RNFL), which is an important parameter for glaucoma assessment.[5,6] In 1995, Schuman and associates showed that the RNFL thickness, as measured by OCT, demonstrated a high degree of correlation with functional status of the optic nerve, as measured by visual-field examination.[5]

Although glaucoma screening has been the most common indication for ONH examination by OCT, imaging of the ONH and RNFL can be useful in other rare and varied neurologic conditions. In this chapter, we go through the common nonglaucomatous conditions in which OCT can be used for imaging.

28.1 Optic Nerve Head

The ONH is vertically oval, with an average diameter of 1.85 to 1.9 mm. The horizontal diameter ranges from 1.70 to1.80 mm. The central excavation in the ONH is the optic cup, and it is horizontally oval. The border between the ONH and the optic cup is the neuroretinal rim. The peripapillary region is divided into the alpha and beta zones (adjacent to disc).

28.1.1 Optic Nerve Head in OCT

The ONH is scanned by the optic disc cube mode in the OCT. It is a 200 × 200 scan. ▶ Fig. 28.1 shows the OCT map of ONH taken in spectral-domain OCT. Scan quality should be checked for every OCT image, with particular attention to the segmentation of RNFL and the signal strength. The value of signal strength ranges between 1 and 10, with 10 representing the best and 1 the worst image signal. Poor signal strength is often related to incorrect scan focus or media opacity. Acquiring a scan with maximal possible signal strength is recommended for RNFL measurement. The scan circle should be centered on the optic nerve center. The central zone shows the average thickness of the nerve fiber layer; next, it shows the quadrant variation in RNFL thickness, followed by the clock hour's variation. The color coding for the distribution of RNFL thickness is given and compared with the normal distribution in the population. The normative display provides a useful reference to determine whether the RNFL measurements are within or outside the normal ranges. Accordingly, green indicates 95% of the distribution of normal values, yellow indicates 5% of the distribution of normal values, and red represents 1% of the distribution of normal values. The lowermost part of the scan map shows the graph comparing patients' RNFL thickness in microns with the normative data distribution. The other modules available in neurologic imaging are advanced visualization, RNFL thickness analysis, and global progression analysis (GPA), which can be used in glaucomatous progression and analysis. OCT GPA is a trend-based analysis with progression analyzed and reported as change over time using serial RNFL measurements. At least

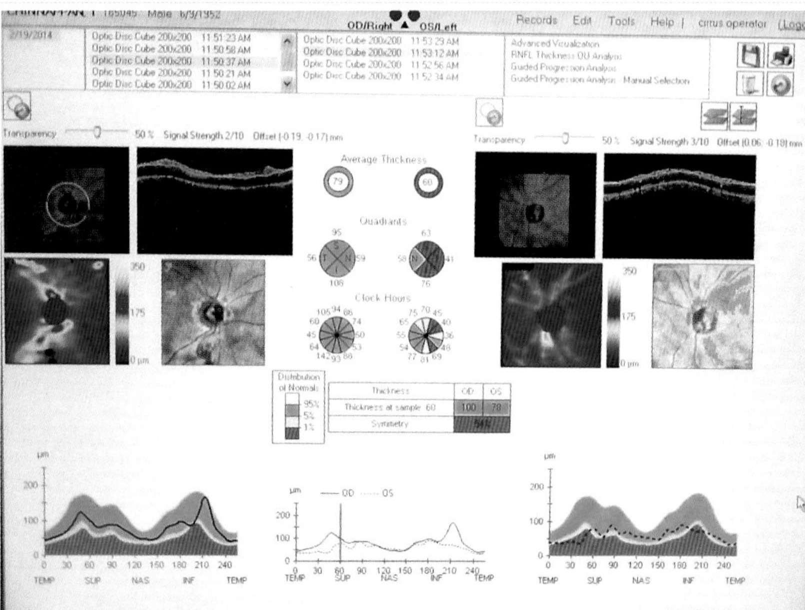

Fig. 28.1 Optical coherence optic nerve head scan as seen in spectral-domain optical coherence tomography. OD, right eye; OS, left eye.

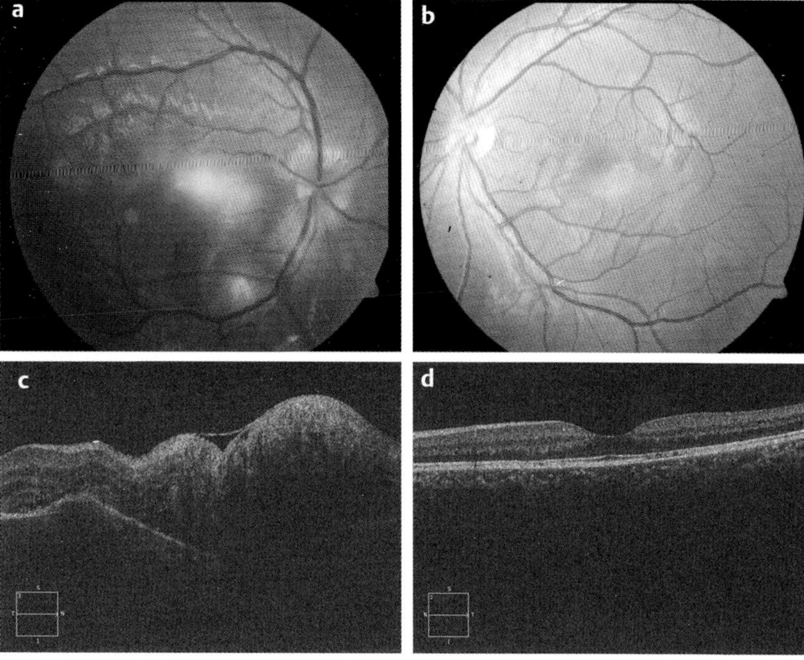

Fig. 28.2 **(a)** Optic neuritis in right eye of an 18-year-old man. **(b)** Normal left eye. **(c)** Increase thickness of retinal nerve-fiber layer (RNFL) in optical coherence tomography noted in the right eye. **(d)** Normal RNFL in the left eye.

four visits are required to generate the GPA report. The GPA overlays serial RNFL thickness profiles and performs linear regression analysis of average RNFL thickness against the duration of follow-up.

28.2 Specific Conditions

28.2.1 Optic Neuritis

Optic neuritis (ON) is an inflammation in the optic nerve (▶ Fig. 28.2), which causes subacute onset of vision loss in children and young adults. The Optic Neuritis Treatment Trial gives the overall scenario of the clinical presentation and management of optic neuritis. OCT provides a noninvasive means to quantify the structural effects of an inflammatory insult to the optic nerve. OCT has been used in patients with multiple sclerosis (MS), who are predisposed to develop ON; it has been shown that thickness of the RNFL was 46% lower in MS eyes relative to control eyes.[7] Atrophy of the RNFL was associated with lower visual evoked potential (VEP) amplitudes, worse log minimum angle of resolution (logMAR) visual acuity scores, reduced visual-field mean deviation, and decreased color vision in ON patients.[8] Trip et al noted that macular volumes were 11% lower in ON eyes compared with control eyes.[8] In addition, a strong correlation was found between OCT measurement of axonal loss and multifocal VEP latency.[9] Recurrent optic neuritis leads to RNFL atrophy; especially in unilateral ON, the changes can be well appreciated. Noval and associates noted an initial increase in RNFL thickness (▶ Fig. 28.3) that resolved by 1.5 months. In ON eyes, they reported a 25% reduction in RNFL thickness at 6 months.[10] Syc et al used OCT to quantify neurodegeneration as an outcome in MS clinical trials.[11] Excellent reproducibility of average and quadrantic RNFL thickness values (▶ Fig. 28.4), average macular thickness, and total macular volume was found using spectral-domain OCT.[11]

28.2.2 Neuromyelitis Optica

Neuromyelitis optica (NMO) is a severe inflammatory process of the optic nerves and spinal cord.[12] In ON eyes, NMO was associated with lower RNFL values compared with MS eyes. The superior and inferior quadrants were more severely affected in NMO than in MS eyes.

28.2.3 Toxic or Nutritional Optic Neuropathy

Toxic or nutritional neuropathy and drug-induced like ethambutol optic neuropathy cause changes in the RNFL. OCT-measured RNFL thickness may be normal or slightly increased nasally on initial evaluation and can become thinned, especially temporally, on long-term follow-up evaluation. Like glaucoma, RNFL thinning occurs, but temporal fibers are involved first in toxic or nutritional optic neuropathy. The inducing factor should be corrected to reduce the progressive RNFL loss.[13]

28.2.4 Compressive and Traumatic Optic Neuropathy

The RNFL is thinned in compressive optic neuropathy, as occurs in patients with band atrophy as seen with chiasmal lesions. In traumatic optic neuropathy, the RNFL measured by OCT reveals such thinning. The location and amount of RNFL thinning are likely to depend on the severity of trauma and the extent of visual loss.[14,15]

28.2.5 Optic Drusen

The optic nerve drusen are often visible on the disc or buried, leading to ONH elevation. There can be damage to nerve axons,

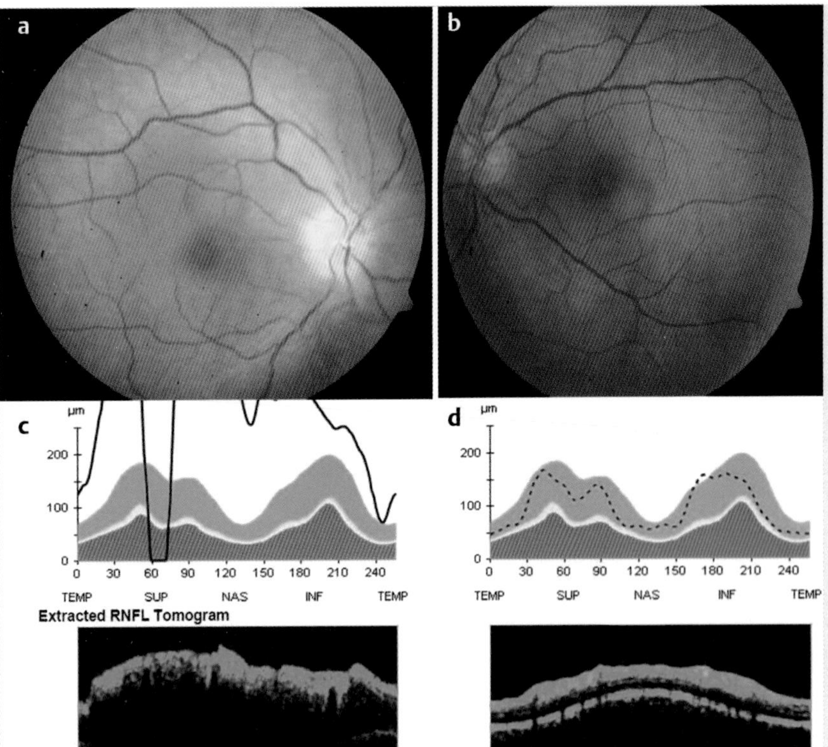

Fig. 28.3 Retinal nerve-fiber layer (RNFL) map in optic neuritis in right eye (OD) shown comparing the normal RNFL thickness map in the left eye (OS).

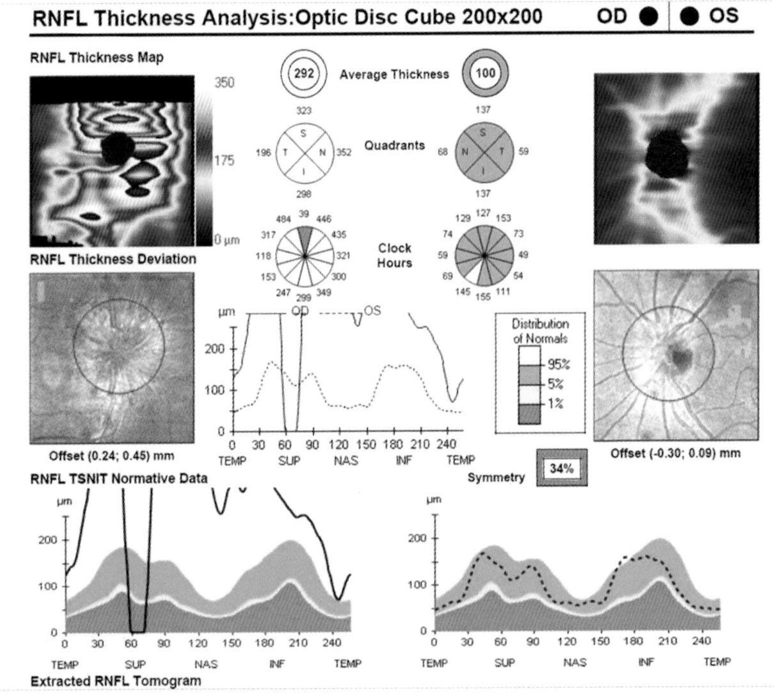

Fig. 28.4 Spectral-domain optical coherence tomography showing the marked difference in the retinal nerve-fiber layer (RNFL) thickness between the right and left eye in an eye with acute optic neuritis in all the zones of the RNFL map. TEMP: Temporal, SUP: Superior, NAS: Nasal, INF: Inferior, TSNIT: Temporal, superior, nasal, inferior & temporal RNFL

which can lead to defects in the nerve fiber layer. The combination of axonal loss resulting from local compression and the possibility of vascular events can lead to RNFL thinning. This thinning of the RNFL is seen in OCT. Roh et al showed significant RNFL thinning in eyes with drusen.[16]

28.2.6 Optic Pit

A small, round optic pit with grayish margins situated on the optic disc can be seen clinically with slit-lamp biomicroscopy. In addition, there can be a well-demarcated circular area of

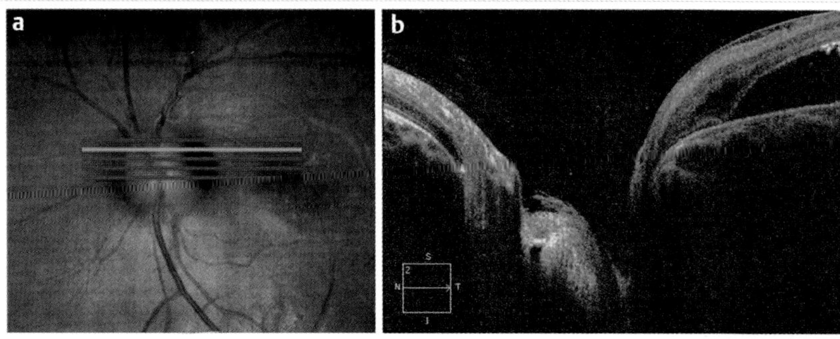

Fig. 28.5 Optical coherence tomography on the optic nerve head showing (a) the depression or (b) optic pit.

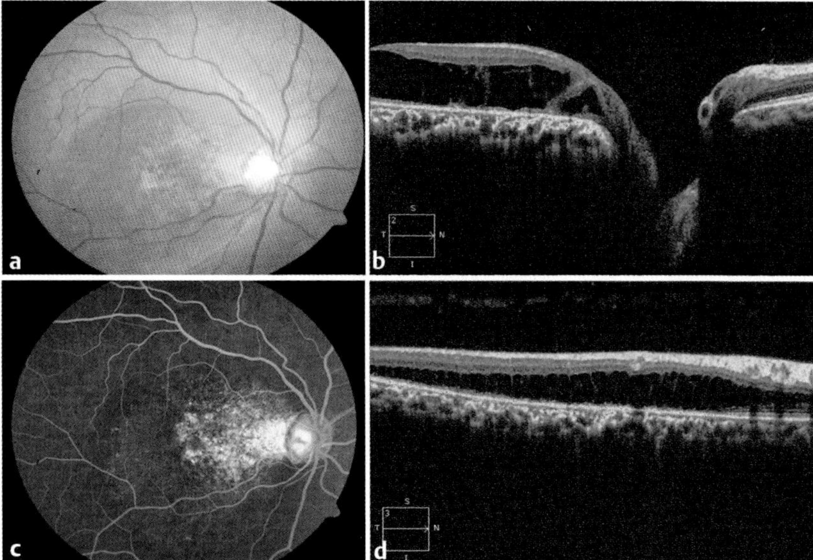

Fig. 28.6 (a) Fundus photograph and (c) angiography (b, d) image showing the macular serous detachment with the continuation track in an eye with optic pit.

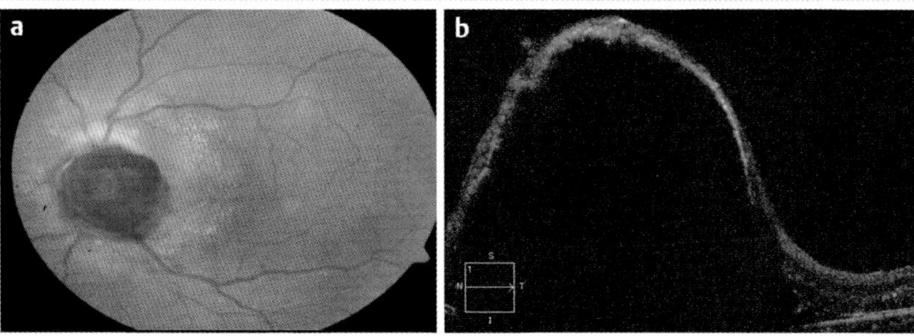

Fig. 28.7 Fundus photograph (a) and (b) Optical coherence tomography of Optic nerve melanocytoms showing nodular elevation.

macular elevation representing either a serous detachment or retinoschisis. OCT on the ONH shows the depression or pit (▶ Fig. 28.5). The OCT macula shows the macular serous detachment with the continuation track (▶ Fig. 28.6).

28.2.7 Optic Nerve Melanocytoma

Melanocytoma is a pigmented tumor arising from melanocytes and is a variant of melanocytic nevus. This pigmented lesion occurs on the optic disc and often extends into the peripapillary retina and choroid. With OCT, one can notice a gradual transition from normal retinal surface to nodular surface. A bright anterior surface is seen owing to marked pigment proliferation, and shadowing, hindering internal details, is noted (▶ Fig. 28.7). OCT can be used for documenting the subretinal fluid and also for assessment of progression of the tumor.

28.2.8 Anterior Ischemic Optic Neuropathy

The RNFL changes in anterior ischemic optic neuropathy (AION) can mimic those of glaucoma; however, early OCT changes are important in diagnosis. Contreras et al OCT-measured RNFL thickness and found that it was increased to 96.4% in the affected eye compared with the fellow eye in the acute phase of AION.[17] According to another report, the RNFL was thinnest superiorly, followed by inferiorly, temporally, and nasally.[18] This pattern of RNFL thinning is likely attributed to the nature of AION that more commonly causes inferior visual-field changes.

28.3 Conclusion

The application of OCT in neuro-ophthalmic disease has grown since its first use in glaucoma and retinal diseases. OCT should be used in conjunction with the ocular examination when evaluating patients who may have nonglaucomatous cupping, with attention to central vision, color vision, and visual-field defects that are not typical of glaucomatous loss and optic nerve pallor disproportionate to cupping.

References

[1] Sakata LM, Deleon-Ortega J, Sakata V, Girkin CA. Optical coherence tomography of the retina and optic nerve - a review. Clin Experiment Ophthalmol 2009; 37: 90–99

[2] Huang D, Swanson EA, Lin CP, et al. Optical coherence tomography. Science 1991; 254: 1178–1181

[3] Fujimoto J, Schumann J, Huang D, Duker JS, Carmen A Puliafito ES. Introduction to optical coherence tomography. In Schumann J, Puliafito CA, Fujimoto J, Duker JS, eds. Optical Coherence Tomography of Ocular Diseases, 3rd ed. Thorofare, NJ: Slack Inc.; 2012:3–25

[4] Swanson EA, Izatt JA, Hee MR, et al. In vivo retinal imaging by optical coherence tomography. Opt Lett 1993; 18: 1864–1866

[5] Schuman JS, Hee MR, Arya AV, et al. Optical coherence tomography: a new tool for glaucoma diagnosis. Curr Opin Ophthalmol 1995; 6: 89–95Review

[6] Burk RO, Völcker HE. Current imaging of the optic disk and retinal nerve fiber layer. Curr Opin Ophthalmol 1996; 7: 99–108 Review

[7] Parisi V, Manni G, Spadaro M, et al. Correlation between morphological and functional retinal impairment in multiple sclerosis patients. Invest Ophthalmol Vis Sci 1999; 40: 2520–2527

[8] Trip SA, Schlottmann PG, Jones SJ, et al. Retinal nerve fiber layer axonal loss and visual dysfunction in optic neuritis. Ann Neurol 2005; 58: 383–391

[9] Klistorner A, Arvind H, Nguyen T, et al. Axonal loss and myelin in early ON loss in postacute optic neuritis. Ann Neurol 2008; 64: 325–331

[10] Noval S, Contreras I, Rebolleda G, Muñoz-Negrete FJ. Optical coherence tomography versus automated perimetry for follow-up of optic neuritis. Acta Ophthalmol Scand 2006; 84: 790–794

[11] Syc SB, Warner CV, Hiremath GS, et al. Reproducibility of high-resolution optical coherence tomography in multiple sclerosis. Mult Scler 2010; 16: 829–839

[12] Naismith RT, Tutlam NT, Xu J, et al. Optical coherence tomography differs in neuromyelitis optica compared with multiple sclerosis. Neurology 2009; 72: 1077–1082

[13] Pasol J. Neuro-ophthalmic disease and optical coherence tomography: glaucoma look-alikes. Curr Opin Ophthalmol 2011; 22: 124–132

[14] Monteiro ML, Cunha LP, Costa-Cunha LV, Maia OO Jr Oyamada MK. Relationship between optical coherence tomography, pattern electroretinogram and automated perimetry in eyes with temporal hemianopia from chiasmal compression. Invest Ophthalmol Vis Sci 2009; 50: 3535–3541

[15] Cunha LP, Costa-Cunha LV, Malta RF, Monteiro ML. Comparison between retinal nerve fiber layer and macular thickness measured with OCT detecting progressive axonal loss following traumatic optic neuropathy. Arq Bras Oftalmol 2009; 72: 622–625

[16] Roh S, Noecker RJ, Schuman JS, Hedges TR III Weiter JJ, Mattox C. Effect of optic nerve head drusen on nerve fiber layer thickness. Ophthalmology 1998; 105: 878–885

[17] Contreras I, Noval S, Rebolleda G, Muñoz-Negrete FJ. Follow-up of nonarteritic anterior ischemic optic neuropathy with optical coherence tomography. Ophthalmology 2007; 114: 2338–2344

[18] Hayreh SS, Zimmerman B. Visual field abnormalities in nonarteritic anterior ischemic optic neuropathy: their pattern and prevalence at initial examination. Arch Ophthalmol 2005; 123: 1554–1562

Index

A

A-scans 16, 25
AC, *see* anterior chamber
adaptive-optics OCT 35
adherent leukoma, keratitis 64, *66*
adherent ocular bandages (AOBs) 110, *111*
aflibercept (Eylea) **183**
- retinal vein occlusion 188
age-related choroidal atrophy **205**
age-related macular degeneration (AMD)
- anti-VEGF therapy 185, *185–186*, **186**
- classification **149**, *151*
- diagnostic methods **170**
- drusen analysis **171**, *172*
- etiologic factors 170
- exudative 174
- geographic atrophy *171*, **171**
- neovascular **174**
-- choroidal, *see* choroidal neovascularization
-- end-stage 174, *177*
-- occult subretinal 174, *175–177*
-- with polypoidal choroidal vasculopathy 174
- phase-variance OCT **27**, *28*
- pigment epithelial detachment **172**
-- central serous chorioretinopathy 174
-- drusenoid 172, *172–173*
-- fibrovascular 174
-- hemorrhagic 174
-- pathogenesis 172
-- retinal angiomatous proliferation 174, *174*
-- serous 172, *173–174*
- tomographic characteristics **171**
- treatment **177**, *178*
- vitreomacular adhesion **176**, *178*
- vitreomacular traction *170*, **170**, **176**, *178*
AION (anterior ischemic optic neuropathy) **237**
AMD, *see* age-related macular degeneration
analysis *7*, **7**
angiography, vs. phase-variance OCT 25
angle evaluation, LASIK patient **40**, *42*
angle-closure glaucoma, anterior-segment exploration 57, *57*
anterior capsulotomy, femtosecond laser **136**, *137*, *139*, **140**
anterior chamber (AC) angle
- cataract surgery 108, *110*
- swept-source OCT 33, *33*
anterior chamber (AC) cells, uveitis **194**
anterior ischemic optic neuropathy (AION) **237**
anterior-chamber (AC) inflammatory reaction in uveitis **194**
- Fourier-domain OCT *196*, **196**, *197*
-- anterior-chamber cell distribution **197**, *198*
-- coefficient of repeatability 197, *197*
-- ordinal scales for cell count *197*, **197**
-- prototype system 196, *196*
-- scanning process 196, *197*
-- time-domain vs. **198**
-- vs. existing methods *198*, **198**
- time-domain OCT *194*, **194**
-- anterior chamber cells **194**
-- aqueous flare **195**
-- automated cell analysis **194**, *195*
-- corneal edema and cell counting **195**, *196*
-- Fourier-domain vs. **198**
-- keratic precipitates *195*, **195**
-- manual vs. automated cell-counting methods **194**, *195–196*
-- membrane **195**, *196*
anterior-segment biometry, spectral-domain OCT **76**
anterior-segment exploration **53**
- angle *57*, **57**
- cornea **56**
-- corneal dystrophies 56, *56*, *61*
-- corneal edema 56, *57*
-- corneal melting *59*
-- descemetocele 56, *56*, *59*
-- intracorneal rings 56, *56*, *59*
-- keratoglobus 56, *56*, *59*
-- LASIK free cap 56, *57*
-- sands of Sahara (SOS) syndrome *61*
-- Terrien degeneration 56, *56*, *59*
- crystalline lens
-- natural **54**, *55*
-- pseudophakic artificial *55*, **55**
- descemetic pathologies *62*
- dynamic evaluation **54**, *55*
- equipment 53, *53*
- future **57**, *58*
- image reconstruction software 53, *54*
- iridocorneal angle *58*
- LASIK
-- flap thickness 58, *58*, *60–61*
-- free cap 56, *57*
- OCT vs. other techniques 53
- pachymetry mapping 58, *58*, *60*
- phakic implants **55**, *56*, *59*
- static measurement *54*, **54**
- time-domain OCT *53*, **53**, *54*
- vertical vs. horizontal internal diameter 54, *54*
anterior-segment OCT
- Descemet membrane detachment **83**, *84*
- glaucoma **211**, *213–214*
- glued intraocular lenses *125*, **125**
- Microphakonit wound *116*, **116**
- swept-source 33
- time-domain and Fourier-domain 10, *11*, **12**, *13–14*
- Visante, *see* Visante anterior-segment OCT
anterior-segment surgery *231*, **231**
- cataract *231*, **231**, *232*
- corneal **232**
- future 231, *232*
- glaucoma *232*, **232**
- refractive *232*, **232**
anti-chamber collapser, Microphakonit 115
anti–vascular endothelial growth factor (anti-VEGF) therapy **182**
- aflibercept **183**
- age-related macular degeneration 185, *185–186*, **186**
- as-needed strategy 182
- background 182
- bevacizumab **182**
- clinical trials **186**
- diabetic macular edema **187**
- future directions **188**
- initiation and maintenance *185*, **185**, *186*
- macular edema from retinal vein occlusion **187**
- pegaptanib sodium **182**
- qualitative analysis **183**, *184*
- quantitative analysis **183**
- ranibizumab **183**
- role of OCT **183**
- treat-and-extend strategy 182
AOBs (adherent ocular bandages) 110, *111*
aqueous flare, uveitis **195**
arcuate corneal incisions, femtosecond laser *137*, *140*, **141**
arteriovenous malformation, retinal **224**
artifacts **7**, *8–9*
- vs. glaucoma *211–212*
Artiflex 50
Artisan hyperopic implant **55**, *56*
astigmatism, ocular residual, glued intraocular lenses 125, **126**, *127*
astrocytic hamartoma, retinal **226**, *228*
astrocytoma, retinal **226**, *228*
Avastin, *see* bevacizumab

B

B-scans 16, 25
backscattering 3, *3*, **7**
BDD (bullous Descemet membrane detachment) 82, *83*
beam splitter 3, *3*
bevacizumab (Avastin) **182**
- age-related macular degeneration 186
- diabetic macular edema 187
BM-scan (multiple successive OCT B-scans) 16, 25
Bowman layer, normal 63
branch retinal vein occlusion (BRVO), anti-VEGF therapy 187
Bruch membrane 145
brunescent cataracts, Lensx femtosecond laser 131, *133*
bullous Descemet membrane detachment (BDD) 82, *83*

C

canaloplasty 232, *232*
capsular bend, cataract surgery 109
capsular block, cataract surgery 109, *109*
capsule changes, intraocular lens tilt **121**
capsulotomy, femtosecond laser **136**, *137*, *139*, **140**
Catalys femtosecond laser system **131**
- anterior-segment landmarks 131, *134*
- automatic mapping 133, *134–135*
- image acquisition 131, *134*
- incision confirmation 133, *136*
- lens tilt 133, *135*
- treatment 133, *137*
cataract surgery **108**
- anterior-segment OCT **108**, **231**
-- anatomical changes *109*
-- anterior chamber angle 108, *110*
-- capsular bend 109
-- capsular block 109, *109*
-- equipment 231, *231*
-- future perspectives 231, *231*
-- measuring anterior segment *108*, **108**
- cystoid macular edema 113, *113*
- femtosecond laser-assisted 108, 112, *112*, **112**
-- macular thickness *113*
-- vs. knife 112, *112*
- foveal thickness 113, *113*
- incision **109**
-- adherent ocular bandages 110, *111*
-- architectural features 109, *110*
-- arcuate configuration 109, *110*
-- biaxial vs. coaxial 110
-- Descemet membrane detachment 111, *112*
-- femtosecond laser vs. knife 112, *112*
-- IOL injection 111
-- raster program *111*, 112
-- sizing arc of contact 110, *111*
- posterior-segment OCT **112**, *113*
- sub-1-mm (700-µm), *see* Microphakonit
cavernous hemangioma, retinal *224*, **224**
CCD (charged coupled device) video camera 4
CCI, *see* clear corneal incision
cellophane macular reflex 166
central corneal thickness (CCT), swept-source OCT 33
central retinal thickness (CRT), and anti-VEGF therapy 183
central retinal vein occlusion (CRVO), anti-VEGF therapy 187
central serous chorioretinopathy (CSCR) 174
central serous retinopathy (CSR) **149**, *150*
charged coupled device (CCD) video camera 4
choriocapillaris 145
chorioretinopathy, chronic central serous, swept-source OCT 35
choroid **201**
- age-related choroidal atrophy **205**
- age-related macular degeneration **203**, *204*
- choroidal coloboma **205**, *206*
- choroidal rupture **204**
- choroiditis **205**, *206*
- closer imaging for posterior structures **202**
- enhanced depth imaging OCT **202**, *203*

- high myopia **202**, *203*
- idiopathic polypoidal choroidal vasculopathy *205*, **205**
- OCT for evaluation **201**
- swept-source OCT 33

choroidal atrophy, age-related **205**
choroidal coloboma **205**, *206*
choroidal hemangioma, circumscribed and diffuse *218–219*, **220**
choroidal lymphoma **223**
choroidal melanoma *216–217*, **218**
choroidal metastasis *221*, **222**
choroidal neovascularization (CNV)
- age-related macular degeneration
-- classification 174, *175*
-- diagnostic methods **170**
-- pathophysiology **203**, *204*
- subfoveal *28*

choroidal nevus **150**, *151*, *215*, **215**, *216*
choroidal osteoma *220*, **221**
choroidal rupture **204**
choroidal tumors **215**
- lymphoma *222*, **223**
- melanocytic *215*, **215**, *216–217*
- metastatic *221*, **222**
- osseous *220*, **221**
- vascular *218–219*, **220**

choroidal vasculature, phase-variance OCT 26, *27*
choroidal vasculopathy, idiopathic polypoidal *205*, **205**
choroiditis **205**, *206*
CHRPE (congenital hypertrophy of retinal pigment epithelium) **225**, *227*
circumpapillary OCT scans *146*, **146**
circumscribed choroidal hemangioma *218–219*, **220**
clear corneal incision (CCI) **109**
- adherent ocular bandages 110, *111*
- architectural features 109, *110*
- arcuate configuration 109, *110*
- biaxial vs. coaxial 110
- Descemet membrane detachment 111, *112*
- femtosecond laser vs. knife 112, *112*
- IOL injection 111
- Microphakonit, *see* Microphakonit
- raster program *111*, 112
- sizing arc of contact 110, *111*

CLR (crystalline lens rise), phakic intraocular lenses *49*, **49**, *50*
CME (cystoid macular edema) *148*, **148**
- cataract surgery 113, *113*

CMM (conjunctival melanoma) **20**, *21*
CNV, *see* choroidal neovascularization
coaptation, Microphakonit incision **116**, *117*
Cogan dystrophy, anterior-segment exploration *61*
coherence *2*, **2**
coherent light *2*, 3
coloboma, choroidal **205**, *206*
color coding 7, *7*, **144**, *145*
combined hamartoma of retinal pigment epithelium and sensory retina **226**, *227*
compensatory plate 3, *3*
complex Descemet membrane detachment 82–83, *83*
compressive optic neuropathy **235**
computer *144*
condensing lens *144*
confocal microscopy 17
congenital hypertrophy of retinal pigment epithelium (CHRPE) **225**, *227*
conjunctiva, invasive squamous cell carcinoma 17
conjunctival intraepithelial neoplasia 17
conjunctival lesions, pigmented **19**
conjunctival lymphoma **21**, *22*
conjunctival melanoma (CMM) **20**, *21*
cornea
- anterior-segment exploration **56**
-- corneal dystrophies 56, *56*, *61*
-- corneal edema 56, *57*
-- corneal melting *59*
-- descemetocele 56, *56*, *59*
-- intracorneal rings 56, *56*, *59*
-- keratoglobus 56, *56*, *59*
-- LASIK free cap 56, *57*
-- sands of Sahara (SOS) syndrome *61*
-- Terrien degeneration 56, *56*, *59*
- intraoperative OCT **232**
- invasive squamous cell carcinoma 17
- normal texture *63*, **63**
- swept-source OCT **33**, *34*
- time-domain and Fourier-domain OCT **12**, *13*

corneal crosslinking (CXL), keratoconus **69**, *70*
corneal curvature, anterior-segment OCT 108
corneal damage, intraocular lens implant **85**, *86*
corneal dystrophies, anterior-segment exploration 56, *56*, *61*
corneal ectasia **68**
- keratoconus **68**
-- corneal keratoplasty *71*, **71**
-- crosslinking **69**, *70*
-- evaluation **68**, *69–70*
-- intracorneal ring implantation **70**, *71*
-- screening *68*, **68**
- keratoglobus **72**, *73*
- marginal pellucid degeneration **72**, *73*
- post-LASIK 46, *47*, *72*, **72**
- risk scoring system in refractive surgery **74**, *75–77*

corneal edema
- and cell counting in uveitis **195**, *196*
- anterior-segment exploration 56, *57*

corneal fibrosis, DSAEK graft detachment with posterior *97*, **97**
corneal flap creation, femtosecond laser **136**, *138–139*
corneal incisions
- clear, *see* clear corneal incision
- femtosecond laser *137*, *140*, **141**

corneal infiltration *67*, **67**
corneal inflammation, *see* keratitis
corneal keratoplasty, keratoconus *71*, **71**
corneal melting, anterior-segment exploration *59*
corneal necrosis, keratitis 64, *65*
corneal pachymetry, time-domain and Fourier-domain OCT **12**, *13*
corneal pathology, LASIK patient **42**, *43–44*
corneal perforation, keratitis 64, *66*
corneal scar
- photoreactive keratectomy **42**, *43–44*
- swept-source OCT of postinfectious 33

corneal thickness
- anterior-segment OCT 108
- swept-source OCT of central 33

corneal topography, LASIK patients 39, *39*, *43*
corneal ulcer, keratitis 63, *64*
corneal volume, swept-source OCT 33
corneal-flap thickness, time-domain and Fourier-domain OCT **12**, *13*
corneoscleral graft, DSAEK graft detachment under prior *96*, **96**
cortical cleaving hydrodissection, Microphakonit 115, *115*
crosslinking (CXL), keratoconus **69**, *70*
CRT (central retinal thickness), and anti-VEGF therapy 183
CRVO (central retinal vein occlusion), anti-VEGF therapy 187
CrystaLens 51, *51*
crystalline lens
- natural, anterior-segment exploration **54**, *55*
- pseudophakic artificial, anterior-segment exploration *55*, **55**

crystalline lens rise (CLR), phakic intraocular lenses *49*, **49**, *50*
CSCR (central serous chorioretinopathy) 174
CSR (central serous retinopathy) **149**, *150*
cup:disc asymmetry 208, *209*
CXL (corneal crosslinking), keratoconus **69**, *70*
cystoid macular edema (CME) *148*, **148**
- cataract surgery 113, *113*

D

deep anterior lamellar keratoplasty (DALK) *71*, **71**
descematotomy, relaxing **84**, *85*
Descemet membrane
- Microphakonit incision **117**
- normal 63

Descemet membrane detachment **82**
- active vs. passive 82
- anterior-segment OCT **83**, *84*
- bullous 82, *83*
- classification **82**, *83*
-- treatment based on **84**, *85*
- clear corneal incision 111, *112*
- complex 82–83, *83*
- Descemet membrane endothelial keratoplasty with glued intraocular lenses **85**, *87*
- diagnosis *82*, **82**
- intraocular lens implant in presence of corneal damage **85**, *86*
- planar vs. nonplanar 82
- relaxing descematotomy 84, **84**, *85*
- rhegmatogenous 82
- tractional 82, *83*

Descemet membrane endothelial keratoplasty (DMEK) 85
- complete detachment *94*, **96**
- detachment requiring air *91*, **92**
- glued intraocular lenses **85**, *87*
- inverted graft *95*, **96**
- predictability for graft attachment 103
- small detachment requiring observation only *90*, **92**
- time-domain and Fourier-domain OCT after 13, *14*
- uncomplicated normal *90*, **92**
- under penetrating keratoplasty *92–93*, **94**
- vs. DSAEK 89
- vs. pre-Descemet endothelial keratoplasty **103**, *104*

Descemet membrane folds
- keratitis 64, *65*
- pre-Descemet endothelial keratoplasty 101, *102*

Descemet stripping automated endothelial keratoplasty (DSAEK) 85
- detachment under prior corneoscleral graft *96*, **96**
- detachment with posterior corneal fibrosis *97*, **97**
- persistent detachment *92*, **94**
- postoperative bullae *91*, **94**
- predictability for graft attachment 103
- uncomplicated normal *90*, **91**
- vs. DMEK 89
- vs. pre-Descemet endothelial keratoplasty **103**, *104*

Descemet stripping endothelial keratoplasty (DSEK) *62*
descemetic dissection *62*
descemetic grafts *62*
descemetic pathologies *62*
descemetocele, anterior-segment exploration 56, *56*, *59*
descemetorrhexis 85
diabetic macular edema (DME)
- anti-VEGF therapy **187**
- time-domain and Fourier-domain OCT 10

diabetic retinopathy
- nonproliferative *147*, **147**
- phase-variance OCT **28**, *29*
- proliferative *148*, **148**

diffuse choroidal hemangioma *218–219*, **220**
DME (diabetic macular edema)
- anti-VEGF therapy **187**
- time-domain and Fourier-domain OCT 10

DMEK, *see* Descemet membrane endothelial keratoplasty
Doppler optical coherence tomography 25
drusen
- age-related macular degeneration 149, **171**, *172*
- optic nerve **235**

DSAEK, *see* Descemet stripping automated endothelial keratoplasty
DSEK (Descemet stripping endothelial keratoplasty) *62*
dye-based angiography, vs. phase-variance OCT 25

E

echo time delay 3
EK, *see* endothelial keratoplasty
ELM (external limiting membrane) 7, *7*, 145

endothelial abscess, keratitis 64, *66*
endothelial alignment, Microphakonit incision *116*, **116**
endothelial clearance, phakic intraocular lenses *48*, **48**, *49*
endothelial inflammation, keratitis 63, *64*
endothelial keratoplasty (EK) **89**
- case studies **91**
- Descemet membrane, *see* Descement membrane endothelial keratoplasty
- Descemet stripping automated, *see* Descemet stripping automated endothelial keratoplasty
- history 89
- intraoperative OCT **89**
-- Haag-Streit iOCT 89, **97**, *98*
- postoperative OCT **90**
-- time-domain and Fourier-domain 13, *14*
- pre-Descemet, *see* pre-Descemet endothelial keratoplasty
- predictability for graft attachment **103**
- preoperative OCT **89**
enhanced depth imaging OCT, choroid **202**, *203*
epiretinal membrane (ERM)
- cellophane macular reflex 166
- defined 165
- diagnosis *166–167*
- epidemiology 165
- Gass grading 166
- IS/OS junction 167
- lamellar macular hole 157, *157*
- macular pseudohole 157
- macular pucker 166
- metamorphopsia 166
- OCT-based classification 166
- pathogenesis 165
- posterior vitreous detachment 166, *166*
- prognostic factors 167
- surgical planning 148, *148–149*, 166, *167–168*
- time-domain and Fourier-domain CT 11
- vitreomacular traction 155, *155*, 166
- vs. vitreomacular traction 168, *169*
epithelial alignment, Microphakonit incision **117**
epithelial ingrowth after LASIK
- spectral-domain OCT *78*, **78**, *79*
- Visante anterior-segment OCT 44, *46–47*
epithelial thickness, keratoconus 68, *68*
epithelial thickness remodeling, refractive surgery **75**, *77*
ERM, *see* epiretinal membrane
external gas-forced infusion, Microphakonit 115
external limiting membrane (ELM) 7, *7*, 145
Eylea (aflibercept) **183**
- retinal vein occlusion 188

F

FA (fluorescence angiography), diabetic retinopathy 28, *29*
FD OCT, *see* Fourier-domain optical coherence tomography
Femto ldv laser 140
femtosecond laser lens and cornea surgery **130**
- arcuate corneal incisions *137*, *140*, **141**
- background 130
- capsulotomy **136**, *137*, *139*, **140**
- Catalys **131**
-- anterior-segment landmarks 131, *134*
-- automatic mapping 133, *134–135*
-- image acquisition 131, *134*
-- incision confirmation 133, *136*
-- lens tilt 133, *135*
-- treatment 133, *137*
- flap creation **136**, *138–139*
- lens fragmentation **136**, *137*, *139*, **140**
- Lensx **130**
-- brunescent cataracts 131, *133*
-- circle scan 130, *131–132*
-- hypermature cataracts 131, *133*
-- line scan 131, *133*
-- scan up to 8.5 mm deep 130, *130*
-- subscapular cataracts 131, *134*
- other imaging technologies **138**
- platforms **130**
- role of OCT in select applications **140**
- Victus **135**, *138*
femtosecond laser-assisted cataract surgery (FLACS) 108, 112, *112*, **112**
- macular thickness *113*
- vs. knife 112, *112*
FFK (forme fruste keratoconus) 39, 68, *68*
fibrinous membrane, uveitis **195**, *196*
filtering bleb, glaucoma 211, *214*
five-line raster 5, *6*
fixation error **7**, *8*
fixed mirror 3, *3*
FLACS, *see* femtosecond laser-assisted cataract surgery
flap creation, femtosecond laser **136**, *138–139*
flap evaluation, LASIK patient **43**, *44–45*
flare meter 194
fluorescence angiography (FA), diabetic retinopathy 28, *29*
focusing error **7**, *9*
focusing lens 4
forme fruste keratoconus (FFK) 39, 68, *68*
Fourier-domain optical coherence tomography (FD OCT) **9**
- anterior segment 10, *11*, **12**, *13–14*
- anterior-chamber inflammatory reaction in uveitis **196**
-- anterior-chamber cell distribution **197**, *198*
-- coefficient of repeatability 197, *197*
-- ordinal scales for cell count *197*, **197**
-- prototype system 196, *196*
-- scanning process 196, *197*
-- time-domain vs. **198**
-- vs. existing methods *198*, **198**
- cornea **12**, *13*
- different methods **10**
- future trends **13**
- history 17
- macular thickness **10**, *11–12*
- nerve-fiber layer **12**
- optics **9**, *10*
- overview 9
- posterior segment 10, *11*
- vs. time-domain OCT in clinical applications **10**, *11*
foveal thickness, cataract surgery 113, *113*
frequency-domain optical coherence tomography, *see* Fourier-domain optical coherence tomography
FTMH, *see* full-thickness macular hole
full-thickness macular hole (FTMH)
- anatomical closure 162, *164*
- cause **157**
- classification *158*
-- Altaweel and Ip 162, *162–163*
-- by cause **157**
-- by size *156*, **156**
-- by status **157**
-- Gass *156*, **156**, 161
-- IVTS Group *154*
- clinical characteristics 161
- complete vitreous detachment *163*
- defined 161
- diagnosis *161*, **161**
- epidemiology 161
- pathophysiology 161
- primary vs. secondary 157
- sequential foveal tomographic images *163*
- size *156*, **156**
- stages 156, *156*
- status **157**
- vitreoretinal traction 162

G

ganglion cell layer (GCL) 7, *7*, 145, *145*
gas-forced infusion, Microphakonit 115
geographic atrophy 149, *151*
- age-related macular degeneration *171*, **171**
glaucoma **208**
- anterior segment **211**, *213–214*
-- angle-closure 57, *57*
- filtering bleb 211, *214*
- intraoperative OCT *232*, **232**
- macula **208**
- masqueraders 210, *212*
- open-angle vs. narrow-angle 211, *213*
- peripheral synechiae 212, *214*
- plateau iris 212, *214*
- retinal nerve-fiber layer analysis **150**, *152–153*, **208**
-- abnormal thinning 208
-- cup:disc asymmetry 208, *209*
-- monitor for progression 208, *210*
-- optic nerve head and lamina cribrosa 208, *212*
- swept-source OCT **32**, *33–34*
- trabecular meshwork and Schlemm canal 211
global pachymetry mapping 38
- LASIK patients 40, *40–41*
global progression analysis (GPA), retinal nerve-fiber layer 235
glued intraocular lenses **124**
- after IOL dislocation 127, *127–128*
- anterior-segment OCT *125*, **125**
- background **124**
- Descemet membrane endothelial keratoplasty **85**, *87*
- ocular residual astigmatism 125, **126**, *127*
- optic position *126*, **126**, *127*
- scleral apposition *127*, **127**
- technique *124*, **124**, *125*
- tilt estimation **125**
- various indications *127*, **127**, *128*
- vs. microscopic tilt in ultrasound biomicroscopy **127**, *128*
- vs. sutured scleral fixated IOLs **128**
GPA (global progression analysis), retinal nerve-fiber layer 235
green disease, glaucoma 208, *211–212*
Groenouw dystrophy *61*

H

Haag-Streit iOCT, endothelial keratoplasty 89, **97**, *98*
hamartoma
- combined of retinal pigment epithelium and sensory retina **226**, *227*
- retinal astrocytic **226**, *228*
hemangioblastoma, retinal *223*, **223**
hemangioma
- choroidal *218–219*, **220**
- retinal cavernous *224*, **224**
hemiretinal vein occlusion, vs. glaucoma 210, *212*
Henle fiber layer 145
history, optical coherence tomography **2**
hypermature cataracts, Lensx femtosecond laser 131, *133*

I

ICRs (indirect choroidal ruptures) 204
idiopathic polypoidal choroidal vasculopathy (IPCV) *205*, **205**
image, factors affecting **6**
image format, phase-variance OCT *26*, **26**
image processing, phase-variance OCT **26**
impending macular hole **157**
incident beam 3, *3*, 4
incoherent light *2*, 3
indirect choroidal ruptures (ICRs) 204
inferotemporal thinning, LASIK patients *39*, 40, *43*
infrared video camera *144*
inner nuclear layer (INL) 7, *7*, 145, *145*
inner plexiform layer (IPL) 7, *7*, 145, *145*
inner segment (IS) 145
instrumentation *4*, **4**, *5*
Intacs corneal implants 70
interference fringes 3
interferometer 2, *3*, **3**, *144*
- Michelson 2, 16
interferometry 2, *3*, **3**
interflap space ulcer, after LASIK 46, *47*
internal gas-forced infusion, Microphakonit 115
interpretation **5**
intracorneal lens, *see* phakic intraocular lenses
intracorneal rings 56, *56*, *59*, **70**, *71*
Intralase laser 140

intraocular lens (IOL) tilt **119**
- advantages of OCT evaluation **123**
- associated changes **121**
-- capsule changes **121**
-- iris shaffing **121**, *122*
-- optic capture **121**
-- pigment dispersion on IOL *121*, **121**
- decentration estimation from 3D reconstruction **120**
- detecting amount **122**
- glued IOLs **125**
- image acquisition **119**
-- high-resolution cornea mode 119, *119*
-- single-scan raw mode 119, *119*
- image analysis 119, *120*
- lens position module **119**
- limitations of OCT evaluation *122*, **122**
- method to calculate *120*
- normal **120**, *121*
- out-patient detection **122**, *123*
- trans-scleral fixation **121**
intraocular lens(es) (IOLs)
- corneal damage **85**, *86*
- Descemet membrane endothelial keratoplasty (DMEK) **85**, *87*
- glued, *see* glued intraocular lenses
- injection effect on clear capsular incision 111
- phakic, *see* phakic intraocular lenses
- piggyback 55, *55*
- spectral-domain OCT **76**
intraocular tumors **215**
- choroidal **215**
-- lymphoma *222*, **223**
-- melanocytic *215*, **215**, *216–217*
-- metastatic *221*, **222**
-- osseous *220*, **221**
-- vascular *218–219*, **220**
- retinal **223**
-- combined hamartoma **226**, *227*
-- of retinal pigment epithelium **225**, *227*
-- retinal astrocytic hamartoma **226**, *228*
-- retinoblastoma **228**, *229*
-- vascular *223*, **223**, *224–226*
intraoperative OCT *231*, **231**
- cataract surgery *231*, **231**, *232*
- corneal surgery **232**
- future 231, *232*
- glaucoma surgery *232*, **232**
- refractive surgery *232*, **232**
intraretinal splitting *157*, **159**
invasive squamous cell carcinoma, cornea or conjunctiva 17
IOLs, *see* intraocular lens(es)
IPCV (idiopathic polypoidal choroidal vasculopathy) *205*, **205**
IPL (inner plexiform layer) 7, *7*, 145, *145*
iridocorneal angle, anterior-segment exploration *58*
iris, glaucoma 212, *214*
iris shaffing, intraocular lens tilt **121**, *122*
iris volume, swept-source OCT 33
iris-trabecular contact (ITC) index *34*
IS (inner segment) 145

K

keratic precipitates, uveitis *195*, **195**
keratitis **63**
- adherent leukoma 64, *66*
- advanced **64**, *65–66*
- advantage of OCT **67**
- assessment for surgery plan **67**
- corneal necrosis 64, *65*
- corneal ulcer 63, *64*
- Descemet folds 64, *65*
- early stages **63**, *64–65*
- endothelial abscess 64, *66*
- endothelial inflammation 63, *64*
- healing stage **64**, *66*
- pathology **63**
- perforation 64, *66*
- prognosis *67*, **67**
- role of OCT **63**
- stromal edema 64, *65*
- vs. normal cornea *63*, **63**
keratoconus **68**
- acute 69, *69*
- classification 69, *69*
- epithelial thickness 68, *68*
- evaluation **68**, *69–70*
- forme fruste 39, 68, *68*
- hyperreflective anomalies 69, *69*
- pan-stromal scar 69, *69*
- risk scoring system in refractive surgery **74**, *75–77*
- screening *68*, **68**
- swept-source OCT 33
- treatments **69**
-- corneal keratoplasty *71*, **71**
-- crosslinking **69**, *70*
-- intracorneal rings 56, *56*, *59*, **70**, *71*
- Visante anterior-segment OCT 40, *41*
- Vogt striae 69, *69*
keratoglobus **72**, *73*
- anterior-segment exploration 56, *56*, *59*
kératoplastie lamellaire antérieure profonde (KLAP) 71, *71*
keratoplasty, penetrating
- Descemet membrane endothelial keratoplasty under *92–93*, **94**
- swept-source OCT 33

L

lamellar macular hole (LMH)
- classification *157*, **157**, *158*
- diagnosis **163**, *164*
lamina cribrosa (LC)
- glaucoma 208, *212*
- swept-source OCT 32
laser-assisted in situ keratomileusis (LASIK)
- complications **44**
- corneal ectasia 46, *47*, *72*, **72**
- epithelial ingrowth
-- spectral-domain OCT *78*, **78**, *79*
-- Visante anterior-segment OCT 44, *46–47*
- epithelial thickness remodeling **75**, *77*
- flap thickness 58, *58*, *60–61*
- free cap 56, *57*
- interflap space ulcer 46, *47*
- sands of Sahara (SOS) syndrome after *61*
- spectral-domain OCT **76**, *78*
- swept-source OCT 34, *34*
- time-domain and Fourier-domain OCT **12**, *13*
- Visante anterior-segment OCT **38**
-- angle evaluation **40**, *42*
-- complication evaluation *43*, **44**, *46–47*
-- corneal pathology **42**, *43–44*
-- corneal topography 39, *39*, *43*
-- flap evaluation **43**, *44–45*
-- global pachymetry mapping 40, *40–41*
-- pachymetry mapping *39*, **39**
-- preoperative evaluation 40, *41*
LASIK, *see* laser-assisted in situ keratomileusis
LC (lamina cribrosa)
- glaucoma 208, *212*
- swept-source OCT 32
lens fragmentation, femtosecond laser **136**, *137*, *139*, **140**
lens thickness, anterior-segment OCT 108
Lensar laser 138
Lensx femtosecond laser system **130**
- brunescent cataracts 131, *133*
- circle scan 130, *131–132*
- hypermature cataracts 131, *133*
- line scan 131, *133*
- scan up to 8.5 mm deep 130, *130*
- subscapular cataracts 131, *134*
leopard spots 223
leukoma, adherent, keratitis 64, *66*
light absorption **6**
light transmission **6**
line-scanning ophthalmoscope 5
linear flap 44, *45*
LMH (lamellar macular hole)
- classification *157*, **157**, *158*
- diagnosis **163**, *164*
low-coherence interferometry 3, *3*
Lucentis, *see* ranibizumab
lymphoma
- choroidal **223**
- conjunctival **21**, *22*
- vitreoretinal *222*, **223**

M

Macugen (pegaptanib sodium) **182**
macula, glaucoma **208**
macular asymmetry analysis, glaucoma *209*
macular cube 5, *5*
macular degeneration, age-related, *see* age-related macular degeneration
macular diseases, *see* vitreomacular interface conditions
macular edema
- anti-VEGF therapy
-- diabetic **187**
-- retinal vein occlusion **187**
- cystoid *148*, **148**
-- cataract surgery 113, *113*
- time-domain and Fourier-domain CT 11, *11*
macular hole
- classification *149*, **149**
- full-thickness, *see* full-thickness macular hole
- impending **157**
- lamellar
-- classification *157*, **157**, *158*
-- diagnosis **163**, *164*
- pseudo-, *see* macular pseudohole
- time-domain and Fourier-domain OCT 11
macular progression analysis, glaucoma *210*
macular pseudohole (MPH)
- classification **157**, *158*
- diagnosis **163**, *165*
- time-domain and Fourier-domain CT 11, *12*
macular pucker 166
macular radial scans **146**
macular raster scans **146**
macular schisis *157*, **159**
macular thickness
- femtosecond laser-assisted cataract surgery *113*
- glaucoma 208
- time-domain and Fourier-domain OCT **10**, *11–12*
marginal pellucid degeneration (MPD) **72**, *73*
melanocytic choroidal tumors **215**
- choroidal melanoma *216–217*, **218**
- choroidal nevus *215*, **215**, *216*
melanocytoma, optic nerve *237*, **237**
melanoma
- choroidal *216–217*, **218**
- conjunctival **20**, *21*
melanosis, primary acquired *20*, **20**
meniscus flap 44, *44*
metamorphopsia, epiretinal membrane 166
metastasis, choroidal *221*, **222**
Michelson interferometer 2, 16
microbial keratitis **63**
- adherent leukoma 64, *66*
- advanced **64**, *65–66*
- advantage of OCT **67**
- assessment for surgery plan **67**
- corneal necrosis 64, *65*
- corneal ulcer 63, *64*
- Descemet folds 64, *65*
- early stages **63**, *64–65*
- endothelial abscess 64, *66*
- endothelial inflammation 63, *64*
- healing stage **64**, *66*
- pathology **63**
- perforation 64, *66*
- prognosis *67*, **67**
- role of OCT **63**
- stromal edema 64, *65*
- vs. normal cornea *63*, **63**
Microphakonit **115**
- advantages of small self-sealing incision **117**
- anterior segment OCT evaluation of wound *116*, **116**
- anti-chamber collapser 115
- cortical cleaving hydrodissection 115, *115*
- features of incision **116**
-- coaptation **116**, *117*
-- Descemet membrane **117**
-- endothelial alignment *116*, **116**
-- epithelial alignment **117**
-- size *116*, **116**
-- stromal hydration **117**
-- with vs. without extension *117*, **117**, *118*
- gas-forced infusion 115

– technique *115*, **115**
MPD (marginal pellucid degeneration) **72**, *73*
MPH, *see* macular pseudohole
multiple sclerosis (MS), optic neuritis 235
multiple successive OCT B-scans (BM-scan) 16, 25
myelinated nerve-fiber layer **150**, *153*
myopia
– choroid **202**, *203*
– sclera **200**
myopic retinal schisis *157*, **159**

N

nanophthalmos, anterior-segment exploration *58*
nerve-fiber layer (NFL) 7, *7*, 145, *145*
– myelinated **150**, *153*
– thickness measurement and analysis **146**
– time-domain and Fourier-domain OCT **12**
neuritis, optic *235*, **235**, *236*
neuromyelitis optica (NMO) **235**
neurophthalmology **234**
– anterior ischemic optic neuropathy **237**
– compressive and traumatic optic neuropathy **235**
– neuromyelitis optica **235**
– optic drusen **235**
– optic nerve head *234*, **234**
– optic nerve melanocytoma *237*, **237**
– optic neuritis *235*, **235**, *236*
– optic pit **236**, *237*
– toxic or nutritional optic neuropathy **235**
nevus **21**, *22*
– choroidal **150**, *151*, *215*, **215**, *216*
NFL, *see* nerve-fiber layer
NMO (neuromyelitis optica) **235**
nodular scleritis **201**, *202–203*
nonglaucomatous optic neuropathies, vs. glaucoma *211*
nuclear layers 7, *7*, 145
nutritional optic neuropathy **235**

O

objective lens 4
OCT, *see* optical coherence tomography
ocular residual astigmatism (ORA), glued intraocular lenses 125, **126**, *127*
ocular surface squamous neoplasia (OSSN) **17**, *18–19*
– vs. pterygium 18, *19*
ocular surface tumors **17**, *18*
– conjunctival lymphoma **21**, *22*
– conjunctival melanoma **20**, *21*
– nevus **21**, *22*
– pigmented conjunctival lesions **19**
– primary acquired melanosis *20*, **20**
– squamous neoplasia **17**, *18–19*
ON (optic neuritis) *235*, **235**, *236*
ONH, *see* optic nerve head
ONL (outer nuclear layer) 7, *7*, 145
OPL (outer plexiform layer) 7, *7*, 145, *145*
optic atrophy **150**, *152*
optic capture, intraocular lens tilt **121**
optic disk cube 5, *6*
optic nerve drusen **235**
optic nerve head (ONH) **147**, **234**
– glaucoma 150, *153*, *212*
– global progression analysis 235
– interpretation of OCT *145*, **145**, 234
– radial scans **146**
– scan acquisition 234, *234*
optic nerve melanocytoma *237*, **237**
optic neuritis (ON) *235*, **235**, *236*
optic neuropathy
– anterior ischemic **237**
– compressive and traumatic **235**
– nonglaucomatous *211*
– toxic or nutritional **235**
optic pit **236**, *237*
optical coherence tomography (OCT) **2**
– analysis *7*, **7**
– artifacts **7**, *8–9*
– backscattering **7**
– coherence *2*, **2**
– factors affecting image **6**
– history **2**
– instrumentation *4*, **4**, *5*
– interferometer 2, *3*, **3**
– interferometry 2, *3*, **3**
– interpretation of output **5**
– principle **2**, *144*, **144**
– scattering **7**
– types of scans *5*, **5**, *6*
– vs. ultrasound imaging **3**, *4*
optometer, Visante anterior-segment OCT 38
Optovue RTVue-CAM 74, *75*
ORA (ocular residual astigmatism), glued intraocular lenses 125, **126**, *127*
OS (outer segment) 145
osseous choroidal tumors *220*, **221**
OSSN (ocular surface squamous neoplasia) **17**, *18–19*
– vs. pterygium 18, *19*
osteoma, choroidal *220*, **221**
outer nuclear layer (ONL) 7, *7*, 145
outer plexiform layer (OPL) 7, *7*, 145, *145*
outer segment (OS) 145

P

pachymetry mapping, corneal, *see* corneal pachymetry mapping
PAM (primary acquired melanosis) *20*, **20**
partially reflecting mirror *144*
PCV (polypoidal choroidal vasculopathy) 174
PDEK, *see* pre-Descemet endothelial keratoplasty
PED, *see* pigment epithelial detachment
pegaptanib sodium (Macugen) **182**
penetrating keratoplasty (PK)
– Descemet membrane endothelial keratoplasty under *92–93*, **94**
– swept-source OCT 33
peripheral synechiae
– anterior 33, *34*
– glaucoma 212, *214*
Peter syndrome, crystalline lens 54, *55*
phacofragmentation, femtosecond laser **136**, *137*, *139*, **140**
phakic intraocular lenses
– Artisan **55**, *56*
– intraoperative OCT *232*, **232**
– posterior chamber **55**, *56*, *59*
– Visante anterior-segment OCT *48*, **48**
–– crystalline lens rise *40*, **40**, *50*
–– dynamic changes of anterior chamber with accommodation **50**
–– endothelial clearance *48*, **48**, *49*
–– preoperative model *50*, **50**, *51*
phakic refractive lens (PRL) 50
phase-variance optical coherence tomography (pvOCT) **25**
– advantages **29**
– applications **26**, *27*
–– age-related macular degeneration **27**, *28*
–– diabetic retinopathy **28**, *29*
– basic principles **25**
– future **30**
– limitations **29**
– technique **25**
–– equipment **25**
–– image format *26*, **26**
–– image processing **26**
– vs. other modalities 25
photodetector *144*
photoreactive keratectomy (PRK), corneal scar **42**, *43–44*
photoreceptor layers 7, *7*
piggyback implant 55, *55*
pigment dispersion
– Artisan hyperopic implant 56, *56*
– intraocular lens tilt *121*, **121**
pigment epithelial detachment (PED) **172**
– anti-VEGF therapy 183, *184*
– central serous chorioretinopathy 174
– drusenoid 172, *172–173*
– fibrovascular 174
– hemorrhagic 174
–– anti-VEGF therapy *184*
– pathogenesis 172
– retinal angiomatous proliferation 174, *174*
– serous 172, *173–174*
pigment epithelial detachments 27, *28*
pigmented conjunctival lesions **19**
PK (penetrating keratoplasty)
– Descemet membrane endothelial keratoplasty under *92–93*, **94**
– swept-source OCT 33
plateau iris, glaucoma 212, *214*
plexiform layers 7, *7*, 145
POAG (primary open-angle glaucoma), foveal thickness after cataract surgery 113, *113*
polypoidal choroidal vasculopathy (PCV) 174
posterior chamber intracorneal lens **55**, *56*, *59*
posterior vitreous detachment (PVD) 154
– anomalous 154
– epiretinal membrane 166, *166*
– vitreomacular traction with incomplete 168, *168*
posterior-segment optical coherence tomography (PS OCT)
– cataract surgery **112**, *113*
– swept-source **35**
– time-domain and Fourier-domain 10, *11*
posterior-segment scan 5, *5*
postinfectious corneal scar, swept-source OCT 33
pre-Descemet endothelial keratoplasty (PDEK) **100**
– correlations and associations **102**
– Descemet folds 101, *102*
– fibrin reaction with shallow detachment 102, *103*
– graft thickness 101, *101*
– graft-host interface haze 101, *103*
– group II detachment 101, *102*
– group III graft detachment 101, *102*
– spectral-domain OCT **101**
– technique *100–101*
– vs. other endothelial grafts **103**, *104*
– well-adhered graft 101, *101*
primary acquired melanosis (PAM) *20*, **20**
primary open-angle glaucoma (POAG), foveal thickness after cataract surgery 113, *113*
principle, optical coherence tomography **2**
PRK (photoreactive keratectomy), corneal scar **42**, *43–44*
PRL (phakic refractive lens) 50
PS OCT, *see* posterior-segment optical coherence tomography
pseudoexfoliation glaucoma (PXG), foveal thickness after cataract surgery 113, *113*
pseudoexfoliation syndrome (PXF), foveal thickness after cataract surgery 113, *113*
pseudophakic artificial crystalline lens, anterior-segment exploration *55*, **55**
pseudophakic bullous keratopathy 85, *87*
pterygium, vs. ocular surface squamous neoplasia 18, *19*
PVD, *see* posterior vitreous detachment
pvOCT, *see* phase-variance optical coherence tomography
PXF (pseudoexfoliation syndrome), foveal thickness after cataract surgery 113, *113*
PXG (pseudoexfoliation glaucoma), foveal thickness after cataract surgery 113, *113*

R

radial scans, through optic nerve head **146**
ranibizumab (Lucentis) **183**
– age-related macular degeneration *185–186*, **186**
– diabetic macular edema 187
– hemorrhagic pigment epithelial detachment *184*
– retinal vein occlusion 187
RAP (retinal angiomatous proliferation) 174, *174*
raster program, clear corneal incision *111*, 112
RDD (rhegmatogenous Descemet membrane detachment) 82
red disease, glaucoma 208, *211*
reference arm 9, 25
– Fourier-domain OCT 9, *10*

- time-domain OCT 9, *9*
reference path 3, *3*
reflection **7**
refractive surgery
- intraoperative OCT *232*, **232**
- spectral-domain OCT **74**
-- anterior-segment biometry and intraocular lens calculation **76**
-- epithelial thickness remodeling **75**, *77*
-- LASIK flap mapping **76**, *78*
-- screening and corneal ectasia risk scoring system **74**, *75–77*
relaxing descematotomy **84**, *85*
retina
- combined hamartoma of retinal pigment epithelium and sensory **226**, *227*
- interpretation of OCT in normal *145*, **145**
retinal angiomatous proliferation (RAP) 174, *174*
retinal arteriovenous malformation **224**
retinal astrocytic hamartoma **226**, *228*
retinal cavernous hemangioma *224*, **224**
retinal detachments, serous 174
retinal diseases **144**
- age-related macular degeneration **149**, *151*
- central serous retinopathy **149**, *150*
- choroidal nevus **150**, *151*
- color coding **144**, *145*
- cystoid macular edema *148*, **148**
- diabetic retinopathy
-- nonproliferative *147*, **147**
-- proliferative *148*, **148**
- epiretinal membrane, *see* epiretinal membrane
- glaucoma **150**, *152–153*
- macular hole *149*, **149**
- myelinated nerve-fiber layer **150**, *153*
- optic atrophy **150**, *152*
- principles of OCT *144*, **144**
- quantitative analysis algorithms **146**
-- nerve-fiber layer thickness measurement and analysis **146**
-- optic nerve head analysis **147**
-- retinal thickness measurement **146**
- retinal topography **147**
- retinal vein occlusions *147*, **147**
- scanning protocols **146**
-- circumpapillary *146*, **146**
-- macular radial **146**
-- macular raster **146**
-- radial through optic nerve head **146**
- uses for OCT *147*, **147**
- vs. normal retina *145*, **145**
retinal hemangioblastoma (RH) *223*, **223**
retinal nerve-fiber layer (RNFL) 7, *7*
- analysis *146*, **146**
- anterior ischemic optic neuropathy **237**
- compressive and traumatic optic neuropathy **235**
- glaucoma 150, *152*
-- abnormal thinning 208
-- cup:disc asymmetry 208, *209*
-- optic nerve head and lamina cribrosa 208, *212*
-- to monitor for progression 208, *210*
- global progression analysis 235
- neuromyelitis optica **235**
- optic nerve drusen **235**
- optic neuritis *235*, **235**, *236*
- swept-source OCT 32
- time-domain and Fourier-domain OCT **12**
- toxic or nutritional optic neuropathy *211*
retinal perfusion images *26*
retinal pigment epithelium (RPE)
- analysis 7, *7*
- combined hamartoma of sensory retina and **226**, *227*
- congenital hypertrophy **225**, *227*
- detachment, *see* pigment epithelial detachment
- interpretation of OCT 145, *145*
- scattering 7
- tumors **225**, *227*
retinal schisis, myopic *157*, **159**
retinal thickness
- central, and anti-VEGF therapy 183
- glaucoma 208
- measurement **146**
retinal topography **147**
retinal tumors **223**
- combined hamartoma **226**, *227*
- retinal astrocytic hamartoma **226**, *228*
- retinal pigment epithelium **225**, *227*
- retinoblastoma **228**, *229*
- vascular **223**
-- retinal arteriovenous malformation **224**
-- retinal cavernous hemangioma *224*, **224**
-- retinal hemangioblastoma *223*, **223**
-- retinal vasoproliferative tumor *225*, **225**, *226*
retinal vasculature, phase-variance OCT 26, *27*
retinal vasoproliferative tumor *225*, **225**, *226*
retinal vein occlusion (RVO) *147*, **147**
- branch 187
- central 187
- macular edema **187**
retinoblastoma **228**, *229*
retinopathy, central serous **149**, *150*
RH (retinal hemangioblastoma) *223*, **223**
rhegmatogenous Descemet membrane detachment (RDD) 82
RNFL, *see* retinal nerve-fiber layer
RPE, *see* retinal pigment epithelium
RVO, *see* retinal vein occlusion

S

Salzmann nodular degeneration 18
sample arm 9, 25
- Fourier-domain OCT 9, *10*
- time-domain OCT 9, *9*
sands of Sahara (SOS) syndrome, anterior-segment exploration *61*
scan types 5, **5**, *6*
scan-depth optical coherence tomography (SD OCT) 10
scattering **7**
Scheimpflug camera, vs. swept-source OCT 33
Schlemm canal
- canaloplasty 232, *232*
- glaucoma 211
Schwalbe's line *201*
sclera **200**
- high myopia **200**
- scleral spur *201*, **201**
- spectral-domain OCT **201**, *202–203*
- swept-source OCT 33
scleral apposition, glued intraocular lenses *127*, **127**
scleral flap enhancement 57, *57*
scleral spur *201*, **201**
- swept-source OCT 33, *34*
scleritis, nodular **201**, *202–203*
SD OCT (scan-depth optical coherence tomography) 10
SD OCT (spectral-domain optical coherence tomography), *see* spectral-domain optical coherence tomography
segmentation artifacts, vs. glaucoma *211–212*
sensory retina, combined hamartoma of retinal pigment epithelium and **226**, *227*
serous retinal detachments (SRDs) 174
signal-to-noise ratio (SNR) **10**
slit-lamp biomicroscope *144*
Slit-Lamp OCT 16
SNR (signal-to-noise ratio) **10**
SOS (sands of Sahara) syndrome, anterior-segment exploration *61*
spectral-domain optical coherence tomography (SD OCT) 16
- case report of advanced *78*, **78**, *79*
- pre-Descemet endothelial keratoplasty **100**
- refractive surgery **74**
-- anterior-segment biometry and intraocular lens calculation **76**
-- epithelial thickness remodeling **75**, *77*
-- LASIK flap mapping **76**, *78*
-- screening and corneal ectasia risk scoring system **74**, *75–77*
- sclera **201**, *202–203*
- vs. phase-variance OCT *26*
spectrometer method **10**, 17
spot size 4
squamous cell carcinoma
- cornea or conjunctiva 17
- in situ 17
squamous dysplasia 17
squamous neoplasia **17**, *18–19*
SRDs (serous retinal detachments) 174
SRNV (subretinal neovascular membrane) 149, *151*
SS OCT, *see* swept-source optical coherence tomography
STAAR intraocular lens *59*
Stratus OCT 16, 53
stromal edema, keratitis 64, *65*
stromal hydration, Microphakonit incision **117**
subfoveal scleral thickness 201
subretinal neovascular membrane (SRNV) 149, *151*
subretinal neovascularization, age-related macular degeneration 174, *175–177*
subscapular cataracts, Lensx femtosecond laser 131, *134*
subtenon injection **199**
- OCT features **199**, *200*
- OCT-assisted *199*, **199**
surface tumors **17**, *18*
- conjunctival lymphoma **21**, *22*
- conjunctival melanoma **20**, *21*
- nevus **21**, *22*
- pigmented conjunctival lesions **19**
- primary acquired melanosis *20*, **20**
- squamous neoplasia **17**, *18–19*
sutured scleral fixated IOLs, vs. glued intraocular lenses **128**
swept-source optical coherence tomography (SS OCT) **10**, 17, **32**
- applications **32**
-- cornea **33**, *34*
-- future directions **35**
-- glaucoma **32**, *33–34*
-- posterior segment **35**
- background **32**
- from time-domain to **32**

T

TD OCT, *see* time-domain optical coherence tomography
TDD (tractional Descemet membrane detachment) 82, *83*
Terrien degeneration, anterior-segment exploration 56, *56*, *59*
time-domain optical coherence tomography (TD OCT) **9**
- anterior segment 10, *11*, **12**, *13–14*, **53**
-- equipment 53, *53*
-- image reconstruction software 53, *54*
- anterior-chamber inflammatory reaction in uveitis *194*, **194**
-- anterior chamber cells **194**
-- aqueous flare **195**
-- automated cell analysis **194**, *195*
-- corneal edema and cell counting **195**, *196*
-- fibrinous membrane **195**, *196*
-- Fourier-domain vs. **198**
-- keratic precipitates *195*, **195**
-- manual vs. automated cell-counting methods **194**, *195–196*
- cornea **12**, *13*
- future trends **13**
- history 16
- macular thickness **10**
- nerve-fiber layer **12**
- optics *9*, **9**
- overview 9
- posterior segment 10, *11*
- vs. Fourier-domain OCT in clinical applications **10**, *11*
toxic optic neuropathy **235**
trabecular meshwork, glaucoma 211
tractional Descemet membrane detachment (TDD) 82, *83*
trans-scleral fixation, intraocular lens tilt **121**
translatable mirror 3, *3*
traumatic optic neuropathy **235**
tumors
- intraocular, *see* intraocular tumors
- ocular surface **17**, *18*
-- conjunctival lymphoma **21**, *22*

-- conjunctival melanoma **20**, *21*
-- nevus **21**, *22*
-- pigmented conjunctival lesions **19**
-- primary acquired melanosis *20*, **20**
-- squamous neoplasia **17**, *18–19*

U

UBM (ultrasound biomicroscopy) 3, *4*, 17
ultrahigh-resolution optical coherence tomography (UHR OCT) **16**
- custom-built 17, *17*
- evolution **16**, *17–18*
- ocular surface tumors **17**, *18*
-- conjunctival lymphoma **21**, *22*
-- conjunctival melanoma **20**, *21*
-- nevus **21**, *22*
-- pigmented conjunctival lesions **19**
-- primary acquired melanosis *20*, **20**
-- squamous neoplasia **17**, *18–19*
ultrasound biomicroscopy (UBM) 3, *4*, 17
ultrasound imaging, vs. optical coherence tomography **3**, *4*
uveitis
- anterior-chamber inflammatory reaction, *see* anterior-chamber inflammatory reaction in uveitis
- vs. glaucoma *211*

V

vascular choroidal tumors *218–219*, **220**
vascular endothelial growth factor (VEGF) 182
vascular retinal tumors **223**
- retinal arteriovenous malformation **224**
- retinal cavernous hemangioma *224*, **224**
- retinal hemangioblastoma *223*, **223**
- retinal vasoproliferative tumor *225*, **225**, *226*
vasoproliferative tumor, retinal *225*, **225**, *226*
VEGF (vascular endothelial growth factor) 182
Vericalc 48
Verisyse intracorneal lens, *see* phakic intraocular lenses
Victus femtosecond laser system **135**, *138*
video camera 4
vignette image 4, **7**
Visante anterior-segment OCT **38**
- conclusion *51*, **51**
- defined 38
- dual-scan mode 38
- enhanced-mode 38
- equipment 53, *53*
- history 16
- image reconstruction software 53, *54*
- keratoconus 40, *41*
- LASIK patients **38**
-- angle evaluation **40**, *42*
-- complication evaluation *43*, **44**, *46–47*
-- corneal pathology **42**, *43–44*
-- corneal topography 39, *39*, *43*
-- flap evaluation **43**, *44–45*
-- global pachymetry mapping 40, *40–41*
-- pachymetry mapping *39*, **39**
-- preoperative evaluation 40, *41*
- light 38
- optometer 38
- overview **38**
- phakic intraocular lenses *48*, **48**
-- crystalline lens rise *49*, **49**, *50*
-- dynamic changes of anterior chamber with accommodation **50**
-- endothelial clearance *48*, **48**, *49*
-- preoperative model *50*, **50**, *51*
- quad-scan mode 38
- standard-resolution mode 38
- uses 38
Visian intracorneal lens, *see* phakic intraocular lenses
Visumax laser 140
vitreomacular adhesion (VMA) *154*, **154**, *155*, *158*
- acute 154
- age-related macular degeneration **176**, *178*
- broad 154, *155*
- concurrent 154
- focal 154, *155*
- isolated 154
vitreomacular interface (VMI) conditions
- classification **154**
- diagnosis **159**
- epiretinal membrane, *see* epiretinal membrane
- macular hole, *see* macular hole
- macular pseudohole
-- classification **157**, *158*
-- diagnosis **163**, *165*
-- time-domain and Fourier-domain CT 11, *12*
- myopic retinal schisis *157*, **159**
- OCT vs. biomicroscopy 161, *161*
- summary *158*, **159**
- vitreomacular adhesion *154*, **154**, *155*, *158*
- vitreomacular traction, *see* vitreomacular traction
vitreomacular traction (VMT)
- advantages of high-resolution OCT 169
- and age-related macular degeneration *170*, **170**, **176**, *178*
- attachment of posterior hyaloid to fovea 168, *169*
- broad 155, *155*
- classification *154–155*, **155**, *158*
- concurrent 155
- defined 168
- diagnosis **168**
- focal 155, *155*
- incomplete posterior vitreous detachment 168, *168*
- isolated 155
- pathogenesis 168
- post-surgery 169
- vs. epiretinal membrane 168, *169*
- with epiretinal membrane 155, *155*, 166
vitreomacular traction syndrome (VMTS), *see* vitreomacular traction
vitreoretinal disease, vs. glaucoma *211*
vitreoretinal lymphoma *222*, **223**
vitreoschisis 155
VMA, *see* vitreomacular adhesion
VMI conditions, *see* vitreomacular interface conditions
VMT, *see* vitreomacular traction
Vogt striae, keratoconus 69, *69*

W

Wavelight laser 140
Weiss ring 154–155
Wyburn Mason syndrome, retinal arteriovenous malformation 224

Z

Zeiss OCT1 16
Zeiss OCT2 16